2nd Edition

MEDICINE
for
DENTAL STUDENTS

2nd Edition

MEDICINE
for
DENTAL STUDENTS

Dr. S.N. Khosla

MD, MAMS, FIAMS
Director, Medical Research Centre, Rohtak
Formerly Prof. & Head, Deptt. of Medicine II
PGIMS, Rohtak (India)

Dr. Amit Khosla

MD
Consultant Physician
Veterans Administration Health Care System
Baltimore, Maryland (USA)

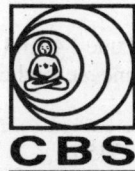

CBS

CBS Publishers & Distributors Pvt. Ltd.

New Delhi • Bengaluru • Chennai • Kochi • Kolkata • Mumbai • Pune

ISBN: 978-81-239-1979-9

First Edition: 2001
Reprint: 2004, 2005, 2006, 2007, 2008
Second Edition: 2011
Reprint: 2012, 2016

Copyright © Authors & Publisher

Published by:
Satish Kumar Jain for CBS Publishers & Distributors Pvt. Ltd.,
4819/XI Prahlad Street, 24 Ansari Road, Daryaganj, New Delhi - 110002
delhi@cbspd.com, cbspubs@airtelmail.in • www.cbspd.com
Ph.: 23289259, 23266861, 23266867 • Fax: 011-23243014

Corporate Office: 204 FIE, Industrial Area, Patparganj, Delhi - 110 092
Ph: 49344934 • Fax: 011-49344935
E-mail: publishing@cbspd.com • publicity@cbspd.com

Branches:
• *Bengaluru:* 2975, 17th Cross, K.R. Road, Bansankari 2nd Stage,
  Bengaluru - 70 • Ph: +91-80-26771678/79 • Fax: +91-80-26771680
  E-mail: cbsbng@gmail.com, bangalore@cbspd.com
• *Chennai:* No. 7, Subbaraya Street, Shenoy Nagar, Chennai - 600030
  Ph: +91-44-26681266, 26680620 • Fax: +91-44-42032115
  E-mail: chennai@cbspd.com
• *Kochi:* Ashana House, 39/1904, A.M. Thomas Road, Valanjambalam,
  Ernakulam, Kochi • Ph: +91-484-4059061-65
  Fax: +91-484-4059065 • E-mail: cochin@cbspd.com
• *Kolkata:* 6-B, Ground Floor, Rameshwar Shaw Road, Kolkata - 700014
  Ph: +91-33-22891126/7/8 • E-mail: kolkata@cbspd.com
• *Mumbai:* 83-C, Dr. E. Moses Road, Worli, Mumbai - 400018
  Ph: +91-9833017933, 022-24902340/41 • E-mail: mumbai@cbspd.com
• *Pune:* Bhuruk Prestige, Sr. No. 52/12/2+1+3/2,
  Narhe, Haveli (Near Katraj-Dehu Road Bypass), Pune - 411041
  Ph: +91-20-64704058/59, 32342277 • E-mail: pune@cbspd.com

Representatives:
• Hyderabad: 0-9885175004   • Nagpur: 0-9021734563
• Patna: 0-9334159340   • Vijayawada: 0-9000660880

Printed at:
India Binding House, Noida (UP)

Preface to the Second Edition

Medicine is an ever growing subject and newer advances are being made constantly as nothing is static. A lot of efforts are required to cope up with these new advances. Since the publication of first edition of the book, newer drugs have been introduced and newer concepts about various diseases have been evolved: To meet all this the need for second edition of the book was felt.

We have revised every chapter of the book and made the necessary changes. Special attention has been given to sections on Peptic ulcer disease, Chronic Diarrhoea, Respiratory and Hepatic Disorders, Diabetes, Osteoporosis, endrocrinal disorders and urinary tract infections etc. Section on Clinical methods has also been revised to make it a compleate section. AIDS is one of the burning problem of the day which affects millions of people all over the world. In section on AIDS, its role in Dental practice and therapy has been discussed thoroughly.

But despite all the changes, the basic concept of the book remains the same so as to meet the needs of Dental Students which we hope they shall find the book a useful guide.

A lot of suggestions were received from friends and well wishers regarding the book. We are thankful to all of them. Thanks also due to M/S CBS Publishers and Mr. B.M. Singh for their efforts to bring the book.

AUTHORS

Preface to the First Edition

The idea of writing this book took shape while interacting with students in their clinical years. Medicine is a vast and expanding field. The students need to read a book which is concise, to the point and yet provides all the essential information about the subject. The dental students face the dilemma of selecting the book even more. This book has been written keeping in view the requirements of the students particularly of the courses like BDS, Pharmacy, B.Sc. Physiotherapy etc.

Medicine is an act of constant learning. Knowledge about the diseases is ever changing and so is the treatment with drugs and the information about other aspects. It has been our endeavour to provide the information in a way which will help the students in acquiring good knowledge about the basic principles necessary in their daily practice and also for consultation of medical problems later on. With this view a chapter on "Cerebro Vascular diseases" has been included since it is a common problem and every doctor should be familiar with it.

In the first part of the book we have dealt with clinical methods; stress however, has also been given to the symptomatology of the diseases in addition to physical examination. A chapter has been particularly included, devoted to common symptoms and signs in medicine.

Every effort has been made to provide the latest information. It is however felt, that the student may read other detailed works to further advance his/her knowledge since it is not possible to give a lot of details in the available space.

Attempt has been made to give useful information in a comprehensive manner. We hope that this book turns out to be a useful guide to the students for the learning of medicine.

The authors are greatly indebted to their many colleagues for their generous help, constant encouragement and invaluable advice.

We are grateful to Dr. A.K. Khurana, M/s Jagson Pal and editors of J.P. Meditimes for kind permission to reproduce some of the colour illustrations.

Our sincere thanks are due to Sh. Vinod Juneja for his painstaking efforts in typesetting the book and our publishers Sh. Satish Jain, Sh. Vinod Jain and their team of dedicated workers Sh. Dharmveer and Sh. B.R. Sharma for valuable help and efforts in bringing out this book:

AUTHORS

Aims of Medicine

Medicine is a vast subject and requires a steadfast, open inquisitive mind to acquire its knowledge through a process of constant exploration and study.

The basic aim of learning medicine is to understand the disease a person is suffering from in a very humane approach.

Patient's ailment or suffering may not be only physical but also psychological. A careful understanding of the psyche of the person coming to the Doctor shall go a long way in reaching the diagnosis and subsequent management. The aim is to learn the subject in a thorough manner to acquire the skill for proper diagnosis and management of the patient to the best of his/her interests.

The present century has made great advances in investigative skills. No doubt advances in laboratory and investigative techniques have revolutionized the concept of medicine and have become a real boon, but still it is very essential to learn basic medicine since any doctor who is bereft of the fundamentals of basic medicine shall never be a complete doctor. Newer diagnostic tools and investigations should only serve as helpful aids and not make or mar the diagnosis of any patient. Those who depend only on these aids shall be doing great disservice to the patient and are liable to misdiagnose the case. So every student of medicine must keep his/her eyes open, and try to learn the subject with zeal and wisdom. One should be receptive to the new ideas but at the same time not discard the old concepts. The art of medicine is an amalgam of old and new wisdom. Our aim is to learn it by being a humble student, and always making endeavors to learn more and more. This is the basic aim of medicine.

In the words of Sir William Osler, a student of Medicine should "Learn to see, learn to hear, learn to smell and know that by practice alone can you become expert. Medicine is learned by the bedside and not only in the class room. Let not your conceptions of the manifestations of diseases come from words heard in the lecture room or read from the book. See and then reason and compare and control. But see first To study medicine without books is to sail an uncharted sea, while to study medicine only from books is not to go to sea at all".

A student of medicine hence, should learn the art of medicine with zeal, constant endeavor, with a balanced outlook and dedication.

Contents

CHAPTER 1

Clinical Methods

1. History-taking
2. General physical examination
3. Gastrointestinal system
4. Respiratory system

5. Cardiovascular system
6. Nervous system
7. Common signs and symptoms
   in medicine

HISTORY-TAKING

Whenever a person presents to the Doctor for his/her ailment, the basic aim is to arrive at a diagnosis of the disease, plan the investigations and outline the treatment.

Diagnosis of any disease shall depend on:

1. History of the patient's illness, present, past and family history.
2. Physical examination (general and systemic).
3. Any relevant investigations (laboratory, biochemical, radiological).

HISTORY OUTLINE

1. Name. Establish the identity of the person.

2. Age. It is important to know the age of the person since certain diseases are more common in certain age groups. Thus degenerative vascular diseases like coronary heart disease, cerebrovascular accidents occur in middle-aged or elderly people while congenital ailments and exanthema shall be seen more in younger age group.

3. Sex. Though there is no hard or fast rule but some diseases occur more in one sex as compared to the other sex. Women before menopause are protected from coronary heart disease because of protective action of female hormones but the incidence in both sexes is the same when a woman reaches menopause. Endocrinal disorders like myxoedema, thyrotoxicosis, Sheen's syndrome, gall stones, and cholecystitis, mammary cancer are known to occur more in females.

4. Occupation. Occupation of a person helps a lot in reaching at a diagnosis in some cases. Thus people engaged in plumbing, paint and varnish works are common victims of lead poisoning. Labourers engaged in coal, and silica mines, asbestos and cotton factories fall easy prey to occupational lung diseases. The incidence of tuberculosis is also higher in such people.

Truck drivers are more prone to suffer from sexually-transmitted diseases including AIDS.

5. Residence. The place from where a patient comes may have an indirect bearing in reaching the diagnosis. There are certain areas in our country where Ancylostomiasis, malaria, guinea worm infestations are endemic and similarly the water supply in some parts contains excess of fluoride (normal permissible limit 1 PP million) and inhabitants of these areas suffer from fluorosis, a debilitating ailment. Again there are certain geographical distribution of diseases. Kala azar is more common in Bihar and other coastal areas of India. Peptic ulcer though universally seen all over the country but the incidence of the disease is higher amongst people of South and mountainous areas like Kashmir valley.

History of present illness. The main object of history taking is to elicit complete information about the patients main complaints along with information about his/her past, family history; One should always be gentle with patient while eliciting the history. Many times the patient may not be able to give a complete history and for this help of his/her close family member may be sought.

One must be thorough in interrogating the patient. In a number of diseases e.g. peptic ulcer, history may be everything while physical examination may reveal nothing. It only highlights the importance of a good history.

Detail the chief complaints in the patients words (like pain in chest: shortness of breath, pain in legs, etc.) in chronological order along with their duration.

It is important to pin point the exact duration of the chief complaints since it shall help in the diagnosis. Thus pain in chest of short duration as compared to that of longer duration has its own significance. An acute pain in chest of short duration may point towards coronary heart disease or pleuritic pain while pain of longer duration shall favour more the diagnosis of myalgia or fibrositis. While interrogating the patient, ask specifically as to when the patient was absolutely fit. This shall help us in pin pointing the start of ailment.

After the person has been interrogated, a summary of his/her ailment be written giving information about the main illness as well as any information gathered by cross questioning or from family members. Each symptom must also be systematically analysed. Thus in a patient with pain in chest, enquire about site of pain, duration accompanying symptoms its radiation factors aggravating or diminishing the pain, the question of previous treatment, investigations, diagnosis must also be recorded. Once a detailed history of the patient's illness has been taken, then stress should be placed on specific questioning of the patient depending on which system appears to be predominantly involved.

Gastrointestinal system. Most of the patients with G.I. symptoms have those related to pain in abdomen or disturbances of bowel habits. In a patient presenting with pain abdomen, enquire about the site of pain, its radiation, nature of pain (whether colicky, continuous or intermittent) accompanying symptoms (like vomiting), its relation to food (in cases of peptic ulcer, food relieves pain in duodenal ulcer while pain of gastric ulcer is increased after meals).

For patients with bowel disturbances, ask about the number of stools passed (their nature—loose, ill-formed, whether any blood or mucus present. If blood present then whether bright coloured (piles) or dark coloured (malaena). Relationship of bowel opening with intake of food (cases of irritable bowel syndrome or neurogenic colon pass loose stools after taking of food)/any pain associated with the act of defecation.

Outline of history

1. Name
2. Age
3. Sex
4. Occupation
5. Residence
6. Chief complaints
7. History of present illness
8. Past history
9. Personal/family history

In cases of liver affections ask for loss or otherwise of appetite (hepatitis) colicky pain and its radiation to shoulder (cholecystitis/gall stones). Vomiting and pain in upper part of abdomen with passage of high coloured urine/clay-coloured stools (infective hepatitis).

Cardiovascular system. History of recurrent sore throats in a young adult/child in a case of rheumatic fever/rheumatic heart disease. Pain in chest, its site, radiation, nature (in Angina pain usually occurs on exertion, is present over the heart and generally radiates to the inner side of left arm and shoulder/neck. Occasionally pain of angina may present with toothache or may be radiated to right arm or even to epigastric region. It is a diffuse, constricting pain and is often relieved by rest).

Palpitation is a very common symptom and is often related to exertion. It is often present in heavy tea/coffee drinkers. Attacks of palpitation occur in cases of paroxysmal atrial tachycardia. Occasionally patient may complain of a sudden missing of heart beat (extra systoles). Breathlessness is a common feature of a cardiac case and especially so on exertion. It indicates poor cardiac reserve. In late stages of heart disease, breathlessness is present even at rest. Attacks of breathlessness coming in early hours of morning (nocturnal dyspnoea) indicate left heart failure.

Respiratory system. History about cough (dry or with expectoration) and its duration. Long duration of cough indicates chronic nature of disease like chronic bronchitis/bronchiectasis/pulmonary tuberculosis. Dry hacking cough indicates malignancy of lung.

Haemoptysis in a chest case can be either due to bronchiectasis/pulmonary tuberculosis/malignancy. Pain in chest (site of pain and its relationship to breathing pleuritic pain increased by respiration). Enquire about appetite and loss of weight (tuberculosis/malignancy lung).

Genitourinary system. History of pain in the lumbar region (renal colic) and its radiation to groin. Pain whether constant or coming in attacks.

Difficulty in passage of urine. Burning during the act of micturition (urinary tract infection).

Increased frequency of micturition (diabetes/enlarged prostate) presence of blood in urine (renal stones/tumour).

History of swelling over the face on getting up in the morning (nephrotic syndrome).

Nervous system. History of any fit (type/nature of fit, any prodromal symptoms, duration of fit, convulsions localised or generalised, history of injury during the fit). One has to distinguish whether the fits are due to any organic ailment (epilepsy, tumour) or hysterical.

Specific history about patient's mental health (social behaviour at home/office/family members/friends). Any abnormal behaviour (suicidal tendency/fits of depression/mania).

For patients coming with paralysis enquire whether acute (coming suddenly—vascular/traumatic/inflammatory) or chronic (prolapsed disc/spinal tumour). In cases of cerebrovascular accidents, history of headache/giddiness.

Haemopoietic system. Specific enquiry about any blood loss from any source (piles). In cases of women, enquire about excessive menstrual blood loss.

History of bleeding from any source (delayed healing of wounds/appearance of petechial spots in cases of thrombocytopenia/bleeding diathesis).

Bones/Joints. Elicit history about pain in the joints (whether single or multiple joints involved as in Rheumatoid arthritis, big joints like knee joint in osteoarthritis). Pain whether constant or fleeting (fleeting joint pain in cases of rheumatic fever). History of painful big toe in a middle aged person shall suggest attack of acute gout.

If pain is in the back and radiating down to leg it favours sciatica/prolapsed disc. Severe stabbing pains in the lower limbs at night might favour diagnosis of syphilitic involvement.

Vague aches and pains in the bones in a child bearing age female will point towards osteomalacia and in a middle aged male towards multiple myeloma.

In short a brief history about specific complaints shall be a pointer towards reaching a diagnosis.

Past history. Information about major illnesses

in the past are very essential. This may include history of any major accident, head injury, previous operations, childhood illnesses like exanthemata. Intake of any drug for long periods. History of recurrent asthmatic attacks in the past or frequent episodes of sore throat are important in diagnosing childhood asthma going on to adult stage in former and rheumatic heart disease in later case. One must pick out the relevant data from the past history and not lay stress on unnecessary facts.

Personal history. In this one has to specially ask about addictions to smoking, alcohol and drugs. The exact quantity of substances consumed and their duration be recorded. This is useful in cases of cirrhosis liver, peptic ulcer, chronic gastritis, polyneuropathy (Alcohol abuse) bronchogenic carcinoma, thromboangitis obliterans (excessive smoking).

Occupation of the patient is also helpful in some cases such as occupational lung disease, lead poisoning etc. Regarding marital status, and family environment a little enquiry is also helpful in telling about any psychological conflicts at home. Similarly in old people there are likely to be some major conflicts because a majority of them may be being neglected by their children.

Family history. There are certain diseases which run in families such as bronchial asthma, diabetes, coronary heart disease, hypertension etc.

So make a note about any major illness amongst the parents/grandparents and their cause of death.

Similarly presence of tuberculosis or any infectious ailment in the patients surroundings may point to the diagnosis.

Physical examination. Physical examination of the patient is important in reaching the diagnosis. *It consists mainly of two forms:*

1. General physical examination
2. Systemic examination

GENERAL PHYSICAL EXAMINATION

It means an overall assessment of the physical characteristics of the patient coming for examination.

It is important to observe the patient acutely (his or her gait, facial expression as the patient enters your office or if lying in bed the posture he adopts and whether he/she is comfortable or not. Thus a patient of renal/biliary colic shall be tossing in bed because of pain while a hemiplegic shall have one limb paralysed and unable to move. Facial expression like twitching (nervous tics, facial palsy, epilepsy) blank face (Parkinsonism) a vacant face with coarse features, lips large and subcutaneous tissue thickened (myxoedema) prominent eyes (exophthalmos) and lid retraction in thyrotoxicosis are important clues.

The built of the person is equally important. Generally there are three types of built.

Asthenic. Thin built, tall and long. More prone to suffer from tuberculosis.

Normosthenic. Normal body built.

Sthenic. Broad shouldered, fat and heavy built likely to fall prey to diabetes, hypertension, coronary heart disease.

IMPORTANT POINTS TO BE OBSERVED

In general, physical examinations are:

1. Eyes. For evidence of pallor (anaemia) congested (chronic cor pulmonale) puffiness of eye lids (nephrotic syndrome).

2. Nose. Pigmentation (in females during pregnancy, disseminated lupus erythematosus, exposure to sunlight). Tip of the nose red in mitral stenosis and heavy alcohol consumers, alae nasi working much in acute chest pathology (lobar pneumonia).

3. Lips. Pale in anaemia. Blue in cyanosis (congenital heart disease, chronic cor pulmonale, exposure to extreme degree of cold).

4. Cheeks. In anaemia there is pallor while butterfly pigmentation occurs in lupus. A bright flush over the malar bones in cases of mitral stenosis.

5. Skull. Size of skull also tells the diagnosis. An unduly small skull is seen in congenital conditions like microcephaly or craniostenosis and an unusually large head is seen in hydrocephalus. In rickets, the head is either oblong or square with

PLATE I

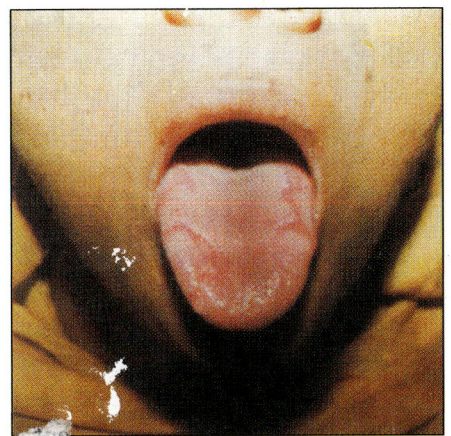

Geographical tongue.

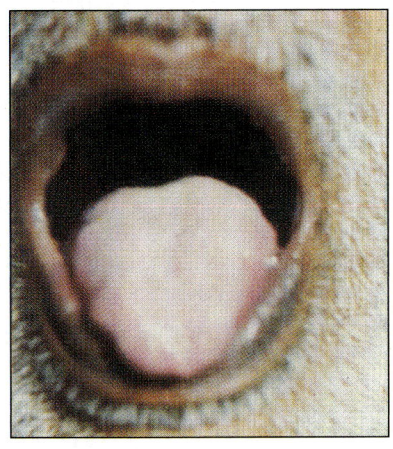

Wasting of tongue in a case of motor neurone disease.

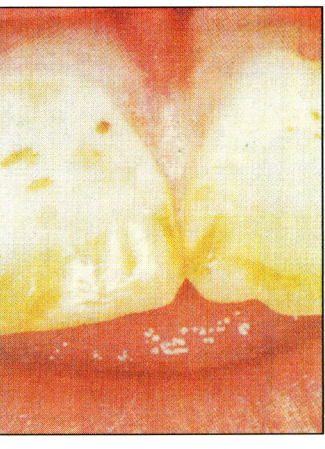

Fluorosis teeth showing yellowish brown staining.

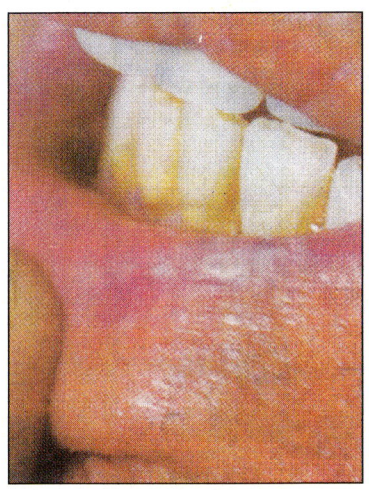

Leukoplakia.

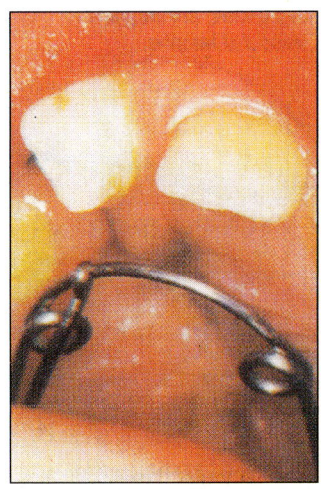

Cleft palate.

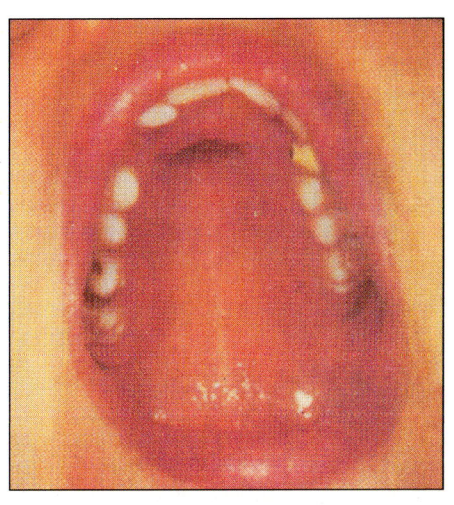

High-arched palate.

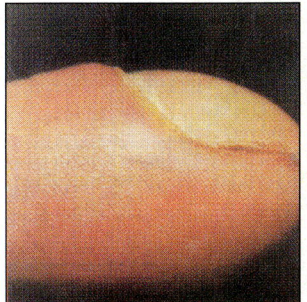

Finger clubbing.

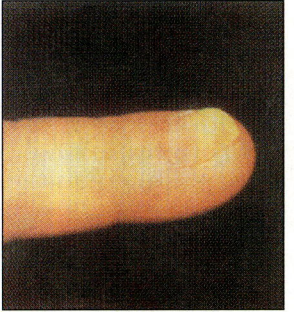

Koilonychia of nails.

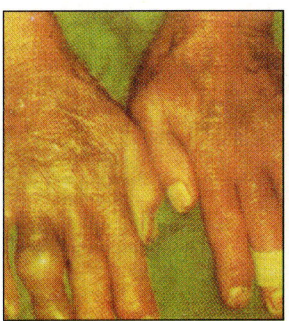

Acrocyanosis. This is as a result of exposure to cold.

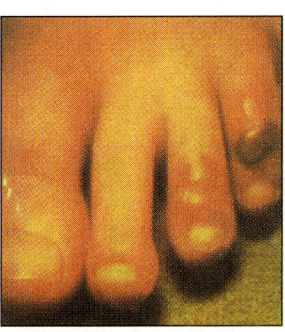

Chilblains on toes.

PLATE II

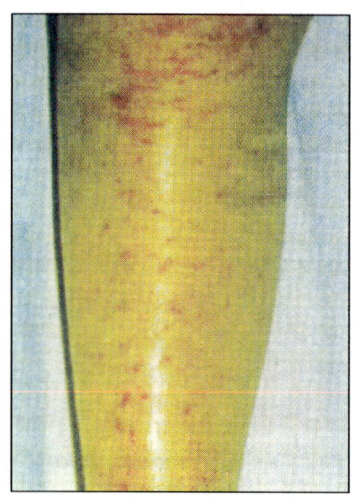

Dermatitis herpetiformis caused by gluten sensitivity in coeliac disease.

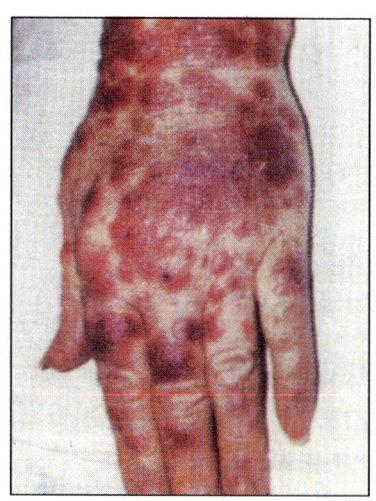

Polyarteritis nodosa manifested by fever, weight loss, arthralgia and vascular lesions.

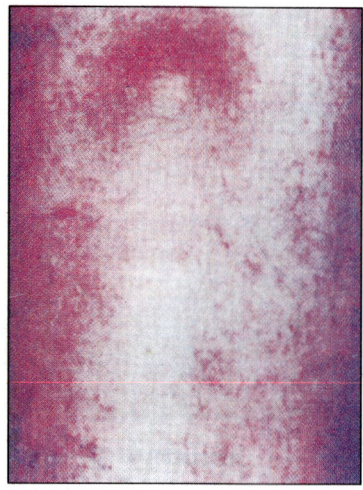

Erythema nodosum characterised by hilar lymphadenopathy, arthropathy and skin lesions.

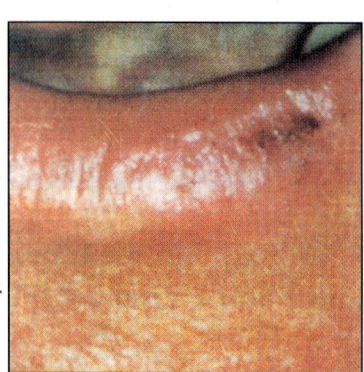

Lichen planus.

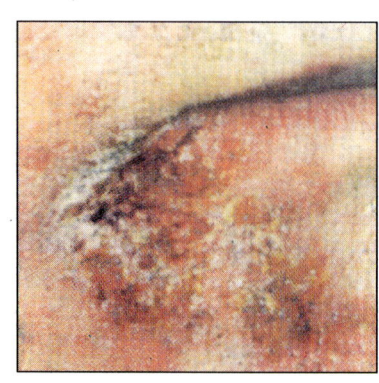

Angular cheilitis.

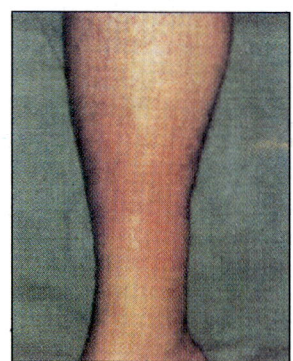

Deep vein thrombosis.

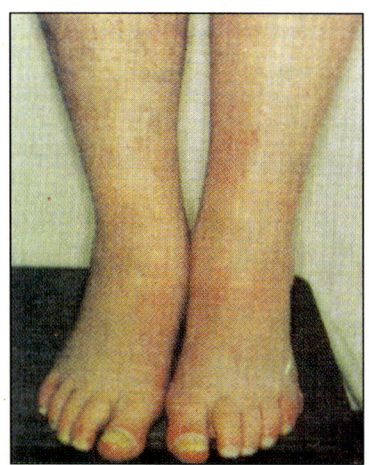

Ankle oedema.

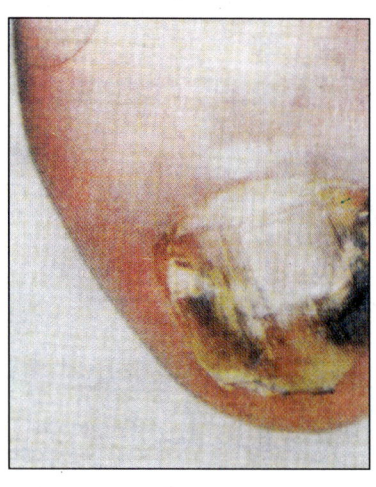

Nail infection caused by trichophyron species.

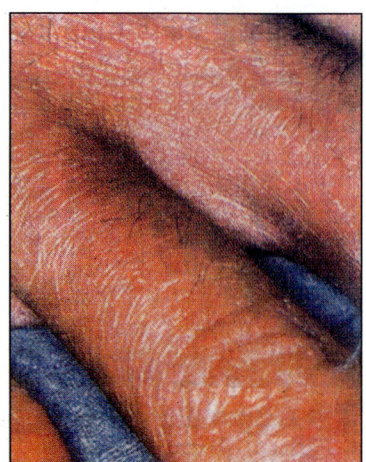

Ringworm of the hand.

cases of dehydration, pale skin in severe anaemia, yellow skin in infective hepatitis, haemolytic jaundice, petechial spots in purpura.

Any lesions on the skin like macules, papules, vesicles, bulla or pustules be observed

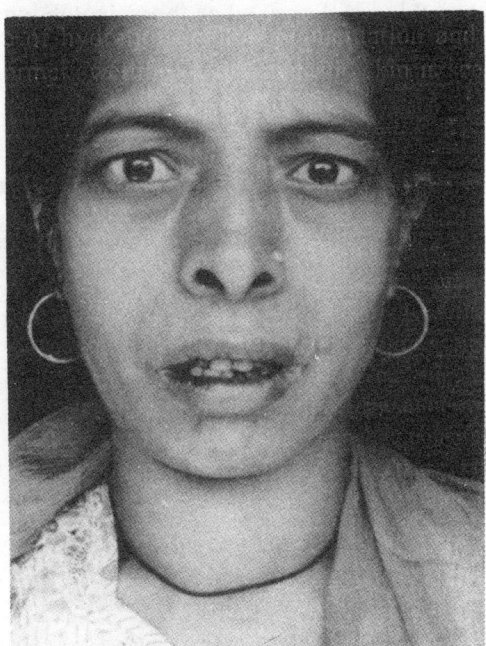

Fig. 1.1. Angular cheilitis and stomatitis.

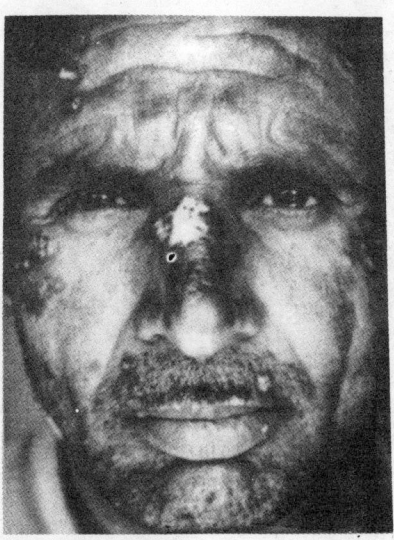

Fig. 1.2. Butterfly pigmentation in a case of disseminated lupus erythematosus.

thickening of the parietal and frontal prominences (bossing of head).

6. Skin. Important observations to be noticed are state of hydration, pallor, pigmentation and any abnormal swelling. A dry inelastic skin is seen in

Grading of clubbing	
Grade I	Swelling of the nail bed. It is soft and there is increased sponginess.
Grade II	The normal angle between the nail bed and nail is lost.
Grade III	Bulbous swelling of the tips of the fingers with convexity of the nails (drum stick or parrot beak appearances)
Grade IV	Grade III + periosteal reaction at the end of long bones (hypertrophic osteoarthropathy).

7. Oedema. Swelling appearing on dependent parts especially on the feet first and then ascending upwards to the legs thighs is seen in congestive heart failure. Swelling on the face especially on the eyelids in the early hours of morning is seen in cases of nephritis/nephrotic syndrome. Compression by growth or glands on the axillary veins or superior vena cava in thoracic region shall result in swelling of neck and arms while obstruction of inferior vena cava shall produce swelling of the lower legs.

8. Hands. Tremors of the hands may be fine or coarse, may be seen in anxiety, senility, thyrotoxicosis, paralysis agitans, alcoholism (delirium tremens) uremia, hepatic coma (flapping tremors). Claw like hand is seen in ulnar nerve palsy and leprosy.

Hands may be large, massive and spatulate in acromegaly.

Colour of nails tells us about anaemia (pallor), cyanosis (blue). Base of nails may become thickened and nail itself becomes convex ultimately taking the appearance of a drum stick (clubbing). Clubbing of nails is either congenital or acquired (pulmonary tuberculosis, congenital cyanotic heart disease, subacute bacterial endocarditis, empyema). In cases of iron deficiency anaemia the nail is thin and the normal convexity is replaced by a concavity (koilonychia).

Causes of clubbing

1. *Congenital and familial*
2. *Pulmonary disease*
   a) Lung abscess
   b) Bronchiectasis
   c) Empyema
   d) Bronchogenic carcinoma
3. *Cardiac diseases*
   a) Congenital cyanotic heart disease
   b) Subacute bacterial endocarditis
4. *G.I. disorders*
   a) Malabsorption syndrome
   b) Ulcerative colitis
   c) Coeliac disease
   d) G.I. malignancies
   e) Cirrhosis of liver
   f) Biliary cirrhosis

Painful nodules on finger tips (Osler nodes) in infective endocarditis, and in osteoarthritis Heberdens nodes at terminal joints of fingers. Swelling and deformity of fingers in rheumatoid arthritis.

9. Neck. Examine the neck for lymph node enlargement (tuberculosis: lymphoma: Hodgkin's disease, secondaries). Presence of sinus indicates tubercular lesion. Thyroid gland if suspected to be enlarged, find out whether uniformly enlarged (goitre) or nodule is felt (nodular goitre). Thyroid swelling will move up and down while swallowing.

Presence of pulsations in the neck especially in the anterior triangle are carotid pulsations seen in cases of aortic incompetence.

Jugular veins will be seen full indicating rise in venous pressure as seen in cases of congestive heart failure. Neck veins may also become prominent and face congested in cases of superior mediastinal obstruction.

10. Respiratory rate. Normal respiratory rate varies from 18 to 20 per minute. In men it is abdominothoracic while in women since the intercostal muscles of thorax play the major part

the breathing is described as thoracico-abdominal. An increase in respiratory rate normally occurs during exertion, excitement but abnormally increases in diseases of the lungs and heart.

A decrease in respiratory rate occurs in opium or narcotic poisoning, in cases of raised intracranial

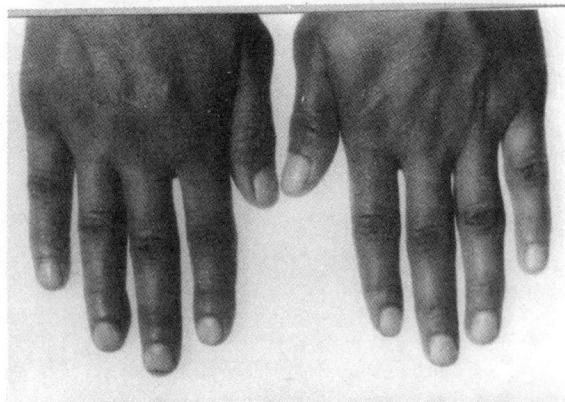

Fig. 1.3. Clubbling of fingers in a case of lung abscess.

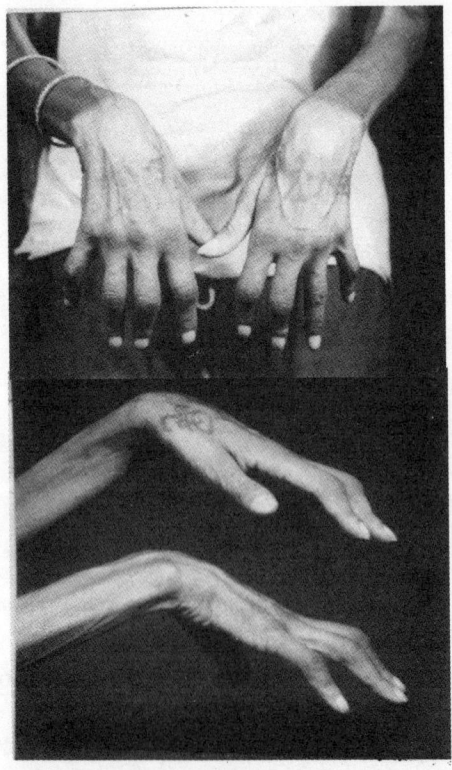

Fig. 1.4-5. Hands in a case of rheumatoid arthritis. There is swelling of fingers and deformity of hands.

tension and diabetic coma. Relationship between respiration to pulse rate usually is 1 to 4 but in cases of lung disease this ratio is disturbed.

11. Temperature. An idea about the temperature of a patient is very essential since it shall tell us about the health of the patient. Roughly temperature may be assessed by placing hand over the forehead. Temperature is recorded by thermometer in the mouth in adults (axilla or groin in children and from rectum in some cases). It can also be recorded by skin thermometers.

The normal oral temperature is 98.6°F (37°C) with a range from 97°F (36°C) to 99°F (37°C), in axilla it is slightly lower 98°F (36.5°C) and in the rectum higher 99.2°F (37.3°C) ranging upto 99.8°F.

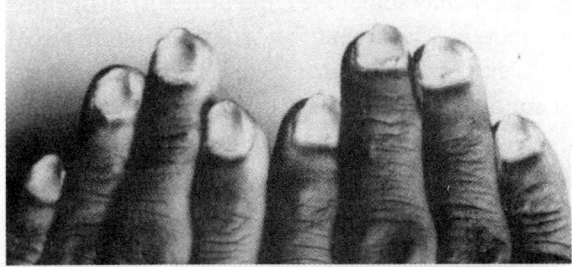
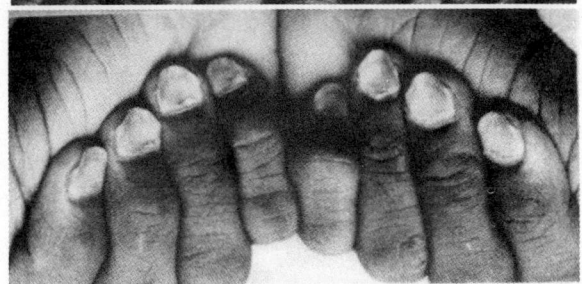

Fig. 1.6-7. Spoon shaped nails (Koilonychia) in a cse of iron deficiency anaemia.

Any rise in temperature above the normal range is labelled as fever or pyrexia. Temperatures going above 106°F is called hyperpyrexia and is considered very dangerous since it can knock out the vital centres in the brain.

Types of fever. Three main types of fever are encountered:

1. *Continuous* when fever does not touch normal at any time during the 24 hours and fluctuations within the day are less than 1½ o Fahrenheit e.g. typhoid.

2. *Remittent* when daily fluctuations are more than 1½° Fahrenheit. The evening temperature is usually higher than the morning e.g. Pulmonary tuberculosis.

3. *Intermittent.* A fever which is present only for few hours during the day e.g. in septic conditions. When intermittent fever occurs daily it is called quotidian, on alternates days tertian, and when after two days interval 'quartan'. Fever may be insidious or gradual. It may come with rigors and chills as in malaria. When fever comes down suddenly it is said to be by crisis. If gradually then lysis.

12. Pulse. Normal pulse ranges from 60 to 80 per minute though on an average pulse rate is 70-75 per minute. Radial pulse is the ideal site for counting the pulse which must be done for one minute. Pulse rate rises during excitement, exertion, in fevers, Thyrotoxicosis, acute infections, atrial tachycardia. Rate above 100 per minute is considered abnormal and similarly pulse rates below 60 per minute.

Athletes may normally show a slow pulse while it is slow in diseases like typhoid, jaundice, raised intracranial tension, viral infections and cases of heart block.

Very slow or very rapid pulse rates indicate pathology in some part of the body and must be looked into.

13. Blood pressure. Recordings of blood pressure form integral part of examination of every patient. Two types of apparatuses are in use, the mercury type (Sphygmomanometer) and anaeroid. The mercury type is the one commonly preferred since it is more accurate and dependable. Blood pressure can be recorded by two methods:

(i) Palpatory technique
(ii) Auscultatory technique

Palpatory method. With the blood pressure cuff round the arm and fingers of one hand placed on radial artery, the cuff is inflated and pressure allowed to come down slowly. The reading at which pulse appears is systolic level and where it disappears is the diastolic pressure. This is a rough method and useful in obese people or where brachial artery is not felt easily.

Auscultatory method. In this after tying the cuff, the pressure is raised generally to a high level and at the same time the chest piece of stethoscope is placed on the brachial artery. The cuff is slowly deflated and the first appearance of sound denotes systolic level and on further deflation when sound becomes muffled it is the diastolic reading.

Blood pressure must be recorded after the patient has rested for at least five minutes. When there is doubt about the recordings at least three readings be taken.

Normally there is a difference of upto 10 mm in the recordings of blood pressure in two arms. Marked difference in the readings in two arms may be due to vascular anomaly, pulseless disease or aortic aneurysm.

Difference between systolic and diastolic levels (pulse pressure) is usually between 30-60 mm. More than 60 mm means wide pulse pressure and occurs in cases of severe anaemia, thyrotoxicosis, aortic incompetence, systolic hypertension and high fevers. Normal blood pressure ranges between 95 to 140 mmHg systolic and 60 to 90 mm Hg diastolic depending on the age of person. Slight rise in systolic pressure occurs due to emotion, excitement, nervous tension while rise of diastolic pressure always indicates organic disease since this level is not effected by any extraneous factor like emotions etc.

Hypotension is diagnosed if systolic levels of blood pressure fall below 90 mmHg. This generally occurs in cases of severe dehydration, vomiting, diarrhoea, acute myocardial infarction, peripheral circulatory failure, shock etc.

GASTROINTESTINAL SYSTEM

The Mouth:

The lips

1. Look for colour of the lips, which may be pale (anaemia) or blue (cyanosis).

2. Swelling of one or both lips will indicate trauma, biting of the lips following an epileptic fit, insect bite, allergy or angioneurotic oedema.

3. Presence of crusts, fissures be looked, cracks at the commissure of lips (angular cheilitis) may be looked. Small painful vesicles over an erythematous surface round about or on lips (herpes febrilis), nose or chin is seen in cases of fever, viral infections of respiratory passages and lobar pneumonia.

Ulcers on the lips commonly are benign as a result of trauma or may be due to tuberculosis or malignancy.

Patient may sometimes find difficulty in opening the mouth. There may be spasm or paralysis of muscles of mastication or there is local pain in cases of arthritis, mumps, tetanus or due to dental problem.

Breath. It may be foul and it tells a lot about many conditions. Common causes shall be poor orodental hygiene, stomatitis, tonsillitis, indigestion, malignancy of upper gastrointestinal tract, bronchiectasis lung abscess and pulmonary tuberculosis. Fruity smell in breath is seen in cases of diabetic coma, starvation or acidosis while patients of uraemia have got ammonical smell. Mousy odour type of breath is seen in cases of hepatic failure (foetor hepaticus).

The tongue. Examination of the tongue tells us about lot of things.

Patient be asked to protrude the tongue. Examine for its coating, mobility and presence of ulcers on the surface and margins.

Normally the tongue is placed in the centre of oral cavity. Deviation to one side may be due to asymmetry of the jaws but more so in hemiplegia it is deviated to the paralysed side. Deviation to one side can also be due to lesions of hypoglossal nerve or facial paralysis. Tremors on the tongue may be seen due to anxiety neurosis, senility, thyrotoxicosis, delerium tremens, parkinsonism. Fibrillary twitchings are present in atrophied tongue following infranuclear or nuclear hypoglossal lesions, motor neurone disease, encephalitis.

Tongue should be examined for its size, colour whether dry or moist and its papillae. A tongue may be enlarged (macroglossia) in acromegaly, myxoedema, cretinism, tumours or inflammatory conditions and malignancy. A small tongue (microglossia) is seen in cases of malnutrition, anaemia, bilateral paralysis of hypoglossal nerve, pseudobulbar palsy.

Normally tongue is greyish red in colour. A pale coloured tongue is seen in cases of severe anaemia. A fiery bright coloured tongue indicates nicotinic acid deficiency while a magenta colour indicates riboflavin deficiency. A bluish tongue is seen in cyanosis and bluish red in polycythaemia vera, and after antibiotics use. Brownish tongue indicates uraemia, dehydration while dark brown patches are seen in Addison's disease.

State of the tongue is a good index of the hydration of the patient. A dry furred tongue indicates dehydration (excessive vomiting, diarrhoea, fever, mouth breathers, coma, uraemia etc). Furring of the tongue is commonly seen in persons who breathe through their mouth, smokers, sufferers from chronic constipation, alcoholics, acute fevers, chronic dyspepsia. Furring of the tongue in the centre and free at the margins has been found to be specific in cases of typhoid fever while a dry brown furred tongue is seen in cases of uraemia.

Fungal infection of the tongue produces a brownish fur and scarlet fever results in a strawberry tongue. Slight furring of the tongue normally is seen on getting up in the morning and after milk drinking.

Examination of the tongue for fissures, pigmentation and papillae is also helpful. Fissures on the tongue commonly indicate vitamin B complex deficiency or congenital fissuring or chronic superficial glossitis.

Atrophy of the papillae results in a smooth bald tongue which is seen in pernicious anaemia, sprue, nutritional macrocytic or microcytic anaemia, deficiency states and gastrointestinal disorders.

Fissuring of the tongue may be seen in the forms of circular or annular zig zag patches giving the tongue the appearance of a geographical tongue. This is congenital anomaly while chronic superficial glossitis or syphilis is also known to produce fissures.

In early phases of deficiency states, the tongue may appear swollen and papillae are prominent and there may be slight swelling but subsequently the tongue assumes a shiny smooth appearance and becomes dusky red in colour.

Whitish patches on the tongue (leukoplakia) may be precancerous or due to syphilis, or after prolonged use of antibiotics.

Margins and under surface of the tongue should be examined for any ulcer, indentations or leukoplakia. A single ulcer may be carcinomatous, tuberculous or syphilitic. Bad dentures or broken tooth may produce small superficial ulcers on the margins of the tongue. They shall be small and non-indurated. A small ulcer on the under surface of the tongue (fraenum) is seen in children suffering from whooping cough. A carcinomatous ulcer seen usually on the side or tip of the tongue is hard, irregular and indurated and painless in early stages. In late stages mobility of the tongue is effected and lymph glands in the distribution become enlarged.

A tuberculous ulcer is commonly seen in case of tuberculosis usually near the tip, is painful, not hard and has undermined edges while syphilitic ulcers are multiple (secondary syphilis) or single (primary) and superficial, painful small, and greyish with punched out bases. Syphilitic ulcers are not commonly seen.

Buccal mucosa. It is important to observe buccal mucosa carefully for pigmentation on the inner surface of the cheeks, palate. Patches of brown or dark streaks of pigmentation can be seen in Addison's disease, severe anaemia especially macrocytic, poisoning with lead, bismuth or arsenic. Koplik's spots (small bluish white spots with erythema at the base) opposite the molar teeth are seen in the early stages of measles in children.

Thrush is sometimes seen in children in the form of small white or greyish white patches adherent to the underlying surface. It is removed with difficulty and leaves behind a raw surface.

Infection of the buccal mucosa leads to the

mucosa becoming inflamed, red and likely to bleed easily. It may not only be acute catarrhal (stomatitis) but may become ulcerative and in rare cases (markedly debilitated and ill patients with poor oral hygiene) lead to gangrene (cancrum oris). There is excessive salivation, tendency to bleed from ulcers and foul offensive breath.

Purpuric/petechiae spots on the buccal mucosa may be seen in cases of haemorrhagic diseases, thrombocytopenia, purpura and in leukaemias. These indicate severe form of disease and should be viewed with caution.

Teeth. There are two sets of teeth. Temporary and permanent. The two lower central incisors are first to appear at sixth to eighth month followed by upper incisors at eighth to tenth month, the lower central incisors and all the front molars at twelfth to fourteenth month. The canines (upper first) come at eighteenth to twentieth month while posterior molars appear at two to two and a half years.

Teeth are important not only for its varied purposes but poor dental hygiene may cause or predispose to diseases such as rheumatoid arthritis, bacterial endocarditis and gastric disorders.

Dentition may be delayed because of rickets, malnutrition cretinism and mongolism. It may become difficult because of anomalous position or impaction of an erupting tooth especially in a small jaw.

Permanent teeth appear by six years of age. First molars are first to appear followed by central incisors at seven year, lateral at eight years, anterior bicuspid at nine years, posterior at ten years, canines at eleven to twelve years. Second and third molars are the last to appear, the former appearing at twelve to thirteen years followed by later between seventeen to twenty five years.

Different forms of anomalies may be observed in teeth. Hutchinson's teeth are specific of congenital syphilis and are seen in two upper central permanent incisors who are peg shaped, widely separated, broader nearer the gum then at the crown, dis-coloured, and have a semilunar notch on the biting edge. Teeth are pitted and discoloured in fluorosis (yellowish brown mottling).

Teeth are projecting and widely placed in Acromegaly. Grinding of teeth is common in young children and result of nervousness, helminthic infection, poor digestion and rickets.

Gums. The colour and health of the gums should be observed.

Pallor of gums is seen in anaemia, blue in cyanosis. Blue line along the margin of the gums is present in lead/bismuth poisoning.

Gums may show hypertrophy in pregnancy and in patients on antiepileptic drugs (Dilantin). Spongy gums with a tendency to bleed are seen in scurvy and conditions like purpura, leukaemias, agranulocytosis, aplastic anaemia, bleeding disorders. The gums are not only swollen and sore but also show bleeding when touched.

Shrinking or atrophy of the gums generally is seen either in senility or wasting diseases. Pus containing pockets involving both teeth and gums are formed in cases of pyorrhoea. The gums are generally retracted and bleed readily. Vincent's disease is a form of acute ulcerative and membranous gingivitis which spreads to involve the oral cavity leading to a peculiar foul odour and infection by fusiform bacilli and spirochetes.

Abdomen. The abdomen is divided into nine regions by means of two vertical and two horizontal lines. These regions help in locating important viscera and landmarks in the abdomen.

The horizontal or transverse lines are drawn. One at the lower border of tenth costal cartilage and the other at the level of anterior superior iliac spines. The vertical lines are drawn upwards on each side from mid inguinal point.

Thus the abdomen has got the following nine segments:

1. *Right hypochondrium* which is the place for right lobe of liver, gall bladder and hepatic flexure of colon.
2. *Left hypochondrium* mainly has got spleen.
3. *Epigastric* is the site of stomach, pancreas and aorta.
4. *Right lumbar* significant for right kidney.
5. *Left lumbar* has left kidney.

6. *Umbilicus.* It is the central part and has omentum, transverse colon.
7. *Right iliac.* Significant structures are caecum, appendix, Ileocaecal junction and right ovary in females.
8. *Left iliac.* Descending sigmoid colon is important organ and left ovary in females.
9. *Hypogastric.* Urinary bladder, prostate in men and uterus in females.

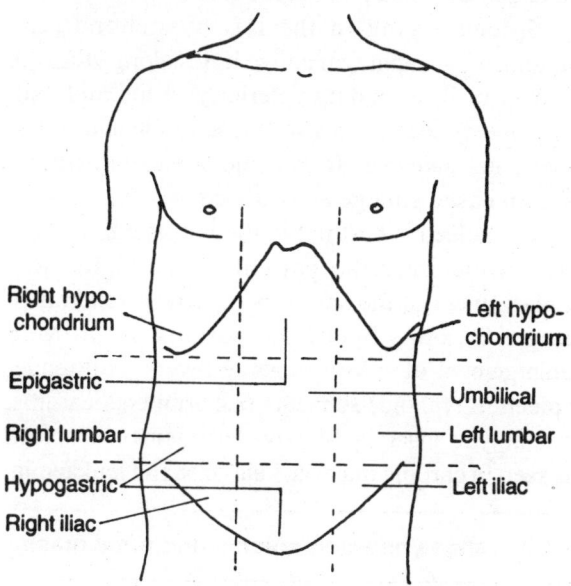

Fig. 1.8. Nine regions of abdomen.

Inspection. Examination of the abdomen be carried out in good light, the patient lying in a recumbent posture.

Look at the shape of the abdomen. Normally the abdomen is flat. A protubrant abdomen may be due to obesity, ascites, intestinal obstruction and pregnancy in females. A retracted abdomen is seen in wasting diseases, malnutrition, tuberculosis and malignancy.

A localised swelling will be due to enlargement of viscera lying in that segment or near by. Prolonged stretching of abdominal skin shall produce linear striae as in cases of pregnancy, obesity, ascites or any abdominal tumour. Purple striae over the abdominal wall are seen in Cushing's syndrome. Aortic pulsations in the epigastric region are visible and are normally seen in thin individuals or may be

transmitted in a case of aortic aneurysm.

Peristaltic waves are sometimes normally seen in a thin person, but visible peristalsis are important and one may have to spend sometime sitting by the bed side to look for these waves. In cases of pyloric obstruction the waves are seen moving from left to right in epigastric region while in cases of intestinal obstruction they are seen moving from right to left.

Examination of the umbilicus is significant. Normally it is indrawn but in abdominal distension, ascites it becomes everted. Bluish discoloration of the umbilicus is seen in cases of intra-abdominal haemorrhage while a cherry red colour is indicative of inflammatory pathology.

Visible veins over the abdomen are abnormal and are seen in intra abdominal growths, portal hypertension, inferior venacaval obstruction. The direction of blood flow in these veins be observed. In intrahepatic portal hypertension the flow is away from the umbilicus while in inferior vena canal obstruction the direction of flow is from below upwards.

The direction of blood flow is measured by emptying a vein with pressure by two fingers and lifting one finger at a time and noting the direction from which the vein is filled up.

Lastly while completing inspection look for any divertication of recti and presence of any hernia (inguinal/umbilical).

Palpation. Palpation of the abdomen should be done by completely relaxing the patient. The examiner sits on the right side and the patient lies with his/her legs flexed in a recumbent position.

Feel for any guarding or rigidity or tenderness. Normal feel of the abdomen is a bit elastic. Marked rigidity is seen in inflammatory conditions of the abdomen like peritonitis. Tenderness on deep pressure may be seen in right iliac fossa (appendicitis), right hypochondrium (tender hepatomegaly, cholecystitis). Deep palpation may be required for palpating deep lying structures. Spleen is best felt in left lateral position. Bimanual palpation is required for palpating kidney, liver and spleen. Doughy feel of the abdomen has been considered significant in cases of abdominal tuberculosis.

Evidence of free fluid in the abdomen (ascites) can be demonstrated by two methods.

Firstly one hand is placed on one side of the abdomen and with the other hand gentle tapping is done on the opposite side. A significant impact is felt. To avoid a false sensation, an assistant may be asked to place the edge of his hand firmly in the middle of the abdomen to damp out any vibrations being transmitted by the abdominal wall.

Percussion. Normal percussion note of abdomen is tympanic and except for liver area or pregnant uterus in females, note is the same all over the abdomen.

Note over the liver area may become tympanitic in cases of air under the diaphragm (intestinal perforation).

Ascites is diagnosed by eliciting shifting dullness on percussion. In a person with moderate amount of ascites on percussion there is dullness in the flanks. On turning the patient to the side the fluid will shift and now the flank shall be tympanitic.

In massive ascites shifting dullness may not be demonstrated and similarly where ascitic fluid is small in amount, fluid thrill may not be seen.

Auscultation. Normal peristaltic sounds are audible on auscultation of abdomen but in cases of peritonitis, paralytic ileus, these sounds may become absent. Absence of sounds over abdomen on auscultation invariably indicates pathology.

IMPORTANT ABDOMINAL VISCERA

Liver. Lying in the right upper quadrant the upper border of liver reaches the fifth interspace while the lower border reaches from right 9th costal to 8th left costal cartilage, the left lobe extends to the epigastric region.

Normally liver is not palpable in the abdomen. When liver is palpable observe by how many fingers or in cms from its border. Observe surface of liver whether smooth or nodular and for presence or absence of tenderness. Upper border of liver should be percussed.

Enlargement of liver occurs in hepatitis, malignancy, congestive heart failure, leukaemia, hodgkin's disease and alcoholic cirrhosis.

Surface of the liver normally is smooth in viral, amoebic hepatitis, congestive failure but it appears granular in portal cirrhosis and nodular in malignancy.

A tender liver means inflammation or congestion while in malignancy liver is non-tender. Liver is pulsatile in Tricuspid incompetence and is best assessed by Bimanual palpation.

Spleen. Lying in the left hypochondrium, bounded by diaphragm above it lies along 9th, 10th and 11th rib extending anteriorly to the mid axillary line. Spleen moves with respiration and is normally not palpable. To become clinically palpable spleen has to enlarge about twice its size.

The spleen is best felt in the left lateral position by rolling over the patient to the right side. Enlargement of the spleen is described in terms of finger breadths below the costal margin. Mild enlargement of spleen in acute fevers (soft tender spleen in typhoid) subacute bacterial endocarditis, haemolytic anaemia. Massive enlargement of spleen is seen in chronic malaria, kala-azar and leukaemia.

Differences between splenic and renal mass

Spleen	Kidney
1. It has a notch	No notch
2. It is directed downwards and forwards towards the umbilicus	Directed towards inguinal region
3. Moves well with respiration	Very little movement
4. Fingers can not be insinuated between the splenic mass and costal margin	Fingers can be easily insinuated between the mass margin
5. Best felt in left lateral position	Not effected, bimanual palpation required
6. It bulges anteriorly	It bulges posteriorly
7. Renal angle is empty	Renal angle full
8. Percussion note over mass dull	Area of resonance on percussion in front of mass

In a palpable spleen look for its consistency whether soft (septicaemia, typhoid, subacute bacterial endocarditis). Firm to hard (chronic malaria, leukaemia, cirrhosis). A notch of spleen is felt and it moves well with respiration.

Many times an enlarged spleen has to be differentiated from an enlarged palpable kidney. A splenic mass has a notch, is directed downwards and forwards towards the umbilicus, moves well with respiration. Fingers can not be insinuated between the splenic mass and costal cartilages. It is dull on percussion. On the other hand a renal mass is rounded, has no notch, is palpated bimanually, has very limited movements on respiration. It bulges into the loin and is bimanually palpable. Renal angle is full and there is area of resonance in front of the mass on percussion. Fingers can be pushed between the kidney mass and costal margin.

Gall bladder. Normally is not felt. It lies at a point opposite to 9th costal cartilage along the outer border of right rectus muscle.

Inflammation of gall bladder produces characteristic physical sign called Murphy's sign. In this when patient takes a deep breath, the examiner pushes his hand at the 9th costal cartilage and when the gall bladder touches the fingers there is a catch in the breath. It is commonly seen in acute inflammation (cholecystitis). Gall bladder may become enlarged and palpable in common bile duct obstruction due to gall stones and malignancy.

Kidneys. Both kidneys lie posteriorly in the dorsolumbar region, the upper poles corresponding to the upper border of 12th thoracic vertebrae, the lower poles almost reaching the iliac crest. The right kidney is lower as compared to left kidney.

Kidney normally is not palpable except in thin individuals. They are felt by bimanual method and move very little with respiration.

Fingers can be introduced between the enlarged kidney and the costal margins. An enlarged kidney tends to bulge forwards, posteriorly renal angle is full. An enlarged kidney may be due to polycystic disease, renal tumour, amyloidosis etc.

Palpation of renal angle is also helpful. In cases of infection of the kidney or of perirenal tissue, tenderness is present at renal angle.

Pancreas. In cases of carcinoma of pancreas when it is grossly enlarged it may be palpable in epigastrium while in mild case of pancreatitis only tenderness is elicited.

Rectal examination. Examination of the rectum is very essential in cases of piles, bleeding per rectum or suspected case of malignancy.

Further help is obtained by proctoscopy and sigmoidoscopy.

RESPIRATORY SYSTEM

Respiratory system constitutes the two lungs, the trachea, bronchi, bronchioles and alveoli. With the manubrium sterni lying in front surrounded by ribs on both sides, the clavicles and scapulae and vertebral spine posteriorly, lungs lie on both sides protected by the bony cage. Though there are numerous land marks on the chest an important one is Louis angle which is the junction of manubrium with the body of the sternum.

Louis angle is the level where trachea bifurcates in its two branches — the right and left bronchus. It is also a land mark from where the ribs and interspaces are counted. It is also the point where the anterior borders of the lungs and the upper border of atria of the heart meet.

Inspection. It is an important part of physical examination and in this one observes:

1. Size and shape of chest
2. Respiratory movements
3. Presence of any abnormal bulge or retraction.

A normal healthy chest is bilaterally symmetrical, smooth without any bulge or retraction except below the clavicles. Normal chest is elliptical in shape, transverse diameter more than anteroposterior in the ratio of 7 to 5.

Chest is to be inspected both from the front and back and from the sides as well as from above the shoulders.

Various forms of abnormal chest have been

described and they range from flat chest, pigeon chest, rachitic chest to barrel-shaped chest.

Flat chest. It is characterised by loss of forward curvature of chest, anteroposterior diameter getting reduced and the chest almost becoming flat. It may be seen in children with rickets or in patients of pulmonary tuberculosis.

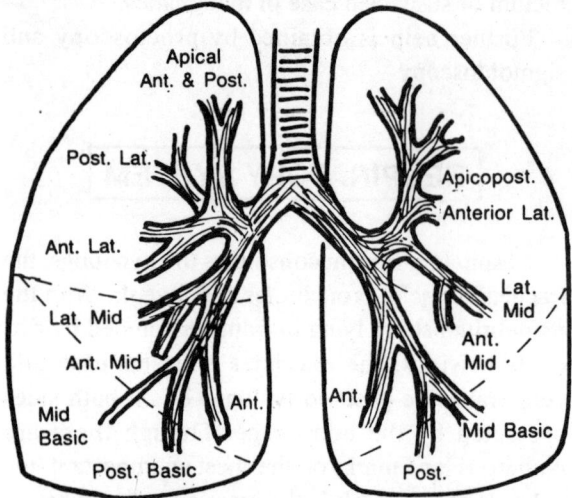

Fig. 1.9. Anatomy of tracheobronchial tree.

Pigeon chest. There is undue prominence of sternum and its adjacent, costal cartilages. The chest loses its normal elliptical shape and assumes a triangular shape. This type of chest may be seen as congenital abnormality or due to rickets in children.

Rachitic chest. *Characteristic features are:*

1. Pigeon shaped chest.
2. Harrison's sulcus which is a transverse groove or depression extending from the sides of xiphi sternum on either side of the chest.
3. Rickety rosary, a form of bead like enlargements of costochondral junctions particularly on the fourth, fifth and sixth ribs. It gives rise to an appearance of 'Beads' on either side of the sternum. This is the typical shape of chest in a child suffering from rickets.

Barrel-shaped chest. This is the chest typically seen in emphysematous case. Here the anteroposterior diameter of the chest increases, the sternum is more arched, ribs are placed more horizontally and the angle of Louis becomes more prominent, the spine becomes more arched and the chest becomes almost fixed in a state of inspiration. The accessory muscles of respiration become prominent and movements of diaphragm are increased.

Asymmetry of chest. Not only one comes across various forms of chest but prominence or bulge of the chest or retraction may be noticed quite frequently.

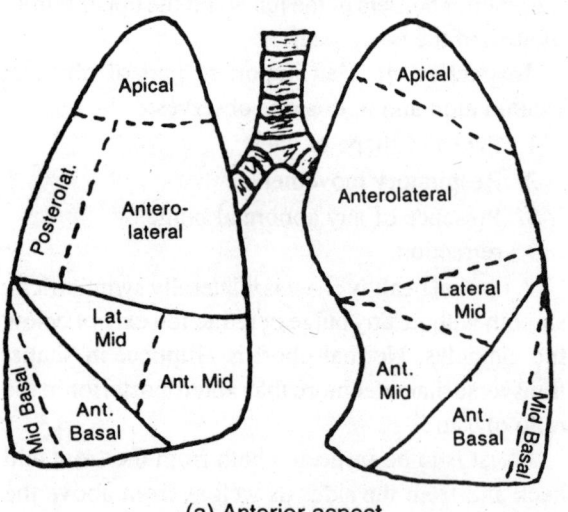

(a) Anterior aspect

(b) Posterior aspect

Fig. 1.10. Segmental anatomy of lungs.

Chest may become prominent on one side in cases of massive pleural effusion. Asymmetry of the spine (kyphosis, scoliosis) shall produce deformity of the thoracic cage due to conditions like Tumours of the lung, mediastinal growths, aortic aneurysm, pericardial effusion, gross enlargement of the heart. Liver abscess & Empyema pointing to surface shall all cause a localised bulging.

Unilateral flattening or retraction may be observed in tuberculosis, fibrosis of lung and adhesions in a case of pleurisy of long standing.

Occasionally an hollow over the lower end of sternum may be observed (pectus excavatum). It may be congenital or due to rickets in children or an occupational hazard as in shoe makers/cobblers.

Respiratory movements. The normal respiratory rate in adults is 18-20 respirations per minute. It increases with exertion, emotion and excitement normally but rapid increase in respiration occurs in persons suffering from fever, cardiac, respiratory or laryngeal ailments.

Breathing involves coordinated movements of intercostal muscles, diaphragm and muscles of the abdomen. Breathing is abdominothoracic in men and children while it is thoraco-abdominal or mainly thoracic in women.

Normal ratio between respiration and pulse rate is 1:4 but in cases of carbon monoxide/narcotic poisoning and respiratory failure the ratio is disturbed.

The normal chest in breathing moves symmetrically on both sides. Bilateral diminution of movements occurs in emphysematous chest ankylosing spondylitis, extensive fibrosis of lung while unilateral diminution of chest movement occurs in the disease confined to that side such as consolidation, fibrosis, pleural effusion. Normally there is intercostal indrawing of the lower spaces during inspiration. Excessive indrawing occurs in bronchial asthma, tracheal or laryngeal obstruction. Diminution or absence of intercostal retraction means massive pleural effusion or in pneumothorax.

Accessory muscles of respiration (sternomastoid, trapezius and short muscles of neck) come into play in cases of extensive lung disease and chronic emphysema. An important type of abnormal breathing is Cheyne-Stokes type of breathing where respiration gets deeper and deeper followed by a period of apnoea followed by another cycle of deepening and diminishing respiration. It occurs in patients of cardiac, respiratory, renal disease, increased intracranial tension and narcotic poisoning.

Another variant of this type of breathing is Biot's type of respiration where breathing is irregular in depth and pauses with occasional sighs. It occurs in cases of meningitis.

In addition to the above, while inspecting chest look for the position of apex beat, any pulsations on the chest (anastomotic pulsations in coarctation of aorta) and about undue prominence of sternomastoid on one side which is indicative of shifting of trachea to that side (pleural effusion).

Palpation. Palpation of the chest is done to confirm the findings of inspection.

Compare the movements of the chest on both sides whether generalized restriction (emphysema) or localised (consolidation, pleural effusion). Position of trachea and displacement of apex beat be observed. Shifting of trachea, and mediastinum away from the affected side occurs in pleural effusion and pneumothorax while its shifting towards the affected side occurs in fibrosis of lung, collapse of one or more lobes of the lung. Vibrations communicated to the chest wall from larynx to bronchi and lungs can be felt on chest wall by placing ulnar border of the hand on chest and patient repeating 'one-two-three'. These vibrations are called 'Vocal fremitus'. It may be increased or decreased depending on the disease of the lung.

Increase occurs in consolidation of lung (pulmonary tuberculosis lobar, pneumonia) pulmonary infarction, collapse of lung with a patent bronchus, a superficial large cavity. Increase in fremitus is because of better conduction of sounds through solid lung tissue to chest wall. Decrease in vocal fermitus occurs in pleural effusion pneumothorax since the relaxed lung fails to convey the vibrations which do not reach the fluid. Sometimes in cases of dry pleurisy a friction rub may be felt over the chest wall.

Percussion. It is an important component of respiratory system examination.

Correct percussion is essential. It must be done from the resonant to the less resonant side, from above downwards. Keep the pleximeter finger in the interspace rather than on the rib, apply firm pressure but do not do heavy percussion. The character and quality of sound produced by the chest wall shall depend on whether there is any pathology underneath or not. Normally the percussion note is tympanitic. It is hyperresonant on emphysematous chest while note becomes impaired in cases of consolidation, fibrosis or collapse. A dull note is seen in consolidation of lung, thickened pleura or carcinoma lung. A stony dullness in note is seen in a case of pleural effusion.

When percussing one must demarcate the borders of lung. Thus on right side the lower border of lung lies over the liver on the sixth rib in the midclavicular line, eighth rib in the midaxillary line and tenth rib in the scapular line posteriorly. Liver dullness gets obliterated in cases of intestinal perforation.

On the left side one encounters area of cardiac dullness and posteriorly there is splenic dullness and of other organs which lie near the spine.

When one gets stony dullness suggestive of pleural effusion the upper border of dullness be demonstrated which is highest in the axilla and lower on the sides. This dullness assumes S-shaped curve and is referred to as Ellis curve.

In cases of hydro pneumothorax, the upper border of dullness is well delineated and remains horizontal. Shift or change in the fluid level is seen with change in the posture of the patient.

Auscultation. It involves demonstration of type of breathing—vesicular or bronchial and its character along with presence or absence of adventitious sounds (crepts, rhonchi) and vocal resonance.

Normal breathing is vesicular and is heard all over the chest. It is low pitched and has a rustling character, the inspiratory phase is prolonged (two to three times more than the expiratory phase), the expiratory phase is lower pitched and there is no pause between the two phases.

Vesicular breathing may be harsh in bronchitis, acute chest infection while it is feeble in a case of pleural effusion. The bronchial breathing is blowing or hollow in character, inspiratory phase equals expiratory phase and there is pause between the two. Bronchial breathing may be low pitched (Cavernous) medium pitched or high pitched (tubular). Low pitched bronchial breathing is heard over moderately large cavities in the lung and in a case of open pneumothorax. High pitched or tubular breathing is heard where consolidation of lung has occurred round small sized bronchial tubes as in consolidation of lung, lobar pneumonia, malignant disease, pulmonary infarction and pleural effusion.

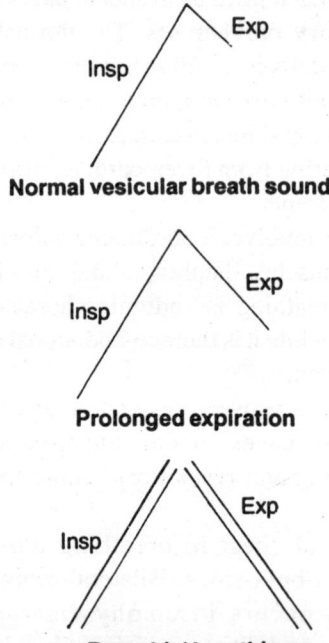

Fig. 1.11. Diagrammatic representation of breath sounds.

Another variety of bronchial breathing is amphoric which is like blowing across a bottle and has a distinct 'echo like' quality. It is heard over a large cavity with smooth wall or in a case of pneumothorax in direct contact with a bronchus. Adventitious sounds comprise of dry sounds (rhonchi), Moist sounds (crepitations), Pleural sounds (pleural rub). These are usually produced in the lung tissue air passages or over the pleura.

Rhonchi are sounds produced as a result of passage through the bronchi which may be narrowed or partially closed because of inflammation, spasm oedema of the wall or thick secretions blocking the lumen of bronchus. Depending on the pitch of sound, rhonchi may be sibilant (high pitched) or low pitched (sonorous). Sibilant rhonchi are whistling squeaking sounds produced in small or medium-sized bronchi while sonorous sounds are deep toned and are heard within the large bronchi. While sonorous rhonchi occur during early part of inspiration or may become continuous, the former variety (sibilant) are heard over the latter part of inspiration or early part of expiratory phase.

Rhonchi are commonly heard in cases of bronchial asthma, chronic bronchitis with emphysema and pulmonary tuberculosis.

Moist sounds also called rales or crepitations are crackling sounds produced as a result of passage of air through secretions in bronchi, bronchioles or alveoli.

Crepitations may be fine, medium or coarse. Fine crepitations tend to occur at the end of inspiratory phase and are due to exudation in the alveoli. They are characteristically seen in early stage of pneumonia, pulmonary tuberculosis and on the bases in cases of congestive cardiac failure.

Medium creptations usually originate from secretions in small and medium bronchi and are heard at end of the inspiration and beginning of expiration. These usually are indicative of more secretions in the alveoli.

Coarse crepitations are bubbling in character and are due to secretions in large bronchi, and heard in both phases of respiration. They are audible in case of bronchiectasis, lung abscess, pulmonary tuberculosis, pulmonary oedema and lung cavity.

Pleural rub. It is a dry sound produced as a result of separation of two inflamed pleural surfaces and occurs during the phase of respiration when the two surfaces are rubbing against each other. Thus a rub appears during part of inspiratory phase and then reappears at the same period of expiration.

Pleural rub characteristically is seen in dry pleurisy and common site is lower part of axilla. Depending on its intensity it may become palpable. It is accentuated by applying pressure by chest piece of stethoscope. Cough does not alter its character. Appearance of fluid in the pleural space tends to make it disappear.

Succussion splash. It is a form of splashing sound, when there is both air and fluid in the pleural space (hydropneumothorax) heard on turning the patient to side, giving him a little shake and listening on the chest wall. It is a very characteristic sound and confirms the diagnosis.

Post-tussic suction. It is a low pitched sucking sound heard over a thin walled cavity in the lung communicating with the bronchus and is produced by re-entry of air. This results in a typical sucking sound.

Vocal resonance. It is the sound heard over various parts of lung when patient speaks rhythmically 'one-two-three'. It may be altered in various pathological processes, increased in consolidation, atelectasis, superficial lung cavity and decreased in pleural effusion, emphysema, pleural thickening.

When spoken words are unusually loud this is called bronchophony and is seen in lobar pneumonia, consolidation pulmonary tuberculosis, pleural effusion (above the level of pleural fluid) and superficial lung cavity.

Whispering pectoriloquy. It is an important diagnostic sign in a large cavity in the lung communicating with the bronchus, consolidation and in pleural effusion at its the upper level. The patient speaks in a whispered tone and these sounds appear to be heard directly in the ear.

CARDIOVASCULAR SYSTEM

It is an important system in the body and consists primarily of heart and the peripheral vessels. Lying in the left side of chest (two thirds to the left and a third to the right of midline) heart maintains the life line by continuous pumping of blood to various vital organs.

Examination of heart consists of inspection, palpation, percussion and auscultation.

Inspection. Area of chest overlying heart is called precordium. Look for its shape, which normally is not bulging or prominent. Bulging of precordium occurs due to deformity of thoracic cage (scoliosis, kyphoscoliosis) or in children due to long standing heart disease or in massive pericardial effusion. Important landmark is Apex beat (Apical impulse or thrust) which lies normally in the 5th inter space, one half to one centimetre inside the left midclavicular line. It is as a result of thrust produced on the chest wall by the apical part of the heart. It becomes forceful in excitement, after exercise, exertion. It may be absent or diminished in persons with thick chest wall, obesity, emphysematous chest or in a weak heart. Apex beat may be displaced in persons with skeletal deformities (scoliosis) and in diseases of surrounding structures where heart is either pushed or pulled from its place. Thus in cases of pleural effusion, pneumothorax apex beat is displaced to opposite side while in lung fibrosis and collapse it is pulled to the same side.

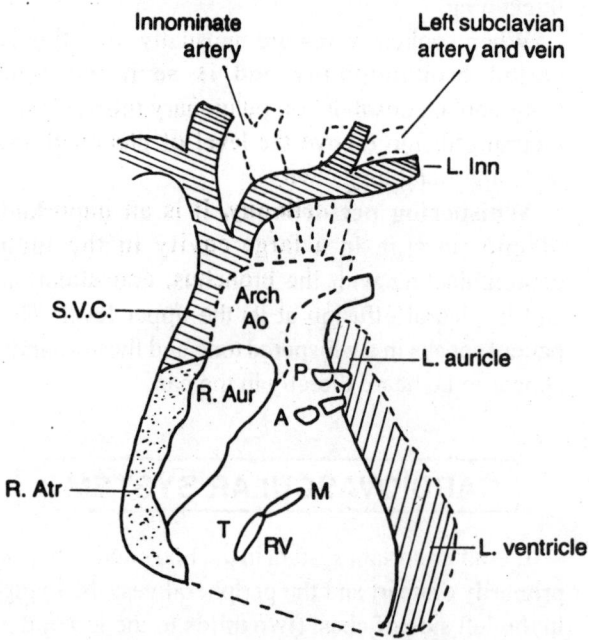

Fig. 1.11. Heart: Its chambers and valves.

Apex beat is displaced outwards and downwards

in left ventricular enlargement due to hypertension, ischaemic heart disease and aortic stenosis, aortic incompetence. In addition to apex beat, one observes for pulsations on the chest wall. Pulsations in the suprasternal notch occur in aneurysm of the arch of aorta or cases of hypertension where aortic arch is raised. Pulsations in the second or third left inter space are due to dilated pulmonary artery. Prominent and pulsating vessels in the interscapular and intercostal regions on the back of chest can be observed in coarctation of aorta.

Causes of absent apex beat

1. Thick chest wall
2. Obesity
3. Apex beat lying behind rib
4. Emphysematous chest
5. Failing heart
6. Pendulous breast in females

Causes of forceful heart beat

1. Excitement
2. Emotions
3. Exercise
4. Thyrotoxicosis
5. Tachycardias
6. Hypertension

Pulsations in the neck are of two forms. Arterial and venous. Pulsations are seen in carotid vessels in excitement, thyrotoxicosis and hypertension while massive pulsations are seen in aortic incompetence. Jugular veins show slight pulsations normally. They become full and distended in right heart failure. In health the height of blood column in jugular vein is at the level of manubrium sterni. This is the level where the pressure in the jugular vein equals that of right auricle in health. Jugular venous pressure is an important index of congestive heart failure. Normally it is 5-10 cm of water. Clinically it is measured when the patient is lying in bed and his/her head at 45° positioned, column of blood in jugular vein is full. With a line drawn parallel to the angle of jaw and the other at manubrium sterni, and a perpendicular line drawn between the two indicates the venous pressure. In cases with severe congestive failure, the column of blood reaches upto the angle of jaw. In superior vena caval obstruction, the neck veins remain constantly full since the venous pressure is not elevated and the cause is mechanical.

Pressure over the enlarged liver or in case of raised intra-abdominal pressure may fill the neck vessels. It is called hepatojugular reflux and may be observed in normal individuals as well in those with right heart failure. Often confusion arises as to whether the pulsations in the neck are arterial or venous. A few differences between the two are worth considering.

Venous pulsations are usually wave like, slow, visible but not palpable, tend to become full during respiration and tend to disappear when the patient sits up in bed. A little pressure over the lower end tends to distend the vessel. In contrast arterial pulsations are sharp, thrust like, coinciding with the apex beat.

Arterial pulsations lie in the anterior triangle of the neck, are not effected either by posture, respiration or abdominal compression.

Besides this look for any prominence of vessels on the chest wall. Prominent veins over the chest are seen in cases of mediastinal growth, inferior

Differences between arterial and venous pulsations in neck

	Arterial	Venous
1.	Present in anterior triangle	Present in posterior triangle
2.	Forceful, sharp, thrust like	Slow, wave like
3.	Palpable	Not palpable
4.	Not affected by respiration	Becomes full during inspiration
5.	No effect of posture	Disappears when patient sits up in bed
6.	No effect of pressure	A little pressure over lower end distends the vessel
7.	No effect of abdominal compression	Pressure over liver distends the veins

venacaval obstruction and in severe degree of right heart failure. Epigastric pulsations can be either cardiac in origin (hypertrophied right ventricle, tricuspid regurgitation), aortic (normal pulsations in thin individuals, aortic aneurysm), hepatic (pulsatile liver).

Jugular venous pressure wave. It consists of three peaks ('a' 'c' and 'v' waves) and two troughs ('x' and 'y' descents). These waves can be observed in jugular vein. 'a' wave is produced by atrial systole as result of increased resistance to ventricular filling. A large 'a' wave is called cannon wave seen in complete heart block. Large 'a' waves occur in cases with right ventricular hypertrophy 'v' wave indicates venous filling of right atrium during ventricular systole. Giant 'v' waves are seen in tricuspid regurgitation. 'y' decent follows 'v' wave when tricuspid valve opens. This is seen in constrictive pericarditis and tricuspid regurgitation.

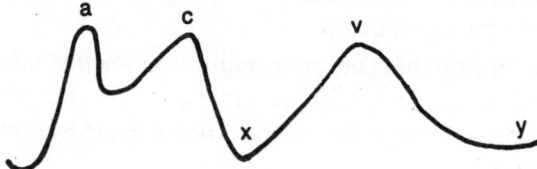

Fig. 1.12. Normal jugular venous wave.

Venous pulsation are obvious on inspection of neck. These pulsations may not be seen in fat persons or when the person is standing.

Palpation. It is an important part of physical examination of cardiovascular system.

First is to locate the apex beat, its exact location and its force. The character of the apical thrust tells a lot. A forceful apex beat may be felt in thin chest individuals, after exertion, thyrotoxicosis and in excitement. A forceful heaving impulse is characteristic of left ventricular hypertrophy as in hypertension and aortic valve disease.

An impalpable apex beat can be present in obese thick chested persons, emphysematous chest, acute myocarditis, failing heart or when apex beat is placed behind the rib.

A sudden forcible tumultous pulsation can be felt in cases of right ventricular hypertrophy.

Any abnormal pulsation felt over the precordium/chest should be observed. Heart sounds are palpated but sometimes an abnormal sensation is conveyed to the hand. This is called thrill. Thrill is produced when the blood passes through a narrowed valve leading to current which sets the surrounding structures into vibration. A thrill must be timed with the apex beat or carotid pulsation.

A thrill which synchronises with the thrust or outward movement of apex beat is systolic whilst the one that occurs during the retraction or indrawing of the apical thrust is diastolic and the one preceding the thrust is presystolic. A thrill is basically an exaggerated murmur. A thrill at the apex is either systolic or diastolic (diastolic in mitral stenosis, systolic in mitral incompetence) and in the second left interspace is either systolic (pulmonary stenosis, atrial septal defect) or continuous (patent ductus arteriosus). A continuous systolic thrill in the third and fourth interspace on left side is felt in ventricular septal defect.

In cases of acute pericarditis, a pericardial rub is felt in the pericardial area. It is differentiated from pleural rub from its site and is not effected by respiration.

Percussion. It is of limited value except that in emphysema, cardiac dullness is obliterated. One can define the cardiac borders by starting percussion for the left border in the fifth interspace from axilla inwards and then for the right border which is right of the right sternal line. Percussion is important in diagnosis of aortic aneurysm and pericardial effusion. In case of pericarditis with effusion, the cardiac area becomes dull assuming a globular shape and the earliest sign is dullness in 2nd and 3rd interspace. Similarly dullness of left border of heart shall extend to the left and downwards in left ventricular enlargement.

Auscultation. Auscultation of heart and detecting various abnormal sounds is an act which is learnt by constant practice.

There are four classical areas of heart where either heart sounds or murmurs are heard.

1. *Mitral area* in the fifth left interspace near the midclavicular line. It represents the apex of the heart.
2. *Aortic area.* 2nd interspace on right side.
3. *Pulmonary area.* Second left inter space on the inner side.
4. *Tricuspid area* at the lower end of sternum near the level of fourth intercostal space on left side.

In addition auscultation is done on carotid vessels to look for aortic murmur which is being conducted along the vessels.

In health two sounds are heard over the various areas. The first sound is produced by the closure of the mitral and tricuspid valves and the second sound due to closure of aortic and pulmonary valves. So quality and character of the sound is best heard in these areas.

Normally only two heart sounds are audible. But sometimes a third heart sound and rarely a fourth heart sound is heard. Third heart sound is soft, short and of low pitch and best heard in the left lateral position.

Heart sounds. One has to define the character intensity duration split and relationship of heart sounds with posture and exercise. Heart sounds may be feeble in thick chested individuals emphysema pericardial effusion myocardial failure.

First heart sound. Its intensity depends on the position of auriculoventricular valve cusps, greater the force of closure more louder is the intensity of heart sound. It is accentuated in cases of mitral stenosis (short, snappy), in fever, thyrotoxicosis and hyperkinetic states while it may be diminished in emphysema, acute rheumatic fever, shock and peripheral circulatory failure. Varying intensity of first heart sound may be heard in partial or complete heart block. Thus in cases of heart block a loud or cannon sound is heard at the apex.

Splitting of first heart sound indicates asynchronous closure of mitral and tricuspid valves and may be heard in healthy elderly individuals and occasionally in bundle branch block.

Second heart sound. Since it is produced by the closure of aortic and pulmonary valves, it is best

PLATE III

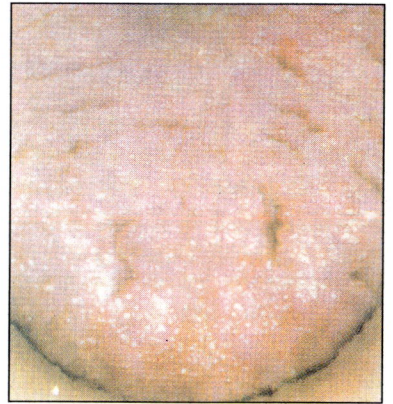

Scrotal tongue.

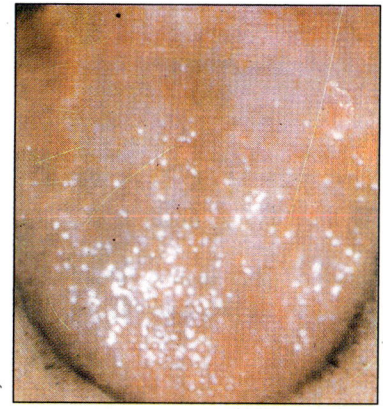

Geographic tongue.

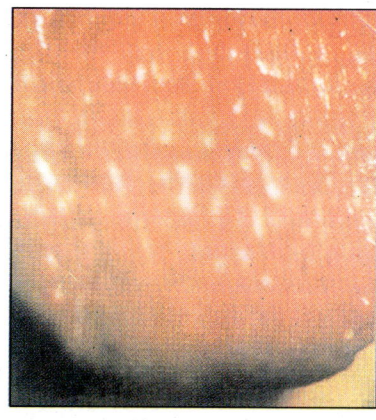

Raw beef tongue in macrocytic anaemia.

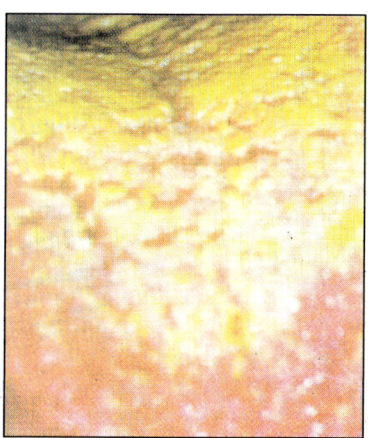

Candida infection. Commonly seen in diabetics and those with reduced immunity and on steroids.

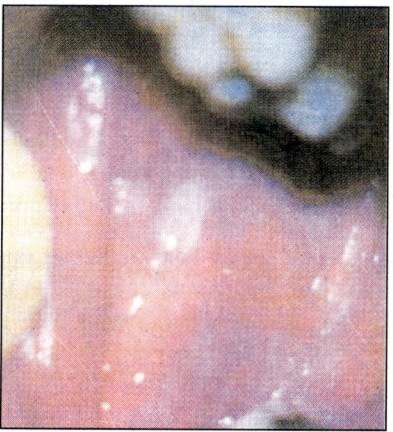

Oral lichen planus.

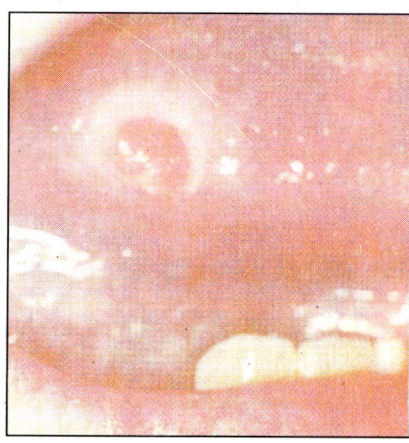

Aphthous ulceration of tongue.

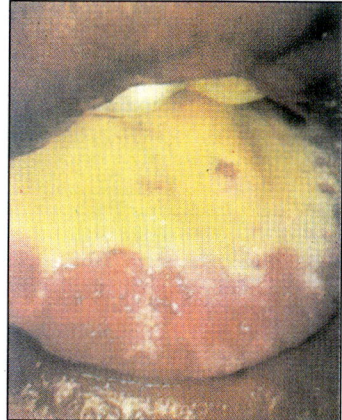

Oral thrush.

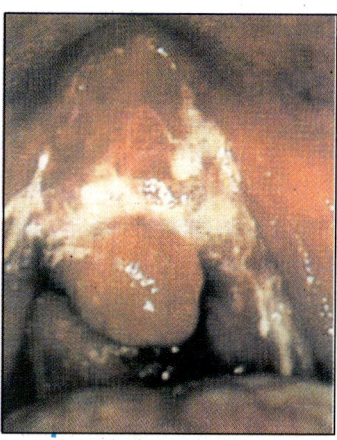

Throat infection. Patient took course of antibiotics for chronic bronchitis. A wide curdy coating over throat was formed. Responded to antifungal drugs.

PLATE IV

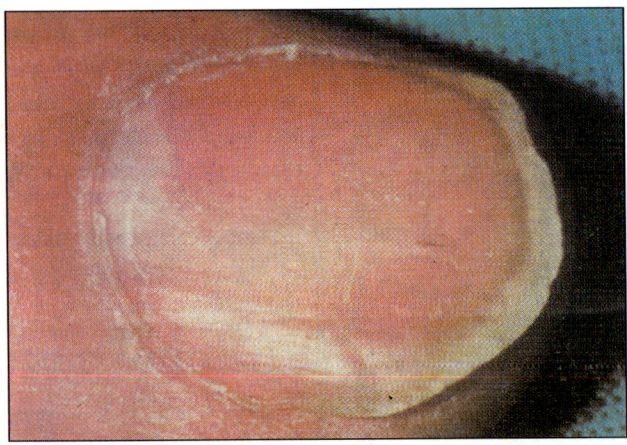

Splinter haemorrhages under the finger nail in infective endocarditis.

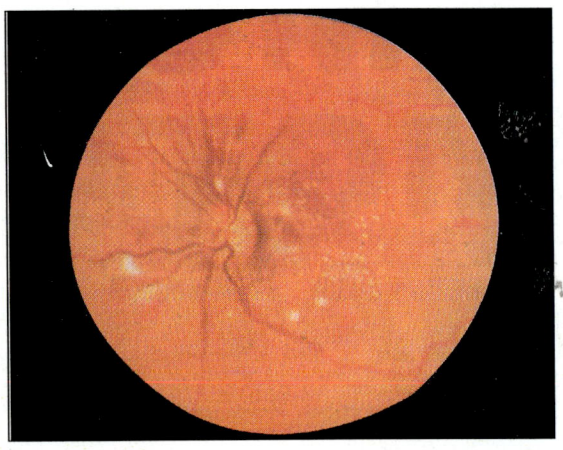

Hypertensive retinopathy (grade III).

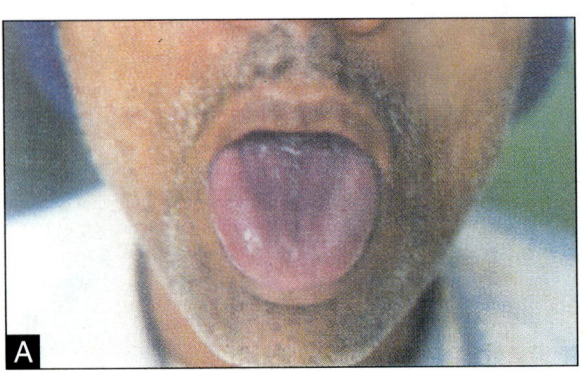

Chronic obstructive pulmonary disease. This is a case of COPD. There is cyanosis (blue tongue—Fig. A).
Nails are clubbed and cyanosed (Fig. B).

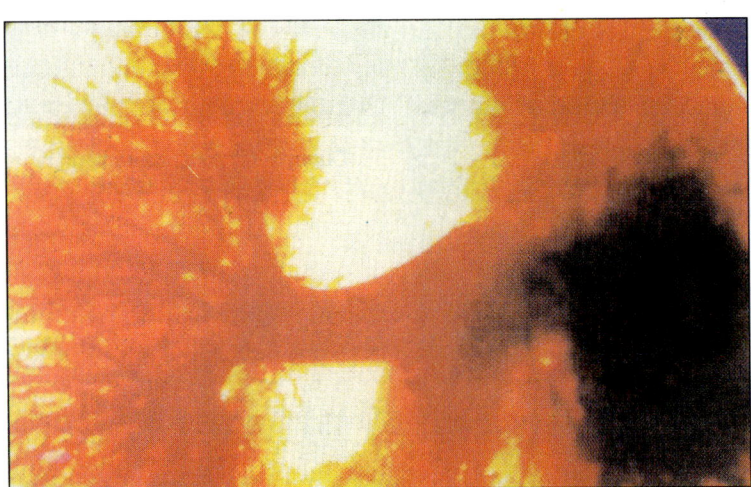

Pulmonary embolism in a case of atrial fibrillation.

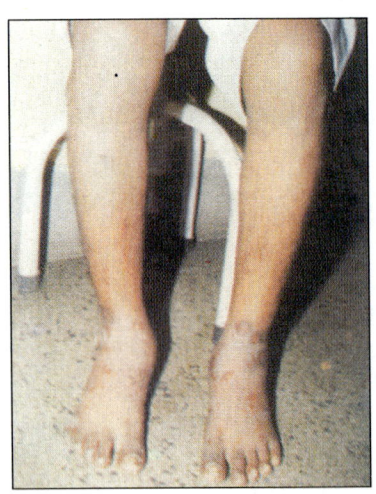

Nephrotic syndrome. Swelling of legs &
feet along with generalised anasarca.

heard at the base, louder than the first heart sound. Asynchronous closure of aortic and pulmonary valves results in splitting of second heart sound. Second sound has two components, the pulmonary and aortic. In health, pulmonary second sound is louder than the aortic: in children and young adults: of equal intensity in middle age while the aortic second sound is louder in elderly people. In disease, aortic second sound is louder in hypertension, aortic dilatation, valvular involvement due to rheumatic heart disease and atherosclerosis while pulmonary second sound is loud and accentuated in pulmonary hypertension, mitral stenosis, congenital heart disease, pulmonary embolism and chronic lung disease (emphysema).

Attenuation or masking of second heart sound may occur in aortic regurgitation, aortic or pulmonary stenosis and atrial fibrillation.

Wide and fixed splitting of second sound occurs characteristically in atrial septal defect. Disappearance of this sign suggests reversal of shunt (right to left) due to pulmonary hypertension.

Triple rhythm. Occasionally in young healthy persons third heart sound which follows the second heart sound is heard early in diastole lying internal to the apex with patient in recumbent position. It tends to disappear or diminish when the patient assumes an upright position, its appearance in disease is ominous. The fourth heart sound is not normally heard in health.

Pathologically third heart sound is loud and accentuated and with the addition of auricular sound, summation of the two sounds may occur. This has been referred to as presystolic or auricular gallop. Protodiastolic or rapid filling gallop and summation gallop. Gallop sound is best heard at the lower end of sternum and signifies left ventricular strain and gross myocardial disease. It is heard commonly in patients of hypertension, myocardial infarction and left heart failure.

Opening snap of mitral. It is the sound midway between second and third heart sound. It is high pitched and snapping in character, heard best at the lower end of left sternal border in 4th intercostal space first sound being short and accentuated.

Opening snap of mitral occurs in a tight mitral stenosis and is not seen in early cases of mitral valve disease and where mitral incompetence or regurgitation is predominant lesion.

Murmurs. These are adventitious sounds and are as a result of vibrations of the valves (endocardial) or walls of the heart and great vessels. They are most often organic in nature except in some cases where alterations in viscosity of blood or increased rate of flow of blood (hyperkinetic state) through the blood vessels may produce a physiological murmur. The production of a murmur depends on the passage of blood from a narrow into a broader stream (mitral stenosis) or backward flow though an incompetent valve (regurgitational murmur) and viscosity of blood or increased velocity of blood stream.

While defining a murmur, one has to time it in relation to heart sound, point of maximum intensity, its radiation or direction of propagation, character (loud or soft) and effect of respiration, posture and physical exercise.

Timing of murmur. Important point is to first time the murmur whether it is systolic or diastolic. Systolic phase starts with the first heart sound and goes upto start of second heart sound. Murmur during this phase is systolic. If it occurs in the whole of systolic phase it is called pansystolic and depending on the phase of systole murmur may be early, mid or late systolic.

Diastolic phase starts from the beginning of second heart sound to the beginning of first heart sound and murmur in this phase is called diastolic murmur. It may be mid, late or early diastolic murmur depending on its phase of occurrence. A murmur present in both systolic and diastolic phases is called continuous murmur (patent ductus arteriosus murmur). Timing of the murmurs is to be done by palpating the apex beat or carotid pulsation since these correspond with ventricular systole.

Localization of murmur at its maximum intensity facilitates in locating its origin and its extent of distribution depending on its loudness (louder the murmur, greater its area of transmission). Sometimes distinctive propagation of murmurs helps in distinguishing the murmur (systolic murmur of mitral regurgitation from mid systolic murmur of aortic stenosis). Similarly systolic murmur of aortic stenosis is conducted to neck vessels while murmur of pulmonary stenosis is conducted only to the left side of sternum.

Character of the murmur also helps in distinguishing it. Murmurs of obstructive origin (mitral stenosis) are rough, rasping while regurgitant murmurs (mitral incompetence) are soft, blowing.

Depending on the degree of intensity of murmurs, *four grades are defined*:

Grade I Faint   Grade III Loud

Grade II Moderate loud Grade IV Very loud

Often the murmurs are described as crescendo type (increasing intensity from its origin) or decrescendo (decreasing intensity from its origin).

Effects of posture, respiration and exercise. Posture has some effect in the audibility of some murmurs. Murmur of mitral origin (mitral diastolic or presystolic murmur) is best heard on turning the patient to left lateral position while aortic diastolic murmur is best heard in sitting position with patient bending forward.

Some murmurs are effected by respiration. This is specially important in murmurs of Tricuspid origin. An organic murmur is faint during inspiration and loud during expiration, while murmurs (systolic and diastolic) in tricuspid incompetence and stenosis display accentuation at the height of inspiration. This character of Tricuspid murmurs distinguishes them from murmurs of mitral origin.

Exercise is also helpful. A faint mitral diastolic murmur shall become accentuated after giving some exercise to the patient. Similarly exercise can differentiate between innocent murmurs and murmurs of organic origin.

Classification of murmurs. There are two main types of murmurs—systolic and diastolic—and these may be further classified into pansystolic, mid- or early systolic, mid-diastolic or early diastolic and depending on the location of murmur and its character, the disease can be diagnosed.

Pansystolic murmur in mitral area or lower end of sternum:

1. Mitral regurgitation
2. Tricuspid regurgitation
3. Ventricular septal defect.

Middiastolic murmur

1. Mitral stenosis
2. Tricuspid stenosis

Midsystolic or early systolic murmur

(*a*) *At aortic valve.*
1. Aortic stenosis   2. Atrial septal defect
3. Aortic dilatation (syphilitic aortitis, hypertension, atherosclerosis, coarctation of aorta).

(*b*) *At pulmonary valve.*
1. Pulmonary stenosis
2. Fallot's tetralogy
3. Anaemia
4. Pregnancy

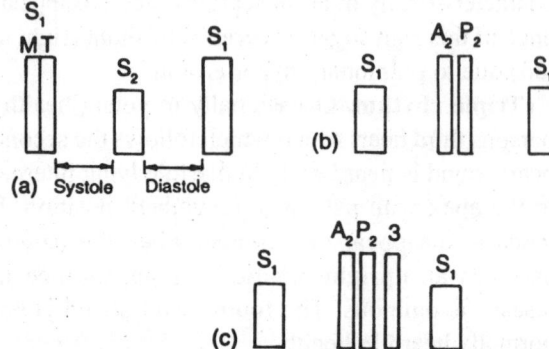

Fig. 1.13. Graphic representation of normal heart sounds. (a) Normal heart sounds over mitral and tricuspid valves, first sound is louder than second and its durations is longer. It is loudest at apex and is produced by closure of mitral and tricuspid valves. (b) Normal heart sounds over aortic and pulomonary valves. Second heart sound is produced by closure of aortic and pulmonary valves. It is louder than first and consists of two components aortic and pulmonary. Systolic interval is shorter than the diastolic. (c) Third sound follows second heart sound and is due to rapid filling of left ventricle in diastole. Normally heard in children and young adults. Best heard at Apex or just internal to it.

Early diastolic murmur

a. Aortic area

1. Aortic regurgitation
2. Aortic aneurysm
b. *Pulmonary area*
   1. Pulmonary regurgitation
   2. Pulmonary hypertension

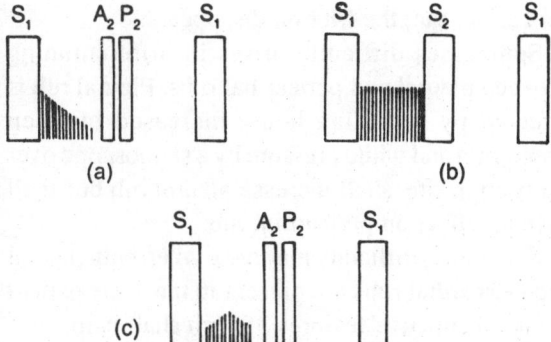

(a)   (b)

(c)

Fig. 1.14. Graphic representation of Murmurs in various valvular defects. (a) Functional (innocent) soft systolic murmur best heard over pulmonary area. (b) Mitral incompetence pansystolic murmur. It embraces first heart sound. It is plateau type. (c) Aortic stenosis ejection systolic murmur (crescendo-decresendo type). It is also called a diamond shaped murmur.

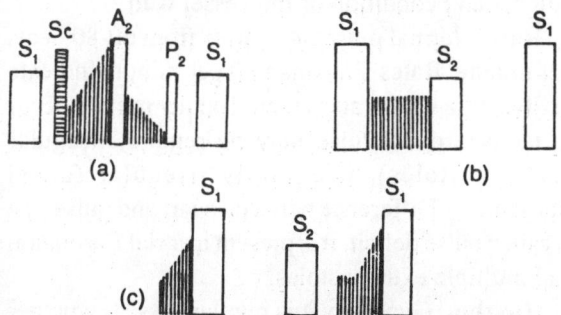

(a)   (b)

(c)

Fig. 1.15. Graphic representation of murmurs in valvular heart disease. (a) Pulmonary stenosis. Ejection systolic murmur with an early crescendo character followed by a larger decreasendo phase. Pulmonary second sound may be delayed soft or absent. Systolic click (SC) may be heard. (b) Tricuspid incompetence. Pansystolic murmur heard at lower end of sternum. The murmur changes its character with respiration. (c) Tricuspid stenosis. Middiastolic rough rumbling murmur crescendo type.

Systolic murmurs. Mitral pansystolic murmur is an important sign of mitral regurgitation. It is loud and blowing and occupies the whole length of systole, often obscuring the first heart sound completely. It is best heard at the apex and is transmitted to the axilla and to the angle of left scapula.

The pansystolic murmur of Tricuspid incompetence is best heard over the lower end of sternum. This murmur is in no way different from the murmur of mitral origin. Distinction can be made by change in character of tricuspid murmur with respiration (maximal during inspiration).

The murmur of ventricular septal defect is a loud and harsh pansystolic murmur usually accompanied by a thrill, best heard in the third and fourth intercostal space on left side. This murmur radiates to the whole of precordium and even to back. In cases of high VSD, the murmur is heard in the second left interspace.

Other causes of pansystolic murmur in mitral area include diseases causing left ventricular incompetence (hypertension, ischaemic heart disease anaemia).

Midsystolic or ejection systolic murmur. Characteristically seen in diseases of aortic and pulmonary valves.

In aortic stenosis, the murmur is rough, loud midsystolic murmur, often called diamond-shaped murmur since it reaches its peak in the mid-systole starting after completion of first heart sound. Classically there is an aortic ejection click after the first sound, a palpable thrill, and the murmur heard over the aortic area, is transmitted to neck vessels.

The murmur of pulmonary stenosis is similar to that of aortic stenosis and ends before the pulmonary component of second heart sound and does not radiate to neck vessels.

Atrial septal defect is characterised by a loud midsystolic murmur heard in the 3rd left intercostal space. There is a wide splitting of second heart sound which is fixed.

Innocent murmur often a soft mid systolic murmur is heard in the pulmonary area on left side in 2nd left interspace or at the base of heart. These murmurs have to be distinguished from organic murmurs and are often labelled as innocent murmurs. These murmurs are soft, are localised and do not radiate to any side and are effected by posture and exercise.

Common causes of these murmurs are anaemia, fever, young adults and during pregnancy.

Diastolic murmurs. These are present in cases of organic heart disease.

Mitral diastolic murmur is mid diastolic, rough rumbling with a presystolic accentuation, best heard at apex and is accentuated on turning the patient to left lateral position and by exercise. First heart sound is short and snappy. The mid diastolic murmur of Tricuspid stenosis is similar in character to that of mitral stenosis and is best heard at the lower end of sternum in the fourth left intercostal space. Murmur is accentuated during inspiration and this distinguishes it from diastolic murmurs of mitral origin.

Aortic diastolic murmur is soft, blowing and present in early diastolic phase. It is generally whiff like and is best heard in 3rd left intercostal space and by asking the patient to bend forward and hold the breath in expiration. The radiation of murmur is variable. It may be transmitted along the left border of sternum and to the apex.

Pulmonary diastolic murmur is early diastolic murmur heard along second and third left interspaces. It is commonly seen in cases of mitral stenosis with pulmonary hypertension (Graham Steell murmur). The murmur of pulmonary incompetence is somewhat like that of aortic incompetence and difference between the two is presence of peripheral vascular signs in aortic incompetence.

Continuous murmurs. A murmur which extends over both the systolic and diastolic phases is called continuous murmur. Diseases producing continuous murmur are patent ductus arteriosus, arteriovenous fistula.

Pericardial rub. A rough scratchy sound heard over the uncovered part of the heart, not corresponding with any event of cardiac cycle but having a to-and-fro character (systolodiastolic). It has to be distinguished from cardiac murmurs which are heard best in areas corresponding to the valve position and they may be related to either systolic or diastolic phase of the heart. Moreover a pericardial rub is effected by the change of posture. Assuming erect position increases intensity of pericardial rub.

Pericardial rub is characteristically seen in pericarditis. When enough fluid collects in the pericardial sac, the friction disappears.

Sometimes difficulty arises in differentiating between pleural and pericardial rubs. Pleural rub is effected by breathing being increased by deep respiration and while pressure by a stethoscope over the friction site, shall increase pleural rub but shall have no effect on pericardial rub.

Sometimes difficulty may arise when both pleural and pericardial rubs are present in the same patient though distinctive features of each shall help.

Arterial pulse. It constitutes an important part of cardiovascular examination and gives important information about state of heart and peripheral vessels.

Pulse is commonly felt at the wrist by placing three fingers of right hand on radial artery.

Pulse is assessed for rate, rhythm, character, volume and condition of the vessel wall.

Rate. Normal pulse rate varies from 60-80 beats per minute. Rates slow than 60 per minute indicate bradycardia while rates above 100 per minute occur in tachycardias. Pulse may be regular, irregular (extra systoles), irregularly irregular (atrial fibrillation). Difference between heart and pulse rate is called pulse deficit. It is present in atrial fibrillation and multiple extra systoles.

Rhythm. Generally it is regular. Assess whether it is irregular and if so regularly irregular or irregularly irregular. An irregular pulse may be due to sinus arrhythmia (pulse rate varying its character with respiration, pulse rate increases during inspiration and slows during expiration. Normally present in children and young adults). Extra systoles (there is regular dropping of beats after every two or three beats). Atrial fibrillation (irregularly irregular pulse. There is pulse deficit present).

Condition of the vessel wall. Normally vessel wall is just palpable but in cases with advanced atherosclerosis vessel wall becomes hard. Palpation of the artery should also be done at other sites like carotids (carotid pulsation diminished in carotid artery occlusion) popliteals, dorsalis pedis, brachial (peripheral vascular disease, coarctation of aorta) and temporal artery (temporal arteritis, collagen diseases).

Volume. Normally pulse is of moderate volume. Poor volume pulse is seen in hypotension, myocardial failure, aortic stenosis and in peripheral circulatory failure.

Good volume of pulse is present in fever, hypertension, aortic incompetence, thyrotoxicosis and after exertion.

Thus a typical pulse in an adult is regular, of moderate volume, vessel wall just palpable with rate between 70-80 beats per minute.

Some varieties of pulse. In addition to the usual description of pulse, one comes across different types of pulse which are helpful in making diagnosis of various physical ailments.

Water-hammer pulse (Corrigan pulse). This is a bounding pulse characterised by a sharp upstroke and a sudden down stroke. This quick rise and fall of the pulse is accentuated by raising the arm. There is a wide pulse pressure (difference between systolic and diastolic levels more than 60). Causes of water hammer pulse are aortic incompetence, severe anaemia, thyrotoxicosis, high fevers, systolic hypertension.

Causes of water-hammer pulse

1. Aortic incompetence
2. Severe anaemia
3. Thyrotoxicosis
4. Systolic hypertension
5. High fevers
6. Patent ductus arteriosus
7. Arteriovenous aneurysm
8. Paget's disease

Anacrotic pulse. Poor volume pulse where a small wave is felt along the upstroke. It is seen in aortic stenosis. When there is presence of both aortic stenosis and incompetence, the pulse wave shows, two equal stroke, it is called pulsus Bisferiens.

Pulsus paradoxus. The pulse changes its character with respiration. Normally there is a slight decrease in pulse volume during inspiration. In pulsus paradoxus, there is exaggeration of normal physiological phenomenon. Pulse volume tends to decrease appreciably or pulse disappear at the end of respiration. This pulse is seen in cases of pericardial effusion and constrictive pericarditis. This pulse is appreciated by asking the patient to take deep breath and then feel the volume of pulse.

Pulsus alternans. There is alternate spacing of strong and weak or large and small beats. It is seen in cases of acute left heart failure (hypertension, myocardial infarction, aortic valve disease). Pulsus alternans is produced in hearts which are severely damaged and there is asynchronous contraction of cardiac muscle fibres.

Pulsus aternans is felt by tying blood pressure cuff around the arm and raising the pressure and keeping it midway between systolic and diastolic levels. The pulse at that time is halved than the earlier one since weak beats have been temporarily obliterated.

NERVOUS SYSTEM

Examination of nervous system in every case is part of systemic examination but special attention has to be paid in patients with neurological disorders. In every case one has to determine the site of lesion and nature of lesion, the pathological process responsible for defect.

A complete neurological examination includes assessment of:

Higher functions. Higher functions include tests for mental state of the patient, mood, memory (of recent past and immediate events), emotional status (elation, depression), flight of ideas, power of concentration and orientation in time and space. Appearance of a patient is important and his/her behaviour shall tell whether there is evidence of apathy, agitation or maniac behaviour. This is significant in psychotic states (Korsakoff psychosis in alcoholics, schizophrenia, mania). Some patients may have erroneous beliefs firmly ingrained in mind despite evidence in the opposite (delusions) while in some there are imaginary aural and visual sensory impressions (hallucinations). There may be disturbed sleep, history of nightmares, fears or phobias.

It is important to always assess the level of consciousness, whether comatose or semicomatose, evidence of delirium confusion, irritability and overall general behaviour.

Speech. It is a higher function of the brain and in disorders of cerebral hemisphere disturbance of speech is referred to as aphasia while involvement of peripheral mechanism resulting in disturbance of articulation and enunciation is called dysarthria.

Speech is controlled by two mechanisms, a producing and a receiving mechanism. The former consists of two parts one responsible for spoken speech and the other for written speech. Similarly receiving mechanism also has two systems—one for spoken speech and other for written. The cortical centres for speech are situated in left cerebral hemisphere in right handed persons and vice versa. Centre for spoken speech lies in lower and posterior part of 3rd frontal convolution also called Broca area while centre for written speech lies in posterior part of second frontal convolution. The posterior half of left superior temporosphenoidal convolution is concerned with the understanding of spoken speech and still further posteriorly for written speech.

Aphasia. In this patient is unable to produce speech (motor aphasia) or unable to understand spoken or written words (sensory aphasia).

Dysarthria. It is disorder of articulation either of tongue, larynx lips etc. and is due to involvement of peripheral organs in contrast to aphasia where the lesion is in cortex. Causes of dysarthria include myopathy, motor neurone disease, parkinsonism, pseudobulbar palsy, chorea.

Nominal aphasia. In this the patient is unable to correctly recall and name the common use objects though he/she may be able to explain the correct use e.g. he may look at a pen and tell that it is meant for writing but may be unable to use correct name

for it. Nominal aphasia is a form of motor aphasia and occurs in lesions of temporal or frontal lobe.

Acalculia. Inability to do mathematical calculations including elementary counting or sums is seen in lesions of parietal lobe.

Apraxia. Inability to perform simple acts such as lighting a lamp or cigarette as a result of extensive involvement of left cerebral cortex or corpus callosum is called apraxia. The patient in this case recognizes the various objects, their use as well but is unable to perform the simple act involving these objects.

Such patients have no motor or sensory paralysis or even ataxia.

Scanning or staccato speech. A form of slow, jerky intermittent speech and patient speaks as with short pauses. Ask him to speak: 'Kurukshetra' or 'constitution' or 'Rashtrapati' and the person will speak in explosive tone.

This type of speech is found in cases of cerebellar disorders and disseminated sclerosis.

Slurring speech. A form of slurred speech and patient speaks as if he/she is in a state of intoxication or inebriation. Slurred speech is met with in cases of general paralysis of insane (G.P.I.) and pseudobulbar palsy.

A feeble form of slurred speech may be seen in cases of myopathy and myasthenia gravis.

Cranial nerves. There are 12 cranial nerves and each has got its specific functions. Examination of cranial nerves is required essentially to locate the lesion in neurological cases.

First or olfactory nerve. It is concerned with the sense of smell which is tested in each nostril separately by use of different types of smell such as oil of peppermint oil of cloves etc. Patient inhales the scent keeping his mouth closed and his/her ability to recognize the smell is noted. Irritating and pungent substances like ammonia should not be used since these act partly by stimulating 5th nerve. Loss of smell (anosmia) occurs in diseases involving olfactory tract (fracture of anterior cranial fossa), tumours, inflammatory conditions such as meningitis (tubercular or pyogenic). When sense of smell is preverted it is called Parosmia in which unpleasant smell has a pleasant odour. This generally follows after head injury.

Second or optic nerve. In this one has to test for (i) acuity of vision, (ii) field of vision, and (iii) colour sense.

Visual acuity is tested initially by rough method, like perception of light and finger counting (hand movements and counting of fingers at varying distance). For finer testing for distant vision, Snellen's chart placed at about 6 metres (20 feet) distance, are employed. The patient is asked to read from above downwards. If he is able to read the lowest line then his vision is 6/6. For near vision, Jaeger chart held at distance of 14 inches is employed.

Depending on vision, different terms are employed. Amblyopia means defective vision and Amaurosis (complete blindness). Blindness may occur gradually and is often due to inflammatory conditions of the eye, optic atrophy. Glaucoma, optic neuritis. Sudden blindness may appear in one eye first or be present in both eyes. Causes include vitreous haemorrhage, retinal detachment, retrobulbar neuritis, retinal artery thrombosis, thrombosis of central retinal vein, alcohol poising and uncommonly in hysteria.

Field of vision. It comprises sum total of objects which eye can see while fixing gaze in one particular direction. In this the person looks not only at the objects at which he is gazing but also at the peripheral limits.

A field of vision is judged by instrument (Perimetry) or by rough method (confrontation). Here both the patient and the examiner sit at same level facing each other at a distance of about 3 feet. For testing field of vision in right eye patient places his hand on one eye (left) while the examiner closes his opposite right eye and with the hand held up and looking steadily into the finger which is moved up and down and sideways in all directions. Towards inner side and when patient says 'yes' on seeing the finger, It maps up the field of vision. This test presumes that the examiners own field of vision is normal, since his field of vision shall act as standard. Defect in the field of vision may be in the form of concenteric or peripheral diminution. It occurs in optic atrophy, bilateral involvement of cortical visual centers, various diseases of retina and hysteria. A defect within visual fluid is called Scotoma which is generally central. Causes of central Scotoma are retrobulbar neuritis, disseminated sclerosis, toxic (tobacco, alcohol) and lesions of visual centre in the brain. Scotoma may be unilateral or bilateral.

Hemianopia. Loss of vision in one half of the visual field in both eyes due to causes other than in retina, is called Hemianopia. Depending on which half of field of vision is effected, the hemianopia is labelled. It is called Homonymous when similar halves of both fields of vision is lost (temporal half of one side and nasal half of the other). Right lateral hemianopia means involvement of right half of the field and left, left half (left lateral hemianopia). Involvement of upper and lower halves of visual fields though not very common are called superior (former) and inferior (latter) hemianopia. Bitemporal hemianopia siignifies involvement of temporal halves or outer fieds of vision and is seen in pituitary tumours or inflammatory lesions of central part of optic chiasma.

Binasal hemianopia (nasal or inner halves of visual fields) is rare and is produced by bilateral disease involving optic chiasma.

Colour vision. This is tested by using coloured cards (Holmgren's wool). Total colour blindness is rare and generally it is red-green blindness, followed by yellow-blue blindness.

Testing of colour vision is important in railway workers, air port traffic controllers, pilots and surgeons.

Ophthalmoscopy. Examination of fundus constitutes an important part of examination of eye. It tells us about the state of optic disc, retinal vessels (arteries and veins) state of retina and macula.

Normal fundus has got orange red colour of surface over which optic disc which is oval in shape can be identified. It has well defined margins and in its center is funnel shaped depression called physiological cup from which arteries and veins emerge. Macula is situated on the temporal or outer edge of the disc, is darker in colour and is devoid of vessels.

Papilloedema. It refers to oedema of optic disc which becomes full and its margins become blurred and there is filling of physiological cup. Arteries are narrowed and veins become congested and tortuous. Papilloedema occurs in cases of raised intracranial tension, chronic nephritis, malignant hypertension, thrombosis of central retinal vein and tumours of the orbit.

Optic atrophy. It may be primary or secondary. The disc is pale white in colour, smaller in size than normal. Primary optic atrophy occurs in diseases involving optic nerve fibres. The disc margins are very distinct and lamina cribrosa becomes visible while vessels appear normal. Causes of primary optic atrophy include degenerative disorders congenital, trauma, and toxins (tobacco, lead, methyl alcohol). Secondary optic atrophy usually follows papilloedema and retrobulbar neuritis, meningo-vascular syphilis.

Optic neuritis. This involves inflammation of the optic disc where swelling or oedema of disc is moderate with hyperemia, blurred margins and exudates and haemorrhages near by in retina. The field defect is central scotoma and loss of vision is out of proportion to changes in the disc. The difference between optic and retrobulbar neuritis pathologically is not much.

Causes include disseminated sclerosis, disseminated myelitis with optic neuritis, orbital infections secondry to infection of nasal air sinuses or dental abscess, meningitis and encephalitis.

Retinal haemorrhages. While examining fundus state of arteries and veins has to be observed. The arteries may be thickened and tortuous while veins may appear congested. Pulsation in the arteries is abnormal. Retinal haemorrahages may be superficial (elongated with flame shaped edges) or deep (dark and blotches) and occur in malignant, hypertension, chronic nephritis, diabetic retinopathy.

Hypertensive retinopathy is characterized by papilloedema, flame shaped haemorrhages, tortuosity and irregularity of the arteries, nipping of veins when crossed by arteries, and exudates. Diabetic retinopathy has got characteristics like that of hypertensive retinopathy except that haemorrhages are deep seated. There are microaneurysms and waxy discrete exudates.

Third, fourth and sixth nerves. These three nerves are examined jointly since their action is concerned with the movements of muscles of eyeball. Third nerve (oculomotor nerve) supplies all muscles of eyeball except superior oblique (4th nerve trochlear nerve) and external rectus (6th nerve, abducent). Third nerve palsy leads to ptosis, divergent squint, inability to move eye upwards, diplopia, dilated pupil, reaction to light or accommodation gone.

Fourth nerve palsy results in impaired downward and outwards movements while in sixth nerve palsy because of external rectus paralysis, there is inability to move the eye outwards. There is diplopia and convergent squint.

These three nerves are tested by asking the patient to look upward and drooping of upper eye lid observed. The movements of eye (to test for muscle paralysis), presence of squint (convergent or divergent) and diplopia have to be tested to find out the involvement of these nerves. Involvement of these cranial nerves occurs in brain stem lesions (vascular, inflammatory, neoplastic) lesions at base of brain (basal meningitis, neoplastic infiltration of meninges, tuberculous or pyogenic meningitis) and infective polyneuritis.

5th nerve (trigeminal nerve). It has got both motor and sensory division which is further divided into ophthalmic, superior maxillary division and inferior maxillary division. Fifth nerve supplies almost whole of face and its paralysis leads to loss of sensation of half of face and scalp including soft and hard palate and nose. Secretions of salivary and lacrimal glands is effected. Trophic lesions on the paralysed side may appear. Taste may be effected on anterior two-thirds of tongue.

Motor root supplies muscles of mastication and it is tested by asking the patient to clench his/her teeth and contraction of temporalis and masseters is felt. Involvement of the nerve will result in weak contractions of muscles as well as deviation of jaw to paralysed side. Trigeminal nerve is involved in post inferior cerebellar artery syndrome, tumours, syringobulbia and fracture of middle cranial fossa.

Facial nerve (7th nerve). It is a purely motor nerve and supplies most of the muscles of face and scalp. The nerve may be effected either at infra-nuclear, nuclear or supranuclear levels.

Paralysis of facial nerve produces loss of expression on the paralysed side. The naso labial fold is less prominent, the eye is difficult to close and may remain open. Patient is unable to raise furrows on forehead and to whistle. Food may collect on the paralysed side and fluids may escape from effected side.

The facial nerve is tested:

1. By asking patient to close his/her eyes tightly and then attempting to open them. Normally the patient resists the attempt but in facial paralysis, the eyelids on effected side are not closed completely and little exertion can open the eye completely.
2. Patient is asked to whistle and to inflate his cheeks and the inflated mouth is tapped by fingers. Firstly patient is unable to whistle and secondly he is unable to inflate the mouth. Air escapes easily from the paralysed side.
3. Patient be asked to show his teeth which he is unable to do. Mouth shall be deviated to healthy side.
4. Ask the patient to look upwards and observe furrowing of forehead which is absent in nuclear and infranuclear type of facial palsy. Let us look at various distinctive features of facial palsy at various levels.

Supranuclear facial palsy. It is primarily unilateral involvement. Main involvement is of lower half of face, upper half of face escapes because of bilateral innervation of upper facial muscles. It is generally associated with Hemiplegia and the lesion commonly is in internal capsule.

Infranuclear lesions. It occurs either at nucleus or when the nerve trunk enters the aqueduct or after emerging from the facial canal or in the facial canal between branching of chorda tympani and nerve to stapedius.

Infranuclear lesions are lower motor neurone type and whole half of face is involved. Lesion of nerve before it has entered the facial canal, produces paralysis of stapedius muscle which results in excessive sensitveness to loud sounds (hyperacusis). If the lesion inside the aqueduct involves the chorda tympani it produces loss of taste sensation in the anterior two thirds of the tongue. Bell's palsy is characteristically seen in lesion of facial nerve when it leaves the skull from stylomastoid foramen.

Causes of infranuclear facial palsy include basal meningitis, cerebellopontine angle tumours, landrys paralysis, vascular lesions while Bell's palsy is commonly due to exposure of the facial nerve to 'cold' often called 'rheumatic'. Other causes include suppurating glands in neck, tumours, encephalitis and infective polyneuritis.

Eighth nerve (auditory nerve). This nerve is concerned with hearing as well as in maintaining equilibrium. It consists of two parts, the cochlear which supplies cochlea and is concerned with the function of hearing while the vestibular division supplies the vestibular and semicircular canals and subserves the function of maintaining equilibrium.

Eighth nerve is involved in chronic otitis media, fracture of skull, acoustic neuroma, and basal meningitis. Cochlear nerve testing includes tests of hearing. Acuity of hearing can be tested by person's ability to hear the whispered or spoken words at a reasonable hearing range.

Further tests are done by tuning fork and these include Rinne's test (normal air conduction is better than bone conduction). A vibrating tuning fork is placed on patient's mastoid and when patient stops hearing it, the examiner holds it over his ear. A person with normal acuity of hearing shall continue to hear for longer period than at bony spot. In middle ear disease the air conduction is decreased. This is rinne's test negative while normally it is positive.

In **Weber's test** a striking tuning fork is placed in the middle of patient's forehead and assess in which ear sound is better heard. In middle ear deafness sound is better heard on the diseased side as compared to normal person where it is heard equally well in both ears. In nerve deafness the sound will be heard in healthy ear while those with bilateral nerve deafness the test is of no use.

Vestibular nerve is tested by caloric and rotation tests which are to be conducted in a laboratory. Involvement of the nerve produces vertigo and nystagmus.

Glossopharyngeal (ninth), vagus (tenth) and eleventh (spinal accessory) nerves. The ninth and tenth nerves are examined together since their functions almost overlap. Ninth nerve supplies posterior third of the tongue, pharynx and carries taste fibres of posterior part of tongue. Isolated lesions of 9th nerve do not occur. Vagus (tenth nerve) is a mixed nerve, the sensory fibres for pharynx, larynx, trachea, oesophagus, heart and abdominal viscera while motor fibres innervate murscles of palate, pharynx and larynx.

These nerves are tested by:

1. Position of uvula which normally is in the center and is deviated to the sound side in paralysis of nerves.
2. Movements of palate: Normally palate moves during speaking (patient says 'a-h'). There is pharyngeal reflex present. In unilateral paralysis there is no elevation of palate on the affected side and uvula is drawn to normal side. In bilateral paralysis, there is no elevation of palate and it remains motionless. Nasal regurgitation is present. Loss of pharyngeal reflex is important sign of tenth cranial nerve involvement since involvement of larynx occurs in vagus nerve paralysis and both sensory as well as motor functions are involved. Unilateral paralysis of the nerve does not produce any symptoms while bilateral paralysis produces loss of voice. Vocal cords lie immobile.

Spinal accessory or eleventh nerve. It mainly supplies trapezius and sterno mastoid muscles and to test for paralysis of trapezius, patient is asked to shrug his shoulders against resistance. There is weakness of trapezius muscle as well as winging of scapula. Sterno mastoid is tested by turning the head against resistance to one side and then to other. In case of paralysis of the muscle the patient is unable to rotate the chin completely from the affected side.

Paralysis of these nerves occur in infective polyneuritis, encephalitis, posterior inferior cerebellar artery thrombosis, syringobulbia and posterior fossa tumours.

Twelfth or hypoglossal nerve. It is a purely motor nerve supplying the tongue.

The nerve is tested by asking the patient to protrude the tongue and note any deviation, movements of the tongue from side to side and observe for any wasting of the tongue and presence of any tremors or fibrillary twitching. Unilateral paralysis causes deviation of tongue to paralysed side. There is atrophy and wasting while bilateral. nerve paralysis make the tongue immobile. There is difficulty in speech and marked wasting with fibrillary twitchings. Causes of nerve involvement include syringobulbia, meningitis, head injury and progressive bulbar paralysis.

Motor system. It comprises mainly body muscles and their function. For assessing motor functions of a patient, the various tests have to be carried for motor power, assessment of muscular paralysis, muscular corrdination, muscle tone, state of nutrition of the muscles and presence of any abnormal muscular movement.

Muscle power of any or group of muscles is carried out individually by doing movement against passive resistance.

Muscle power is graded as per the following:

Grade 0	No contraction
Grade 1	Flicker or trace of contraction
Grade 2	Patient can move the limb with gravity eliminated
Grade 3	Limb can be moved against gravity
Grade 4	Movement against gravity and moderate resistance
Grade 5	Normal power

Various muscles in the body are assessed for their weakness and power. Loss of muscle power results in partial weakness (paresis) or complete (paralysis). There may be paralysis of one limb (monoplegia) one side (hemiplegia), diplegia means paralysis of two limbs either upper or lower, paraplegia, weakness of lower part of body and quadriplegia signifies weakness of all four limbs.

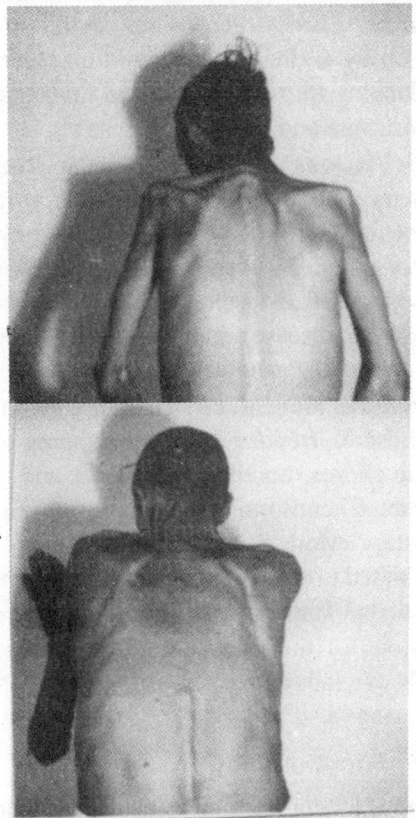

Fig. 1.16-17. Winging of scapula. This is characteristically seen in paralysis of nerve to serratus anterior: Winging of scapula becomes prominent when patient applies thrust against wall.

Next to muscle power is muscle tone where two impulses (excitation and inhibition) exert opposite action on the muscle tone. Muscle tone is tested by assessing resistance to passive movements. Increased tone is called hypertonia which occurs in upper motor neurone lesions while decreased tone (hypotonia) means lower motor neurone lesion.

Clasp knife rigidity is spastic form of tone where initially resistance is felt on passive movement of limb, but with the continuation of further movement the resisitance suddenly disappears. It is seen in pyramidal tracts involvement (upper motor neurone lesion). When resistance to passive movement is

present in all direction it is called lead pipe rigidity and when there is jerky rigidity it is cogwheel type. This occurs in cases of extra pyramidal tract involvement (parkinsonism). In hysterical rigidity the patient exhibits resistance to passive movement in proportion to the effort made by the examiner. Moreover hysterical rigidity follows no typical pattern.

Muscle coordination is important in a way it depends on postural sense, vestibular and cerebellar function. Lack of muscular coordination results in ataxia and this is tested commonly by finger nose test, heel-knee test pronation-supination test, and threading a needle test.

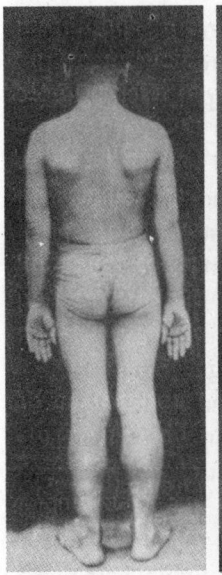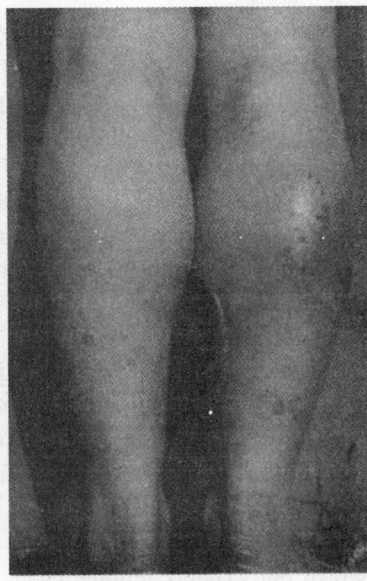

Fig. 1.18-19. A case of pseudo hypertrophic muscular dystrophy. Note well developed calf muscles.

Nutrition of muscles depends on the person's age, general health, body build and exercise the person has been doing. When muscle becomes small, bulk of muscle is lost it is called atrophy. Muscular atrophy occurs in lower motor neurone lesions. Motor neurone disease and peripheral nerve involvement. When muscle increases in bulk, hypertrophy occurs (body builders, wrestlers) but in cases of pseudohypertrophic muscular dystrophy, there is increase in bulk of calf muscles but diminished strength, it is called pseudo hypertrophy.

Abnormal muscular movements. Abnormal muscular movements may be localized or widespread. Spasm is an exaggerated involuntary muscular contraction. It may be tonic (continuous muscular contractions, brief in duration) or clonic (Repetitive short contractions with brief periods of muscular relaxation). Tonic and clonic contractions generally occur in epilepsy. When these become wide spread they are called convulsions.

Myoclonus. It is jerky form of contraction occurring in a muscle or a limb. It may be repetitive occuring in 10 to 60 contractions per minute having no definite pattern.

Myoclonus generally occurs in epilepsy and encephalitis.

Tetany. There are intermittent spasms of the peripheral muscles because of increased excitability of peripheral nerve. It occurs in patients with low levels of calcium in the body and alkalosis. Tetany may be elicited by tapping of facial nerve in front of ear (Chvostek's sign) and by tying a cuff around the arm and raising pressure. Positive test (Trousseau's sign) means the hand going into a corpopedal spasm.

Torsion spasm. It means extensive involvement of limb which shows abnormal grotesque picture. It may be seen in cases of encephalitis lethargica.

Hemiballismus. A violent form of movement localized to one side of the body. It occurs in lesions of subthalmic region.

Tremors. These are rhythmic movements of a part of body (hand, tongue, head, lips) where there are alternate contractions by a group of muscles and then by the opposing group.

Tremors may be fine or coarse. They are accentuated by asking the patient to do some activity like stretching the hands in front or lifting some object. Fine tremors occur in thyrotoxicosis, anxiety states. Tremors in Parkinson's disease are pill rolling type (rhythmic, coarse and slow rotatory type).

Senile tremors occur in old age and are mid way between fine and coarse tremors.

Intention tremors indicate cerebellar disorder where the tremors are coarse and are brought on by person doing some voluntary movement and the tremors become marked at the later part of movement.

Flapping tremors. Flapping movements like the birds wings occurring at metacarpophalangeal and wrist joints. These tremors are coarse and are brought on by asking the patient to extend his/her arms. Flapping tremors are seen in hepatocellular failure, uraemia and respiratory failure.

Fasciculations. These are seen as irregular, involuntary repetitive contractions of single or bundle of muscle fibres visible on naked eye and often brought on by mechanical stimulation like tapping of muscle. Muscle fasciculations occur in motor neurone disease and in diseases where there is anterior cell degeneration.

Choreiform movements. These are involuntary semipurposive, irregular jerky movements seen in rheumatic chorea, huntingtons chorea, and chorea gravidarum. Choreiform movements are diminished by voluntary effort. Sometimes these movements may be limited to one half of the body (hemichorea).

Athetosis. These are slow coarse contortive contractions of the muscles of the extremities, especially of hands and feet and are seen in diseases of basal ganglia.

Sensory Functions

A number of functions connected with sensation are tested. Appreciation of sensations depends on adequate stimulation of receptors present in skin, muscles, tendons and joints and conveyed to higher system through sensory fibres.

Sensory functions include power to appreciate light touch and pressure (Tactile sensibility), pain and thermal sensations, two point discrimination, tactile localization and deep sensibility (Joint sensation, pressure pain, vibration sensation, appreciation of size, shape and form of objects, weight sense).

Tactile sensibity. Here light touch in the form of cotton swab is used as a stimulus and applied on various parts of the body and areas of loss of sensations are mapped out. Pressure touch shall be appreciated when the part of body is touched by a blunt object, may be with fingers.

When sensibility to touch is lost it is called anesthesia. Loss of sensations will indicate involvement of peripheral nerves and also a lesion in the spinal cord corresponding to spinal segments.

Pain sensibility. It is tested either by a pinprick (superficial) or by applying pressure on deep structures, like muscles or bones (pressure pain).

When there is absence of pain, it is called analgesia and an exaggerated sense of pain is called hyperalgesia. Absence of pressure pain (elicited by pressing on tendo Achilles) is an important sign of tabes dorsalis).

Thermal sensibility. Thermal sensations are conducted by fibres that closely follow that of pain. It is tested by using two tubes containing cold and hot water on different parts of body and any diminuation or loss of this is mapped out. When there is preservation of touch but absence of pain and temperature sensations, it is called dissociated anaesthesia. It is characteristically seen in conus medullaris lesion and syringo myelia.

Tactile discrimination. It is tested by using two pins and touching the skin of palms and soles. These pins are sufficiently at a distance where the patient can appreciate double contact. Patient can normally distinguish points 1.5 to 2 cm apart. Disturbances of tactile discrimination occur in lesions involving sensory motor cortex in parietal area.

Sense of position and movement are closely related and should be appreciated at the same time. In this patient is asked to recognize the movement and direction of his/her limbs. Involvement of postural sensibility is due to a lesion involving sensory motor cortex.

Recognition of size shape and form. These faculties are tested by placing common objects like pencil, scissor in the patients hand. Failure to do this is called ASTEROGNOSIS and is seen in lesion of post central gyrus and parietal lobe.

Appreciation of vibration and joint sense. Vibration sense is tested by placing a vibrating tuning fork on a bony point. This sense is lost in tabes dorsalis, peripheral neuritis and diseases involving the post columns.

Joint sense. Identification of passive movements of a joint depends on the integrity of post columns. This sense is lost in all diseases like tabes dorsalis, subacute combined degeneration of the cord etc.

Abnormal sensations. Hyperpathia describes condition where pain threshold is increased while parasthesia refers to various sensations like pin pricks, insects crawling over the body. There is absence of any outward stimulus. Parasthesia occurs commonly in cases of diabetes neuropathy.

Reflexes

There are three main type of reflexes:

1. Superficial
2. Deep
3. Organic

Superficial reflexes.

1. Corneal reflex (Cranial nerve V and VII). The stimulus for this reflex is light touch upon the cornea with a thin piece of cotton/wool. Response is bilateral blinking. The reflex is mediated through the first division of 5th cranial nerve (afferent) and the seventh cranial nerve (Efferent). Loss of this reflex is early sign of involvement of 5th cranial nerve. It is also seen in a case of cerebellopontine angle tumour.

2. Conjunctival reflex (cranial nerves V & VII). This is elicted by touching the conjunctive with a wisp of cotton. Result is reflex contracture of the orbicularis palpebraum. Again both V (sensory) and the VII (motor) mediate the reflex. Lesions of the 5th nerve shall result in the loss of this reflex.

3. Palatal reflex (cranial nerves V, IX, X). There is elevation of soft palate when it is touched. The reflex is lost in diseases involving the nucleus of vagus nerve. When only one vagus nerve is involved the uvula is displaced to the normal side. Fifth and IX cranial nerves are concerned on the affarent side while vagus / spinal accessory controls the efferent side.

Pharyngeal reflex. (Cranial nerves IX and X). Reflex consists of constriction or gagging of the posterior part of the pharynx when it is touched or tickled. The reflex is controlled by IX (afferent) and Xth nerves. (efferent). Lesions of the vagus nuclei result in its loss.

Abdominal reflexes (upper or epigastric T6 - T9. Mid abdominal T9 - T11 and lower or hypogastric T11 to LI).

Here the abdominal wall is stroked from costal margin to downwards. It is a superficial reflex and is elicited at three levels - below the costal margin, at umbilicus and lower levels when there is brisk contraction of the segment of the abdominal wall which has been stroked. The reflex is dependent on the integrity of pyramidal tract. Loss of reflexes indicates involvement of pyramidal tracts. Before eliciting the reflex, proper relaxation of the abdominal wall must be ensured. Abdominal reflexes normally are absent in obese flaccid abdomens and in females with repeated pregnancies who have a loose abdomen.

Abdominal reflex are also lost in cases of disseminated sclerosis, and lesions of pyramidal tracts.

Cremasteric reflex (L1 - L2). It is closely related to the abdominal reflex. Here inner side of thigh is stroked and result is drawing upwards of testicle on the side thigh is stroked. The reflex is diminished or abolished in lesions of the pyramidal tract.

Gluteal reflex (L4 & L5) A scratch on the buttocks produces contraction of the glutei.

Anal reflex. (S4 & S5) stroking of skin around the anus produces contraction of the anal sphicter.

Bulbo cavernous reflex (S2, 3 & 4). Squeezing of the glans penis results in contraction of the bulbocavernous muscle. The reflex is effected in cases of tabes dorsalis and lesions of sacral nerve roots. (Cauda Equina).

Plantar reflex (L5, S1 & S2). It is an important reflex and normally is elicited by stroking against the lateral border of foot by means of a blunt object (like key or pencil). Normally there is plantar flexion of the toes. In lesions of the pyramidal tract, the plantar reflex becomes extensor when there is spreading of the toes and the big toe extends upwards (Babinski response). An extensor plantar response may normally be seen in infants from 6 to 12 months but in adults it is always due to organic disease except in cases of deep coma when plantar is bilateral extensor. Transient extensor plantar response has been observed in patients of epilepsy following a fit. Other methods of eliciting babinski include:

CHADDOCK'S sign where lateral malleolus is stroked.

OPPENHEIM'S sign. Here firm pressure is applied along the anterior surface of tibia and lastly

GORDON'S reflex where by squeezing or pinching of the tendoachilles. Babinski-like response is achieved.

Deep Reflexes. These are usually elicited by delivering a sharp blow on the tendon which reacts by causing sharp contraction of the muscle. A deep reflex is due to the activity of a reflex arc consisting of both. excitatory and inhibitory impulses. Eliciting of a reflex depends on the state of the muscle and muscle tone. Diseases of the lower afferent and efferent neurones make the reflex diminished Or absent. This happens in cases of tabes dorsalis and peripheral neuropathy where both motor and sensory fibres are affected.

When a deep reflex is exaggerated, it is always associated with upper motor neurone lesion. Here the upper motor neurones exert an inhibitory influence on the reflex arc and are responsible for maintaining muscle tone. When this control is cut off the muscle tone increases and the tendon reflexes are either increased or exaggerated.

Sometimes it may be difficult to elicit a deep reflex. If so then a process called reinforcement is employed. For reflexes in lower limbs the patient is asked to reinforce by hooking the fingers of both hands and then exerting pressure. For reflexes of upper limb, clenching of teeth is done to reinforce. Exaggerated reflexes always indicate lesions of the pyramidal tract or motor cortex. Sometimes slightly brisk reflexes may be observed in tense or hysterical individuals.

Jaw jerk (mid pons). Normally the jerk is absent or sluggish. It is elicited by striking at the lower jaw while keeping the mouth slightly open. Contraction of muscles closing the jaw results.

Exaggeration of the reflex indicate upper motor neurone lesion.

Biceps reflex (C5, C6). A strike on the patients biceps tendon produces flexion of the forearm with a jerk.

Triceps jerk (C6, C7). Patient flexes the semi prone arm and a tap on the triceps tendon above the olecranon process elicits extension of the elbow.

Supinator jerk (C5, C6). A blow on the styloid process of the radius in the semi prone position of forearm produces flexion of the fore arm.

Knee jerk (L2, L3, L4). A blow upon the patellar tendon produces extension of the knee. The reflex can be elecited both in sitting and supine position.

Ankle jerk (L5, S1, S2). A tap on the tendoachilles results in sharp contraction of the calf muscles and plantar flexion of the foot.

Significance of reflexes. Normally all reflexes are elicited and are equal on both sides. They are diminished or absent in lower motor neurone lesion (peripheral neuropathy), myopathy and anterior horn cell involvement. Inequality in the reflexes on the two sides points to pathological lesion of the nervous system.

Reflexes are exaggerated in upper motor neurone lesions (Pyramidal tract or motor cortex involvement). In case deep reflexes are diminished or absent, reinforcement be done before declaring the reflex absent.

Clonus. It is a pathological form of reflex where slight pressure on the dorsi flexed foot produces rhythmic repetitive contractions of the calf muscle. This phenomenon lasts as long as the pressure is maintained on the foot. It is called ankle clonus and is sign of pyramidal tract involvement.

A sustained clonus is referred to as true but if the phenomenon dies out after a few jerks, it is called false or pseudo clonus. This type of clonus is seen in neurotic individuals.

Besides Ankle clonus we have also a **patellar clonus** which is elicited by suddenly pushing down the patella and clonic contractions of the quadriceps muscle are observed. Patellar clonus is also a sign of pyramidal tract involvement.

Organic reflexes. These are mainly concerned with the functioning of anus and urinary bladder. The activity of anal sphincter is controlled by sacral fourth and fifth segments.

Urinary bladder has got nerve supply from both sympathetic (T11, 12, L1) and parasympathetic pathways (S2-S4). There may be retention of urine, incontinence or overflow incontinence and in some cases hesistancy or precipitate micturition depending on the site of lesion. Very often the transverse lesions of spinal cord or paracentral lobes or internal capsule produce various types of bladder symptoms.

Cerebellar functions. Cerebellum plays an important part in maintaining voluntary movements and posture. Involvement of cerebellum and its tracts results in muscular contraction becoming weak and delayed. There is an abnormal posture especially in unilateral cerebellar lesions and often patient may be unable to stand as there is hypotonia and ataxia.

For cerebellar functions the various tests include:

1. *Dysmetria.* The range of movement and coordination of muscles is involved and there is difficulty in performing certain acts.

2. *Adiadokinesia.* It is ability to carry out repeated rapid movements (supination and pronation). When these movements become irregular or clumsy it is called dysdiadokinesia.

3. *Rebound phenomenon.* This is disturbance of movement due to muscular hypotonia. Patient flexes his arm against resistance and if the examiner suddenly releases the forearm the hand suddenly flies, patient striking his face. Normally the hand is arrested by contraction of opposite group of muscles.

4. *Walking in straight line.* In cerebellar lesion the patient is unable to walk on a straight line and tends to fall towards the affected side.

5. *Abnormalities of reflexes.* Superficial reflexes are unaffected in cerebellar disease. But deep reflexes show specific signs. Pendular knee jerk is very characteristic.

6. *Disorders of articulation and phonation.* It means a scanning, jerky and explosive speech. At the same time some syllables tend to slurr.

7. *Nystagmus*. It is present in horizontal plane but occasionally it may be rotatory.
8. *Pointing test*. There is deviation of finger when patient is asked to move the limb in a given plane and in unilateral cerebellar disease the patient may past point towards the affected side.
9. *Acute and chronic cerebellar dysfunction*. Acute cerebellar dysfunction follows commonly a vascular lesion or inflammatory in nature while chronic lesions are slowly progressive and commonly are either degenerative or due to a tumour.

Gait

Observing gait of the patient and the way he walks shall tell a lot about muscular coordination, any deformity and also any local disease interfering with normal walking (osteoarthritis, ankylosing spondylitis). Various forms of gait have been described and most of these are due to a neurological defect.

Hemiplegic gait. Characteristically seen in cases of cerebrovascular accidents, it is spastic type of gait where patient drags the paralysed limb sideways and forward in semicircular fashion almost forming an arc.

Scissors' gait. It is characteristically seen in children suffering from cerebral diplegia. The legs are spastic, cross each other in walking and remain approximated.

Ataxic gait. Seen in cases of cerebellar ataxia and other forms of cerebellar disease. Patient has a 'reeling' gait and walks as if in a drunken state.

Sensory ataxic gait. Present in tabes dorsalis, subacute combined degeneration of the cord sensory neuropathy. Patient raises his limbs very high and then brings them down in a stomping manner. This gait becomes very much marked when the patient closes his eyes.

Shuffling gait. Characteristically seen in cases of Parkinsonian disease. It is also called Festinant gait. It is slow, shuffling and patient takes small steps while keeping himself bent forwards. Arms do not swing. Patient is unable to stop quickly when pushed either forwards or backwards.

High stepping gait. Commonly seen in patients of polyneuritis, peripheral neuropathy. Patient raises his foot abnormally high and then drops it to the ground with force. There is foot drop and wasting of peripheral muscles of the lower limbs.

Waddling gait. Wide based with lordosis the patient walks like a duck. The body is tilted backwards and sways from side to side while walking. Normally it is seen in late stages of pregnancy but is otherwise seen in myopathy, muscular dystrophy, congenital dislocation of hip and osteomalacia.

Hysterical gait. A gait which fits into no known pattern and has got bizarre presentation. Person appears to be healthy and changes his/her style of walking in the presence of friends/relatives.

Prognosis in a patient. This is very important from the patient and his/her family members view point. *It depends on a number of factors:*

1. Disease from which the patient is suffering. In benign diseases prognosis is good while it is not good in persons suffering from malignancy. Again in an acute case, like acute myocardial infarction, prognosis should be given in guarded manner.
2. Stage at which the patient presents.
3. Type of disease
4. Type of treatment given.
5. General care of the patient and lastly it shall be very important to know whether a correct diagnosis has been arrived at by appropriate investigations since prognosis shall be directly proportional to the way the patient's diagnosis has been arrived at and the line of treatment instituted. Response of the patient to treatment instituted also governs the prognosis.

When patient's relatives ask the attending physician about the prognosis of their patient, always give a guarded prognosis. If patient is suffering from an incurable disease, the prognosis should be explained to the family members in a discrete manner but all unpleasant things should be kept away from the patient. But in an incurable disease like malignancy, AIDS, the diagnosis of the disease and its ultimate prognosis should be gradually told to the patient and the situation explained.

Treatment. Treatment of any patient and of his/

her illness depends on the competence of the attending physician. Only if a correct diagnosis has been arrived at, the right treatment can be instituted. Treating any illness is an art. Medicine is a continuous process of self-learning and every patient is treated individually depending on the acumen of the physician. *Treatment is to be done under two headings:*

1. General line of treatment which means general nursing care. Care of bowel and bladder. Maintenance of proper hydration and nutrition.
2. Specific treatment: Depending on the underlying disease, specific treatment is instituted.

COMMON SIGNS AND SYMPTOMS IN MEDICINE

Anorexia (loss of appetite)

It means loss of appetite and there is lack of desire to eat. Anorexia is a common symptom of number of conditions which may be mild in nature while in some it may indicate a serious ailment.

Anorexia occurs mainly in gastrointestinal disorders but may also occur in other conditions.

1. Emotional disturbances like anxiety, depression, anorexia nervosa.
2. Acute infections like septicaemia, fever, toxaemic conditions.
3. Cardiac Congestive heart failure, subacute bacterial endocarditis.
4. Renal. Renal failure, uraemia, nephritis.
5. Liver. Infective hepatitis, cirrhosis of liver. In hepatitis, loss of appetite and aversion to food is one of the earliest symptoms.
6. Gastrointestinal. Gastritis (acute or chronic), malabsorption syndrome.
7. Respiratory: Pulmonary tuberculosis, chronic respiratory failure, chronic cor pulmonale.
8. Malignancy anywhere in the body like carcinoma lungs, carcinoma stomach, liver, Hodgkin's disease, lymphomas, reticulosis.
9. Endocrinal causes like myxoedema, Addison's disease.
10. Drugs such as digitalis, ampicillin, amoxicillin, diuretics, analgesics.
11. Chronic alcoholism.

Diagnosis of the cause of anorexia shall depend on a good clinical history, physical examination and relevant investigations.

Management is of the underlying cause.

NAUSEA AND VOMITING

Nausea and vomiting are almost interrelated symptoms. Nausea often precedes vomiting. In nausea, the person has a feeling of discomfort and there is a desire to vomit which constitutes the act of bringing out the stomach contents. Severe form of vomiting is accompanied by retching.

A number of causes operate in the causation of vomiting. These may be either toxic, obstructive central or reflex.

Common causes are:

1. *Gastrointestinal causes.* Acute or chronic gastritis, pyloric obstruction, post-gastrectomy (dumping) syndrome. Carcinoma of stomach, intestinal obstruction, viral hepatitis, cirrhosis of liver, acute cholecystitis, acute pancreatitis or chronic recurrent pancrealitis.
2. *Systemic causes.* Renal colic, uraemia, pregnancy (first trimester) fever, diabetic, acidosis, food poisoning, chronic alcoholism, radiation sickness.
3. *Drugs* especially digitalis, cytotoxic drugs; Antitubercular drugs (rifampacin, pyrazinamide), pethidine, morphine, indomethacin, metronidazole, chloroquine, quinine.
4. Neurological disorders, migraine, brain tumours, brain abscess, cerebral concussion, meningitis (pyogenic, tubercular), intracranial haemorrhage, Mèniére's disease, encephalitis, vertigo.
5. Pschogenic. Unpleasant site or smell, hysteria, acute shock.

Let us look at some of the common causes of vomiting:

Emotional factors. Various emotions particularly those of disgust or fear may result in vomiting especially in neurotic people. Hysterical vomiting is common in women and represents a physical defense against some intolerable situation. This is generally at a subconscious level, is effortless and usually occurs during or immediately after meals and is not accompanied by nausea. Stomach in such women is only partially emptied so that nutrition is maintained. Such women require a patient hearing and going into their personal as well as marital history.

Habit vomiting. It is a strange form of vomiting which is rarely under control of will. This may occur as cyclical vomiting of children. The habit of vomiting persists even after the organic cause has been treated such as whooping cough in children.

Reflex vomiting. Painful stimulation of any afferent nerves particularly those of abdominal viscera such as in biliary and renal colic cause reflex vomiting. Vomiting of Meniers disease, sea and air sickness is caused by a reflex arising from excessive stimulation of the semi circular canals.

Toxic vomiting. Toxic products produced in the body in diseases like uraemia, diabetes, cirrhosis of liver may initiate vomiting. Toxins formed in acute infections such as pneumonia, septicaemia and toxaemia excite vomiting by action on the gastric mucous membrane and on the vomiting center. Toxic vomiting differs from central vomiting (cerebral tumours, meningitis, encephalitis, raised intracranial tension) as it is always preceded by nausea.

Local causes. Gastric irritiation due to diverse causes such as toxins, decomposing or contaminated food, inorganic or organic poisons, and drugs induce vomiting. Strong alcoholic drinks or consumption of spicy foods or over distension of stomach with food after heavy meals, expectorant mixtures and strong salt water are also responsible.

Clinical approach to a case of vomiting.

In order to reach the diagnosis of cause of vomiting a number of factors have to be considered:

1. A vomiting of short duration may be due to food poisoning or acute gastritis while of longer duration may be caused by chronic gastritis, pyloric obstruction, subacute intestinal obstruction and gastric malignancy.

2. Abdominal pain either accompanying or preceding vomiting occurs in renal or biliary colic, pancreatitis, acute gastritis, acute appendicitis.

3. A history of drugs being consumed especially chloroquine, digitalis, cytotoxic drugs etc. shall be helpful.

4. Headache or vertigo will be pointer towards neurological cause of vomiting.

5. Projectile vomiting in pyloric obstruction.

6. Vomiting in the first trimester of pregnancy in women. Young women in apparently good health and suffering from vomiting of some duration shall be either due to hysteria or functional cause.

7. Physical examination for jaundice (hepatitis), hepatomegaly (cirrhosis, hepatitis), tenderness at Macburny's point (appendicitis), murphy's sign (cholecystitis), epigastric tenderness (pancreatitis, gastritis), reversed peristalsis in abdomen (pyloric obstruction), mass in abdomen (malignancy), neck rigidity (meningitis, encephalitis, head injury), impairment of consciousness (cerebral haemorrhage, hepatic coma, meningitis, encephalitis), Kussmaul breathing (uraemia, acidosis), fetor hepaticus (hepatic coma).

8. Examination of vomitus is also helpful. Large volumes in acute dilatation of stomach. Bright blood in carcinoma of stomach. Presence of food particles consumed earlier favours pyloric obstruction.

9. Investigations of a case of vomiting shall include all tests keeping in mind the aetiological factors. These shall include barium meal study of stomach and duodenum, endoscopy, C.T. scan skull to exclude neurological causes. Blood chemistry like S. bilirubin (hepatitis), blood urea, creatinine (renal failure), blood sugar (diabetic coma), serum electrolytes (for electrolyte imbalance).

Management of a case of vomiting means treatment of underlying cause since vomiting is a symptom and not disease itself. *General principles of management are:*

1. Maintain adequate hydration, regulate electrolytes.
2. For symptomatic relief injection Metoclopramide to be given stat. For motion sickness promethazine theoclate (Avomine) 25 mg tablet 1-2 hours before taking journey is helpful.

HAEMATEMESIS

Haematemesis means bringing out of blood from the stomach or the lower oesophagus. This blood is generally dark coloured because of effect of acid on the blood and may be mixed with food contents while malaena is the passage of dark coloured blood in stools.

Common causes of haematemesis are:

1. *Gastric.* Peptic ulcer, gastric carcinoma, acute gastric erosion.
2. *Liver.* Portal hypertension cirrhosis of liver. Bleeding from oesophageal varices is an important aetiological factor.
3. *Blood disorders.* Thrombocytopenia, purpura, haemophilia, leukaemias, aplastic anaemia.
4. *Drugs.* Aspirin induced haematemesis is common. Other drugs like corticosteroids, NSAIDs (non steroidal antiinflammatory drugs) are also known to cause.
5. *Uncommon causes* include Mallory-Weiss syndrome where due to strong retching a tear may occur at lower end of oesophagus and bleed occurs.

Telengactesia in stomach is another source of haematemesis and sometimes may be very massive. Occasionally a case of haemoptysis may swallow blood and get malaena.

Diagnosis of haematemesis and malaena depends on the aetiological factor. A patient of peptic ulcer will give history suggestive of ulcer while in portal cirrhosis in addition signs of portal hypertension shall be present. A recent history of drug intake like aspirin will suggest drug induced haematemesis. In blood disorder there will be tell tale signs of bleeding at various sites, Splenomegaly may be present.

Further confirmation is made by barium meal study, endoscopy and study of haemtological profile (total and differential count, platelet count, bleeding and clotting time, prothrombin time, factor V and VII).

Treatment of a case of haematemesis shall be:

General

1. Put the patient to bed.
2. Arrange fresh blood transfusion.
3. Maintain nutrition and hydration.
4. Pass a Ryle's tube and do constant suction. In a case of suspected peptic ulcer, an antacid in gel form be given every 2 hourly. Alongwith H_2 receptor antagonist (INJ Ranitidine 50 mg *l*/V 6 hourly).

For bleed from oesophageal varices, Sengastaken tube, vasopressin and subsequent sclerosis of varices.

Specific

1. Treat the underlying condition appropriately.
2. Once the acute crisis is over and bleeding subsides then treatment is to be planned according to the basic disease. Drug-induced haematemesis shall require only symptomatic treatment and caution not to use such drug in future.

Haemoptysis

Bringing out of bright coloured blood with expectoration constitutes haemoptysis. It is very important to differentiate haemoptysis from haematemesis since confusion may arise in some people when expectorated blod is swallowed and patient may present with malaena.

Blood in haemoptysis is bright coloured, mixed with sputum and may be frothy while in haematemesis, blood is dark coloured clotted and may be mixed with food particles. *Common causes are:*

Pulmonary. Pulmonary tuberculosis, bronchiectasis, bronchogenic carcinoma, pneumonia, bronchial adenoma.

Cardiac. Mitral stenosis, pulmonary infarction, congenital cyanotic heart disease.

Blood diseases. Purpura, haemophilia, leukaemias.

Miscellaneous causes. Trauma to the chest. Penetrating injury of chest. Rupture of an amoebic liver abscess into lung and patient bringing out an anchoy coloured sputum. Sometimes an aortic aneurysm may leak into the lung through a bronchus or rupture. Rarely malingering individuals may produce haemoptysis.

Methods of enquiry. In a young adult, common causes shall be bronchiectasis, lung abscess, mitral valve disease and pulmonary tuberculosis while in a person above the age of 50, causes shall be bronchogenic carcinoma, pulmonary infarction, pulmonary tuberculosis, bronchiectasis, pnumonia. Quantity of blood expectorated shall vary from person to person and the extent of disease. Haemoptysis may be profuse in pulmonary tuberculosis, mitral stenosis, bronchiectasis and sometimes it may be so profuse that patient may choke himself to death.

A chronic history of cough with mucoid sputum favours bronchiectasis while low grade evening rise of temperature, weight loss, anorexia and poor health suggests pulmonary tuberculosis. In bronchogenic carcinoma there is dry hacking cough and a currant jelly type of sputum. Presence of valvular lesions suggests mitral disease and coexistence of bleeding from other sites a blood disorder. History of injury (blunt or penetrating) to the chest wall shall clinch the cause to be trauma.

Diagnosis of aetiological cause of haemoptysis can be based on radiology of chest, bronchography and haematology for exclusion of any blood disorder. Sputum may be examined naked eye as well as for AFB and malignant cells.

Treatment. A case of massive haemoptysis may sometimes go into shock. Since patient is losing large amount of blood fresh blood transfusion and plasma may be given. In addition supportive measures like keeping respiratory passages clear so that the patient does not choke, in his secretions and Prophylactic use of antibiotics. Once the acute crisis has been managed, appropriate treatment for the underlying pathology be instituted.

OEDEMA

Excessive accumulation of fluid in tissue spaces of the body constitutes oedema which may be localized or generalized.Oedema is caused by an increase in the amount of interstitial fluid due to increased permeability of the capillary walls, increased hydrostatic pressure in the capillaries and decreased colloid osmotic pressure of plasma proteins. Thus there is passage of fluid from the capillaries to the tissue spaces and there is accumulation of fluid in the subcutaneous tissues as well as serous spaces (pleura, peritoneum, pericardium).

A number of causes can produce generalized swelling (anasarca). *Out of these common are:*

Generalized oedema

1. Cardiac.Congestive heart failure, Constrictive pericarditis.
2. Renal. Acute nephritis, Nephrotic syndrome
3. Nutritional. Hypoproteinemia, deficiency state, beri-beri, malnutrition
4. Hepatic. Cirrhosis of liver
5. Endocrinal. Myxoedema

Localized oedema

1. Allergic. Angioneurotic oedema
2. Inflammatory. Cellulitis
3. Congenital. Milroy's disease
4. Lymphoedema. Filariasis
5. Venous. Inferior vena caval thrombosis

1. Cardiac. Any condition which leads to a ventricular failure (hypertension, ischaemic heart disease, rheumatic heart disease etc) is subsequently going to produce swelling of body where oedema of feet and dependent parts is the first to appear. If the patient is confined to bed, swelling appears over gluteal and sacral regions. Ascites is invariably present though it may vary from minimal to severe and often occurs late. Patient has history suggestive of progressive dyspnoea, more marked on exertion or it may be nocturnal suggestive of early left heart failure. By the time, the patient shows generalized swelling there are quite distinct physical signs which include oedema, ascites, engorged neck veins etc. There is evidence of cardiac involvement in the form of cardiomegaly, heart murmurs, gallop rhythm etc. Blood pressure may be elevated depending upon the cause of the failure. Liver is enlarged and tender.

Lungs show signs of bilateral congestion (rales at the bases). There may be hydrothorax.

Another important cause in this group is constrictive pericarditis. The swelling is mainly present on face, neck, and feet. Orthopnoea is commonly present but acute pulmonary oedema practically never occurs. Ascites often precedes oedema (ascites precox) which is massive, persistant or recurring. Heart may not be enlarged and shows only a triple rhythm with a loud third sound in early diastole (i.e. pericardial knock). Pulse volume is low and is typically of pulsus paradoxus type. The distended veins collapse suddenly during diastole which is an exaggeration of the normal descent. Diagnosis can be made by showing poor cardiac pulsation on screening. Electrocardiogram frequently shows low or poor voltage graph with flat or inverted 'T' waves and atrial fibrillation in one third of cases. Pericardial calcification can be seen in about half of cases on X-ray chest.

2. **Renal.** Nephrotic syndrome is one of the commonest causes of anasarca and is characterised by swelling present all over the body, more marked on face, hands and abdomen. Ascites usually is severe. Evidence of cardiac and hepatic involvement is lacking. Neither liver nor heart are enlarged. There may be hydrothorax. Diagnosis can easily be established by the presence of massive albuminuria reduced serum protein levels and hyper-cholesterolaemia.

Important causes of nephrotic syndrome are primary glomerular disease (e.g. mimimal change, focal and segmental, membranous and proliferative glomerulopathies), infection (post-streptococcal glomerulonephritis and malaria), drugs (e.g. organic gold, mercurials, penicillamine and probenecid), neoplastic (e.g. Hodgkin's disease) systemic lupus erythematosus, diabetes mellitus and preeclamptic toxaemia.

A case of acute nephritis does have generalized swelling but of less severe degree as compared to nephrotic syndrome. Swelling is generally confined to face and extremities, more apparent when the patient gets up in the morning. Blood pressure is elevated and the heart may occasionally be enlarged.

Urine examination shows albumin in traces with red blood cells and RBC casts. Acute nephritis usually follows an attack of infection with group A B haemolytic streptococci. It can also occur during the course of a wide variety of other bacterial and viral infections with deposition of immune complex in glomeruli responsible for the usually transient damage that occurs.

Diagnosis of this entity shall entail recognition of abrupt onset of haematuria and proteinuria accompanied by evidence of azotaemia and salt and water retention.

3. **Hepatic.** Cirrhosis of the liver is common factor to be considered. These patients have swelling marked over the feet which generally follows appearance of ascites which is often very severe and is recurrent. Patient may have history of jaundice in the past while in great majority of patients, history is not available Liver, which is enlarged in initial stages, shrinks in due course of time. Spleen is palpable in most of the cases. In majority of patients, one should look for signs of hepatocellular failure like spider naevi, palmar erythema, gynaecomastia, testicular atrophy. Bleeding from various sources etc. A history of haemetemesis, alcoholism, nutritional deficiency shall be further pointer towards establishing the diagnosis.

Investigation like liver biopsy, barium swallow, and endoscopy for oesophageal varices shall help in confirming the diagnosis.

4. **Nutritional.** Nutritional deficiency states are important factors responsible for the production of generalized swelling especially in under developed countries. Swelling due to hypoproteinaemia is usually generalized but may remain confined to the lower extremities from where it starts first. Ascites is usually present but is of mild to moderate degree. There are signs of nutritional deficiency. Skin is inelastic. There is anaemia. Hydrothorax may be present. There is characteristic absence of evidence of cardiac or renal pathology. Factors indicating either poor intake of diet or poor absorption can be elicited to clinch the diagnosis.

Blood shows severe degree of anaemia with marked lowering of serum proteins. In the same group we have patients of generalized swelling where oedema occurs because of war or famine conditions. It should not be difficult to arrive at a convenient diagnosis in such patients.

Beri-beri (wet or mixed type) may have the picture of generalized swelling where oedema and ascites appear almost together. Cardiac enlargement or even congestive failure may be seen. Hydrothorax may occur. Cases of beri-beri may be seen in epidemic form and some have history of poor dietary intake. Presence of peripheral neuropathy substantiates the picture. Therapeutic response to vitamin B1 is the best way to confirm the diagnosis.

5. **Endocrinal.** Of the endocrinal causes, obesity and myxoedema have to be considered. Any person who starts rapidly putting on weight may complain of generalized swelling. A thorough examination must be done in such patients to exclude the basis of any organic ailment.

Myxoedema is characterized by generalized swelling which is non-pitting in character. In addition, these patients have typical myxoedema facies, hoarse voice, loss of hair over the outer third of eye brows, slugghish deep tendon reflexes with delayed relaxation i.e. myxoedema reflex. Further confirmation of diagnosis can be made by EKG (poor voltage graph with flattening of T-waves), estimation of PBI and radioactive iodine uptake.

Diagnosis. It is arrived at by a thorough history with appropriate physical examination. Sudden onset of oedema especially over the face in early morning with oliguria and smoky urine points to a renal pathology. History of haematemesis, alcohol intake suggests cirrhosis while in cardiac oedema, there is progressive history of palpitation, breathlessness, suggestive of underlying heart disease. Specialized investigations ranging from blood chemistry, liver and kidney biopsy, barium swallow for oesophageal varices and oesophagogastric endoscopy shall be further helpful aids.

Treatment of any case shall depend on the underlying cause and institution of appropriate dietetic and drug therapy.

Localised oedema. Localized oedema is generally confined to a small part and various factors already enumerated shall be operative according to aetiology. An allergic reaction shall produce angioneurotic oedema, a familial and hereditary tendency in young females producing oedema over legs and feet in Milroy's disease, venous obstruction or occlusion giving rise to oedema over dependent parts or in filariasis or inflammation oedema may be confined to one limb.

Malaena

Passage of dark coloured blood in stools constitutes malaena. A patient having malaena need not be having haematemesis since in such cases the blood passed is dark coloured, stools become tarry. This is because in patients having malaena the bleed is generally lower down in the intestines. At the same time bleed from gastric, duodenal ulcer, oesophageal varices the blood is passed lower down and presentation is that of malaena. Common causes are:

- Peptic ulcer
- Portal hypertension
- Typhoid fever
- Malignancy GI tract
- Ulcerative colitis
- Bleeding diathesis, purpura, hemophilia, leukaemias.

Management. Diagnosis should be made with relevant investigations and appropriate treatment instituted.

WEIGHT LOSS

It is a common symptom and number of causes may be operative. Thus we have weight loss where appetite is normal but there is weight loss and in other category where appetite is impaired or patient is unable to take food because of secondary factors. These include diseases of mouth, larynx, tongue where patient has difficulty in swallowing. In this category are also diseases of oesophagus like achlasia, malignancy, mediastinal growths producing pressure symptoms on oesophagus.

After excluding secondary causes, let us look at endogenous factors where weight loss occurs rapidly.

1. Diabetes mellitus primarily juvenile or insulin-

dependent, thyrotoxicosis, Addison's disease.
2. Malabsorption, post gastrectomy syndrome, peptic ulcer.
3. Cirrhosis of liver, malignancy liver
4. Pulmonary tuberculosis, bronchogenic carcinoma, chronic lung disease (bronchiectasis, lung abscess)
5. Renal failure, malignancy, AIDS.
6. Cardiac cachexia, subacute bacterial endocarditis.
7. Coeliac disease, regional enteritis, abdominal tuberculosis.
8. Psychiatric disturbances, anorexia nervosa, depression.

Clinical assessment. Weight loss is a serious problem and relevant investigations should be carried out depending on clinical impressions. Management depends on the underlying disease process.

PALPITATION

It has been defined as awareness of the heart's action, and often is a cause of worry to a person since palpitation is presumed to be indicative of heart dysfunction. But this may not be so. Palpitation is experienced by a normal person engaged in strenuous physical activity, after exercise, during period of acute emotional stress, anxiety and tension. Similarly palpitation may occur in both cardiac and non-cardiac conditions.

Non-cardiac or extrinsic factors

1. Acute fevers, severe anaemia.
2. Exertion, excitement, exercise.
3. Heavy drinkers of tea, coffee, alcohol, smoking,
4. Cardiac embarrassment due to massive pleural effusion, pneumothorax, ascites, cardiac temponade.
5. Anxiety neurosis, cardiac neurosis (De costa's syndrome)
6. Diaphragmatic hernia, gastric distension
7. Thyrotoxicosis, pheochromocytoma, hypoglycemia.
8. Convalescence from acute illness.

9. Drugs like nifedipine, ephedrine, salbutamol, adrenaline, eltroxin etc.

Cardiac or intrinsic factors:

1. Disturbances of cardiac rhythm, extrasystoles, paroxysmal atrial tachycardia, atrial fibrillation or flutter, ventricular tachcardia.
2. Hypertension
3. Valvular heart disease

Method of enquiry. Palpitation may be major symptom in a case of acute anxiety in an otherwise healthy person. A careful assessment of a person suffering from non-cardiac causes for any drug intake, excessive tea, coffee drinking, alcohol, smoking and other innumerable causes should be carefully carried out and diagnosis established.

For cardiac factors, history of isolated jump or skipping of heart beat shall favour extrasystoles while attacks of tachycardia coming suddenly and disappearing, point towards paroxysmal supraventricular tachycardia. In atrial fibrillation or flutter, there is already a pre-existing cardiac ailment. Ventricular tachycardia, a life threatening ailment comes at a stage when patient is very ill and palpitation may not be the predominent complaint.

Associated factors like loss of weight, tremors, excitement shall be present in thyrotoxicosis while cough, breathlessness, fever are present in cases with pleural effusion, pneumothorax.

When palpitation is the outstanding complaint, all suspected organic causes must be excluded. For suspected cardiac irregularities a simple electrocardiogram and Holter monitoring shall be able to pin point the cause.

Management. In a case of palpitation due to non-organic causes, assurance to the patient shall suffice. If necessary antianxiety drug like Alprazolam (0.25-0.5 mg) twice a day be prescribed. If patient does not improve then Tab. Propranolol 20 mg twice a day be given.

For organic causes of palpitation, appropriate treatment depending on the disease be prescribed.

HEMATURIA

Passage of blood in the urine is called hematuria. A

systemic disease producing bleeding from mucous surfaces may produce blood in urine but commonly any lesion in the urinary tract from kidney to urethra is the cause of hematuria. Red-coloured or smoky urine of hematuria must be distinguished from red-coloured urine produced as a result of certain dyes and drugs (Dindevan, nalidixic acid). Common causes are:

1. **Lesions of the urinary tract.** Polycystic kidney, acute nephritis, trauma, tuberculosis of kidney, papilloma of the renal pelvis, renal stone, ureteric stone, cystitis of urinary bladder, papilloma and carcinoma of bladder, stone in urinary bladder, bilharziasis and prostatitis.

2. **Disorders of the adjacent organs.** Diseases of the viscera lying adjacent to the ureter and bladder may involve them and produce hematuria. In this category are carcinoma of rectum and cervix uteri involving the bladder.

3. **General disorders.** Blood disorders like hemophilia, purpura, scurvy, leukaemias. Hematuria may also occur in subacute bacterial endocarditis, hypertension, renal infarction, black water fever, Dengue etc.

Approach to a patient of hematuria. Hematuria generally denotes different aetiological factors at different age groups. In children cause of hematuria may be acute nephritis, acute hemorrhagic fever, bladder stone, blood disorders while in adults common causes shall be renal calculus, tuberculosis of kidney, renal tumours and in elderly people commonly it is prostate disease or malignancy of urinary tract.

History is suggestive in most of the cases. Attacks of renal colic suggest calculus, painful hematuria, tuberculosis of the kidney and painless hematuria malignancy. Rupture of kidney producing hematuria has history of trauma of the abdomen. Hematuria is profuse in tumours of kidney or bladder.

Examination of urine on naked eye is very helpful in localizing the site of urinary tract from where hematuria is taking place. A bright red-coloured urine indicates bleeding either from urinary bladder or lower urinary tract. In diseases of the urethra or prostate, urine is blood-stained only at the beginning of micturition. When bleed is from higher level i.e. from kidney or upper part of ureter urine is evenly mixed with blood. When blood comes out after the bladder has been evacuated it means that blood is coming from urinary bladder (cystitis, tumour).

Pain during micturition is present in calculus in any part of urinary tract, growth of bladder or when blood clot is passing through the urinary tract. Frequency of micturition is increased in urinary tract infection (cystitis, pyelitis). In acute nephritis, hematuria is accompanied by hypertension, fever and swelling over the body while in systemic diseases (blood disorders, leukaemias) there shall be evidence of bleeding from other sources especially on mucous surfaces.

Diagnosis of causes of hematuria shall be made on basis of history and relevant investigations including urine examination, plain X-ray abdomen, intravenous pyelography, ultrasound of abdomen and computed tomography (CT scan) especially for tumours of the kidney, urinary bladder.

Treatment and management shall be governed by the aetiological cause of hematuria.

ABDOMINAL PAIN

Pain in abdomen, a frequent complaint, may be mild, moderate or severe in nature which may require urgent management. It may be superficial or deep. But there are mainly two types—somatic when pain arises from structures constituting the abdominal wall or peritoneum while visceral pain arises from abdominal viscera due to their distension, spasm, obstruction or ischemia. Occasionally pain may be referred to abdomen from disease elsewhere and classic example of this is pain in a case of acute myocardial infarction being referred to epigastric region. Similarly in diseases of the thorax and spine pain may be referred to abdomen.

Causes of abdominal pain.

Anatomically abdomen is divided into nine compartments and it is easier to locate the cause of pain considering its site. Further to consider the differential causes as (i) those arising from abdominal wall, (ii) extra-abdominal and intra-abdominal.

a. **Abdominal wall.** Fibrositis, myalgia, neuralgia, herpes zoster.

b. **Extra-abdominal.** Myocardial infarction, pneumothorax, diaphragmatic pleurisy, angina pectoris.

c. **Intra-abdominal.**

1. *Epigastrium.* Gastric ulcer, gastritis, carcinoma stomach, hiatus hernia, duodenal ulcer, pancreatitis (acute or recurring), amoebic hepatitis or abscess, congested liver.

2. *Right hypochondrium.* Amoebic hepatitis or liver abscess, viral hepatitis, passive congestion of liver, cholecystitis, empyema of gall bladder.

3. *Left hypochondrium.* Splenic infarction, splenic rupture or abscess, diseases of splenic flexure of colon.

4. *Right lumbar/left lumbar.* Renal colic, infection of urinary tract, ureteric colic, diseases of colon, diverticulitis.

5. *Right iliac fossa.* Acute appendicitis, amoebic colitis, carcinoma colon, acute salpingitis or oophritis in females, regional ileitis (Crohn's disease).

6. *Left iliac fossa.* Amoebic colitis, ulcerative colitis, diverticulitis, carcinoma colon.

7. *Umbilical.* Mesenteric artery thrombosis. Tubercular enteritis, appendicitis, lymphadenopathy, organic diseases of small intestines.

8. *Hypogastrium.* Urinary bladder stone, prostatitis, cystitis.

Approach to patient with abdominal pain. Approach to a patient with abdominal pain is primarily towards the pain, its site, character, severity, radiation and referral to any site, along with accompanying symptoms and how relieved.

Physical examination of abdomen is equally important. In gastric or duodenal ulcer tenderness is in the epigastric region; in acute cholecystitis, there is tenderness to the right of costal margin with catch in breath (Murphy's sign), tenderness at Macburny's point in acute appendicitis. Similarly in renal pathology, renal angle is tender. Abdomen in peritonitis is rigid and liver dullness may be obliterated in perforation of the gut.

Presence of an acute pain of recent origin points towards a more serious ailment while chronic pain in abdomen is generally due to inflammatory conditions. Pain in renal, ureteric stone or gall stones is colicky in nature, generally of short duration and is relieved after the acute attack and patient may have symptom-free period. A chronic pain lasting for weeks accompanied with weight loss and poor health points to the possibility of malignancy.

Radiation of pain is equally important. Pain of acute cholecystitis is referred to shoulder or angle of scapula, pancreatitis pain to back and renal or ureteric pain to the groin.

Some cases especially of gastric or duodenal ulcer have relationship with food. While pain in gastric ulcer is increased after ingestion of food the pain of duodenal ulcer is relieved after taking food. A fatty meal may trigger an attack of acute cholecystitis.

Associated symptoms like vomiting (appendicitis, cholecystitis, pancreatitis), dysuria and hematuria (renal, urteric colic) when present helps in making a diagnosis. Tenderness in lower abdomen is present in diseases of the female genitalia (salpingitis, oophoritis). On auscultation abdomen is silent in peritonitis.

A patient with abdominal pain shall require a number of investigations. Presence of leucocytosis (high total leucocyte count with rise in polymorphs) will be seen in inflammatory conditions of abdomen like perforation, pancreatitis, pelvic inflammatory conditions. Urinalysis for sugar and ketone bodies (diabetes) and porphyrins in porphyria.

Blood for serum bilirubin (hepatitis), serum amylase (pancreatitis), blood sugar (diabetes), blood urea, creatinine levels. Plain X-ray abdomen for presence of fluid and air levels (paralytic ileus, peritonitis), gas under the diaphragm (perforation), stones (gall stones, renal or ureteric colic).

Ultrasound of abdomen for hepatomegaly, gall stones, pancreatitis, renal stones and for other inflammatory or malignant conditions.

In cases where disease of stomach and duodenum is suspected (ulcer, gastritis, malignancy) barium meal study of gastrointestinal tract is advised. Oral and intravenous cholecystography for gall bladder diseases, ERCP for pancreatitis or pancreatic calculi, pyelography for renal pathology, barium enema for diseases of colon, gastroendoscopy and colonoscopy may be done where indicated.

Let us look briefly now at some of the common ailments of abdomen responsible for abdominal pain.

Gastric ulcer. Pain in epigastrium, diffuse or gnawing starts half to two hours after a meal relieved by antacids or vomiting.

Duodenal ulcer. Pain in epigastric region more to right side. Comes 2-3 hours after a meal. History of pain at night. Pain relieved by food.

Chronic gastritis. Discomfort, sense of fullness and burning sensation in epigastrium shortly after meals.

Perforation of peptic ulcer. Sudden acute pain in abdomen with patient going into shock. Peritonitis sets in and abdomen becomes rigid.

Carcinoma stomach. Dull constant pain or discomfort in epigastric region. Loss of appetite and weight common. A mass may be felt in late stages. Virchow glands when palpable clinch the diagnosis.

Acute pancreatitis. Sudden pain in epigastrium accompanied by vomiting, radiating to back. Shock may be present. Often patient is suffering from gall bladder disease.

Chronic or relapsing pancreatitis. Recurrent attacks of pain accompanied by vomiting in epigastric region, weight loss and loss of appetite common. Complicated by diabetes and pancreatic calcification.

Carcinoma head of pancreas. Dull constant pain to start with. Later on pain becomes very severe, radiation of pain to back. Obstructive jaundice, progressive weight loss and cachexia.

Acute cholecystitis. Attacks of colicky pain in right hypochondrium near tip of ninth costal cartilage. Pain accompanied by vomiting radiates to shoulder or tip of scapula. Murphy's sign present.

Amoebic hepatitis or abscess. Dull constant pain in right hypochondrium, Liver enlarged and tender. Intercostal tenderness on right lower chest on deep percussion. Low grade fever, toxaemia and ill health.

Abdominal angina. There may be referred pain of acute myocardial infarction in epigastric region. Pain may be very severe, accompanied by shock.

Vascular spasm of mesenteric artery or vessels supplying abdominal viscera may sometimes produce severe pain simulating angina like symptoms.

Hiatus hernia. Epigastric pain or discomfort related to posture. More when patient lies down after meals or when bending forward. Heart burn and belching common complaints.

Diaphragmatic or basal pleurisy. Sharp stabbing pain in upper part of abdomen aggravated by deep breath. Fever, cough and toxaemia are other features of this condition. Pain may be referred to back or shoulder.

Miscellaneous. Obstruction of hollow viscus like gall bladder produces colicky pain. Pain of kidney pathology is in lumbar region and often colicky and goes down along the ureter to groin.

Pain in diseases like porphyria, diabetes, uremia, lead poisoning is of varying nature ranging from dull constant type to severe forms.

Of the neurologic causes, diseases involving sensory nerve roots supplying the abdominal wall may produce severe lancinating or knife like pain. Conditions like herpes zoster, diabetes, herniated discs or neurofibromatosis are the common aetiological factors.

Uncommonly a young person may have chronic abdominal pain varying in intensity and of no fixed pattern. This pain typically is seen in hysterical or neurotic persons. But before one labels any pain in abdomen of psychogenic origin, all organic causes must be excluded by meticulous examination and investigations.

LOW BACK PAIN

It is a very common complaint and often produces distressing symptoms. Pain in the low back may vary in intensity from mild to severe, varying with physical activity or movements of the back and often relieved by lying down in bed or physical rest.

Causes of low back pain are variable and may

range from benign condition like sprain of the back muscles to spinal tumours.

1. Lesions of the vertebaal column: Prolapsed Disc, Spondylosis, osteoarthritis, ankylosing spondylitis, rheumatoid arthritis, tuberculosis of spine, osteomalacia, pagets disease, spinal carcinomatous deposits.
2. Lesions of soft tissues: Muscular sprain, fibrositis, lumbar strain, trauma.
3. Lesions of spinal cord: Benign tumours (menin-gioma, neuroma, osteoblastoma) maligant (secondaries spine, multiple myeloma, Hodgkin's disease, lymphoma).
4. Non-skeletal disorders producing back pain: Pelvic disorders (pelvic inflammatory diseases, cervical erosions, uterine fibroids) retroperitoneal tumours, aortic aneurysm, pancreatitis, gastric ulcer penetrating deep and producing pain in back.
5. Psychogenic.

Approach to the patient. Any patient with low back pain should be specially asked for site of pain, its relationship to posture and movements of spine. Neurologic pains radiating from back favour a spinal tumour. The pain of prolapsed disc is generally localized to one space and may go lower down to other joint spaces. Recurrent attacks of pain occur and tend to be more and more severe. Ankylosing spondylitis pain produces more of a stiff bamboo like spine with movements of spine severely restricted. Peripheral involvement of small joints occurs in rheumatoid spine. A dull constant pain with ill health in women should favour possibility of pelvic inflammatory disease. Symptoms become worse during mensturation. Pain of pancreatitis or a penetrating gastric ulcer is associated with abdominal complaints with gnawing pain going to the back.

Pain of secondaries spine or tumour when present is severe and excruciating not relieved even by strong narcotics. Pain of disc prolapse though aggravated by movements and exertion, is relieved by rest.

Diagnosis of cause of low back pain shall depend on a good clinical history analysing the symptoms. Investigations include blood for ESR, rheumatoid factor, X-ray of spine (both PA and lateral view) and CT of spine.

A vaginal examination in women is essential. In women suspected of osteomalacia history of repeated pregnancies, malnutrition, disturbances of serum calcium and phosphorous levels, X-ray of pelvis showing osteoporosis with pseudo fractures shall confirm the diagnosis.

Management of a case shall depend on the underlying condition. For benign conditions like muscular sprain, back exercises, analgesics and diathermy is helpful. For specific conditions treatment on specific lines has to be instituted. A spinal tumour may be delineated by myelography and CT scan. Surgical removal is the only course. For secondaries spine chemotherapy has to be given.

A case of prolapsed disc if not relieved by conservative line of therapy and is producing neurological symptoms, surgical removal or excision of the disc may have to be undertaken.

Chest pain

Pain in chest is a common complaint and can be due to number of causes ranging from mild and reversible ailments to serious illnesses often with grave prognosis. Depending on the cause, the prognosis shall vary. Often the pain in chest especially on the left side is of coronary heart disease. A case with chest pain requires thorough history, and detailed investigations.

Classification of causes:

Diseases of the musculoskeletal system. Myalgia, myositis, myofibrositis, local trauma, fracture of rib, costochondral arthritis (Teitz's syndrome), intercostal neuralgia, osteoarthritis of spine, spinal cord tumours, metastasis in ribs.

Diseases of nerve roots. Herpes zoster, neurofibromatosis, pressure on nerve roots, intercostal neuralgia.

Disorders of cardiovascular system. Angina pectoris, myocardial infarction, coronary artery disease, aortic stenosis, syphilitis aortitis, myocarditis, pericarditis (tuberculous, rheumatic, viral), postmyocardial infarction pericarditis, dissecting aneurysm of aorta.

Diseases of respiratory system. Pneumonia, pleurisy (tuberculosis, viral), pneumothorax, pulmonary malignancy, pulmonary infarction, mediastinitis, mediastinal tumour.

Diseases of gastrointestinal system. Oesophagitis, cardiac achlasia, oesophageal reflux, peptic or oesophageal ulcer, carcinoma oesophagus.

Miscellaneous causes. Chronic mastitis, premenstrual pain, cardiac neurosis, anxiety neurosis, hysteria.

Methods of enquiry. Enquiry has to be made of site of pain, its radiation, nature (discomfort, choking, heaviness), duration of pain, aggravating and relieving factors. Is the pain continuous or comes in attacks or on exertion.

Pain in coronary heart disease is generally present in precordial region radiating to neck, shoulder or jaw. It may be dull or choking in nature. Patient is unable to pin point it. Anginal pain is brought on by exertion and relieved by rest. In myocardial infarction there are accompanying symptoms like sweating and breathlessness.

Muscular skeletal pain is present in youg adults in any part of chest and has no particular radiation. Pain of costochondritis is localized to 2nd or 3rd costal cartilage and is often aggravated by local pressure. Nerve root pain is always in the distribution of nerve roots and generally radiates from back to front. It is increased by movements of spine, neck or trunk and often pain can be located to some spinal segment. Herpes zoster pain is severe and is in the distribution of dorsal nerve roots. There are vesicular eruptions.

Pain of angina pectoris is often retrosternal radiating to the left arm but uncommonly to both arms, neck, jaw or epigastrium. Pain is often constricting, choking and oppressing lasting for a few minutes. It is often brought about by exertion, cold, emotional factors and is relieved by rest or nitrates. Electrocardiogram is usually normal. When pain of angina pectoris lasts for more than 15-20 minutes, is not relieved by rest, nitrates, possibility of myocardial infarction is considered.

Pain in cases of myocardial infarction is severe, crushing, constricting accompanied by sweating, weakness, pallor and often patient may collapse. Sometimes a patient of myocardial infarction may have cardiac arrhythmias or acute left heart failure complicating the condition. Electroacardiogram is diagnostic.

Pain in pericarditis is commonly frequent over the pericardial region and may be either sharp or dull continuous type lasting for few days. Signs of cardiac embarrassment like cough, dyspnoea may be present. Pericardial rub when present is diagnostic.

Pleural pain is sharp stabbing or cutting. Pain increased by deep inspiration or coughing is suggestive of pleurisy. Presence of pleural rub, fever cough, breathlessness clinch the diagnosis. X-ray of chest is helpful in diagnosing the condition.

Aortic aneurysm is commonly syphilitic in origin. It is generally a middle aged person who comes complaining of pain in sternal or parasternal region radiating to back. Anginal pain may coexist. There is abnormal bulging over the chest wall and pulsations of aneurysm itself may be palpable. Patient has a brassy cough, hoarseness of voice and breathlessness as a result of pressure of aneurysm. X-ray and flouroscopy shall demonstrate a pulsatile mass. Pain in case of dissecting aneurysm of aorta is generally present anteriorly and then spreads to back. It is severe and gives a tearing sensation in the chest. Pain is often accompanied by breathlessness, shock, prostration and is continuous, severe, not relieved by usual analgesics. Radiology of chest and electrocardiography are helpful in diagnosing the condition.

Often pain in chest especially in retrosternal region may be due to oesophageal spasm or oesophagitis. It is a burning type of sensation, related to meals. There may be difficulty in swallowing and regurgitation of food. Cases of hiatus hernia have pain coming up from epigastric region going towards the chest more marked after a heavy meal, bending forward or in recumbent position. Pain in a case of hiatus hernia is often mistaken for pain of coronary heart disease. Distinction can be made by meticulous history about relationship of pain to food and posture.

Often pain in cardiac area is cause of anxiety even when it is not due to cardiac in origin. Persons with cardiac neurosis have pain over precordial region, localise to a spot with vague radiation to different sites. There is palpitation, anxiety and complaints of tremors, faintness. A pain of cardiac neurosis should not be ignored and patient reassured after all the tests including electrocardiogram (resting and after exercise), TMT, radiology of chest are normal.

While considering pain in chest region one must consider precipitating or aggravating factors. Pain of pericarditis, pleurisy is increased by deep breathing coughing, oesophageal pain by swallowing especially spicy food. Pain due to muscular myalgia or myositis by movements or contraction of the muscles.

Thus pain in chest encompasses number of diseases and it is not difficult to reach diagnosis if due attention is paid to all the factors responsible for causing pain.

SHOCK

It is a serious emergency in clinical practice and may be defined as a condition in which there is wide spread reduction in tissue perfusion with cellular hypoxia leading to acute circulatory collapse and reversible cellular injury which if allowed to progress may lead to irreversible damage. A patient in shock has a pale, cold and clammy skin. Arterial pulse is rapid thready and even impalpable with marked fall of blood pressure (systolic levels below 90 mmg), a rapid and shallow respiration. There is oliguria (urinary output less than 400 ml in 24 hours) or anuria. Patient is anxious, restless and his/her itellectual functions may be clouded.

Causes. A number of factors are responsible for producing shock. These may be inadequate cardiac output (cardiogenic shock) inadequate blood volume (hypovolemia) or mechanical obstruction to venous return (extra-cardiac obstructive shock) and peripheral vasodilatation (distributive shock).

   a. Cardiogenic shock. It is a very serious condition and causes include acute myocardial inf-

arction, myocarditis, ventricular tachycardia or fibrillation, rupture of a ventricular septum or aneurysm, massive pulmonary embolism, air/fat embolism, and ball valve thrombus in mitral valve disease.

Other causes are acute cardiac temponade (haemopericardium following blunt or penetrating injury to chest, massive pericardial effusion) constrictive pericarditis, cardiac rupture following acute myocardial infarction.

   b. Inadequate blood volume (oligaemic shock). Severe blood loss following injury, surgery, ante-partum or post-partum haemorrhage. Medical emergencies like acute gastro enteritis, cholera, celphos poisoning, haematemesis and malaena from bleeding peptic ulcer or oesophageal varices in portal hypertension are important causes. Other causes include acute addisonian crisis, plasma loss in extensive burns, crush syndrome.

   c. Peripheral vasodilatation (distributive shock). Septic shock (gram-negative septicaemia), bacterial toxins (meningococcal, pneumococcal, streptococcal, staphylococcal, shigella), anaphylactic shock (drugs, sera, incompatible blood transfusion), snake bite, sting bite by bees, scorpion, electric shock, neurogenic shock are important causes in this group.

   d. Mechanical obstruction to venous return (extra-cardiac obstructive shock). Inferior vena caval obstruction. Portal vein thrombosis, pericardial temponade form main causes in this group.

Clinical features. Clinical signs in a case of shock to a large extent depend on the aetiological factor. In hypovalemic shock patient is cold, pale. There is tachycardia, increased sweating, low blood pressure, Tachypnoea and oliguria or anuria. Patient is restless and often shows signs of confusion. In cardiogenic shock, in addition to other features of shock there may be signs of myocardial failure in the form of engorged neck veins, gallop rhythm and basal crepitations in lungs. Patients with septic shock have features of severe toxaemia, high fever, rigors, rapid bounding pulse while those in anaphylactic shock show signs of allergic reaction (urticaria, bronchospasm, restlessness and fall of blood pressure).

Most of the times a case of shock has mixed features and classical signs of any group may not be present.

Management. First approach to a patient with shock is to revive him/her and keep the vital centers functioning.

The general guidelines are:

1. Put the patient to bed and keep him warm.

2. Oxygen be administered.

3. Maintain adequate fluid balance in shock caused by massive bleeding either due to injury or bleed from an ulcer or varices. Rush one to two pints of fresh blood rapidly. The total amount of blood to be transfused shall depend on assessment of blood loss. Till further blood is available, plasma or plasma substitutes (low molecular weight dextran) may be given.

In cases of water loss due to dehydration, diarrhoea, vomiting, first pint of normal saline is adminstered rapidly followed by the second and third bottle in next 1/2 to 1 hour. For acidosis, sodium bicarbonate (1.5% solution) or molar lactate is to be administered. Normal saline is to be alternated with 5% glucose or glucose saline solution.

Amount of fluid to be administered shall again depend on the assessment of fluid loss. Care must be taken to prevent volume overload since it carries with it the risk of pulmonary oedema. Ideal method is to monitor central venous pressure by using a manometer system.

Since electrolytes have been lost, a close monitoring be done and their replacement done. In patients with anuria or oliguria, potasium supplementation is contraindicated.

For patients with primary shock, sympathomimetic pressor amines are the drugs of choice.

Noradrenaline, an alpha adrenergic agonist, is usually administered (one ampule contains 1 mg per ml, 2-4 ml in a bottle of 5% glucose saline) slowly intravenously. It is a powerful vasoconstrictor and its effect manifests quickly. Blood pressure must be monitored and drip maintained so that systolic levels are above 100 mmHg. It is of value in cases of shock where there is peripheral pooling of blood. Care must be taken that the drug does not leak into subcutaneous tissues since it produces tissue necrosis and gangrene at that site.

Mephentine sulphate acts by increasing the cardiac output as well as by peripheral vasoconstriction. It has been used both intramuscularly and intravenously. Dosage is 1 ml (15 mg) to be given intramuscularly and followed by 15-30 mg every 1-2 hours. For acute emergency intravenous injection (60 mg) may be administered immediately followed by infusion of 0.1% mephentine in 5 % dextrose.

Mephentine is primarily indicated for shock accompanying severe medical illness, hypotension during surgical procedures or following spinal anaesthesia.

Dopamine, a naturally occurring amine, acts on alpha and beta adrenergic receptors with a positive inotropic effect on heart. Intravenous infusion of the drug raises cardiac output and systolic blood pressure with little effect on diastolic levels. Renal and hepatic blood flow improves with resultant increase in urinary output. It is mainly used in shock caused by hypovolemia, septicaemic shock and cardiogenic shock.

Dose is 2-50 µg/kg/minute by slow intravenous infusion. Dose can be increased to 100 µg/kg/minute. In cases with hypovolaemia producing shock, hypovolaemia must be corrected before administering dopamine.

Side effects include nausea, vomiting, tachycardia, palpitation, anginal pain, headache and vasoconstriction.

Another drug of use is Dobutamine. It is akin to dopamine but produces greater improvement in cardiac output and reduces systemic resistance thus improving cardiac performance. It is the drug of choice for a case of cardiogenic shock.

Dosage. 2.5-10 µg/kg/minute in intravenous infusion (50 mg/ml). Special care should be taken while giving the drug in a patient of acute myocardial infarction. Side effects include cardiac arrhythmias.

For shock due to endotoxins, septicaemia, antibiotics in high dosage should be started parenterally. Steroids are also beneificial in this type of shock.

In anaphylactic shock: Injection Adrenaline is administered intramuscularly immediately (0.5-1 ml is the usual dosage). In addition Dexamethasone (4-8 mg) intravenously is to be given. Antihistaminics are also administered parentcrally but their role is limited.

For cases with cardiogenic shock, especially following myocardial infarction, therapy is directed towards salvaging the myocardium (thrombolytic therapy, oxygen, dobutamine, steroids, intravenous infusion). Ventricular tachycardia, fibrillation shall require appropriate treatment with Lignocaine and defibrillation. Pericardial temponade due to massive pericardial effusion or haemopericardium requires immediate pericardial tapping and relieving the mechanical factors.

In case of massive pulmonary embolism producing shock, in addition to supportive measures, anti-coagulation and emergency surgery like pulmonary embolectomy may be required.

COMA

It is a state of unconsciousness from which the patient is unarousable and does not respond to external stimuli. Depending on the state of consciousness, it may be graded as deep coma. Coma is not a disease but rather a symptom of number of serious diseases and requires urgent management.

Causes. Various causes ranging from cerebro vascular accidents to diabetes shall be operating and have to be promptly looked into:

1. Cerebrovascular causes: Cerebral thrombosis, haemorrhage, subarachnoid haemorrhage, cerebral infraction (arterial, venous).
2. Head injury: Intracerebral bleed, rupture of aneurysm or arteriovenous malformation.

3. Infections: Meningitis (viral, tubercular), encephalitis, cerebral malaria.
4. Metabolic causes: Diabetic coma, uraemia, hypoglycemia, myxoedema.
5. Hepatic coma
6. Poisons: Barbiturates, alcohol, cellphos poisoning, opium.
7. Physical causes: Heat stroke, hyperpyrexia, electric shock.
8. Hypertensive encephalopathy.
9. Chronic respiratory insufficiency with decompensation
10. Status epilepticus.

Degree of coma. A lot depends on the degree and state of coma. Thus a patient may be in stupor when he responds to painful stimuli by opening the eyes or some bodily movements. Further on the state of semi coma may be present in some patients while some patients shall be in deep coma. Here the patient is unresponsive to all forms of stimuli. The pupils react poorly and are often dilated and fixed. Breathing is usually shallow and often laboured.

Investigations of a case of coma

History. It is the most important part. An history of diabetes, accident (Head injury) high fever, intake of drugs shall be pointer towards important causes. Type of onset is important. It is sudden in cases of cerebro vascular accidents, cerebral haemorrhage but gradual in case of liver failure, uraemia, diabetic coma etc. Preceding symptoms such as fits, headache or vomiting shall be present in cases of meningitis, encephalitis. Exposure to heat or sun shall be present in a suspected case of sunstroke. Previous history of fits and convulsions shall be helpful in making a diagnosis of status epilepticus.

Physical examination

General physical examination. Patient lies listless with laboured breathing. He is flushed when alcohol is responsible. There is icteric tinge in hepatic coma. Patient of diabetic coma and uraemia have acidotic ammonical odour in their breath while hepatic failure patient has got a mousy odour. Pungent smell is present in cellphos poisoning

Skin: Cold and sweaty in shock, diabetic coma and poisoning.

Head: Depressed fracture. Bleed from ears suggests fracture of base of skull.

Neck: Rigidity in meningitis, encephalitis, intra cranial haemorrhage.

Pupils: Unequal in intracranial lesion. Constricted pupils in opium poisoning.

Respiration: Deep in diabetic coma. Slow in increased intracranial pressure, cheyne stokes in uraemia.

Cyanosis in poisoning, chronic respiratory insufficiency.

Organomegaly: Palpable spleen in Hepatic coma, cerebral malaria.

Blood pressure: Raised in hypertensive encephalopathy, cerebrovascular accidents, uraemia.

Temperature elevated in hyperpyrexia, cerebral malaria, pontine haemorrhage. Low grade in cerebrovascular accidents. Subnormal in diabetic coma.

Investigations

1. Fundus examination for Papilloedema. Look for changes of diabetic retinopathy and hypertensive encephalopathy.
2. CT skull for assessing cerebro vascular accident. Cerebral haemorrhage / infarction / Head injury
3. Blood sugar: Serial estimations to exclude diabetes.
4. Blood urea
5. Blood smear for malarial parasites.

Management

1. Immediately establish a clear air way. Do gentle suction. In presence of cyanosis administer 50% to 100% oxygen with or without 5% CO_2. If required, endotracheal intubation and artificial ventilatory support be instituted immediately.
2. Start intravenous, line immediately and administer fluids. Draw blood for various biochemical tests. Restore acid base balance.
3. Monitor pulse, blood pressure and respiration.
4. Care of the bowel and bladder.

5. Start sunction of any secretions in respiratory passages.
6. Make a correct diagnosis and treat the underlying cause since coma is a symptoms of a serious ailment.

Vertigo

It is a sense of rotation either of the patient or his/her surroundings. As compared to vertigo, we have dizziness where patient does not have a feeling of turning but a sense of loss of consciousness secondary to cerebral ischaemia.

In humans there is a sophsticated mechanism of balance dependent upon visual, proprioceptive and superficial sensory function which is integrated in the central nervous system and controlled by the coordinated working of reticular formation, extrapyramidal system, the cerebellum and the cerebral cortex. Vertigo may be induced by alterations in the complex system including postural maintenance control mechanism.

Vertigo may be physiological or pathological. In physiological from of vertigo there is mismatch of various stabilizing influences on the vestibular functions of the brain. This occurs most commonly in cases of sea sickness, height vertigo and car sickness.

Pathological form of vertigo is due to many causes and include:

1. **Otological causes:** Otitis media, Meniere's disease, infection of upper respiratory tract, labrythinitis, chronic middle ear disease, otosclerosis.
2. **Neurologic causes:** Cerebral arterosclerosis, vertebral basilar artery insufficiency, intracranial tumour, raised intracranial pressure, acoustic neuroma, meninigitis, encephalitis, Ramsay-Hunt syndrome.
   Metabolic causes: Hypoglycemia, hyperventilation, hyperthyroidism.
3. Tumours: Meningeal tumours, secondaries, lymphomas.
4. Haematological: Anaemia: Hyperviscosity syndrome.
5. Drug intoxications: Digitalis, Quinidine.

6. Positional vertigo. Here vertigo is precipitated by position of the head and is worsersed by turning the patient's head either to left or right. Sometimes it follows head injury.

7. Psychogenic vertigo. This is a very common form and occurs in patients fear of height, crowds etc.

Evaluation of patient of vertigo

A detailed history is very important. In cases of meniers disease where there is often a sense of uneasiness accompanied by nausea and vomiting. Once the acute attack subsides patient has got a feeling of ringing noises in the ears.

Cases of vertebro basilar artery insufficiency have atherosclerotic vessels. Cases of labrynthitis shall have features of viral infection. An examination of vestibular tests is essential to demonstrate any abnormality. CT scan and MRI may help in some cases to make a diagnosis. But often they are not of much help. Standard test is electronystagmography (ENG) to test the vestibular functions.

Treatment of acute vertigo consists of bed rest and use of antihistaminics (Betahistine 8 mg three times a day) Promethazine Theoclate (25 mg twice a day) Prochorperazine Maleate (5mg three times a day).

For vertigo due to vascular causes, vasoldilators are employed (Pentoxi fylline 400 mg three times a day).

In cases with anxiety tranquilizers are employed and are found beneficial. Diazepam and Lorazepam are commonly used.

But let us not ignore the fact that vertigo might be just symptom of a more serious ailment and should be treated accordingly.

Constipation

It is one of the commonest ailments of gastro-intestinal tract which affects almost every individual in various age groups at some time or the other in their lifetime. It may be defined as a bodily dysfunction where the bowels are emptied at long/infrequent intervals with or without difficulty.

The frequency of bowel motion depends to a large extent on the nature and type of food being consumed. In addition the problem of lack of physical activity also potentiates the condition.

There are innumerable causes where a person can be a victim of constipation. Many times the constipation is due to the quality of diet, intake of soft foods, lack of fibre containing foods like fresh fruits and green vegetables. Inadequate intake of fluids is another important factor. Life style of a person also plays an important role. Thus lack of physical activity, exercise, leading a sedentery life and a life dependent on push button gadgets all predispose to the development of the condition.

Besides diet and life style factors one must also consider other possible causes which could be responsible for chronic condition. Some of the commonly used drugs like iron supplements, calcium, diuretics, calcium chemical blockers etc. are known to cause constipation. In addition constipation when associated with anaemia may indicate a gastro-intestinal malignancy. This is especially so in elderly person. Other important causes include hypothyroidism, spastic colon, pyloric stenosis. Irritable bowel syndrom, diverticular disease, anal fissure, perianal abscess, carcinoma colon, etc. So in every case of constipation besides going into the details of the food habits, physical activity and toilet habits, investigations into the history of drug intake (Laxatives, iron and calcium supplements, diuretics, etc.) history of weight loss and any bleeding from anal canal should be taken. Further investigations should exclude any specified organic disease. Colonoscopy is a must in any case of chronic constipation with unexplained anaemia and weight loss. This is especially required in a middle aged or elderly person to exclude malignancy of the colon. Management of a case of chronic constipation shall be guided by a number of factors.

Firstly exclude any organic cause of chronic constipation and if there is one it should be treated accordingly. Secondly in a person where constipation has no underlying cause, different guidelines should be followed e.g.

1. Take diet which consists of roughage like salads fresh fruits and green vegetables.

2. Cultivate regular meal times, do not skip the meals.
3. Cut on soft foods like sweets, ice cream, cakes, pizzas highly spiced and greasy foods.
4. Take adequate quantity of fluids at least 5–6 glasses of clean pure water daily.
5. Lead an active physical life. Take part in outdoor activities and games.
6. Maintain regular habit of going to toilet every day in the morning. To facilitate movement of the gut one can take a cup of tea or glass of water on getting up in the morning.
7. For those whose constipation is not responding to general measures, a mild laxative may be advised to break the habit. Laxatives which increase the bulk and thus supplement the insufficient dietary roughage are useful since they produce their effect by increase in bulk, holding small amounts of water and thus soften the faeces with resultant expulsion. In this category ISPAGHULA (ISPAGOL Husk) is very good and generally two to three teaspoonfuls either at bed time or in the early hours of morning are quite useful.
8. Other laxatives include liquid paraffin, milk of magnesia, DULCOLAX (BISACODYL), senna, PURSENIDE and LACTULOSE (a semi-synthetic dissaccharide of fructose and lactose). These are all mild laxatives and generally preferred. Strong purgatives include magnesium sulphate castor oil etc. These are irritants to the intestines and also lead to loss of electrolytes and fluids from the body. Strong purgatives should be avoided in pregant women, elderly and debilitated individuals. To sum up constipation should be treated according to the causative factor. Most of the patients respond to diet, exercise, change in life-style and regular toilet habits.

Diseases of Gastrointestinal Tract

DIAGNOSTIC APPROACH IN GASTROINTESTINAL DISORDERS

Gastrointestinal disorders are of common occurrence and involve a great degree of distress to the patients. Most patient come with vague abdominal symptoms of dyspepsia and ill health while in some there is specific history of pain abdomen, anorexia and weight loss.

The first principle in any patient presenting with G.I. symptoms is to listen carefully to the patient, analyse the complaints thoroughly questioning the patient minutely about his/her complaints and trying to reach a conclusion. A thorough and detailed history shall go long way in reaching the diagnosis. In this example of a case of peptic ulcer should suffice where history is everything while physical examination is nil.

Investigation of the patient about his/her ailment shall vary according to the complaints. A thorough clinical examination is a must. In patients with diarrhoea, chronic contipation and change in bowel habits, a digital examination of rectum be done to exclude any pathology in the rectum.

Investigations in cases of alimentary disorders:

Examination of faeces. A simple naked eye examination of faeces is very important. Look at the amount of stools passed, their colour, consistency, odour and presence of any abnormal constituents. Presence of bright coloured blood indicates that blood is coming from lower part as in piles while dark coloured blood means that it is from upper part of G.I. tract like a bleeding peptic ulcer, intestinal haemorrhage or from large intestines as in ulcerative colitis.

Mucus is present in irritable bowel syndrome and chronic amoebiasis or malabsorpation syndrome. Clay-coloured stools are seen in cholestatic or obstructive jaundice.

Microscopic examination should be done to identify protozoa such as *Entamoeba histolytica*, *Giardia lamblia*. Other abnormalities such as helminthic ova and larvae, pus cellular exudate, blood and undigested food particles be looked.

Benzidin test is often employed for detecting occult bleeding form a source in G.I. tract. Prior to carrying this test, it is essential to exclude iron-containing drugs, green leafy vegetables and red meats from the diet for 2 to 3 days.

In this test a small amount of faeces is taken by means of a glass rod from the centre of stools and smeared on a slide. A few drops of the benzidin solution are run on the smear. A blue or blue green colour developing within a minute indicates a positive test.

Microbiological examination of stools for identifying bacteria fungi and viruses are required in epidemics of diarrhoea or cases of chronic diarrhoea.

Gastric acid analysis. Earlier on fractional test meal using a gruel meal was done to estimate free and total acidity of the stomach. But the test has been replaced by augmented histamine test and pentagastrin stimulating tests. These are more specific and give reliable information.

Augmented histamine test. Patient is fasting overnight. In the morning, a ryles tube is passed and constant suction is done. This is done for 15 minutes and juice discarded. After this collect juice every 15 minutes for 60 minutes. This constitute basal collection.

At 60 minutes give injection Mepyramine maleate 50 mg by i/m injection. Continue suction for next 30 minutes and discard this. At 90 minutes give Inj. histamine acid phosphate 0.04 mg/kg body weight (1.25 mg) by subcutaneous injection. For next 60 minutes collect 4 specimens at 15 minute intervals. These specimens after histamine tell about amount of maximal acid output.

Basal acid output varies from 1.3-4 mEq/hr while maximal acid output ranges form 17.2-22 mEq/hr.

Pentagastrin test. In this the procedure is almost identical. At the end of one hour of basal juice collection injection pentagastrin in a dose of 6.0 µg/kg body weight is given either intramuscularly or subcutaneously and stimulated secretion collected for next 1 hour.

The basal output ranges from 2.1-3.6 mEq/hr while maximal acid output is in the rang of 13.5-21.5 mEq/hr. Out of these tests, augmented histamine is contraindicated in patients of coronary heart disease and hypertension. Pentagastric test is comparatively safe and no serious side effects are observed except occasional headache, tiredness and nausea.

Histamine fast achlorhydria is seen in cases of pernicious anaemia while increased acidity is seen in duodenal ulcer. Cases of gastric ulcer are often associated with low secretions of acid. Very high acid values are seen in Zollinger-Ellison syndrome.

Tests of intestinal absorption and malabsorption:

D-Xylose test. The patient fasts over night and empties the bladder in the moring. After this 5 gramme of D-xylose dissolved in a glass of water is given to the patient to drink. Over the next five hours when the subject is still kept fasting, 1-2 glasses are given to ensure good urinary output and the urine passed is collected in a bottle. At the end of 5 hours, urine is collected and xylose estimated colorimetrically. Normal excretion of D-xylose is more than 1 gm in 5 hours.

Faecal fat estimation. Patient is given 50 gm of fat in the diet for 4 consecutive days. This amount is in addition to the normal fat intake. The stool specimens are collected for 3 days and fat is estimated.

A normal person passes less than 15 gm of fat in 3 days (5 g per day) while fat more than 18 gm (6 g per day) indicates steatorrhoea.

Radioactive labelled triolen (C14) is administered orally. This is hydrolyzed. Labelled glycerol is absorbed and metabolized by the liver. The $14CO_2$ produced is exhaled and is measured hourly for 6

°hours in the expired air. Normally more than 3-5 per cent of the administered labelled fat appears in the breath per hour.

Lactose tolerance test. In this 50 g of glucose is given orally and blood glucose levels measured half hourly for next two hours. A flat glucose tolerance curve indicates malabsorption.

Breath tests. In this radio labelled substances like $14CO_2$, hydrogen and lactulose are given and their excretion in breath estimated. Increased excretion in breath indicates bacterial over growth in the intestines.

Schilling test. It is done to look for vitamin B_{12} malabsorption. Patient fasts overnight and empties his bladder. Small dose of radioactive labelled vitamin B12 CO58 dose (1 mc in 100 ml of water) is given orally followed 2 hours later by a large dose of non-radioactive vitamin B_{12} dose (1000 μg), the flushing dose. All urine is collectd for 48 hours. In normal subjects radioactive Vitamin B_{12} is excreted in the urine during the nest 24 hours. Normal range 200-1000 μμg/ml while in severe dificiency of vitamin B_{12} it is less than 80 μμg/ml.

Figlu test. It is a test to detect folate deficiency. A loading dose of histidine is given (15 g histidine hydrochloride in glass of water) and urine collected for 8 hours. Urinary excretion of figlu is estimated. Figlu is an intermediate product in the breakdown of histidne to glutamic acid and is excreted in the urine when further metabolism is blocked by folate deficiency. Normal excretion of figlu is 17 mg or less in the 8 hours.

Biopsy. Sometimes a biopsy from G.I. tract is required to confirm the histological diagnosis.

In case of stomach, a gastroendoscope is passed and biopsy taken under direct vision. For small intestines, a Crosby capsule attached to a thin suction tube is passed in a fasting state. Its position in the intestines is guided by screening under fluroscopic control. Once the capsule is in position, the knife of the capsule is moved by suction and biopsy obtained. By this method biopsy can be obtained from jejunum and ileum. Biopsy obtained is studied by dissecting microscope and histology studied after proper staining.

Complication from the use of the biopsy capsule are minimal. Sometimes perforation of the intestines may take plase.

The specimen when studied under the microscope for malabsorption may show following appearances.

Group I   Finger like villi which are slender and cylindercal.

Group II   Leaf like villi. Villi are broad and flattened in one of their transverse axis and elongated in the other.

Group III   Convoluted villi when villi are fused into a continuous series of convoluted ridges.

Group IV   Flat mucosa. There are no mucosal contours at all.

Appearances in group III and IV are suggestive of malasorption.

Rectal and colonic biopsies. These are done either through a sigmoidosocope or a colonoscope. These are required to confirm the diagnosis in disease of the colon and rectum as in ulcerative colitis, Crohn's disease.

Cytology. Cytological examination of exfoliated cells from the oesophagus, stomach, and colon is an important and useful test for diagnosis of malignant lesions.

Radiology. Radiological examination of the gastrointestinal tract is useful aid in diagnosing a number of pathological conditions.

Plain X-ray abdomen. It is useful in various ways. Size of the various abdominal organs may be assessed. Air under the diaphragm indicates performation of the abdominal viscera.

Calculi in the gall bladder, bile duct or urinary tract may be seen. Calcification in the pancreas is seen in cases of chronic pancreatits. Occasionally calcification may be seen in adrenals in Addison's disease, in abdominal glands in tubercular lymphadenopathy.

Intestinal obstruction or paralytic ileus is diagnosed by presence of multiple fluid and air levels in the dilated loops.

Barium contrast studies. Barium swallow for

visualising diseases of oesophagus like oesophageal varices, strictures, neoplasma, achlasia done both by conventional method and double contrast when high accuracy of lesions in stomach and duodenum is obtained.

Barium meal study of stomach and duodenum is obtained. Barium study of stomach and duodenum is especially required in cases of peptic ulcer, chronic gastritis and malignancy of stomach. All patients with vague abdominal discomfort and dyspepsia must be submitted to a barium study.

Barium meal follow through is required for studying small bowel diseases like malabsorpation syndrome, tuberculosis of the gastrointestingal tract and malignancy. Barium enema is done when it is required to study the large intestines. The patient is prepared before hand by a laxative and colon washed. On an empty colon, barium sulphate is given as enema and pictures of barium filled colon are taken and after evacuation of barium.

Double contrast studies give better diagnostic help. Barium enema is indicated in diseases of colon (ulcerative colitis, Crohn's disease, diverticulosis, tuberculosis, malignancy, strictures and polyposis) as well as of caecum and ileoceacal junction.

Ultrasound. It is a useful non-invasive technique and helpful in assessing organomegaly in abdomen and presence of a mass, abscess, calculi and any major pathology. But it has its limitations. It can not help in diagnosing an ulcer, varices and a small malignancy.

C.T. scan (computed tomography). This is a better technique than ultrasonography and can help in detecting any mass, abscess and fistula.

Gastrointestinal endoscopy. Introduction of fibroendoscopy is of significant help is diagnosing diseases of gastrointestinal tract.

Upper gastrointestinal endoscopy is done by both forward oblique and side viewing endoscopes. It is very useful in detecting oesophageal varices, strictures, malignancy and diseases of stomach and duodenum. Not only the disease is examined under direct vision but biopsies and cytological examination of lesions can be carried out. Endoscopy is also employed for injecting sclerosing

agent in varices, removing foreign body and dilating stricutres.

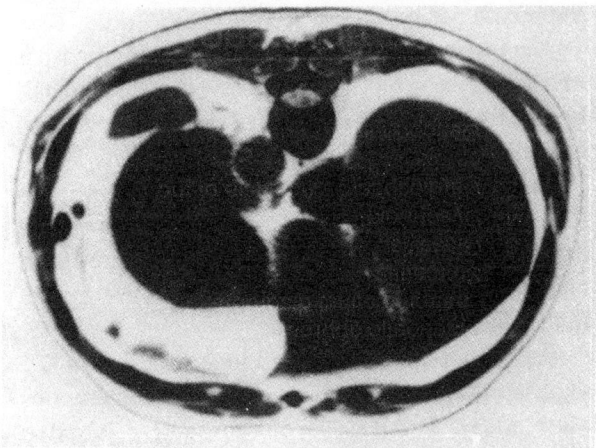

Fig. 2.1. C.T. Scan. Shows liver and spleen.

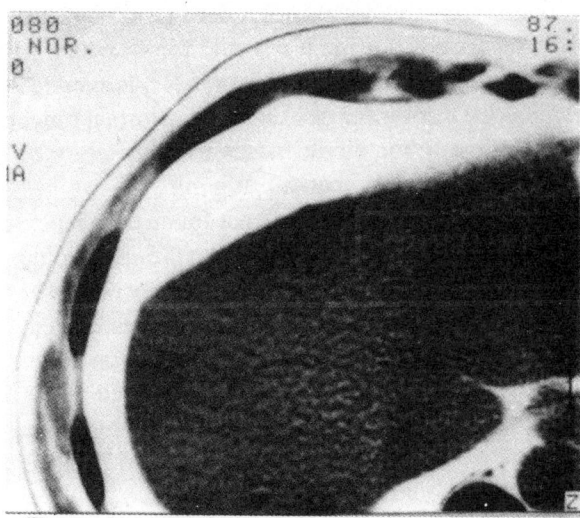

Fig. 2.2. C.T. Scan. Shows magnified view of liver.

Colonoscopy. It allows good visualization of the colon and ileoceacal areas. Not only the area is examined under direct visualization but biopsies are also taken from various sites. Colonoscopy is also used for removal of polyps. Complications of colonoscopy mainly include perforation of the colon.

Endoscopic retrograde cholangiopancreatography (ERCP). This technique is useful in diagnosing disease of the pancreas and hepatobiliary system. Here papilla of water is cannulated and a contrast medium is injected, when pancreatic ducts and hepatobiliary system are visualized. The procedure is done under fluoroscopic control. Complications include pancreatitis, peritonitis, perforation and bleeding.

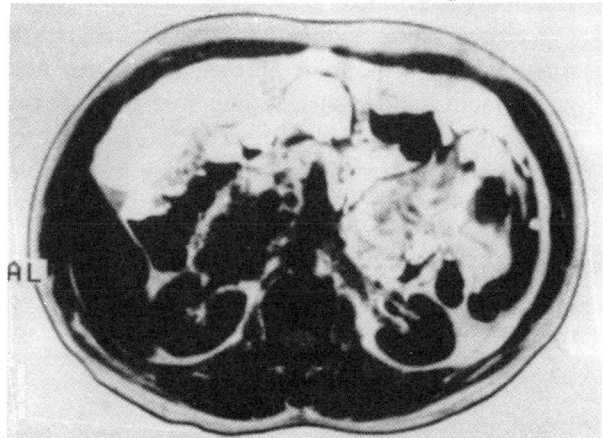

Fig. 2.3. C.T. Scan. Shows both kidneys.

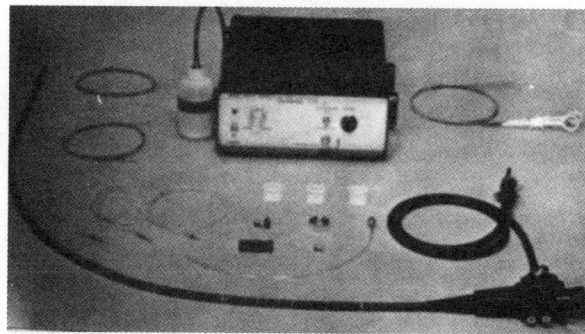

Fig. 2.4. Gastroduodenoscope with accessories.

Sigmoidoscopy. It is an important investigation for visualization of the disease in descending colon and rectum. It may form part of routine examination in diseases of the colon. No preparation is required. Left lateral position is the usual one adopted for passing the instrument which is generally flexible. While passing sigmoidoscope, undue force must not be employed. Mucous membrane of the colon should be carefully examined for vascular pattern, presence of ulcers and inflammation. Somttimes a polyp may be seen.

In ulcerative colitis, mucosa is hyperaemic, oedematous and bleeds easily. Ulcers may be seen.

Other diseases which can be looked by sigmoidoscopy are Crohn's disease (areas of inflamed mucosa with normal intervening areas, cobblestone mucosa), caricinoma (hard irregular friable mass) and polyps.

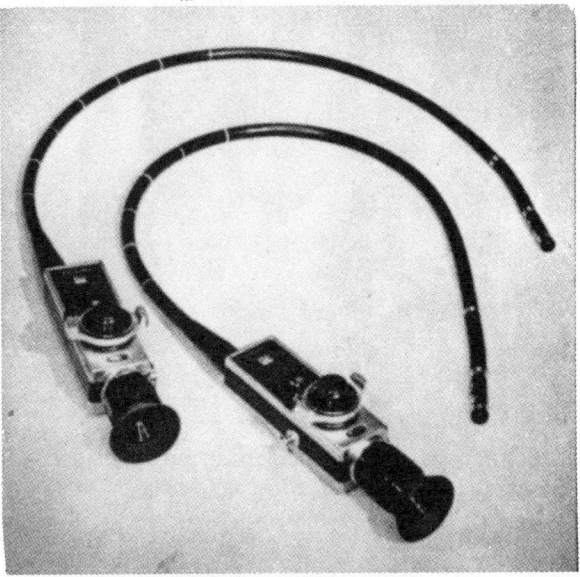

Fig. 2.5. Gastroscopes

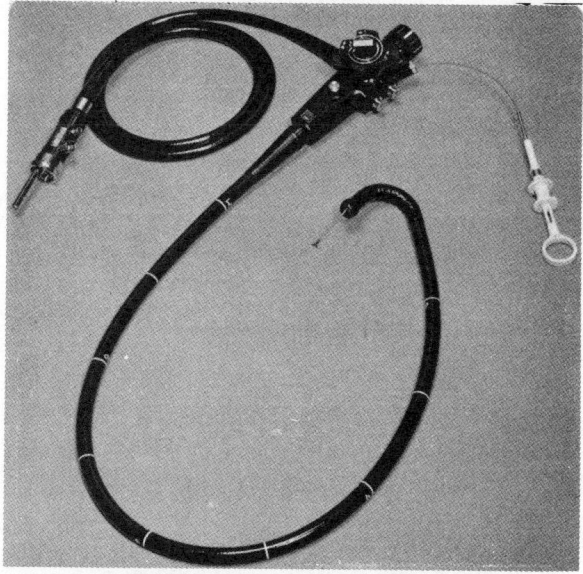

Fig. 2.6. Photograph of clonofiberscope

Peritonoscopy. This is the method employed to study the peritoneal cavity. A peritonoscope or laparoscope is employed to study the abdomonal structures.

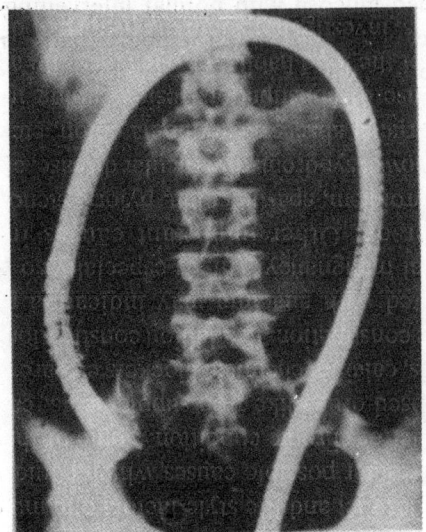

Fig. 2.7. X-ray picture of colonoscope in position. It is reaching the caecum.

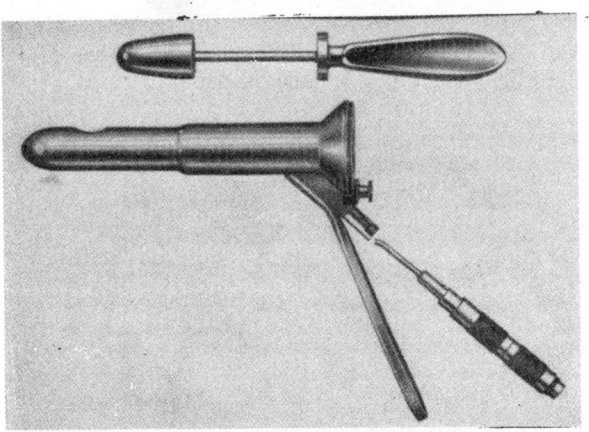

Fig. 2.8. Proctoscope.

The examination is usually performed under local anaesthesia with aseptic precautions. After introducing air into the peritoneal cavity. Laparoscope is inserted into peritoneal cavity through a small incision in the abdominal wall. By this method, lapratomy is avoided.

Laparoscopy is required for studying diseases of the liver, gall bladder, spleen, intestines and peritoneum. Upper surface and free edge of the organ is studied under direct vision and any pathology observed. **Biopsies are also** taken from suspicious lesions.

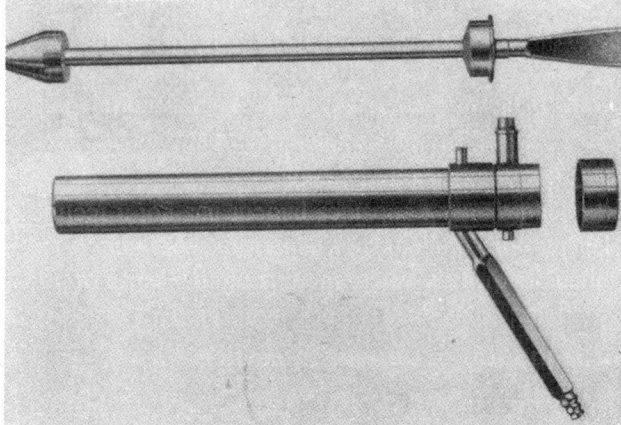

Fig. 2.1.9. Sigmoidoscope.

Minor surgical **procedures can also** be carried via laparoscope. Presence of infections in the peritoneal cavity, adhesions of viscera to anterior abdominal wall, bleeding diathesis and cardiac disorders are contraindications to the procedure.

It is a safe procedure in experienced hands. Complications which can occur include haemorrhage infection, perforation of organs and air embolism.

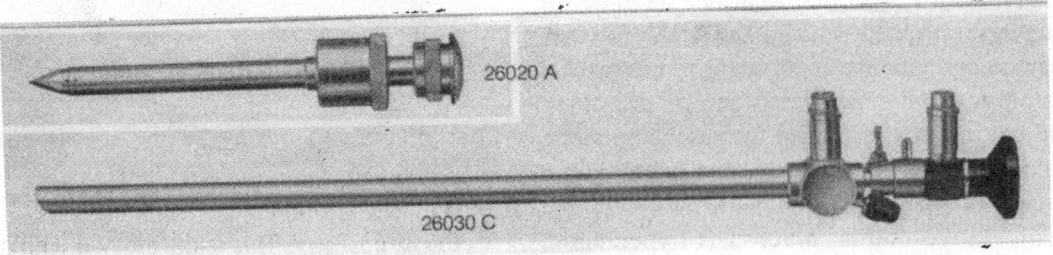

26020 A

26030 C

Fig. 2.10. Peritonoscope.

STOMATITIS

It means inflammation of the mouth and is caused by bacterial, viral, fungus infections in persons with poor oral hygiene or in systemic illnesses such as leukaemia, blood disorders, agranulocytosis, diabetes, uremia, Crohn's disease, deficiency states and AIDS HIV disease. Heavy metals like mercury, bismuth, anticancer drugs. Gold therapy and trauma are also aetiological factors in some cases.

A common form of stomatitis (catarrhal) develops in ill-nourished children and in adults during fevers, having septic teeth and badly fitting dentures. People who do not maintain proper oral hygiene especially during serious ailments, their lips, tongue and gums are affected which become inflamed, swollen and painful. Tongue is furred and there is foul smell.

Bacterial stomatitis. It is common in our population and generally occurs as a result of streptococcal haemolyticus infection, spreading from inflamed throat to buccal mucosa leading to inflamed buccal mucosa with red looking angry ulcers. Mouth is sore and there is excessive salivation.

Vincent's stomatitis is a severe form of ulceromembranous stomatitis and is caused by anaerobic organisms which are normally colonizing in the subunginal area. Onset of the disease is sudden and usual location is gingiva. There is bleeding, sloughing followed by ulceration of gums which are painful. A foul breath emanates. There is greyish exudate and ulceration of gingival mucosa between the teeth. Signs of toxaemia like fever, tachycardia, lymphadenopathy are present. Tender painful gums make eating difficult and painful. Vincent's stomatitis generally occurs especially in children who are ill-nourished and have poor oral hygiene.

Gangrenous stomatitis (Cancrum oris). It is a fulminating form of ulceromembranous stomatitis and generally occurs in children or young adults who are severely malnourished and are recovering from a debilitating illness or acute fever (typhoid) or exanthemata like measles etc. It occurs in the form of a sloughing ulcer inside the cheek or gums which rapidly spreads to buccal mucosa, teeth, gums and mandible. Teeth may fall out and there is perforation of cheek even leading to the sloughing of mandible. Breath has a putrid smell and there are constitutional symptoms like high fever, toxaemia, rapid thready pulse, bronchopneumonia and in severe fulminating cases death may result. In some cases, the disease process may be halted and remission may take place leaving behind a disfiguring defect.

Viral infection. Various types of viral infections produce aphthous or vesicular type of stomatitis. The lesion consists of small vesicles surrounded by erythema. These generally rupture quickly leaving behind grey ulcers with crust and red margins. They are extremely painful present on the inner surface of lips and cheeks, and margins of the tongue. Patient generally a child or a young adult has features of toxaemia like fever, malaise. Breath is foul and often cervical lymphadenopathy is present. There is often acute gingivitis. Various viruses responsible are:

a. *Herpes simplex virus type I.* Here mainly lips and oral mucosa are involved. Ulcers tend to heal spontaneously unless there is presence of secondary bacterial infection.

b. *Herpes zoster.* There may be reactivation of varicilla-zoster virus and is in the form of unilateral vesicular eruption and ulceration in the 5th nerve distribution and may involve cheek, tongue gingiva, and palate.

c. *Hand, foot and mouth disease (Type A Coxsackie virus).* There is involvement of oral mucosa, pharynx with sudden rise of fever, headache and veiscles in the mouth which ulcerate and become painful. Lesions heal spontaneously.

d. *Epstein-Barr virus, infectious mononucleosis (glandular fever).* A disease of young adults which often occur in epidemic form. The characteristic features are sore throat, fever, headache, cervical lymphadenopathy and marked fatigue. Multiple petechial spots and ulcers appear on palate many days before appearance of lymphadenopathy. Diagnosis can be made by detecting the presence of atypical mono-nuclear cells in peripheral blood. Paul-Bunnell reaction is positive in second week of the disease. The disease is self limiting and recovery takes place early. Lesions in the mouth tend to disappear during convalescence.

HIV disease and AIDS. It produces all types of lesions of the oral cavity involving palate and oropharynx. It may be ulcerative acute necrotizing, pseudo membranous associated with lympha-denopathy and febrile illness. Recurrent aphthous ulcers are common.

Fungal infections. Commonest is candidiasis caused by *Candida albicans*. It is in the form of white membranous patchy lesions involving gums, buccal mucosa and palate. The greyish patches can be wiped leaving behind red bleeding surfaces.

Patients who are suffering from diabetes mellitus, AIDS, malignancy or receiving broad-spectrum antibiotics or on high dose of steroids, are very ill and in immunocompromised state are liable to suffer from candida infection of the mouth which may even spread downwards into G.I. tract.

Actinomycosis though not very common may involve the jaw and adjacent structures like submandibular region, lymph glands and floor of the mouth. It produces a swelling which is tender, not very hard and shows soft spots at certain places resulting in abscesses and multiple sinuses which contain characteristic granules called sulfur granules (gram-positive mycelia).

Organisms of actinomycosis normally reside in the mouth and invade the mouth via a carious tooth, after extraction, from gums, periodontal membrane and fracture of jaw. It is a slow growing disease process though it may occur in acute form. Generally the disease process lasts from months to years. Diagnosis is confirmed by looking at the pus or excised gland for mycelium. In an uncomplicated case prognosis is good but when secondary infection takes place, the chances of complete eradication of the disease become uncertain.

Miscellaneous causes:

Deficiency diseases. Deficiency diseases like pellagra, beri-beri, iron-deficiency anaemia and pernicious anaemia involve the mouth and alimentary tract.

Pellagra which is a chronic disease due to deficiency of members of vitamin B complex group like riboflavin, pyridoxine but mainly nicotinic acid is characterised by dermatitis over the areas exposed to sunlight, diarrhoea, dementia and mucosal abnormalities. Tongue becomes red, swollen and inflamed. Buccal mucosa may show the same changes along with gums, palate and mucosal surface of lips. Hot and spicy food increases burning sensation in the mouth.

A combination of deficiency of nicotinic acid with vitamin B_1 produces the same picture of stomatitis and glossitis along with picture of beri-beri (pellagrous beri-beri).

Iron-deficiency anaemia and pernicious anaemia produce achlorhydria, atrophic gastritis, glossitis (tongue reddened and inflamed in early stages with vesicles appearing; later on papillae are effected resulting in a bald tongue). Stomatitis appears in late stages, inflammation of the buccal mucosa is general and the angles of the mouth are effected. This is called angular stomatitis.

Recurrent aphthous ulcers. Sometimes single or multiple painful superficial ulcers occur on the mucous surfaces of the mouth, tongue and buccal mucosa. These ulcers are small (1-2 mm in diameter) and have erythematous borders. These ulcers generally occur during second decade and persist into adulthood but become less frequent with advancing age. Females are involved more than men.

The exact cause of these ulcers is not known. Majority of adults experience the condition at some time or the other during their life time. Local trauma, heredity, deficiency states and gastrointestinal disorders are some of the risk factors.

Depending on their size, aphthous ulcers may be classified as minor (less than 1 cm in diameter) and major (upto 3 cm). To start with there is a small painful red macule or papule at the site of minor mucosal injury. A burning or tingling sensation may be felt before ulceration. Ulcers may be single or multiple. These are sharp, discrete and may be oedematous. Big ulcers on healing may leave behind white depressed scars.

Histologically varying degree of epithelial ulceration and inflammatory cells are seen. Course of ulcers is variable. They are often cause of great distress and even may make eating difficult. Minor ulcers may heal spontaneously in a week to 10 days. It is the major forms of ulcers which are resistant to treatment and persist for long periods. They heal with scarring.

Treatment of aphthous ulcers is mainly topical. Nystatin tablet dissolved in glycerine is applied three to four time a day over the ulcer.

Other remedy is to give Tetracycline in retention form orally (contents of the capsule of tetracycline suspended in water and held in the mouth for 15 minutes) two times a day. When ulcer is not responding to treatment, cauterization with silver nitrate (AgNO3) stick will help and accelerate the process of healing.

Sometimes topical steroids are also employed.

Stomatitis in blood diseases. Cases of acute leukaemia will show haemorrhage in the palate and buccal mucosa and subsequently there is necrotic ulceration. Gingival hyperplasia with ulceration and haemorrhage develops and in later stages it is complicated by infection.

Similar type of lesions in the oral cavity are present in lymphomas, purpura, agranulocytosis, haemophilia and other bleeding disorders.

Stomatitis following chemotherapy. Administration of cytotoxic drugs like fluracil, methotrexate produce inflammation of the oral mucosa and soft tissue structures in the mouth. In fact almost all type of anticancer drugs are known to produce stomatitis which is dose related and depends on the duration of time the drug has been administered.

In early stages the patient shows redness and swelling of buccal mucosa which progresses to ulcer formation, bleeding and secondary infection.

Tongue is involved in majority of the cases. Mouth ulceration and stomatitis make eating difficult and painful. Healing of ulcers after stoppage of chemotherapy takes at least 7 to 10 days.

Stomatitis in systemic diseases. A number of systemic diseases varying from bacterial (steptococcal, tuberculosis, syphilis, Vincent's infection), viral (herpes simplex, herpes zoster, varicella, variola, Coxsackie A, primary HIV infection), fungal (candida, histoplasmosis), nutritional deficiencies (pellagra, beri-beri, scurvy, pernicious anaemia, iron-deficiency anaemia), blood disorders and malignancies (leukaemia, lymphomas, agranulocytosis, purpura), heavy metal poisoning (bismuth, lead, mercury, silver), skin disorders (lichen planus, pemphigus, lupus erythematosus, erythema multifome, Behcet's syndrome), metabolic disorders (diabetes) to renal diseases (uremia) are responsible for producing stomatitis. In addition stomatitis may complicate or is produced as a result of intake of various drugs like anticancer drugs, sulfonamides, chloramphenicol.

Tuberculosis. Tubercular lesions in the mouth may involve nose, cheek, gums, palate and pharynx. Sometimes it is in the form of a solitary nodule which may ulcerate forming an irregular ulcer with undermined edges. The lesions in the mouth most of the time accompany skin form of tuberculosis (lupus) or in a person suffering from extensive pulmonary tuberculosis when it is painful, bleeds easily and may be complicated by secondary infection.

Syphilis. All forms of syphilis (primary, secondary and tertiary) may produce stomatitis. Primary syphilis involves the mouth at the point of entry (lips, tongue) and is in the form of a rapidly developing painless ulcer with indurated borders. It heals in 1-2 months. Secondary syphilis is marked by maculopapular lesions of oral mucosa, palate with greyish membrane covering them. Tertiary syphilis is in the form of a gumma which involves mainly the palate and tongue. Gumma may ulcerate and leave behind fibrosis and perforation of palate. There is atrophy of papillae of tongue resulting in a bald tongue.

STOMATITIS IN SKIN DISEASES

Lichen planus. It most commonly affects the oral mucosa in the form of white spots and streaks. These lesions may occasionally ulcerate and often produce a sensation of rawness in the mouth. There is associated erosive gingivitis. Skin is often involved. There are polygonal purplish flat topped papules on wrists, thighs, skin, palms, calves ankles and soles. White striae appear and spots of pseudoscaling. Resolution of the lesions results in pigmentation.

Erythema multiforme. It is a reaction of hypersensitivity to bacterial, viral infections and some commonly used drugs (cotrimoxazole).

Primarily lesions occur on the mucous surfaces of the lips and mouth and skin. It is a rapidly progressive disease often preceded by malaise 24-48 hours before the lesions appear.

The lesions are polymorphic and various forms varying from papulo vesicular, macular to bullous forms occur. The bullae rupture with haemorrhage in between. Skin lesions show exudation, brownish red discoloration while in the mouth erosion occurs more rapidly forming a uncerative pseudomem branous lesion which is painful. Patient shows signs of toxaemia in the form of arthralgia and albuminuria.

The Stevens-Johnson syndrome is severe form of erythema multiforme characterised by extensive bullous, exudative lesions which ulcerate and produce distressing symptoms. Mouth and lips are extensively involved showing haemorrhagic crusts.

Pemphigus vulgaris. It is in the form of a bullous eruption which may occur anywhere in the mouth and skin. There are number of bullae both small and large which rupture leaving behind raw areas from which serum oozes. Secondary infection may occur. These lesions generally occur on the pressure spots of skin. Oral lesions are in the form of ruptured bullae which are ulcerated, denuded covered by a white exudate. The mucous surface of the lips, tongue, cheeks, and roof and floor of the mouth are extensively involved. Patient has a feeling of rawness in the mouth and has difficulty in eating.

It is a progressive disease with occasional remissions followed by fresh outbreaks which are much more severe than the early attack.

Behcet's syndrome. It is a rare disease characterized by multiple ulcers in the mouth, eyes, ulceration of the genitalia, and inflammatory bowel disease. Ulcers may appear in the mouth or eyes, months or years before the full fledged disease appears. Nodules on the skin may be present. Ulcer persist for several weeks and heal spontaneously.

Diagnosis. Diagnosis of stomatitis should pose no problem if the various aetiological factors are considered and the disease investigated.

Treatment:

1. General
2. Specific

General. It includes care of the mouth hygiene. Tongue should be kept clean. Teeth be cleaned carefully and antiseptic gargles and mouth washes be used two to three times a day.

To prevent irritation and soreness of the mouth, glycerine be applied locally on the mucosa. A soothing medication containing choline salicylate, cetakonium chloride in ethyl alcohol in the form of gel (Gelora) may be applied 3 to 4 times a day.

For secondary bacterial infection, appropriate antibiotics in the form of Penicillin/Ampicillin/Amoxycillin be employed by parenteral route.

General nutrition of the patient be taken care of. In case of severe form of stomatitis where there is difficulty in eating, parenteral nutrition be employed.

Specific:

Bacterial. Since commonly it is streptococcal stomatitis injectable Penicillin/Amoxycillin/Ampicillin is to be employed.

For Vincent's stomatitis, metrogyl 200 mg three times a day for 5 days.

Fungal. Candida stomatitis is treated locally by Nystatin, dissolved in glycerine and applied locally. Nystatin, amphotericin or miconazole given orally is useful.

Fluconazole a bis-triazole antifungal drug is effective against systemic and mucosal candidiasis.

Dose is 200 mg on first day followed by a 100 mg once a day for 2-3 weeks. Special precautions have to be taken while administering this drug in immunocompromised patients and in those with liver dysfunction. Side effects include nausea, headache, abdominal pain, vomiting, diarrhoea and skin rash.

Viral. Commonest viral involvement of mouth occurs due to herpes simplex and herpes zoster virus. Most of the time ulcers heal spontaneously within a week or so but secondary infection delays the healing.

Acyclovir, an antiviral drug, is effective for management of mucocutaneous herpes simplex, herpes zoster and chickenpox.

For herpes simplex producing stomatitis, dosage is 200 mg 5 times daily at 4 hours interval for 5 days and for herpes zoster drug has to be continued for 7 days. For prophylaxis or suppression of the symptoms dose is 200 mg 4 times daily.

Side effects include headache, nausea. Special precautions should be taken in persons suffering from renal impairment.

Acyclovir cream may be applied locally for cutaneous lesions due to herpes simplex or zoster virus but it is not to be used for buccal or mucosal lesions.

Actinomycosis. Most patients respond to high doses of Penicillin given parenterally for 4-6 weeks followed by oral penicillins or tetracyclines (chlortetracycline, doxycycline or oxytetracycline). Total duration of therapy ranges from 2 to 4 months.

Dermatological causes producing stomatitis. These cases follow protracted course having periods of remissions and relapses. Acute episodes may be tided over by parenteral steroids. Long-term oral prednisolone is helpful. Hydrocortisone pellets may help locally in relieving symptoms. In advanced stages patient suffers from cachexia, weight loss and infection which may prove fatal.

Infectious mononucleosis. In majority of patients no specific treatment is required and oral lesions disappear early. Where there is severe involvement of nervous system like encephalitis or thrombocytopenia, corticosteroids are helpful.

Causes of stomatits

1. *Bacterial*
   a. Streptococcal stomatitis
   b. Vincent's stomatitis
   c. Gangrenous stomatitis
   d. Syphilis
   e. Tuberculosis

2. *Viral*
   a. Herpes simplex
   b. Herpes zoster
   c. Hand, foot and mouth disease (type-A coxsackie-virus)
   d. Glandular fever
   e. HIV infection and AIDS

3. *Fungal*
   a. Candidiasis
   b. Actinomycosis

4. **Stomatitis due to heavy metals**
   a. Lead
   b. Bismuth
   c. Mercury
   d. Silver

5. **Stomatitis in deficiency states**
   a. Pellagra
   b. Scurvy
   c. Pernicious anaemia
   d. Beri-beri

6. **Blood disorders**
   a. Haemophilia
   b. Thrombocytopenic purpura
   c. Leukaemia
   d. Agranulocytosis
   e. Lymphomas
   f. Malignancy

7. **Skin disorders**
   a. Lichen planus
   b. Pemphigus
   c. Lupus erythematosus
   d. Erythema multiforme
   e. Behcet's syndrome

8. *Miscellaenous*
   a. Diabetes
   b. Uremia
   c. Drug toxicity

Miscellaneous causes. Where stomatitis is due to deficiency states like pellagra (nicotinic acid), scurvy (vitamin C), beri-beri (vitamin B_1), heavy doses of these vitamins correct the stomatitis.

Stomatitis as a result of blood disorders, malignancies requires no specific treatment except of the underlying condition.

Cases of lead poisoning require use of chelating agents such as Dimercaprol, Edetate calcium sodium (EDTA) and Penicillamine while mercury poison is best treated by the use of Dimercaprol and Penicillamine.

Stomatitis as a result of bismuth toxicity characterized by the appearance of blue line at the gum margin does not necessarily require treatment except for stoppage of use of the drug and maintaining good oral hygiene. In advanced cases of stomatitis where extensive ulceration is present, Dimercaprol (B.A.L.) use is recommended. In cases where stomatitis follows chemotherapy, progress of the lesions can be halted by halting further administration of the drugs.

GLOSSITIS

It is inflammation of the tongue accompanied by soreness and redness. A number of factors may be responsible for this and these range from excessive abuse of alcohol, spices, smoking, tobacco chewing, vitamin B complex deficiency, megaloblastic anaemia to metabolic disorders like diabetes mellitus. Use of dental prostheses, ill-fitting dentures, inflamed gums or ill-spaced teeth can all cause excessive salivation and tingling sensation in the tongue.

Generally the tongue is of normal size and is neither large nor too small. It is moist, greyish red in colour with normal papillae on the surface.

Tongue may become large (macroglossia) in endocrine disorders (acromegaly, cretinism, myxoedema), metabolic disorders (primary amyloidoses), tumours (haemangioma, lipoma, lymphangioma), inflammations (acute inflammation, abscess of tongue), allergic (insect bites, angioneurotic oedema) and developmental conditions such as Down's syndrome. A small tongue (microglossia) may be seen in malnutrition, facial hemiatrophy and in cases of pseudobulbar palsy. Scrotal tongue is somewhat bulky tongue but it does not indicate any disease.

A pale or white tongue is commonly seen in cases of anaemia while cases of nicotinic acid deficiency (pellagra) have a bright red, beefy fiery tongue with rawness at the margins.

Strawberry or raspberry tongue is characteristically seen in scarlet fever and is due to hypertrophy of fungiform papillae. Blue tongue is found in cyanosis and polycythemia while magenta tongue is characteristic of riboflavin deficiency. A brown coated tongue is present in uremia, grey tongue in high fevers, thrush, while a black tongue is seen in fungal infections and after excessive use of antibiotics. Patchy pigmentation of tongue in the form of dark brown patches may be seen in Addison's disease.

Glossodynia. It is pain arising from the tongue and is symptomatic of irritation due to excessive heat, trauma, avitaminosis, electrogalvanism, tobacco and alcohol. Sometimes in people who have no teeth, abnormal stress on temporomandibular joint may produce glossodynia.

Geographical tongue

Often called benign migratory glossitis it is asymptomatic, idiopathic condition where there is rapid loss of superficial filiform papillae and their regrowth resulting in reddened denuded areas giving zig-zag appearance on the surface of the tongue. These red and white areas on the tongue may remain fixed or wander across the surface of the tongue. This typical appearance of tongue is called geographical tongue.

About 2% of the population has this condition. It sarts in young age and persists for life. Its etiology is unknown. Histologically there is hyperkeratosis at the edge of tongue and spongiosis. There is migration in the epidermis of polymorphonuclear cells and lymphocytes forming sometimes micro abscesses while in the dermis there may be nonspecific infiltration.

Geographical tongue is a benign condition and has often been associated with vitamin B complex deficiency. Though there are no symptoms yet often a feeling of soreness of tongue is complained of. Geographical tongue requires no treatment except reassurance. If avitaminosis is suspected adequate dosage of vitamin B complex are given.

ACUTE GLOSSITIS. Deficiency of nicotinic acid is notorious for producing acute glossitis where the tongue is scarlet red, fiery and angry-looking. Tip of the tongue and margins are reddened and raw. If left untreated, deep ulcers may appear on the sides and dorsum of the tongue which is covered by a thick greyish membrane on a red base. Secondary infection may occur. Further extension may occur to the mucous membrane of the mouth, palate, gums and lips. Mouth is sore and tongue painful. Hot spicy foods produce burning sensation.

Treatment is by giving nourishing non-irritating diet including milk, fresh fruits and vegetables. Nicotinic acid in tablet form is effective. Daily dose is 500 mg for the first 10 days and then decreased to 200 mg per day. Untreated and uncontrolled diabetes produces a large, red, glazed and fissured tongue which is sore and sometimes painful when secondary infection or fungal infection complicates the glossitis.

Treatment is control of diabetes, proper oral hygiene and use of antifungal drugs.

ATROPHIC GLOSSITIS. Atrophy of papillae on the surface of the tongue produces a smooth bald tongue. It is commonly seen in cases of nutritional macrocytic anaemia and iron-deficiency anaemia where there is associated atrophic gastritis and achlorhydria. In early stage the tongue is swollen diffusely, painful and bluish red in appearance. There is soreness and painful burning sensation. Small erosions may appear on the surface. As the disease progresses the tongue becomes smooth, pale and glazed.

Treatment of atrophic glossitis is treatment of underlying cause. In addition non-specific treatment in the form of mouthwash and application of soothing lotions is advised. Sometimes painful condition of tongue responds to antifungal drugs (Nystatin dissolved in glycerine)—local application three to four times a day.

SCROTAL TONGUE (FISSURED TONGUE). It is a congenital malformation in the form of deep fissures or furrows running in different directions on the surface of tongue. It is a normal variation of the tongue and is considered not indicative of ill health. Its incidence is estimated to be 5% of the population and is a common finding in otherwise healthy individuals. Lesions are called fissures which are related to deep valleys in the dorsal tongue that do not involve the mucosal epithelium and therefore are not painful.

Sometimes food debris collect in these fissures and cause irritation and soreness of the tongue. Treatment is to maintain careful hygiene of the tongue and clean the various fissures and furrows by a soft wool tipped probe. Fissured tongue though a benign condition persists throughout life and the condition becomes exaggrated with the passage of time.

GLOSSITIS RHOMBOIDEA MEDIANA (MEDIAN RHOMBOID GLOSSITIS). It is a congenital anomaly of the tongue where there is a raised lozenge-shaped elevation with denuded area in the median posteror part of the tongue. The patient generally has no symptoms except when candida infection superimposes. Often this elevation is mistaken for cancerous growth.

An uncomplicated glossitis of this type requires no treatment except when there is fungus infection superadded. Antifungal drugs given orally as well as applied locally helps.

HAIRY TONGUE. In this type of tongue there is hypertrophy of the filiform papillae on the dorsum of the tongue especially in its anterior third and there is failure of keratin layer to desquamate normally. This gives the tongue a black-brown discolouration. This colour is further aggravated by use of antibiotics, tobacco, betal nut or *pan* chewing, sweets containing dyes, fungi and chromogenic organisms. No treatment is required except to maintain adequate hygiene of the oral cavity and treating the underlying cause.

STRAWBERRY/RASPBERRY TONGUE. This is the type of tongue seen in cases of scarlet fever. In early stages there is hypertrophy of fungiform papillae giving appearance of red dots over the grey surface of tongue (strawberry tongue). As disease progresses there is exfoliation as well as hypertrophhy of both fungiform and filiform papillae forming large dots on the surface of tongue (raspberry tongue).

SYPHILITIC GLOSSITIS. In the modern era of antibiotics syphilitic glossitis is very uncommon but sometimes an occasional case may be seen.

Primary form of syphilis presents as chancre while in the secondary stage there are mucous patches and multiple small shallow ulcers over the dorsum of tongue. Localized gummata may be seen in tertiary stage. It may ulcerate and is in the form of a deeply embedded painless swelling.

Sometimes a white, firm, smooth plaque may be seen over the surface of the tongue. It is called leukoplakia. Though it is painless to start with but may become fissured and painful subsequently. Leukoplakia may be seen in treating form of syphilis. It is a precancerous condition and requires regular follow-up and management.

MOELLER'S GLOSSITIS. It is a rare form of glossitis and is predominantly an affection of women. There are pleomorphic lesions. There may be denuded red patches of filiform papillae or a bald smooth glazed tongue or white leukoplakic nodules. There is burning sensation in the tongue and feeding becomes painful

Treatment is by heavy doses of vitamin B complex and nicotinic acid.

DYSPHAGIA

It means difficulty in swallowing and cause may be either a local pathology or it is part of a generalized systemic disease. Very often the patient points to the exact position of obstruction in the oesophagus. *Causes of dysphagia can be divided into two main categories:*

1. Diseases pertaining to oesophagus and its surrounding structures.
2. Dysphagia in neurological disorders.

Diseases pertaining to oesophagus. *Causes can be better classified according to the site of* obstruction:

1. Upper end dysphagia (pharyngo-oesophageal dysphagia)
2. Diseases of mouth and tongue like stomatitis, pharyngitis, glossitis, webs, rings (Plummer-Vinson syndrome), pharyngeal pouch, hysterical, corrosive strictures, goitre, malignancy.

Mid-oesophageal dysphagia. Commonly present in oesophagitis which may be bacterial, viral or fungal. Other causes are carcinoma oesophagus, pressure by mediastinal tumour, enlarged mediastinal glands (lymphoma, Hodgkin's malignancy), aortic aneurysm, enlarged left atrium.

Lower oesophageal dysphagia. It is the commonest form of dysphagia and common causes are achlasia of the lower end of oesophagus, malignancy, strictures following either peptic oesophagitis or corrosive substances, lower oesphageal rings (Schatzki rings).

Dysphagia in neurological disorders. Dysphagia is a common manifestation of organic neurological disorders and is because of involvement of either muscles involved in the act of swallowing or damage to the swallowing centre in the medulla. The various causes are:

1. Post-diphtheritic paralysis
2. Myasthenia gravis
3. Motor neurone disease
4. Acute bulbar paralysis
5. Bulbar polio
6. Infective polyneuritis
7. Scleroderma and other related collagen disorders

Investigations of a case of dysphagia:

History. A number of factors in history shall help in making a diagnosis of the causative factor:

1. Age. Post-diphtheritic paralysis commonly occurs in children and young adults, while in young females cause can be cricoid webs (Plummer-Vinson syndrome), hysterical or achlasia. Carcinoma of oesophagus in middle-aged or elderly persons.

2. Onset. An acute onset favours neurological disorder like bulbar polio, infective polyneuritis,

PLATE V

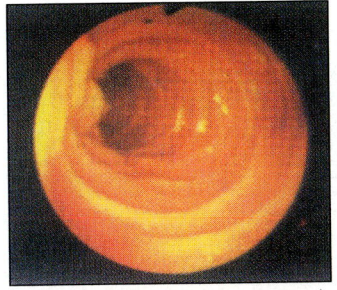

Normal duodenum.

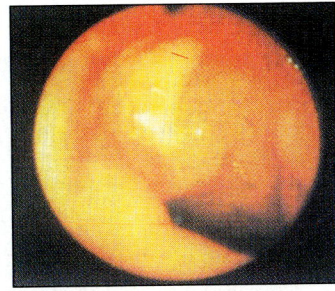

Duodenal ulcer.

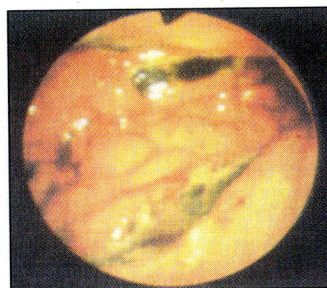

Acute gastric ulcer.

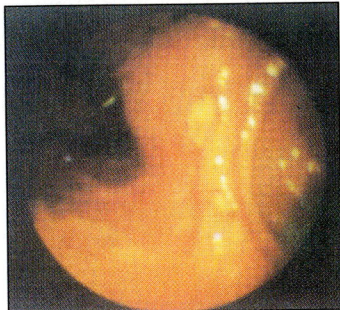

Ulcer at gastric angle.

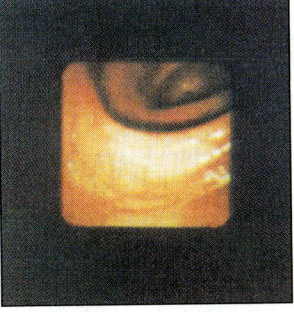

Semilunar folds of normal sigmoid colon.

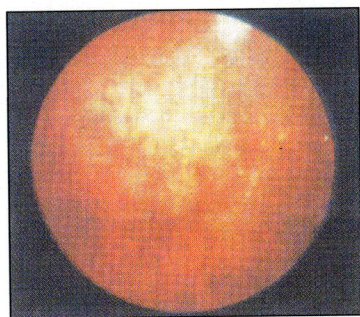

Ulcerative colitis.

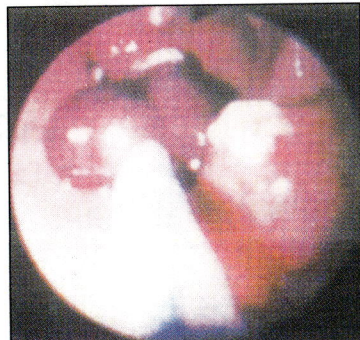

Large bowel polyps.

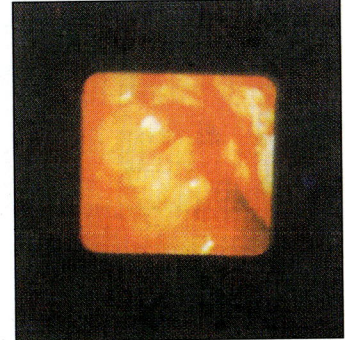

Colonic carcinoma. Large ulceration surrounded by nodular haemorrhagic wall.

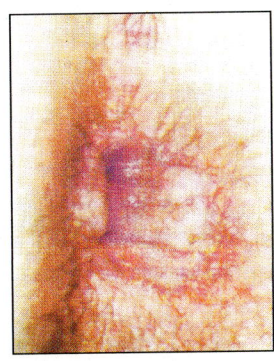

Crohn's disease. Anal and perianal lesions.

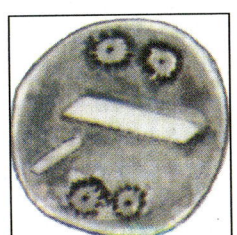

Saline preparation.

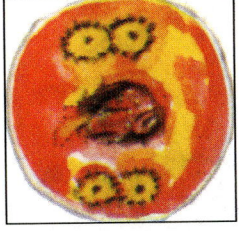

Iodine preparation.

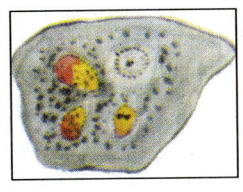

Trophozoite (active) form of *E. histolytica*.

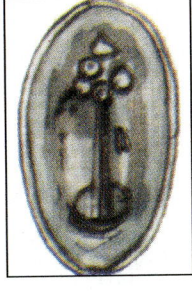

Cysts.

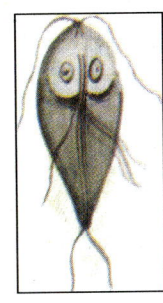

Active (vegetative) form.

CYSTS OF *ENTAMOEBA HISTOLYTICA*

GIARDIA INTESTINALIS

PLATE VI

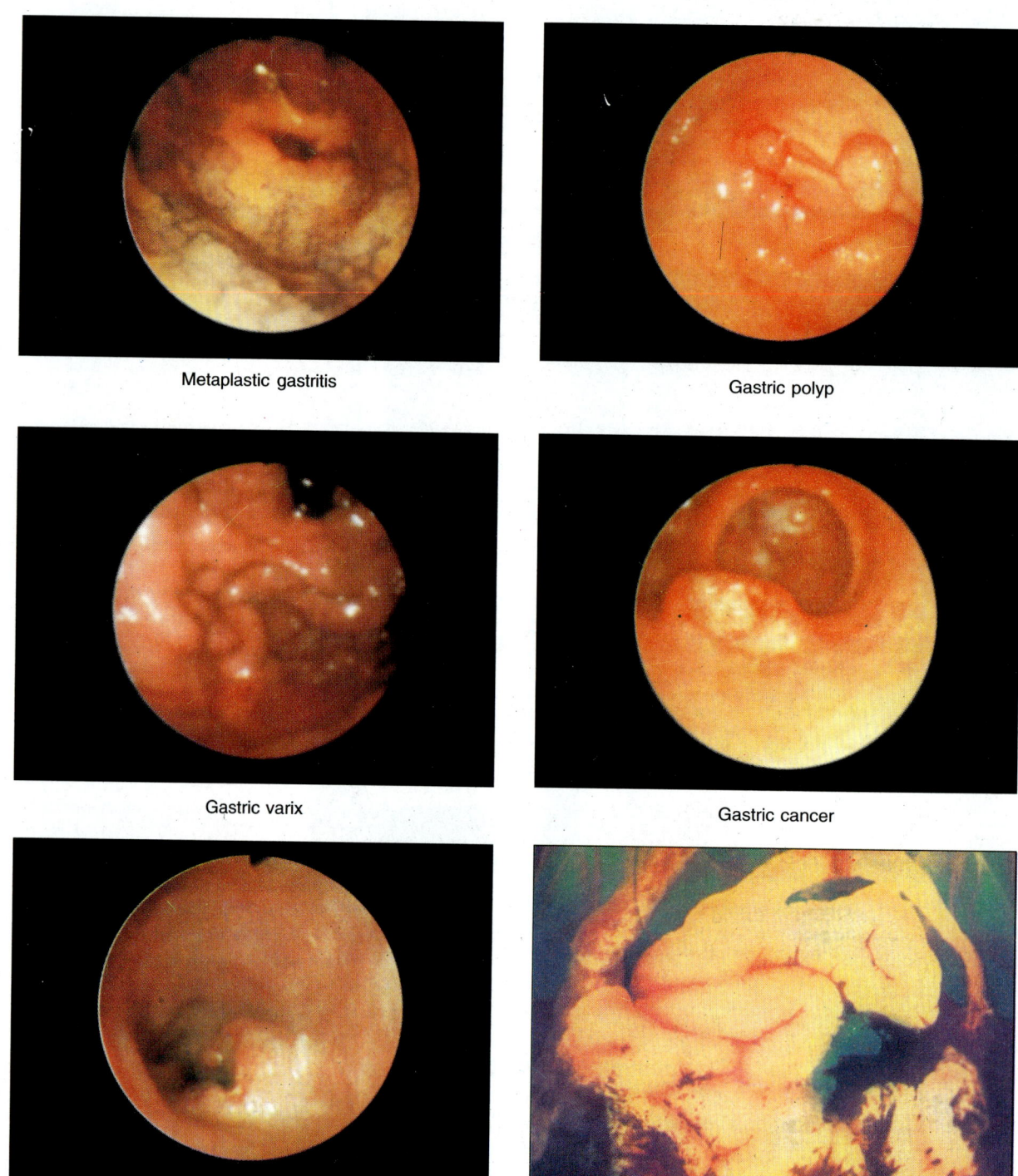

Metaplastic gastritis

Gastric polyp

Gastric varix

Gastric cancer

Esophageal cancer

Crohn's disease: Multiple strictures

acute bulbar paralysis, and foreign body while a slow progressive course favours malignancy or achlasia. Episodic dysphagia of long duration indicates a benign disease. Transient dysphagia of short duration favours an inflammatory process like oesophagitis, but an onset of dysphagia going on from weeks to months must be viewed with suspicion.

If there is history of swallowing of some corrosive substance it shall point to a stricture of oesophagus.

3. Duration and progress. The type of food causing obstruction also helps in making a diagnosis. Diffculty in swallowing only solid foods occurs in mechanical dysphagia which subsequently also is with liquids. In cases of achlasia cardia and oesophageal spasm, obstruction to both solids and liquids is present from the onset while symptoms of dysphagia are intermittent. Progression of symptoms of dysphagia without any remission is present in carcinoma of oesophagus and it is worse with solids. Pain at the site of lesion if localized will be a pointer to the disease. Epigastric burning or something sticking there occurs in peptic oesophagitis or achlasia. Hoarseness of voice suggests involvement of left recurrent laryngeal nerve by carcinoma of oesophagus or laryngeal carcinoma.

Regurgitation of food contents, haematemesis and malaena shall be other features of carcinoma oesophagus.

In myasthenia gravis, dysphagia increases in severity as the day passes and sometimes there is spontaneous improvement especially when rest has been given to muscles of deglutation while in motor neurone disease, the dysphagia is slowly progressive and there is no change in its course.

Change of posture is helpful in reaching a diagnosis in hiatus hernia when patient gets relief by sitting up and the symptoms worsening off in lying position. Patients with scleroderma and other collagen disorders have difficulty with liquids in the recumbent posture but not in upright position.

Physical examination. It is important pointer towards the various oesophageal factors:

Presence of anaemia, koilonychia and a glazed tongue in a young female shall suggest Plummer-Vinson syndrome. Examination of mouth, throat for evidence of stomatitis, glossitis malignancy and evidence of pharyngeal disease, neck for enlarged thyroid gland and chest for mediastinal tumour, aortic aneurysm, cardiac enlargement be carried out.

In addition look for signs suggestive of motor neurone disease, bulbar palsy, myopathy and myasthenia gravis. Skin examination is helpful in excluding scleroderma and other collagen disorders.

Investigations. In every case of dysphagia in addition to routine investigations following investigations are important:

1. *Haemoglobin and peripheral blood film for type of anaemia.*

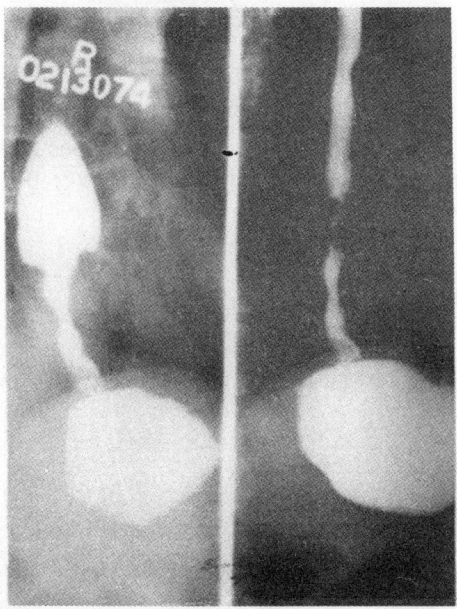

Fig. 2.11. Showing carcinoma in the middle of oesophagus

2. *Radiology.* Barium swallow is the most important diagnostic tool. It will show the presence of stricture—its site and length. A hiatus hernia will also be seen in a head down position. A small web may be seen in upper part (cricopharyngeal region) or in the lower part (web-like annular constriction at oesophagogastric junction). X-ray chest for mediastinal widening, and aneurysmal dilatation, or cardiac enlargement.

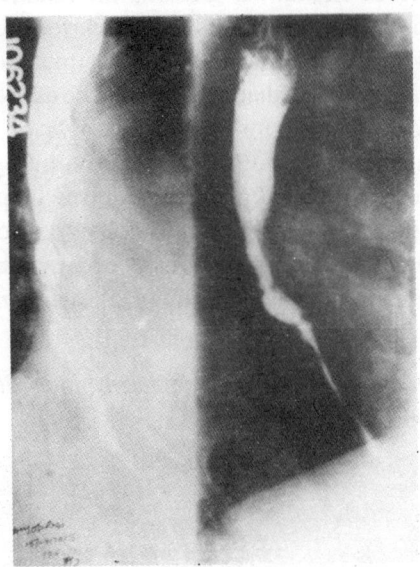

Fig. 2.12. Barium meal study of oesophagus showing carcinoma involving middle and lower third of oesophagus

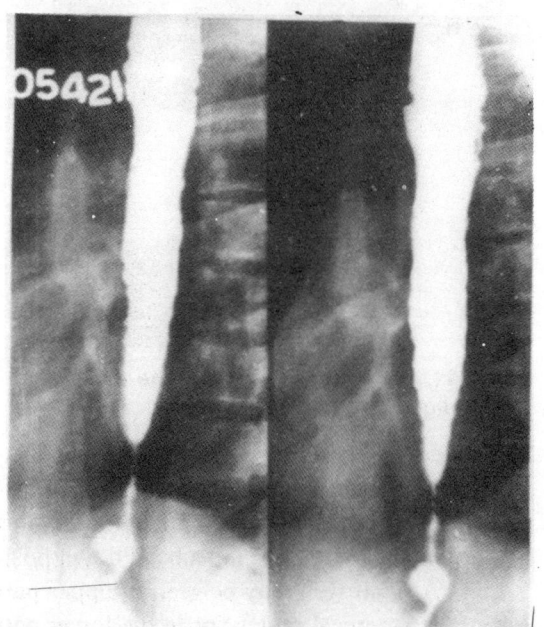

Fig. 2.13. (a) Barium meal study showing carcinoma in lower third of oesophagus.

Note. Complete narrowing of the lower end of oesophagus.

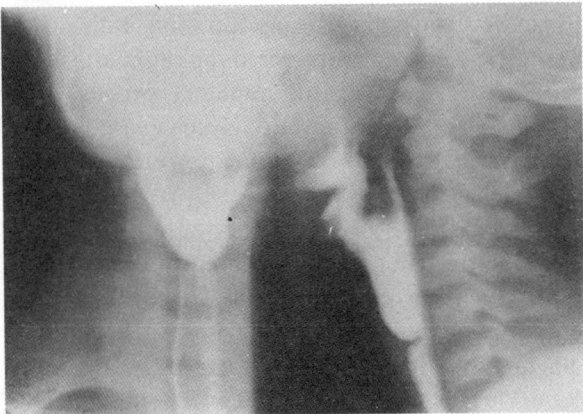

Fig. 2.13. (b) Cricold webs in a case of Plummer-vinson syndrome. This is characterised by anaemia, koilonychia and dysphagia)

3. Oesophagoscopy. Fibreoptic oesophagoscopy is an important test and combined with biopsy from the site of lesion must be performed in every case.

4. Oesophageal motility. These studies are helpful in diagnosing cases of achlasia of the oesophagus, motor and neuromuscular disorders of the oesophagus, diffuse oesophageal spasm but are of no value in cases of dysphagia due to mechanical factors.

Treatment. Dysphagia is a symptom complex of a number of diseases both local as well as general. Hence treatment has to be planned depending on the aetiological factors. Cases of plummer vinson syndrome require treatment by means of good nutrition and heavy doses of iron. Carcinoma of oesophagaes shall be managed by surgery while neuromuscular disorders producing dysphagia require conservative line of management.

CARDIOSPASM: ACHLASIA OF THE CARDIA

A disease which affects both sexes but more in women especially in middle age in which the muscular activity of body and lower end of oesophagus are disordered.

The main complaint is difficulty in swallowing which is most troublesome with solids but subsequently it is with liquids as well. Patient feels as if something is sticking at the lower end of sternum. When pain is produced it is severe and of burning quality. It is retrosternal or in epigastric region and is radiating to the chest and arm.

Patient may voluntarily try to induce vomiting immediately after taking meals to relieve himself of the discomfort. Regurgitation may take place and this is more with liquids than with solids. This may prevent the patient from taking adequate quantities of food. Initially symptoms of achlasia last for a short period but gradually no interval free period is left and the patient is left with permanent feeling of obstruction. Marked weight loss occurs.

Course of the disease can be divided into three phases. In the first phase patient has pain, difficulty in swallowing frequent regurgitation of food and is afraid to take full amount of food.

In second phase there is improvement of symptoms giving the patient a false sense of well-being. Actually the oesophagus is dilated now and the passage of food through the cardia may take place slowly.

Third phase is the final phase which occurs at a late stage. There is weight loss, loss of appetite and respiratory complications may occur either because of pressure from the large dilated oesophagus or there may be regurgitation of oesophageal contents into respiratory passages causing aspiration and infection.

Diagnosis. It is made by barium swallow which shows a dilated oesophagus extending to oesophagogastric junction at which there is a narrow conical termination in a string fashion.

Oesophagoscopy shows mucous membrane at lower end of oesophagus to be chronically inflamed and there may be erosions. It is equally important to exclude an obstructing lesion and carcinoma at lower end of oesophagus. Manometry is helpful. It may show a normal or elevated basal lower oesophageal sphincter pressure.

Treatment. General management includes maintenance of nutrition by giving patient soft semiliquid or liquid nutritious foods. In case the oesophagus is dilated markedly, it should be regularly emptied. In diet avoid ice cold food, spices and alcohol. Use of antacids is helpful. But treatment with antispasmodics, anticholinergic and octyl nitrate inhalations is unsatisfactory. Calcium channel antagonists like Nifedipine may help in some cases.

Main line of treatment is by balloon dilatation or by use of bougies. Major complications in this procedure are perforation, bleeding and rupture of lower end of oesophagus.

In case of failure with dilatation, Heller's operation of cardiomyotomy is performed. It is equally effective. Main complication is stricture formation.

Prognosis. It apparently is good if patient comes at early stage. In cases of long standing, chances of developing malignancy and respiratory complications are high which carry poor prognosis.

OESOPHAGITIS. Inflammation of the oesophagus which may be either acute or chronic, is a result of number of factors:

Causes of acute oesophagitis:

1. *Chemical irritants*. Alcohol, corrosive substances (strong alkalis/acids), spicy foods drugs (Aspirin, potassium chloride, steroids, NSAIDS).
2. *Acute bacterial infections*. Diphtheria, scarlet fever, sterptococcal throat infection.
3. *Viral infections*. Herpes simplex, varicilla zoster virus, cytomegalo virus, human immunodefeciency virus.
4. *Fungal infections*. Candida
5. *Radiation* of lung or mediastinum
6. *Skin disorders*. Pemphigus, Stevens-Johnson syndrome.

In acute form of oesophagitis, irritants which may be in the form of alcohol, spicy foods, corrosive substances and drugs like aspirin, potassium chloride, steroids and especially those belonging to NSAID (non-steroidal anti-inflammatory drugs) group act as causative agents. Other causes include infections due to viruses, bacteria or fungi and this is more so in patients who are immunocompromised.

Acute infections may spread from pharynx down to oesophagus as in scarlet fever, diphtheria, acute pharyngitis. Other causes include viral oesophagitis due to herpes simplex virus, varicella zoster virus, cytomegalovirus and human immunodeficiency virus; candida oesophagitis due to candida; radiation oesophagitis following radiation of lung or mediastinum for malignancy; corrosive oesophagitis following ingestion of strong alkalis or acids accidentally or suicidal purposes, and oesophagitis may be seen in skin disorders like pemphigus, Stevens-Johnson syndrome.

As compared to acute oesophagitis chronic oesophagitis is generally as a result of reflux of acid contents at the oesophageal mucosa when the normal mucosal defense of oesophagus fails. Chronic oesophagitis may also be continuation of the same factors which operated in acute stage.

Symptoms in acute case are in the form of a burning sensation behind the sternum, dysphagia and often chest pain which may sometimes simulate angina like pain. Deglutation is very painful and the patient may be afraid to even drink water or swallow his saliva. Any attempt to swallow produces a reflex spasm. In cases of cardiac achlasis, stasis of food at lower end of oesophagus may produce not only ulceration but peptic strictures. Patients complain of constant heart burn and there is often history of reflux vomiting.

Diagnosis of oesophagitis is based on history, barium swallow, oesophagoscopy and mucosal biopsy. A normal barium swallow or oesophagoscopy does not exclude the diagnosis. In some cases barium swallow shows either a stricture or ulcer formation while oesophagoscopy may reveal erosions, stricture or ulcer formation. In patients with normal oesophagoscopy, mucosal biopsy shall clinch the diagnosis.

Treatment. It shall be general and specific. Cases of acute oesophagitis should be managed on general lines like giving of small feeds at frequent intervals in the form of demulcents. Head end of the bed be raised. Patient should avoid alcohol, smoking, spicy foods, tea, coffee, carbonated drinks and fruit juices.

Milk is a good food which not only shall help in alleviating symptoms but also reduce acidity and be given every 3-4 hourly.

Specific therapy includes drugs. Antacids preferably in liquid form (15-20 ml four times a day) be given. H2 blocking agents (Ranitidine 150 mg twice a day). Proton pump inhibitors (Omeprazole/ Lansoprazole once a day) along with drugs like Metoclopramide or Cisapride to raise oesophageal sphincter pressure and help in gastric emptying can be employed. For patients with viral aetiology, Acyclovir (800 mg twice orally) candida (Ketoconazole 200 to 400 mg in a single dose or Tab. Nystatin (every 6 hourly) and for bacterial causes appropriate antibiotics (Penicillin/ Ampicillin/Amoxycillin).

Treatment of both acute and chronic oesophagitis should be continued for sometime after the subsidence of symptoms. Cases of chronic oesophagitis/reflux oesophagitis may require treatment for 3 to 6 months or even longer.

There may be a small percentage of cases of reflux or chronic oesophagitis which fail to respond to medical treatment and there is formation of stricture and once the stricture is formed it has to be treated either by dilatation or resection.

GASTRITIS

Gastritis means inflammation of the gastric mucosa which may be either acute or chronic. A number of factors ranging from bad eating habits, excessive alcohol consumption, infections, poisons to drugs may be important aetiological factors. Diagnosis of gastritis is based on history, clinical examination and histologic features in a case whether acute or chronic.

Acute catarrhal gastritis. It is an acute process where irritants like strong acids or alkalis, drugs like salicylates, steroids, NSAIDs Indomethacin, poor eating habits, condiments, strong tea/coffee, alcohol, tobacco, poor oral hygiene, swallowing of infected sputum or secretions from sinuses, throat, gums act as a source of constant irritation, the degree of gastritis varying with the intensity and duration of irritation. In some cases toxic products of bacterial activity such as salmonella, staphylococci, acute physical and mental stress may produce features of gastritis.

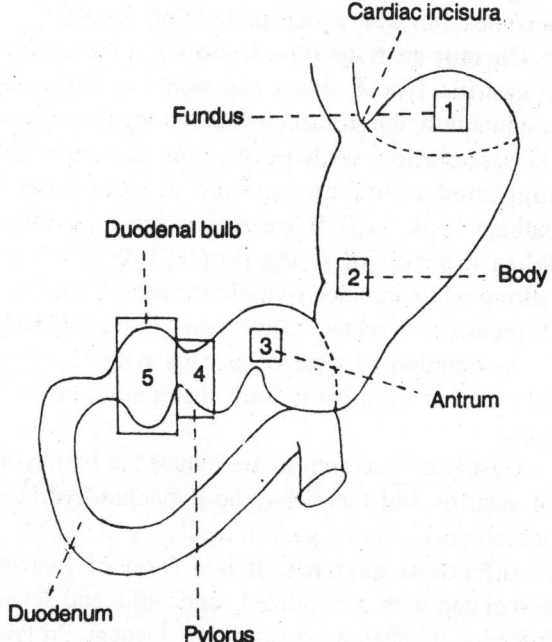

Fig. 2.14. Diagrammatic representation of stomach.

Helicobacter pylori, a short, spiral-shaped gram-negative bacillus, is another important cause of acute gastritis though mostly it is associated with chronic form of gastritis.

Acute erosive gastritis or haemorrhagic gastritis. It is an acute process characterized by breakdown of gastric mucosal barrier and there is not only erosions but also inflammation and haemorrhages in the gastric mucosa. These lesions may be distributed diffusely throughout the gastric mucosa or be localized to the body or antrum of the stomach. Most of the time the erosions are superficial confined to the gastric mucosa but sometimes may extend deeper. Acute erosive gastritis most commonly develops in seriously ill patients suffering from septic shock, extensive burns, severe infections, trauma, septicemia,

respiratory and renal failure. Drugs like aspirin, NSAIDs group and ethanol are other substances known to disrupt gastric mucosal barrier causing an erosive gastritis.

Symptoms in an acute gastritis generally are in the form of an acute pain or burning sensation in the stomach. There is upper abdominal discomfort, nausea and vomiting. Appetite is lost. Vomiting often brings relief.

In cases of erosive gastritis there is haematemesis or malaena in addition to other symptoms.

Physical examination shows an ill-looking person with dry coated tongue. Fever is present in patients with infective cause. Upper abdominal tenderness and signs of blood loss in the form of pallor, tachycardia and hypotension may be present.

Physical signs and symptoms shall vary depending on the aetiological factors. Thus symptoms shall be mild in those cases of gastritis resulting due to poor eating habits, lack of teeth, improper chewing of food and bolting of indigestible food.

Diagnosis of acute gastritis depends on history (like infections, drug intake, poisoning by alcohol, ingestion of iriritants, tea, coffee, spicy food, etc). Leucocytosis is present in persons with infection. Upper gastrointestinal endoscopy shall confirm the diagnosis by demonstrating congestion, erosions, easy friability and haemorrhages in the gastric mucosa.

Treatment. General measures include maintenance of fluid and electrolyte balance. In patients who are repeatedly vomiting, gastric lavage may help. In cases of severe haematemesis or malaena, fresh blood transfusion has to be given.

Antacids (aluminium-magnesium hydroxide preparation) 30 ml every two hourly orally to start with and on improvement the dose may be shifted to 4-6 hourly.

H2 receptor antagonist (Ranitidine) be given intravenously every 4-6 hours initially and then switched on to oral preparation of either H2 receptor antagonist (Ranitidine/Famotidine) or proton pump inhibitor (Omeprazole/Lansoprazole). Pain can be relieved by anticholinergics.

Initially rest to the stomach is advised by

withholding oral feeds except sips of water. As condition improves milk in small quantities is given every two hourly and subsequently soft, non-irritating food is introduced in the diet. All substances which act as irritants or where aetiological factor is located must be treated accordingly. Removal of irritant substances should be a permanent feature to prevent recurrence.

Most of the patients of acute gastritis do well with conservative line of treatment. In very rare case where massive haemorrhage is taking place and this is not controlled by conservative line of therapy surgery is advocated but surgery has its own hazards and carries high degree of morbidity and mortality. So it is better to carry out surgery only when absolutely essential.

Chronic gastritis. It is probably continuation of the same process which caused acute gastritis and there may be number of factors responsible for it. Chronic gastritis is diagnosed not only by clinical examination, radiology but mainly by histological examination of gastric mucosa. *Various forms of chronic gastritis include:*

1. Chronic superficial gastritis
2. Atrophic gastritis
3. Hypertrophic gastritis
4. Infectious gastritis
5. Eosinophilic gastritis
6. Granulomatous gastritis
7. Chronic active gastritis

Chronic superficial gastritis. It is an early stage of chronic form of gastritis and diagnosis is based on histological examination where there are inflammatory changes in the lamina propria (lymphocytes and plasma cells) with atrophy of superficial part of the gastric glands, and decrease in mucus in mucous cells of the gland.

Chronic atrophic gastritis. This is further progression of chronic superficial gastritis and develops as the disease process progresses. The inflammatory infiltrate goes into deep portions of the mucosa and there is dislocation of the glands. Mucosal cells atrophy partially or completely resulting in variable thinning of the mucosa. Gastric epithelium may undergo metaplasia and is converted into intestinal type of epithelium which may be patchy or diffuse.

Gastric atrophy is the final form of chronic gastritis. There is atrophy of gastric mucosa, glandular structures are lost and there is little or complete absence of inflammatory cells. Mucosa becomes thin and reveals underlying vessels.

Chronic gastritis type A and B. Of these forms of gastritis, type A is less common, involves body and fundus of the stomach while sparing the antrum. Its association with pernicious anaemia has suggested either an immune or autoimmune pathogenesis. Type B gastritis is more common. When it occurs in young people, it involves the antrum while in elderly whole stomach is effected. Its incidence is related to age, being more in elderly.

Association of type B gastritis with H. pylori infection is significant from therapeutic point of view.

Gastric acid secretions are reduced in both types of gastritis and there may be hypochlorhydria or achlorhydria. Serum gastrin levels are elevated.

Infectious gastritis. It is a form of gastritis associated with generalized septicemia and severe infection with streptococci, staphylococci, Proteus, E. coli, Herpes, cytomegalovirus etc. Immunocompromised patients fall easy prey to this form of gastritis.

Eosinophilic gastritis. It is an uncommon form of gastritis characterized by eosinophilic infiltration of the stomach wall. It complicates eosinophilic gastroenteritis.

Granulomatous gastritis. Granulomatous diseases like tuberculosis, syphilis, candida, Crohn's disease, and histoplasmosis may involve the stomach producing ulceration and ultimately stricture formation.

Aetiological factors. All types of factors operating in acute gastritis which progress to a chronic stage produce chronic gastritis in its various manifestations. *Thus the factors shall be:*

1. Repeated injury to the gastric mucosa over a period of time by strong tea, coffee, alcohol, spices and tobacco.

2. Presence of infection in the throat, teeth, gums, sinuses and swallowing of infected sputum in a fulminating case of pulmonary tuberculosis, bronchiectasis and lung abscess.
3. Chronic use of anti-inflmmatory drugs like salicylates, indomethacin, NSAIDs.
4. Regular use of very hot beverages. Improper mastication of food especially in those using ill-fitting dentures.
5. Circulating parietal cell antibodies and autoimmune pathology in cases of iron-deficiency anaemia and pernicious anaemia.
6. Reflux of duodenal contents into the stomach following partial gastrectomy causing chronic gastritis.

Symptoms. Common symptoms of chronic gastritis are those of chronic upper abdominal pain, dyspepsia, nausea, flatulence and loss of appetite. Sometimes the symptoms resemble like those in a chronic peptic ulcer. There is pain related to meals and a sense of fullness or burning sensation. Patients of chronic gastritis show increased sensitivity to alcohol, strong tea, coffee and other irritants like smoking, spicy food. Chronic ill-health, chronic constipation accompanied by intermittent periods of diarrhoea may persist for a long time.

Physical examination shows a chronically ill patient with a furred tongue. Tenderness is present in the epigastric region. Signs of malnutrition, anaemia (iron deficiency/megaloblastic anaemia) are present.

Diagnosis. In addition to history, physical examination following investigations are carried out:

1. *Haemoglobin, haemogram*, peripheral blood film for type of anaemia.
2. *Gastric acid studies*. A histamine fast achlorhydria is present in chronic atrophic gastritis especially in those having associated pernicious anaemia. In early stages of chronic superficial or hypertrophic gastritis, acid secretions may be increased but as the disease progresses, and atrophic gastritis appears, hypochlorhydria or achlorhydria appears.
3. *Serum gastrin levels*. These are increased in chronic gastritis.

4. *Radiology*. Barium meal study of stomach generally is not very helpful. In hypertrophic form, gastric rugae may become prominent abnormally while in atrophic gastritis, rugae markings are absent or markedly diminished

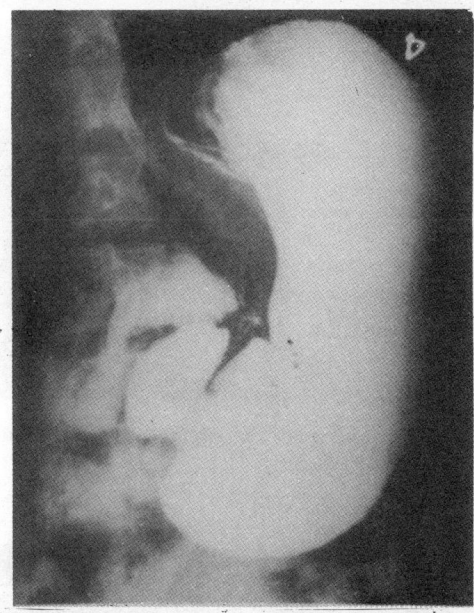

Fig. 2.15. Barium meal stomach and duodenun Normal appearance.

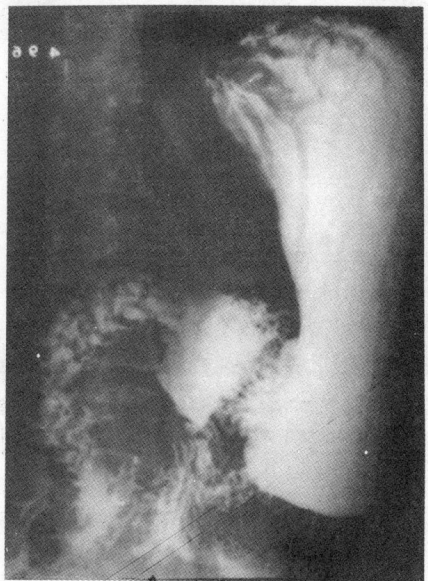

Fig. 2.16. Barium meal showing mucosal folds Normally seen.

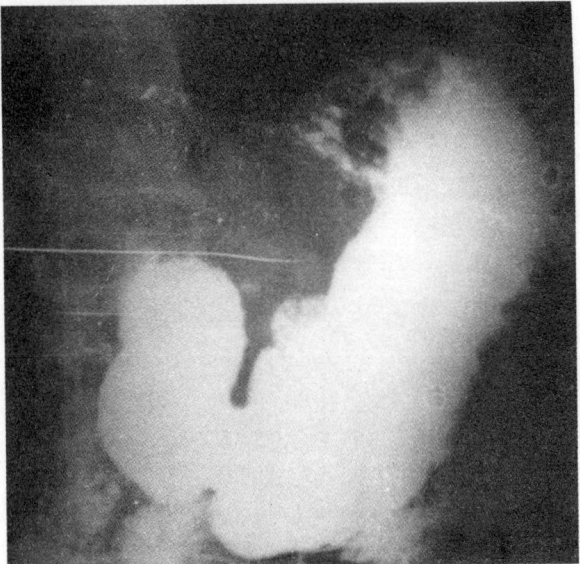

Fig. 2.17. Barium meal - Mucosal folds prominent in a case of chronic gastritis.

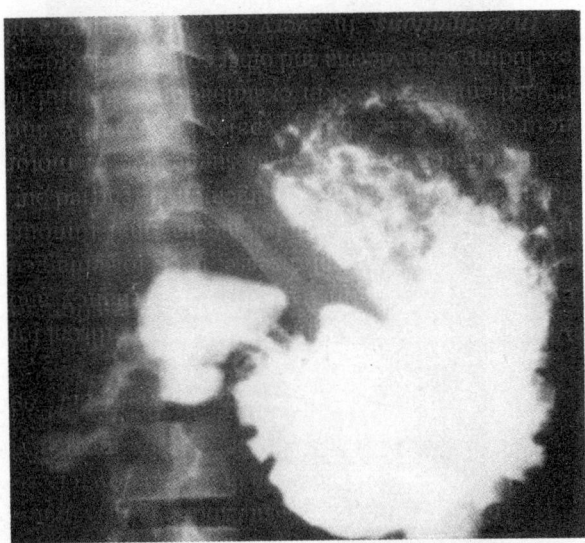

Fig. 2.18. Barium meal - Case of chronic hypertrophic gastritis. Observe abnormal prominence of gastric mucosal folds.

along the greater curvature and fundus giving the stomach a bald appearance. But there is no good correlation between radiological and histological findings.

5. Gastroscopy. It may or may not be very help-

ful. In hypertrophic gastritis, rugae are very much hypertrophied while in atrophic gastritis or gastric atrophy, mucosa is smooth, pale and thin and through it vessels can be seen.

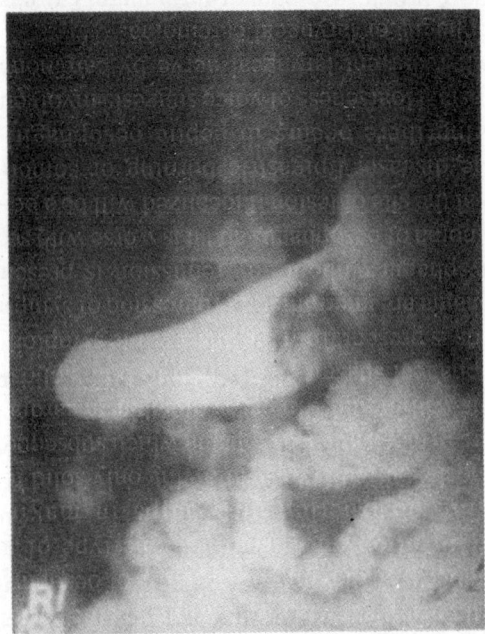

Fig. 2.19. Barium meal - Case of gastric carcinoma. Note filling defect in stomach.

6. Gastric biopsy. It is an important tool and if biopsies from gastric mucosa are taken at multiple sites, histological diagnosis of gastritis in its various stages is established.

Treatment. All factors which are acting as chronic irritants should be removed. All sites of infection and sepsis should be treated with appropriate antibiotics. Patient be directed not to take very hot or cold drinks. Food be chewed properly and taken in small morsels.

Milk in small amounts be given every 4 hourly in the presence of acute symptoms.

For symptomatic relief of pain in chronic superficial gastritis, antacids (20-30 ml) every 4 hourly along with anticholinergics are useful.

Patients of pernicious anaemia shall require parenteral vitamin B_{12} while in those with iron deficiency heavy doses of parenteral iron have to be given.

Cases of infectious gastritis have to be managed on appropriate parenteral antibiotics and supportive measures. In eosinophilic gastritis, response to steroids is favourable.

H. pylori gastritis previously been managed with a combination of amoxycillin, bismuth subsalicylate and metronidazole. But now slight modifications in this regimen are advocated. A combination of Omeprazole 20 mg + Amoxycillin 750 mg + Metronidazole 400 mg thrice a day or Clarithromycin 250 mg + Metronidazole 400 mg + Omeprazole 20 mg twice a day for period ranging from 7 to 14 days has been found to be useful. Success with these regimens is about 90%.

Campylobacter pylori infection

Campylobacter pylori infection has been incriminated as one of the commonest of chronic infections in man. There is a positive correlation between C. pylori colonization and inflammatory changes in the stomach and between eradication of C. pylori and reduction of duodenal ulcer relapse.

Colonization of C. pylori is very common and almost half of the world population carries the organism in their stomach. Its prevalence increases with age suggesting that there is a constant exposure to the organism in the community. On a rough estimate 90-100% of duodenal ulcer patients and over 75% of gastric ulcer patients have this infection.

The natural reservoir of C. pylori is not known. Probably it is present in both animals and humans. Its incidence is highest amongst people who handle animals like meat workers and veterinary surgeons. Transmission from man to man also occurs. It can be transmitted during instrumentation like endoscopy and staff handling gastroscopes have higher incidence.

Pathology: C. pylori infection plays an important role in the aetiology of gastritis and there is close association between the presence of C. pylori on the gastric mucosa and histologically confirmed type B chronic active gastritis. Ninety percent of patients with C. pylori infection have gastritis where as less than 5% of patients with normal mucosa are colonized. Interestingly C. pylori only colonizes gastric type of mucosa and does not colonize the intestinal type mucosa in the stomach.

C. pylori is a gram negative spiral bacterium responsible for chronic active type B gastritis. It produces inflammatory reaction in the mucosa with the production of polymorpho nuclear and mononuclear cell infiltration. Evidence is also accumulating to support the role of this organism in addition to gastritis in cases of non-ulcer dyspepsia. The bacilli live under and in mucous layer covering the gastric epithelium and mainly inhabit the antrum and body of stomach.

Infection with the organism once established is difficult to eradicate. It possesses many enzymes including a powerful urease which assists its colonization in an acid medium.

Symptomtology. C. pylori causes the same clinical picture as a case of acute and chronic type B gastritis like substernal discomfort, pain epigastrium etc. Its exact role in the occurrence and maintenance of peptic ulcer disease is not very clear though there is enough evidence to incriminate it as one of the aetiological factor.

Diagnosis

A number of tests are advised. These include urease test, histology and culture.

14C, Urea breath test is an important test. Monoclonal antibodies have been developed for rapid diagnosis. Determination of urea concentration or ammonia content of gastric aspirate are more anecdotal techniques.

Gram staining of brush specimen of gastric mucosa is another sensitive test.

An unbuffered one minute urease test provides a sensitivity of 98% and is the quickest method to make a diagnosis. Confirmation is done by taking a biopsy specimen and doing histology as well as culture.

Serodiagnosis of C. pylori infection depends on the presence of specific antibodies in the serum. Such an antibody response is demonstrated by complement fixation test, haemagglutination and ELISA, Out of these ELISA is emerging as the most commonly applied technique.

Treatment. When a case of chronic gastritis / peptic ulcer is not responding to conventional line of therapy, suspicion of c. pylori infection must be considered. Its eradication not only relieves the symptoms but also leads to prolonged remission especially in cases of peptic ulcer.

Patients with C. pylori infection are preferably given triple therapy with Bismith, amoxycillin and metronidazole. Dosage of colloidal bismuth (Tripotassium Dicitrate bismuthate) is 480 mg daily in 2 divided doses, (1 tablet 120 mg) and should be taken half hour before meals. It generally colours stools and tongue black and is contraindicated in children, pregnant women and patients of renal disease. Amoxycillin 500 mg 8 hly and metronidazole 500 mg thrice a day are to be combined with bismuth preparation, all the drugs are to be given for 2 weeks. Eradication of the organism takes place in 9 out of 10 cases.

PEPTIC ULCER

It is universally present all over the world, the incidence varying from region to region, country to country. Peptic ulcer comprises a group of ulcerative disorders of the upper part of gastrointestinal tract involving mainly the stomach and duodenum. It derives its name not from any pathogenic role of pepsin but from the fact that ulcer can occur only in the presence of acid and pepsin. For the development of ulcer, there has to be disturbance of balance between gastric acid secretions and factors which comprise mucosal defence. Peptic ulcer is found only in those parts of the digestive tract where there is constant exposure to acid-pepsin or in places where there is presence of gastric mucosa i.e. lower end of oesophagus. Stomach, upper part of duodenum, small intestines anastomosed to the stomach and rarely at the junction of a Meckel's diverticulum with the small intestines. Of the various anatomic sites where peptic ulcer can occur the gastric and the duodenal areas are the most important.

Peptic ulcer is a disease of middle-aged adults though it is known to occur in young people as well.

Both gastric and duodenal ulcers occur with equal frequency in men and women though duodenal ulcer is much more common. Vast majority of gastric ulcers are found along the lesser curvature and duodenal ulcers in the first three inches of the duodenum (duodenal bulb).

Incidence. It is difficult to define the exact incidence of the disease since it is universally present. Its distribution is global and no particular race or community is exempt. In India ulcer is commoner in the south, in the hilly areas like Kashmir and along the coastal regions. But it does not in any way mean that ulcer is uncommon in north and rest of country.

About one in 10 people are supposed to suffer from peptic ulcer like symptoms at some time or another. The disease itself is characterized by periods of remissions and relapses.

Age and sex. All ages are known to be effected by ulcer but on an average the onset occurs in second or third decades going upto the fourth or fifth decade. Both sexes are effected. Duodenal ulcer is about four times more common in men than in women. Women have a relatively less incidence of the disease especially during the reproductive years of life and this immunity declines with the start of menopause. Probably female hormones are acting as protective factors in women.

Social class. Duodenal ulcer occurs with greater frequency than gastric ulcer in higher social grade though this does not hold in Indian population where it is equally prevalent amongst the poor labourer class especially in South India and hilly areas. But professional and business class, executives who are more ambitious and are always in rat race to reach the top, are the people who are work conscious, meticulous and are always on the go. They are the one who have made the grade or just about to make it and they feel that there is no going back. So such class of people pay their own price and result is that they not only become more susceptible but also get ulcers. It is the make up and temperament of an individual which is an important factor.

Emotions and stress. Stomach is one organ which is a good barometer of an individual's emotions whether they are of anxiety, happiness or depression, since all these emotions are reflected on the gastric mucosa as well as secretions of the stomach.

Tensions may be of different kind either at home or at work and to a large extent they persist in the subconscious mind as well. Thus the rapid industrialization and urbanization in its wake has brought the stresses of a big metropolitian city life and this is evident in a poor migrant worker who has shifted into the city and now there is more stress of not only of the job but also of making both ends meet.

An ulcer patient is often worked up about something, feels and grumbles about everything whether it is his job, family or even the society in general. This is one man who always finds some fault or the other in everything and tries to achieve perfection. This type of personality of an ulcer prone individual is characterized by rigidity in behaviour, over consciousness and intolerance. People with ulcer are the one's who seem to reflect disturbances in their inner self than in the outside world. The effects of stress at place of work, as well as the one asociated with living conditions have a bearing on the problem of ulcer. Men in uniform who have to be away from their homes for very long periods at a stretch are always more prone to get ulcers.

It would be difficult to say whether there is really an ulcer personality except that such people are abnormally anxious, aggressive, have an excessive obsessional trends, are more prone to anxiety, dependance, guilt feelings and become extremely tense under slightly difficult situations.

Familial and genetic factors. The incidence of peptic ulcer in first degree relatives of ulcer patients is three times as high as in general population. An increased incidence of HLA-B5 antigen and elevated serum pepsinogen levels are seen in patients of duodenal ulcer and persons with this trait have more chances to develop an ulcer.

Diet. It has an important bearing on the production of ulcer. The incidence of ulcer in those who take hot spicy food is very high. Similarly people whose diet is rich in carbohydrates but poor in proteins are prone to develop ulcers. The temperature of food eaten also is important since food or beverages taken very hot act as thermal irritants.

Not only it is the type of diet like consumption of hot food, chillies, spices, condiments and excessive use of sugar, tea, and coffee but the way food is eaten. The eating habits of a person may act as important factor in the aetiology of disease.

One hypothesis is that in people of north who masticate or chew their food properly as compared to the people of south who take sloppy diets like rice, sambhar, idli, dossa etc. there is secretion of a large volume of saliva of a high buffer capacity which protects the acid bathed mucosa. Similarly masticatory diets have inhibitory effect on bile flow while the sloppy diet promotes a free bile flow which abets the production of ulcer by its alkalinity dissolving the resistance formed by mucin. But this hypothesis is self-contradictory since ulcer is equally prevalent in north Indians where people masticate their food as compared to southerners who take sloppy diets like rice sambhar etc.

Another interesting theory is that it is the excessive consumption of refined carbohydrates like sweets, chocolates and confectionary and a diet low in protein content which may predispose to ulcer formation because of lack of buffering action of proteins on gastric juice.

Thus poor nutrition, thermal and chemical irritation due to the excessive and liberal use of chillies, condiments and spices along with hot food and beverages go a long way in the causation of peptic ulcer.

Tobacco, alcohol. These two factors have an important bearing on the problem. Smokers have an higher incidence of ulcer, and have higher mortality from the disease. Ulcer in smokers take longer time to heal. In fact healing is delayed by smoking. Habit of eating and chewing of tobacco is another factor. Though smoking does not increase gastric acid secretions yet it inhibits pancreatic bicarbonate secretion, thus accelerating the process of ulcer formation. Alcohol especially of high spirit content not only produces direct inflammation and injury to the gastric mucosa but subsequently increases gastric acid secretions, thus increasing proneness to ulcer formation.

Blood groups. A relationship between blood groups and ulcers has been established. The risk of duodenal ulcer in blood group O subjects as compared to other blood group is higher.

Similarly a relationship between the ability to secrete ABO blood group antigens in saliva and other body fluids in cases of duodenal ulcer has been established. ABH non-secretors (H substance, a mucopolysaccharide) have greater chance of developing ulcer while blood group antigens in secretors give protection against duodenal ulceration.

Association between peptic ulcer and other diseases. Certain diseases run the higher risk of developing a gastric or duodenal ulcer and these include chronic gastritis, hiatus hernia, chronic emphysema with or without cor pulmonale, hyperparathyroidism, biliary cirrhosis and an acute ulcer called Curling's ulcer following extensive burns.

Pathogenesis of peptic ulcer. Peptic ulcer ococurs only in the presence of acid pepsin and when there is disturbed balance between gastric acid pepsin secretion and mucosal resistance.

Gastric acid secretions are regulated by chemical, neural and hormonal factors and gastrin released from antral mucosa is a strong stimulant of gastric acid secretions. Major stimulation to gastric acid secretion is ingestion of food, coffee, alcohol and other irritants. These secretions are controlled by gastrin and vagal stimulation.

The exact mechanism by which mucosal resistance takes place may not be defined but this defence is monitored by gastric mucus secreted by gastric mucosal cells present in gastric glands, bicarbonate ions secreted by non-parietal gastric epithelial cells, mucosal blood flow and luminal hydrogen ions. Prostaglandins E present in gastric mucosa inhibits gastric mucosal injury.

Thus a number of factors ranging from injury to the gastric mucosa, lowered mucosal resistance, dietary and nutritional factors, heredity, emotions, gastric acid secretions, defective mucosal resistance and gastric hormones play their role in the pathogenesis of peptic ulcer. In short it is 'acid pepsin' versus 'mucosal resistance'.

Symptoms. The onset of the disease is gradual spread over a period of months. The earliest symptom is pain which varies in intensity from mild to severe, having a gnawing or burning character. It is generally located in the epigastric region and may radiate upwards or to the back. Pain invariably disappears after sometime and may be relieved by vomiting.

Pain character and rhythm distinguishes between gastric and duodenal ulcers. In gastric ulcer pattern is FOOD-PAIN-RELIEF. Pain comes 15 minutes to 2 hous after meals depending on the site of ulcer. In ulcers situated near the cardia, the pain begins immediately after meals and in prepyloric ulcer it is about 2-3 hours after meals. The pain generally disappears after about an hour and is relieved either by vomiting or by alkalis. When pain increases in severity, a small quantity of acid fluid along with food may be brought up often induced by the patient to get relief.

Sometimes there is blood brought out in the vomit, it is mixed with food and is coffee colored. There is malaena. Occult blood is invariably present in stools in early stage while in late stages malaena may occur, the stools becoming tarry.

Appetite is good in the beginning but fear of pain may make the patient take less food and the result is weakness, and loss of weight.

In duodenal ulcer pain is a common symptom. There is generally a sense of discomfort or fullness after a large meal. This is gradually replaced by pain (sharp, boring or burning) which occurs between 2 to 4 hours after every meal. Food always brings relief in pain. The pattern of pain is PAIN-FOOD-RELIEF-PAIN. Ingestion of food brings part neutralization of gastric acid secretions. Patient of duodenal ulcer has often to get up at night because of pain especially if the last meal was finished less than 3 hours before going to sleep.

Pain is located in the epigastric region slightly to the right side of middle line. It may radiate to the right side or to the back when ulcer is penetrating deep.

Initially pain of duodenal ulcer may be associated with hunger pain since it is relieved quickly by taking food. The disease is invariably characterized by periods of remissions and relapses. Episodes of pain lasting for some weeks or months alternate with periods of more or less complete freedom from symptoms. Cases of duodenal ulcer worsen in cold weather and the attacks of pain may be brought on by anxiety, exposure to cold, acute infections, excessive smoking or drinking and indiscretions in food.

Physical examination. Except for tenderness present at the site of lesion on palpation, there may

---

Diagnosis

1. Typical history of epigastric pain related to food. Remission and relapses.
2. Conventional barium meal positive in 70-80% of cases.
3. Double contrast barium study positive in 90% of cases.
4. Gastric acid secretion studies.
5. Gastroduodenoscopy.
6. Serum gastrin assay in those where surgery planned or gastrinoma suspected.

---

be no physical signs. A case of gastric or duodenal ulcer is better diagnosed by a good history of the disease.

Diagnosis. Cases of peptic ulcer are diagnosed by a detailed history since physical examination does not reveal much. Once the diagnosis is made, confirmation be done by further tests.

Investigations:

1. **Fractional test meal**. A gruel meal is given to stimulate the gasric secretion. Both free and total acidity are estimated. A rising curve suggestive of hyperchlorhydria is seen in cases of duodenal ulcer.

   Augmented histamine test is more specific. Here 1.25 mg of histamine is injected sabcutaneously to act as a stimulant (dosage is 0.04 mg/kg body weight). Both basal and maximal acid output are measured (normal values of basal acid output 1.4-3.4 mEq/L and MAO 17.2-22 mEq/L). This test is contrain-

dicated in cases of coronary heart disease, hypertension, cerebrovascular accidents and elderly people. Acidity levels when raised are helpful in establishing the diagnosis. Pentagastrin test is another test. It is more safe.

2. **Barium meal examination** of upper gastrio-inestinal tract to demonstrate the presence of ulcer. Gastric ulcer may be seen in the form of crater along the lesser curvature while in cases of duodenal ulcer not only is there ulcer crater in the proximal part of duodenal bulb but in chronic cases there is deformity of the duodenal bulb.

   Routine barium examination does not give very high positive results but with double contrast barium meal examination detection of ulcers may be upto 90 per cent.

3. **Gastroendoscopy**. Fibreoptic endoscopy gives the confirmatory evidence about idientifying the ulcer and its activity. In case of doubtful lesions, biopsy from the site can be taken.

   Gastroendoscopy not only helps in making the diagnosis but is also useful as a tool to assess the ulcer healing.

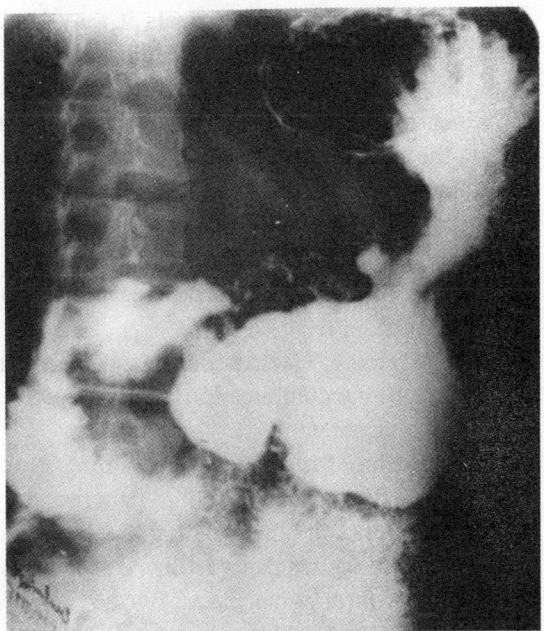

Fig. 2.20. Gastric ulcer. Barium meal showing a large ulcer on lesser curvature of stomach.

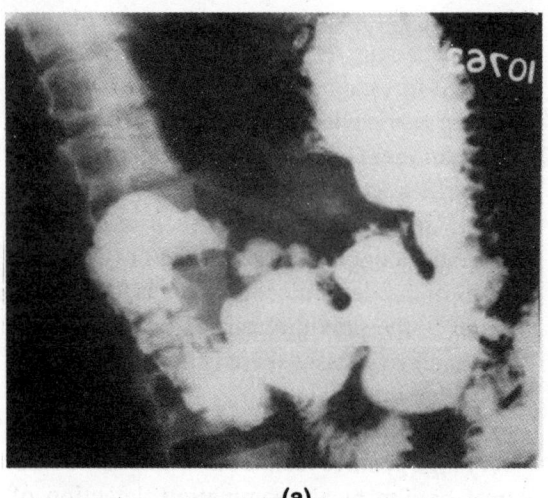

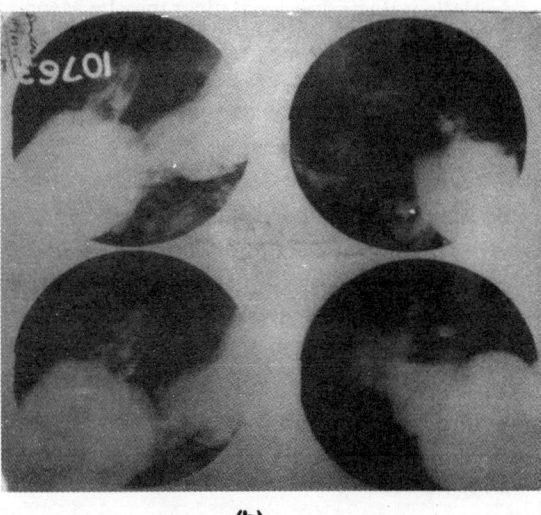

(a)　　　　　　　　　　　　　　　　(b)

Fig. 2.21 (a) **Duodenal ulcer.** There is mucosal hypertrophy of stomach Dudenal cap is deformed with an ulcer crater. (b) Duodenal ulcer. Double contrast barium meal study showing deformed duodenal bulb and persistent ulcer crater.

Complications of ulcer. Various complications in peptic ulcer which may develop at some stage of the disease are:

1. **Pyloric obstruction.** It is a common complication of duodenal ulcer present in post-bulbar region. As the ulcer heals it may leave behind a cicateral scarring resulting into stenosis. Cases of pyloric obstruction present with projectile vomiting, the vomitus containing the gastric contents of food taken earlier on. In early cases of pyloric obstruction, medical treatment may help but in late stages only surgery can help.
2. **Perforation.** of ulcer produces picture of acute peritonitis.
3. **Haemorrhage.** Haematemesis and malaena. It is a serious complication and requires urgent management.
4. **Penetration of ulcer** into surrounding structures and deep penetration into pancreas may produce constant boring pain in the back and picture simulating pancreatitis. Dense adhesions may form at the site.
5. **Malignancy** in an ulcer is a late and an uncommon complication.

Principles of ulcer treatment

1. Diet
2. Antacids
3. H_2 receptor antagonists
4. Proton pump inhibitors
5. Mucosal coating agents
6. Anticholinergics
7. Sedatives/tranquilizers/anti-depressants
8. General measures

Management of an ulcer patient. An ideal approach in the management of a case of peptic ulcer is to give relief from the discomfort of pain and to promote quick healing of an ulcer with an eye towards prevention of recurrence and complications. *The line of treatment can be divided into:*

1. Diet
2. Physical and mental rest
3. Drugs
4. Role of surgery

Diet. The basic principle of diet in an ulcer patient is to reduce quantity and quality of gastric juice by food which acts as a buffering substance and thus serves also as an effective antacid.

Medical treatment. Major objectives:

1. Relief of pain
2. Ulcer healing
3. Prevention of ulcer recurrence and complications

Milk is an eminently satisfactory antacid because its proteins act as buffering substance and fat content inhibits gastric secretions and motility. Milk taken repeatedly at short intervals buffers acid and acts as part of programme designed to neutralize the gastric juice during working hours and at night. Main aim of milk diet has been to reduce gastric acidity, suppress motor activity of the stomach and maintain mucosal resistance.

Food stimulates the secretion of acid in the stomach depending on its quantity and composition and the way it is eaten.

Milk is a relatively poor stimulant of acid secretions, is a good buffer to acid, soothens the gastric mucosa and is also good for its nutritive value and convenience of taking.

In acute stage the stomach is kept in a state of relative rest. As the most vigorous contractions of stomach occur when it is empty and the next most vigorous contractions are encountered as the stomach tries to empty its contents after a meal, so hourly or two hourly feeds of liquid or semi solid consistency are advised to induce periods of relative stomach rest as well as decrease in motor activity.

Food acts as a soothing agent and often relieves the pain. In acute stage a strict diet regimen of milk and bland semisolid diet at frequent intervals is advised. But as the condition improves, cream, vegetable puree, custard, pudding and jelly, are added slowly and gradually over a period of weeks to months, the quantum of diet is increased and method devised by which a bland, non-spicy, not hot and a high protein (cheese, boiled or steamed fish, chicken, milky puddings) rather than a high carbohydrate diet is substituted.

There are no hard and fast rules about diet in cases of peptic ulcer but a broad outline can be suggested.

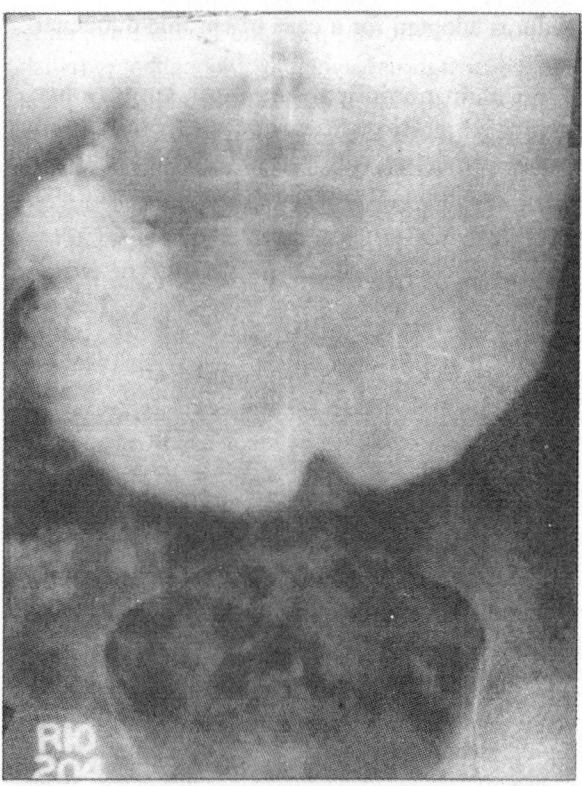

Fig. 2.22. Barium meal study stomach: Note dilated stomach. There is very little barium in rest of G.I. Tract. This is suggestive of pyloric stenosis.

Strict dietary regimen is only advocated till the patient has acute symptoms and pain.

Diet must be such as it suits the likes and dislikes of the patient. Bland food means that which is not chemically, mechanically or thermally irritating. Thus orange juice or other fruit juice or ice cold drink taken on an empty stomach shall have a damaging effect on the gastric mucosa. Similarly fried, spicy foods, salads and uncooked vegetables may act as powerful mechanical irritants.

Very sweet or sour foods are to be avoided. Bread and chapaties of refined wheat, toast, rice are advised but hard and tough cereals like jowar, bajra and maize have to be avoided. Corn flour, sago, dalia are good substitutes.

Food which is tough, fibrous and may irritate mechanically be avoided. Vegetables should be well cooked, preferably boiled soft and mashed like potatoes, cauliflower, peas and beans. Raw, under cooked or fibrous vegetables like cabbage, radish, tomatoes with skin on, fried vegetables and palak or sarson-ka-sag be avoided.

Of the fruits, bananas, apples (without their skin), mangoes, chiku, papaya (ripe) and pears are permitted while sour oranges, unripe papaya, guavas, pineapple and raw or hard fruits of any kind are better left alone.

Meat should be soft like chicken (boiled or steamed), tender mutton and boiled or baked fish, liver, brain but fried and seasoned meat be avoided. Eggs should preferably be taken as either boiled or poached but not fried.

Cut on spicy food. Pickles, chutneys and condiments have to be avoided. Indian food is generally hot and spicy but for an ulcer patient it should be made non-spicy and bland.

Of the sweets, excessively sweetened confectionary, chocolates, sweets, cake, pastries have to be avoided. Preference should be for custard, jellies, sweet curd, yogurt, ice cream containing less of cream.

Very hot or cold foods have to be avoided and these include caffeine containing beverage like coffee, tea and cola drinks.

Smoking and alcohol are other dangerous portents for an ulcer patient. They are to be avoided since they not only prevent the healing of ulcer but also increase the acidity. The important thing in the dietetic management of ulcer is to ensure that the gastric acid is constantly neutralized. Hence the desirability of frequent small feeds. Long intervals between meals are to be avoided. Stomach should not be without food for more than two to three hours. Small snacks in between two principal meals and preferably a cup of milk on retiring at night.

In addition to advice about the diet to be followed in an ulcer patient, patient should be advised to eat food slowly and neither to hurry it down nor to skip it. Stomach should not be over loaded. Food be chewed slowly and eaten in relaxed atmosphere. Nervousness or tension shall harm the ulcer healing. In other words dietary discretion is desirable for an ulcer patient. Whatever controversies may be there about role of diet in management of an ulcer patient, it can not be denied that diet has a role to play, a strict dietary regimen in acute stage and gradual relaxation in diet with certain precautions as healing of ulcer takes place.

Physical and mental rest. Most of the people with ulcer are always tense and consciously or subconsciously harbouring certain fears and have lot of problems on their mind.

Guidelines for an ulcer patient

1. Adopt a positive attitude towards life.
2. Keep your cool.
3. Take adequate rest.
4. Have regular feeds (small and frequent).
5. Take small feeds of milk at regular intevals. It shall soothe your stomach.
6. Avoid smoking, alcohol, carbonated drinks (colas), strong tea and coffee.
7. Avoid fried or spicy foods.
8. Diet should be soft and bland.
9. Avoid taking aspirin and other drugs of NSAIDs group.
10. Keep off tensions.
11. Avoid raw under-cooked or fibrous vegetables, fruits with skin. Gravies, cakes, pastries be avoided. Prefer refined foods, well-cooked and soft vegetables.

It is essential for a person with an ulcer to take proper periods of rest both at work and at home. Person should be advised to cultivate philosphical attitude both towards work and life.

Regularity of living habits has to be cultivated. The person should not unnecessarily worry over which he has no control and the pin pricks of daily life should be borne with fortitude.

Fatigue is a great enemy of ulcer subjects and prevents the healing of ulcer. Patient should be advised not to fatigue himself and his work schedule be adjusted in such a manner that there is always sometime for rest and relaxation. Relaxation is essential not only for the body but also for the mind.

In short there should be no better advice for the patient than to cultivate complete relaxation of both

PLATE VII

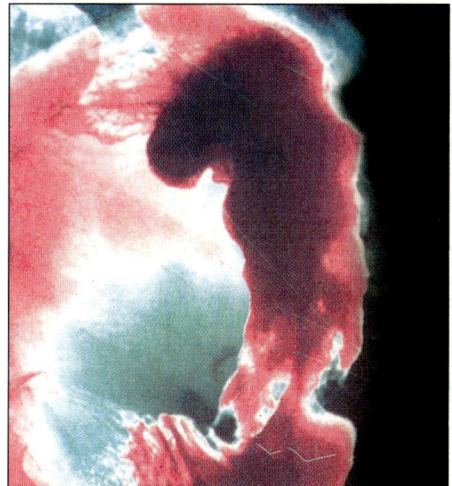

Carcinoma stomach

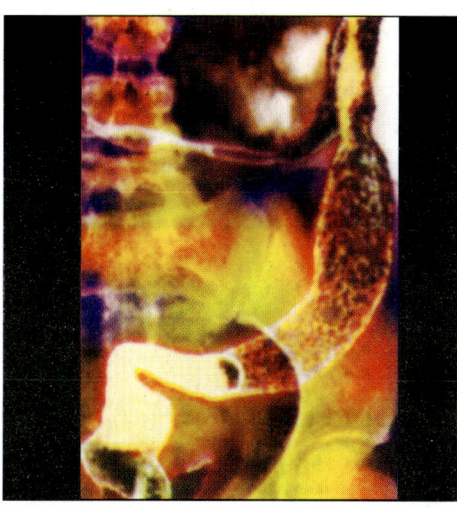

Ulcerative colitis. Note extensive involvement of colon

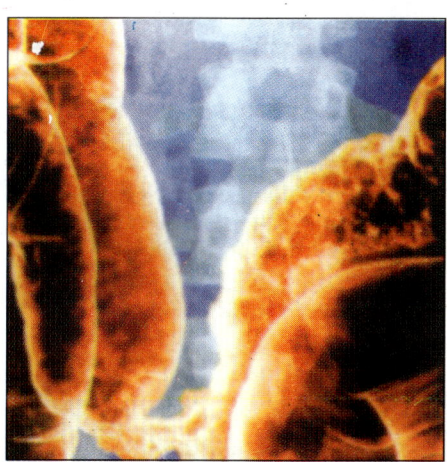

Strictures in a case of Crohn's disease

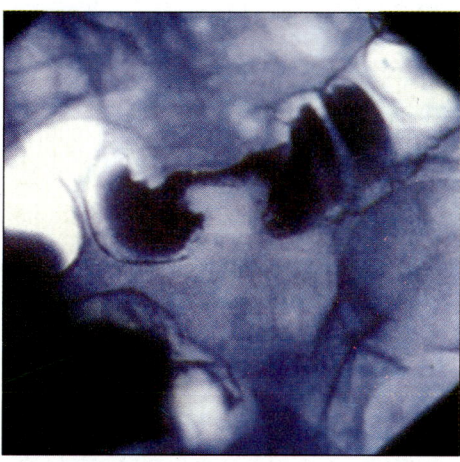

Carcinoma colon. Barium enema showing filling defect in colon

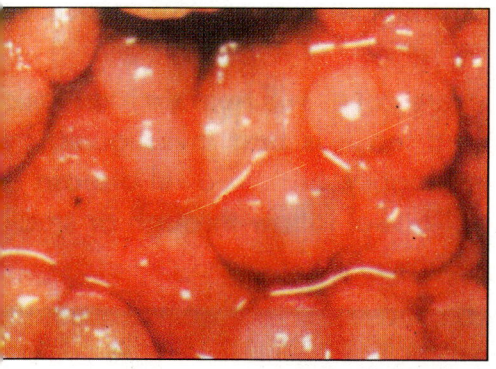

Crohn's disease: Cobblestone appearances

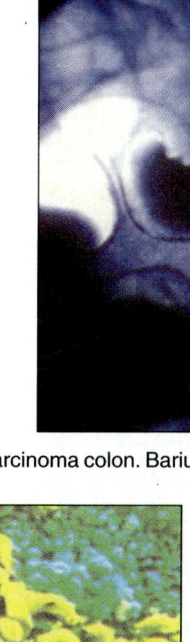

H. pylori in the stomach

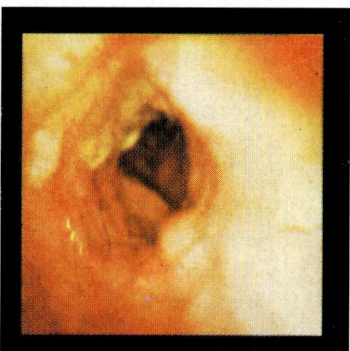

Colonoscopy in a case of ulcerative colitis showing scattered polyps

PLATE VIII

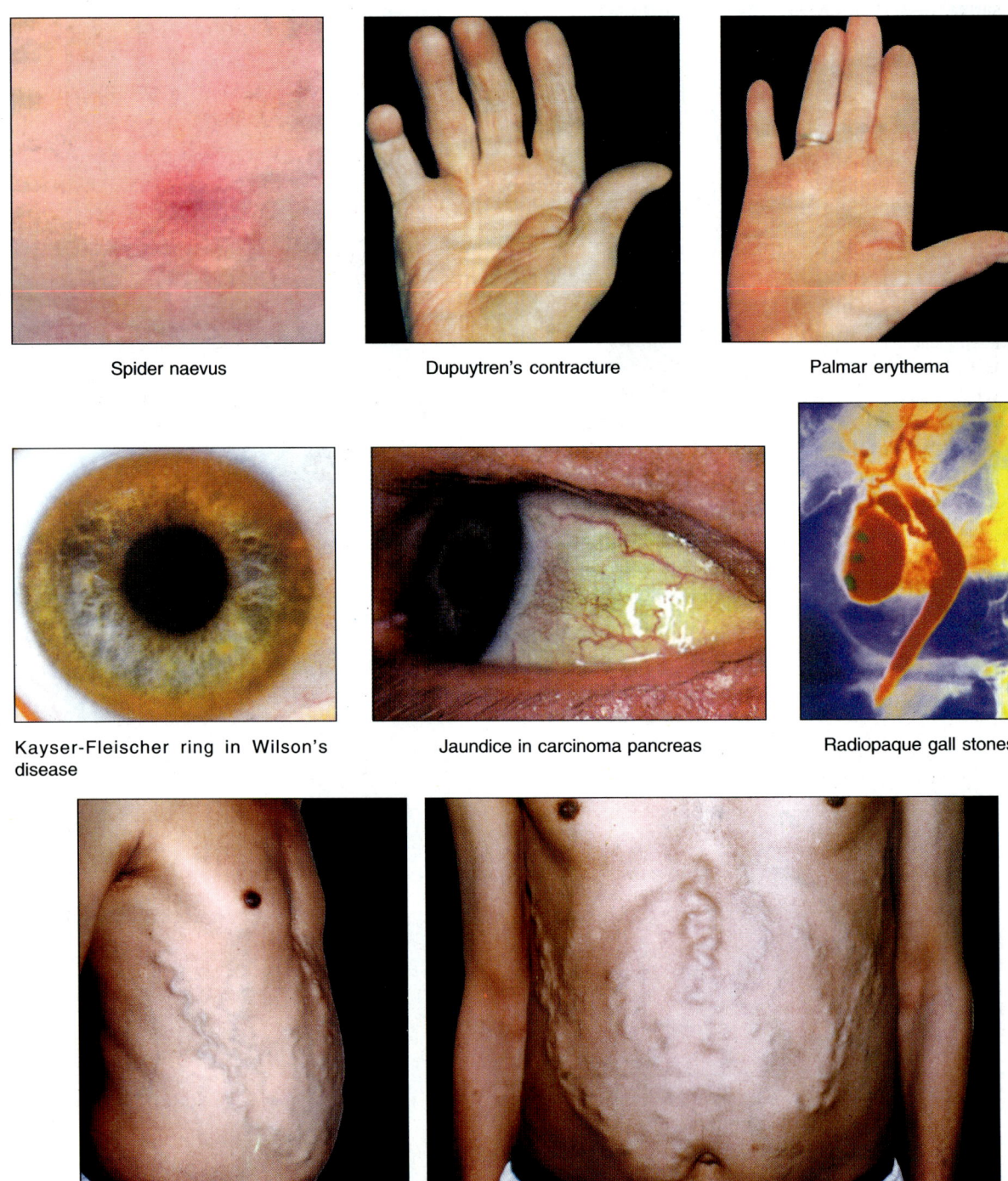

Spider naevus

Dupuytren's contracture

Palmar erythema

Kayser-Fleischer ring in Wilson's disease

Jaundice in carcinoma pancreas

Radiopaque gall stones

Figs. (a) and (b) showing dilated abdominal veins in venacaval obstruction

mind and body coupled with the development of saner living and eating habits.

In ulcer patients who are overanxious Alprazolam (0.25 mg) twice a day is helpful and where depressive symptoms are overshadowing the picture, Trimipramine (25 mg) two tablets at bed time are helpful.

Drugs. These include antacids, antisecretory drugs and antispasmodics.

Antacids. Antacids form major tool in the treatment of ulcer and have been used since long. Although an ideal antacid is one which exerts a prolonged neutralizing effect on gastric acid, which is not absorbed from the gastrointestinal tract and which is non-toxic, free from side effects, cheap and palatable does not exist but for therapeutic purposes, a number of antacids are available which give a satisfactory response.

Sodium bicarbonate though a strong acid neutralizer is unsuitable for routine protracted antacid therapy. It liberates carbon dioxide in the stomach and there is risk of alkalosis. Though it gives fastest relief but it lacks demulcent effect and affords no protection to the gastric mucosa.

Among the non-absorbable antacids Aluminium hydroxide is preferred. It has moderate neutralization but good demulcent action. There is no alkalosis and neither acid rebound. Its regular use produces constipation and phosphate depletion from the body.

Magnesium trisilicate is also a good antacid since in addition to slow acid neutralization it acts as adsorbent and because of its gelatinous consistency it adheres to gastric mucosa and yields prolonged neutralizing effect. It has very little side effects.

Magnesium hydroxide is a strong neutralizer of acid and only a small percentage of the salt is absorbed in the small intestines. It produces loose stools or diarrhoea.

Calcium carbonate. It is inexpensive and a strong acid neutralizer. There is acid rebound after use of this drug. A small percentage (10%) of the drug is absorbed from the proximal part of small intestines.

Prolonged use of this antacid shall produce alkalosis and picture like that of milk-alkali syndrome.

In short every antacid has its plus and negative points. Aluminium as well as calcium salts cause constipation while magnesium cause diarrhoea. So a combination of these salts is preferred. Ideally antacids should be given in gel form every four hours since these have a more rapid action. Tablets have to be chewed and are easy to carry. Antacids should be given at 1½ and 4 hours after a meal since this is the time when gastric acidity is maximum. Dosage is 10-15 ml or 1 tablet every four hourly. A last dose of antacid must be given at bed time to control nocturnal acidity.

Drugs blocking acid secretions:

H₂ receptor antagonists. These are the most frequently employed therapeutic agents and inhibit gastric acid secretions both at basal and maximal stimulated secretions level. Various drugs in this group are:

Cimetidine. It is a selective histamine antagonist which blocks the H2 receptor in the gastric mucosa thereby inhibiting histamine mediated hydrochloride secretions.

Side effects include gynaecomastia, leucopenia, thrombocytopenia, mental confusion, lethargy, interstitial nephritis, elevation of transaminases and creatinine levels, pancreatitis, bradycardia and hypotension especially in elderly.

Drug interaction is with diazepam, propranolol, phenytoin and warfarin.

Dosage. Tablet (200 mg)—one tablet thrice a day and 2 at bed time for 6 weeks. Most patients have recurrence of symptoms and have to be given the drug for longer periods.

Ranitidine. It has the same half-life as cimetidine but is six times more potent than cimetidine. Dosage (150 mg tablet) two times a day or 300 mg at bed time.

There are less side effects. Occasional adverse reactions include headache, dizziness, thrombocytopenia, leucopenia, confusion and rarely hepatitis. Special precautions in hepatic and renal failure cases should be taken.

Ranitidine produces faster healing of ulcer and there are less chances of recurrence. It is safe in long-term use.

Famotidine. It is a potent. H2 antagonist and is 8 to 10 times more potent than Ranitidine in reducing nocturnal acid secretions. It is potent and long duration of action makes it an excellent therapeutic agent. It reduces the acid and pepsin content as well as the volume of basal, nocturnal and stimulated acid secretions.

Dosage. One tablet (40 mg) twice a day or two tablets at bed time for 4 to 6 weeks.

Side effects. Headache, dizziness, constipation, diarrhoea, nausea and anorexia.

Drug interactions. It does not interfere with the administration of drugs like warfarin, propranolol, phenytoin.

Precaution. The drug should be used with caution in pregnancy and nursing mothers or those with renal failure.

Antacids

1. Ideal antacid should be potent in neutralizing acid, inexpensive. Not absorbed from G.I. tract and contain negligible amounts of sodium.
2. Combination of two antacids (aluminum hydroxide/magnesium trisilicate/hydroxide) preferable.
3. Give gel/liquid 15 ml preferably one hour and three hour after meals and at bed time.
4. Antacids may act as placebo but do give relief.

Roxatidine acetate hydrochloride. It is also a potent and selective H2 receptor antagonist and markedly inhibits both basal as well as stimulated gastric acid secretions. Absorption of the drug is not effected either by food or antacids.

Dosage. One tablet (75 mg) twice a day for 4-6 weeks. It should be used with caution in cases of hepatic and renal insufficiencies.No drug interaction has been seen.

Side effects include gastrointestinal disturbances, dizziness, restlessness, visual disturbances, drowsiness.

Proton pump Inhibitors:

Omeprazole. It acts on the final step of acid production and thus inhibits intragastric acidity irrespective of stimulus. Because of its antisecretory activity both basal as well as stimulated acid secretions are inhibited.

Dosage. 20 mg once daily for 6-8 weeks it should be used with caution in patients with hepatic and renal insufficiency.

Side effects. Skin rash, nausea, diarrhoea, headache.

Drug interaction with warfarin, phenytoin, aminophylline, diazepam.

Lansoprazole

It has the same effect as omeprazole and by its highly selective mechanism of action it produces inhibition of the enzyme H+K+ATPase in the parietal cells and effects the final stage of gastric acid formation. Thus both basal and maximal stimulated secretions are inhibited.

Dosage. One capsule (30 mg) daily preferably at bed time.

Drug interactions with Diazepam and Phenytoin.

Side effects. Headache, skin rash, diarrhoea.

Pantoprazole. It is a proton pump inhibitor and inhibits specifically the gastric H^+ K^+ ATPase enzyme which is responsible for acid secretion in the parietal cells of the stomach. It gives symptomatic improvement and healing of both gastric and duodenal ulcers as well as reflux oesophagitis.

Dose 40 mg tablet per day either during or before breakfast. The drug is to be given for two weeks in a case of duodenal ulcer and 4 weeks in gastric ulcer.

Side effects include Headache, diarrhoea, Pruritis, Dizziness and rarely skin rashes.

Esmoperazole. It is also a proton pump inhibitor and works by decreasing the amount of acid produced by the stomach. Esmoperozole is one of two stereo enantiomers in omeprozole.

It is specially indicated in the treatment of oesophageal reflux disease, healing and maintenance of healed erosive oesophagitis. It is also indicated for eradication of H. Pylori in combination with antibacterial agents. Dose 20-40 mg once daily for 4 to 8 weeks. Side effects include Headache, diarrhoea. Abdominal pain nausea and increase in levels of creatinine, uric acid, Bilirubin and alkaline phosphatase. If used for long periods, esmoperazole may interfere with the absorption of drugs because of its effects on gastric pH.

Rabeprazole Sodium. It is also called proton pump blocker. It suppresses gastric acid secretion by the specific inhibition of H^+/K^+ ATPase enzyme at the secretory surface of the gastric parietal cells. Dose 10-20 mg to be taken once daily in the morning. Drug is specially recommended for active duodenal and benign gastric ulcer, erosive gastro oesophageal reflux disease (GORD) and their long term management. Side effects include headache, Diarrhoea, nausea, asthenia, dizziness and flu syndrome.

Precaution should be taken to exclude gastric or oesophageal malignancy before starting the drug. Drug interacts with ketoconazole and digoxin.

Mucosal coating agents. These are the drugs which act as mucosal protecting agents. They do not have any effect on gastric secretions i.e. of inhibition or neutralization of gastric juice.

Carbenoxolone sodium. A synthetic preparation of liquorice root. It has been shown to prolong life span of gastric mucosal cells thus altering quality of gastric mucus and increasing mucosal resistance from acid pepsin attack. Healing properties of the drug are substantial.

Side effects include sodium retention, hypokalemia with resultant oedema and hypertension, muscle weakness. Because of these side effects the drug is not much used.

Sucralfate. It is a complex combination of aluminium hydroxide and sulphated sucrose. It is maximally absorbed and is similar to antacids and H-2 receptor antagonists in its effectiveness in ulcer patients. It acts locally by binding to the ulcer site and preventing contact of gastric juices with the mucosa. It also produces endogenous Prostaglandins E-2 and thus increases local mucosal defence. It is effective in the treatment of duodenal ulcer and preventing its recurrence.

Dosage. One tablet (1 gm) four times daily one hour before meals and at bed time for 4-8 weeks.

An antacid should not be taken half hour before or after sucraflate. Special care has to be taken in patients with renal impairment.

Side effects include G.I. symptoms like constipation, abdominal distension.

Drug interaction with tetracyclines, phenytoin, H-2 blockers, digoxin, warfarin, theophylline.

Anti-spasmodics, anticholinergic agents. Anticholinergic drugs act by inhibiting the vagal influences governing the secretion of hydrochloric acid and the effects of acetylcholine on muscarine cholinergic receptors. These drugs decrease the gastric acid secretions and diminish gastric motility and are good adjuvants to other therapy like antacids, H_2 receptor antagonists.

Belladonna group of drugs are the earliest one to be in use. These give relief to pylorospasm which is bound to occur in every case of ulcer. The decrease in gastric acidity, reduction in volume of gastric secretions and inhibition of gastric motility are major beneficial effects in a case of ulcer.

Earlier on tincture belladonna 5-10 ml was used but now synthetic preparations are preferred.

Propantheline (Probanthine). Dose 15 mg thrice a day and at bed time.

Oxyphenonium Bromide (Antrenyl) 5 mg thrice a day.

Side effects include dry mouth, blurred vision, constipation, difficulty in micturition, suppression of sweat and saliva, cardiac arrhythmias.

Drug is contraindicated in patients with glaucoma, prostatic hypertrophy, coronary heart disease, impaired gastric emptying.

Prognosis. If a patient of an ulcer follows strictly the diet regimen, avoids offending substances, takes adequate physical and mental rest along with proper dosage of drugs (antacids, H2 receptor antagonists, etc), the chances of healing of an ulcer are good.

But there may be few cases where:

a. There is failure of medical treatment
b. Development of complications like haemorrhage, pyloric obstruction, perforation or suspected malignancy
c. Recurrence of ulcer.

In all such cases surgery is contemplated.

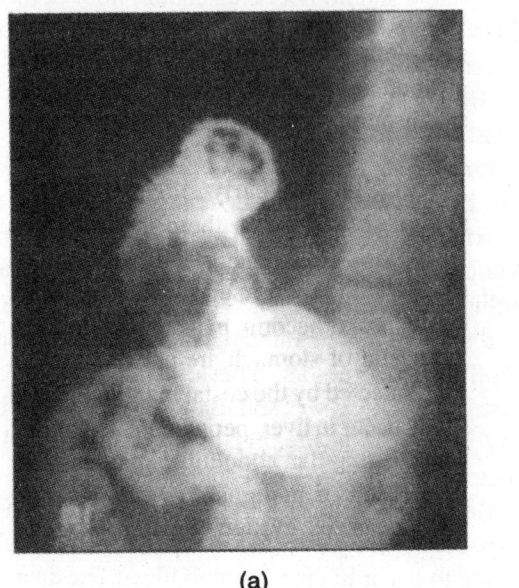

(a)

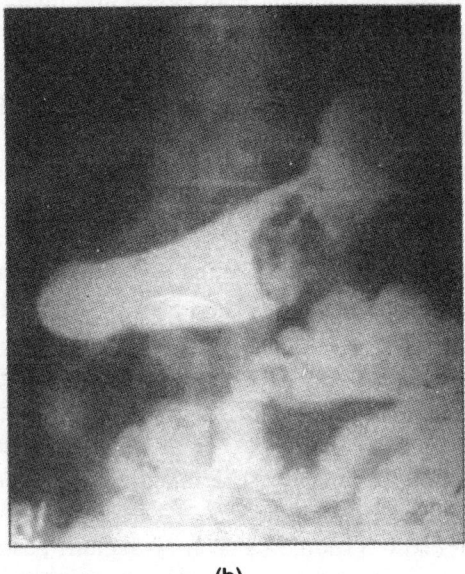

(b)

Fig. 2.24. Barium meal stomach and duodenum in carcinoma stomach. Note Filling defect

Type of surgery:

Billroth type I or partial gastrectomy is recommended for patients with gastric ulcer where lower part of stomach is removed and anastomosed with duodenum.

Vagotomy with antrectomy, vagotomy with pyleroplasty or highly selective vagotomy are the procedures adopted for a case of chronic duodenal ulcer.

The main complications after surgery are recurrent ulceration, diarrhoea, afferent loop syndrome presenting with vomiting, reflux gastritis, dumping syndrome, steatorrhoea, malabsorption and anaemia.

Carcinoma of the stomach

It is the commonest form of growth of the gastio-intestnal tract, which affects men more as compared to women. It is common in the age group of 50 to 65 years though it does occur at younger age also.

Aetiology

1. Heredity. Some families are more predisposed to suffer from it. It is probably related to its increased incidence in patients of blood group A.

2. Predisposing factors. These include chronic gastritis, gastric ulcer, gastric polyps and atrophic gastritis.

The most frequent type of growth arises from glands in the stomach and generally is an adenocarcinoma. It may arise from a preexisting peptic ulcer. The growth is irregular with hard raised edges. Other forms include a soft fungating polypoid or scirrhous type of disease. The last produces leather bottle type of stomach.

The spread of growth takes place in any direction. It is by direct spread, lymphatics or blood stream. Most commonly it is by direct spread and involves the lower part of oesophagus producing dysphagia as well as the greater and lesser omentum and may even spread to pancreas and transverse colon. It is by way of lymphatics that carcinoma stomach spreads to distant, sites such as liver, mediastinum and produces metastases. Involvement of supra-clavicular glands (Virchow's glands) is important site of spread of metastases. Blood spread is responsible for production of hepatic metastases.

Symptomatology

The earliest symptom is epigastic discomfort, which is in the form of pain immediatel, or soon after meals. After a time the pain become continous but is still increased after meals. At the same time patient starts having loss of appetite which is associated with loss of weight and anaemia. There are bouts of vomiting which are associated with a growth at the pyloric end.

Often the pain of carcinoma stomach resemble that of a peptic ulcer and it being related to food and relieved by antiulcer regime makes, the delay in diagnosis. Substernal oppression and dysphagia occurs when the malignancy is at the upper end of stomach and is involving the lower end of oesophagus. Diarrhoea is uncommon and is associated with gastric stasis. When metastases occur in abdomen and liver, ascites may become apparent. Thrombophlebitis is another less common feature.

Physical signs. In early stages there are no physical signs but later on there is tenderness in epigastric region. A mass may be felt there. It is more so in growths at the pyloric end which lie just right to the umblicus and become palpable while growths of the upper end of stomach are not often palpable as they are protected by the costal margin. Secondary deposits may occur in liver, peritoneum and omentum giving rise to irregular abdominal masses. Ascites occurs as a result of malignant peritonitis. Distant spread of disease is evident by involvement of virchows glands in the left supraclavicular region. A rectal examination may reveal metastases in recto vesical or rectovaginal pouch.

In advanced cases patient is very emaciated and anaemic. There is loss of subcutaneous fat, and elasticity of the skin. Oedema appears over dependent parts.

Diagnosis. It is based primarily on clinical history and investigations. Any person above the age of 40, who has vague abdominal complaints with loss of appetite and weight, Suspicion of gastric malignancy must be entertained and person be investigated.

Most important is Barium meal study of stomach and duodenum. A space-occupying lesion shall be seen. There may be destruction of mucosa, irregularly of the folds and loss of distensibility at the site. Leather bottle stomach shall be suggestive of diffuse growth.

Endoscopy combined with gastric biopsy shall be of importance in making the diagnosis. Gastric secretary tests do not have much role but AHT shall show achlorhydria. A simple gastric aspirate may show mucus and sometimes blood. Exfoliative cytology may be of some use but best way to make diagnosis is by endoscopy and gastric biopsies from various sites of suspected growth.

Treatment. It is mainly surgical but most of the times when a diagnosis is made the growth is inoperable and then only palliative measure have to be adopted.

Subtotal gastectomy is the standard approach for all patients of carcinoma stomach. Here about seven eighth portion of stomach is removed along with both the greater and lesser omentum. Reconstruction of stomach is by polya method. This operation has low mortality. Immediate results are good while long term results are bad.

Total gastrectomy is advocated by some but it carries high degree of mortality and morbidity. Intestinal continuity is restored by anastomosis between the lower end of oesophagus and a Roux loop of intestine.

Prognosis

It depends on the time of making the diagnosis. Earlier the diagnosis better the chances of survival. Involvement of peritoneum and presence of distant metastases carries poor prognosis. Growths in the pyloric region carry favourable prognosis. Type of growth is equally important. Prognosis is very poor in infiltrating type of malignancy.

DIARRHOEAL DISEASES

It may be acute or chronic of long standing. These account as a major cause of morbidity in tropics and are due to number of causes ranging from bacterial, viral, to protozoal ones.

The enteropapthogenic bacteria produce diarrhoea by their ability to invade the intestinal mucosa and to produce enterotoxins or both. The clinical picture produced by these organisms depends on these factors and the level of intestinal tract involved. The intestines respond to enterotoxins by hypermotility which also results from mucosal invasion by these organisms. Once invasion has occurred these bacteria release endotoxins which have potent local and systemic effects. As compared to these vibrio cholera is the classic non-invasive agent producing diarrhoea. Exposure of the intestines to enterotoxins of these organisms results in massive secretion of fluid and electrolytes into the intestines which exceeds the rate of absorption which also continues on. Result is hypermotility of the intestines and watery diarrhoea.

ACUTE DIARRHOEA

It is of varied aetiology. Causes range from infectious causes (bacterial, viral) Protozoal (Amoebiasis, giardia) to non-specific causes like Traveller's diarrhoea, dietetic in indiscretions.

Acute bacterial diarrhoea is associated with inflammation and superficial ulceration of the mucosa of the colon. There is sudden passage of loose ill formed stools with colicky abdominal pain. Of the various organisms responsible Sh. Shigae, Sh. Flexneri, Sh. Boydii' B. dysenteric Sonne, E. coli, Salmonella, Staphylococci accounts as major organisms.

Common organisms responsible for acute diarrhoea

Sh. shigae
Sh. flexneri
Sh. boydii
B. dysenteric sonne
E. coli
Salmonella
Staphylococci
Vibrio cholera
Clostrtidium welchii
Clostridium botulism
Viruses (norwalk, rotavirus)
Protozoal (E. histolytica, giardia)

Most cases of diarrhoea in these cases are of sudden onset with illness coming acutely generally following consumption of contaminated food or water. There is malaise, fever, headache, vomiting, chills, lower abdominal cramps along with severe watery diarrhoea. Cases with insidious onset do not come for several days. As the disease process increases toxaemia becomes apparent. With fluid loss, patient becomes dehydrated, tongue becomes dry, pulse is rapid and muscular cramps appear.

Salmonella group of organisms cause diarrhoea after ingestion of contaminated food. There is headache, fever, malaise, nausea, vomiting and liquid stools often containing mucus and blood. Staphylococal infection initially produces vomiting which is very severe as well as diarrhoea.

Causes of acute diarrhoea

1. *Bacterial.* Invasive: Shigella, Salmonella, Yersinia vibrio parahemolyticus, E. coli (invasive)
   Non-invasive: E. coli, Cholera vibrio, Klebsiella, Clostridium, Staph. aureus, B. cereus
2. *Viral.* Parvoviruses, norwalk, hawaii, echo type 1 & 18.
3. *Protozoal.* E. histolytica, Giardia
4. Toxic and systemic causes
5. Drugs (broad-spectrum antibiotics)
6. Non-specific

Enterotoxin producing strains of E. coli also account for a number of cases of acute diarrhoea where neither bacterial or protozoal organisms are detected. Often diarrhoea may be viral in origin. Various viruses incriminated include Echo group, rotavirus, enteric adenovirus, norwalk and related viruses. Symptoms include fever, vomiting, headache, diarrhoea and general malaise. Many times the disease is self-limiting.

The source of infection in all these type of acute diarrhoeas remains the reservoir in man and animals. Food, milk and water become infected from contamination and infection may be carried by flies. This malady becomes more in summer and rainy months and in people who do not follow the elementary rules of hygiene. Susceptibility also increases in people with poor nutrition and those suffering from chronic debilitating illnesses.

Vibrio cholera is an important cause of profuse severe diarrhoea in our country. It generally occurs in epidemic form though sporadic cases are often seen. Any natural calamity like flood, famine or places where people congregate like fairs and festivals are harbingers of the epidemic of cholera. Some people are more susceptible as compared to others. Thus starvation, excessive exhaustion, poor health, alcoholism and use of excessive purgatives especially during epidemics makes a person an easy victim to the disease. The whole disease process develops in a period spread over few hours to few days. Vibrio cholera is a non-invassive organism which releases large amounts of isotonic fluid from intestinal mucosal cells by its enterotoxins. In moderate to severe cases, there is abrupt onset with painless watery diarrhoea and vomiting which is effortless. Stools contain very little faecal matter and have a classical 'rice water' appearance due to presence of mucus and large number of organisms. Person soon becomes moribund. There is abundant loss of fluid and soon there is electrolyte imbalance and dehydration. Extreme thirst and marked restlessness appears and soon the patient may go into a state of shock and collapse with subnormal temperature. Renal failure preceded by oliguria may be terrminal event.

Food poisoning is much more frequent cause of acute diarrhoea than is generally supposed. There is history of persons taking food from a common source as in an institute or a community feast and large number of people fall ill at the same time. Often some cases have mild symptoms and may be missed. It is the more serious ones which get noticed.

It is not difficult to arrive at the conclusion that the diarrhoea in a particular person is due to food poisoning since several people who took of a meal have either acute gastroenteritis or signs of toxaemia. Generally the infection is either by Salmonella, staphylococcal or Clostridium welchii organisms. The source of infection is generally stale contaminated food. Even stored food which has not been kept under proper refrigeration will produce food poisoning. This is more likely to occur with milk products, and non-vegetarian foods like fish and meats since such foods get rotten early without adequate storage and refrigeration.

Botulism is rather a serious and often fatal form of food poisoning due to organism Clostridium botulinum. Meats, vegetables and fruits which have been preserved incorrectly in tins generally harbour the organism. In such cases the tin is generally swollen up or broken indicating the presence of toxins. Food shows alteration in colour, consistency, smell and taste. Most of the persons consuming such type of food show up with symptoms of illness within 24 to 48 hours after taking the infected food. Vomiting is very common followed by nausea, abdominal distension and cramps associared with diarrhoea. Gradually nervous system gets involved, the heart rate goes up, blood pressure falls and death may follow soon.

Travellers' diarrhoea is another form of acute diarrhoea which effects travellers all over the world who go outside their place of residence. It is especially so in people travelling to Africa, Arabic, Latin American countries and tropics. This is an acute diarrhoea which often incapacitates the person soon after his arrival in that country. There is repeated passage of watery loose stools without any blood, abdominal colic and signs of general ill-health, malaise, headache, weakness. Travellers' diarrhoea is probably due to change in environment and climatic conditions vis-à-vis acquired immunity in local population. Since no specific organisms have been idientified it is presumed that these people suffer from either E. coli or viral infection (Norwalk and Rotavirus).

Hill diarrhoea is another form of diarrhoea which is close to travellers' diarrhoea and occurs in people who visit hill stations during the hot season. Again it is typically confined to tropics, highlands of Sri Lanka, Europe and South America and occurs in people coming from planes who visit hill stations situated at 6000 ft or above. A number of causes ranging from exhaustion, immunity, to protozoal infection have been incriminated yet infection with pathogenic organisms cannot be ruled out. Patient has symptoms of dyspepsia, flatulence, abdominal distension and morning diarrhoea. The person passes four or five stools urgently before noon and surprisingly after that he is comfortable. Stools are large, pale, frothy and do not smell much. An episode of hill diarrhoea lasts only for a few days and subsides of its own.

Acute diarrhoea may commonly be due to dietetic indiscretions and often part of acute anxiety states. It is a common symptom as a side effect of drugs especially antibiotics like ampicillin, amoxycillin and cephalosporins.

Probably one of the commonest causes of diarrhoea in our country is infection with Protozoa like Entamoeba histolytica and giardia. Acute amoebic dysentery generally starts insidiously without much general symptoms. The sufferer generally passes three to four stools with pain and tenesmus in abdomen. In the more severe form there is acute diarrhoea with griping pain and frequent passage of loose motions containing blood and mucus. To start with the stools may be liquid with mucus and blood having a foul odour. Generally there is no fever but in the presence of superadded infection signs of toxaemia appear. In most cases amoebic dysentery can be diagnosed in the presence of tenesmus associated with diarrhoea.

Diagnosis in acute diarrhoea.

1. *History*
   a. Enquire about quantity, frequency consistency and number of stools.
   b. Fever, malaise, vomiting, abdominal cramps.
   c. Recent travel
   d. Food consumed
2. *Physical examination.* Look for evidence of dehydration, pulse, blood pressure.
3. *Stools.* Naked eye and microsopic examination for parasites, RBCs, pus cells.
4. *Stool culture* for bacteria, viruses.
5. *Complement fixation test.*

Giardia, a parasite of worldwide distribution, is often responsible for producing acute diarrhoea in children and young adults. It produces loose illformed yellowish stools containing mucus but no blood. Diarrhoea often alternates with constipation. Symptoms of abdominal colic, nausea, loss of weight, flatulence, fatigue and weight loss may be present.

Diagnosis of acute diarrhoea is based on history in a large number of cases. Dietetic indiscretions, drug intake and moving to another place or hilly areas shall tell the diagnosis of aetiological factors.

Diarrhoea following within 10-12 hours after ingestion of food will more likely be bacterial. Viral diarrhoea mainly effects children and young adults. Vomiting precedes diarrhoea. Cholera is charactrised by passage of watery rice-coloured stools and extreme degree of prostration.

Assessment of dehydration and fluid deficit in a case of diarrhoea:

Mild dehydration:

General appearance	Thirsty, alert, restless
Pulse and BP	Normal
Skin	On pinching, retracts immediately
Mucous membrane	Moist
Urine flow	Normal
Estimated fluid deficit	40-50 ml/kg

Moderate dehydration:

General appearance	Thirsty, alert, giddiness with postural changes
Pulse	Rapid and weak
Respiration	Deep. May be rapid
Blood pressure	Normal or low
Skin	On pinching retracts slowly
Eyes	Sunken
Urine	Dark-coloured, amount reduced
Fluid loss (estimated)	60-90 ml/kg

Severe dehydration:

General appearance	Ill appearance, cyanosis, extremities cold and sweaty, muscle cramps
Pulse	Rapid feeble, often impalpable

Respiration	Deep and rapid
Blood pressure	Low, may be unrecordable
Skin	On pinching retracts very slowly
Mucous membrane	Very dry
Urine	Very little amount passed
Fluid deficit	100-110 ml/kg

Further confirmation can be done by examination of stools for ova and cysts of E. histolytica, giardia. Stools culture for vibrio cholera, shigella, salmonella, staphylococcal and viruses should be done to confirm the aetiological agent.

Viral diarrohea

It persists for a period of 1-3 days Diagnosis supported by absence of polymorph leucocytosis as well of erthrocytes in stools.

Demonstration of virus in stools by electron microscopy. Rise in complement fixing antibody titres. Direct demonstration by ELISA test.

Treatment. In all cases of acute diarrhoea, main thrust is to maintain adequate hydration, electrolyte balance and nutrition.

Treatment of acute diarrhoea:

1. *General.* Rest, maintenance of fluid balance and nutrition (oral/IV fluid), electrolyte replacement.
2. *Drugs.* Specific, non-specific.

Fluid therapy.

– Loss of water and electrolytes from the body in stools, vomit, urine, sweat and insensible losses, matched with fluid intake.
– Oral rehydration therapy useful in only mild to moderate dehydration.
– Progress of rehydration therapy should be assessed after one hour and then every 1-2 hours.
– Assess for number and volume of stools passed. Number of vomits.
– Presence of dehydration: Assess whether rehydration fluids (oral or I/V) are being given in adequate amounts and successfully.

Fluid replacement is to be done to correct the dehydration in the patient. **Dose in a mild to moderate water and electrolyte imbalance.** In mild to moderate cases oral rehydration solution should be given (ORS). This contains sodium (90 mmol/litre) potassium (25 mmol/litre) chloride (80 mmol/litre), bicarbonate (30 mmol/litre) and glucose (111 mmol/litre). An oral solution prepared by dissolving in one liter of water is given at frequent intervals in a dose of 50-100 ml/kg body weight within four hours. Maintain with 100 ml/kg body weight per day till diarrhoea stops. **For patients suffering from severe dehydration or circulatory collapse**, intravenous fluids (5% dextrose, 5% dextrose saline and ringer lactate solution) have to be administered. These are to cover loss of fluid in stools, vomit, and perspiration. Fluid intake should be monitored by level of hydration, pulse rate and blood pressure levels as well as amount of urine passed.

For cases of cholera, the basis of treatment is maintenance of biochemical equilibrium, correction of acidosis and replacement of fluid loss as well as electrolyte balance. Rapid transfusion of hypertonic saline and alkaline hypotonic solution be done. One pint of fluid in 15-20 mts and then 1 litre of saline every 2-4 hours is given at the rate of 50 ml per minute till the pulse is restroed. Infusion (glucose, glucose saline) may reach 18-20 litres. Since there is going to be acidosis because of loss of bicarbonate soda bicarb 100 cc 10% solution I/V twice a day is given. It is important to monitor urinary output, serum sodium, potassium and bicarbonate levels and these be corrected accordingly.

Antimicrobial therapy. Mild to moderate cases of acute diarrhoea may be self limiting and require only general supportive measures like fluid and electrolyte correction along with symptomatic therapy.

Antimicrobial therapy is helpful only where bacterial infection is suspected and it is essential to shorten the course of the disease and to decrease the excretion of causative organisms.

Nalidixic acid is bactericidal to most of the common gram negative organisms like Salmonella,

Shigella, E. coli and Proteus. Dosage is 1 gm 6 hourly for 5-7 days. Special precautions in patients of hepatic and renal insufficiency be taken.

Norfloxacin, a quinoline penetrates into the bacterial cells readily than nalidixic acid exerting a potential bactericidal effect by inhibiting A subunit of bacterial DNA gyrase. For bacterial diarrhoea, hill and travellers diarrhoea, the drug is effective. Dosage is 400 mg twice a day orally for 5 days. It may be combined with Tinidazole 300 mg twice a day for 6 days. Norfloxacin should be used with caution in patients predisposed to seizures and renal insufficiency.

Cases of viral diarrhoea are generally self limiting. For cholera, Injection Tetracycline 500 mg I/M four times a day along with Injection Metrogyl 500 mg I/V 8 hourly for 5 days are effective in addition to fluid therapy. Cases of acute amoebic dysentery or giardia should be treated with Metrogyl 200 mg three times a day x 6 days or Tinidazole 300mg twice a day for 6 days.

For all cases of acute diarrhoea, symptomatic relief by use of anti motility drugs (diphenoxylate-atropine, loperamide) are helpful but these drugs interfere with the excretion of pathogens from the intestines and should be used with caution in the presence of severe toxaemia. Special precautions should be taken in their use in elderly and those suffering from glaucoma, and urinary bladder neck obstruction.

Diet in any case of diarrhoea if there is no vomiting should preferably be liquid and semi solid. Adequate amounts of fluids (ORS) should be given to combat dehydration.

CHRONIC DIARRHOEA

It means diarrhoea persisting for weeks or months, commonly of more than three months duration. Such patients complain of disturbed bowel functions and in majority there may be periods of passing loose stools alternating with constipation. In some there may be general complaints of weight loss, anaemia, malnutrition dyspepsia and abdominal distension.

Chronic diarrhoea may be due to either small bowel involvement or large bowel. In the former group shall be cases of lactase deficiency, malabsorption syndrome, sprue, pancreatic insufficiency due to chronic pancreatitis, bacterial over growth in small intestines, as in diverticulosis, intestinal carbohydrate dyspepsisa, steatorrhoea, post gastrectomy diarrhoea, intestinal tuberculosis, while chronic diarrhoea due to large bowel involvement predominently occurs in ulcerative colitis, irritable bowel syndrome, chronic amoebiasis, diverticulitis and Crohn's disease. In addition endocrinal diseases like hyperthyroidism, diabetes mellitus and adrenal insufficiency are also cause of chronic diarrhoea.

Let us look at some of the common causes of chronic diarrhoea.

Causes of chronic diarrhoea

Small bowel diarrhoea

1. Lactase deficiency
2. Malabsorption syndrome
3. Sprue
4. Pancreatic insufficiency
5. Bacterial overgrowth (diverticulosis, blind loop syndrome)
6. Intestinal carbohydrate dyspepsia
7. Steatorrhoea
8. Post-gastrectomy diarrhoea
9. Intestinal tuberculosis

Large bowel diarrhoea

1. Ulcerative colitis
2. Irritable bowel syndrome
3. Chronic amoebiasis
4. Diverticulitis
5. Crohn's disease
6. Endocrinal disorders. Hyperthyroidism, diabetes mellitus, Addison's disease.

Intestinal carbohydrate dyspepsia. Most of these patients suffer from a feeling of discomfort and distension in the lower part of abdomen. This is because of excessive fermentation of carbohydrates resulting in production of carbondioxide and acetic and butyric acids. In addition there is increased motor activity of the intestines. Large amount of gas collects in the abdomen and during night it passes lower down increasing discomfort, resulting in loss of sleep. Diarrhoea is mild. Large amount of gas is passed with stools which because of increased acid content may cause burning sensation round anus. Stools are foul swelling and contain undigested food and vegetables particles.

Lactose deficiency. A form of disease which occurs in infancy but may be acquired late in life. It is inherted as an autosomal trait. Most such people complain of abdominal discomfort, watery diarrhoea and cramps especially within a short time varying from a few minutes to hours after the ingestion of milk and milk products.

Lactose intolerance. Common in children. Starting in adult life equally common.Compatible with good health.

Patient complains of abdominal discomfort. Flatulence, colicky pain and diarrhoea within one or two hours of taking milk. Diagnosis confirmed by giving 50 g of lactose which should reproduce the symptoms and give a flat blood glucose curve. Management by lactose-free diet.

Milk intolerance is very common amongst the Indian population and one rough estimate puts that probably one out of every tenth Indian is experiencing intolerance. It is due to lactose intolerance as well as deficiency of disaccharide enzyme in intestines; the acuteness of the problem depending on the degree of lactase deficiency. Impressions about lactose intolerance being responsible for causing chronic diarrhoea are not difficult to make when the history is there.

Lactase deficient patients get fullness, nausea, abdominal cramps and diarrhoea after drinking milk or taking any food containing lactase. The whole picture depends on the degree of lactase deficiency and the amount of lactose ingested. Stools of these patients are frothy and have a peculiar sour odour.

Coeliac disease. It is a form of disease which begins in early childhood and is characterized by sensitivity to gluten in wheat/cereals and the person suffers from passage of frequent, pale, frothy and foul-smelling stools. There is wasting and growth is effected. Rickets may appear. Patient improves when gluten containing cereals are withdrawn from the diet.

Sometimes the disease may persist throughout childhood. It may disappear completely or diminish by the time the person reaches adolescence. It may reappear in third or fourth decade. Attacks of diarrhoea may be precipitated by intercurrent illnesses or excessive intake of fatty foods. In addition to severe diarrhoea, weight loss and marked weakness are present. Stools are watery semi-formed, frothy and have a peculiar rancid smell. Since these stools contain excess of split fat they often float in water and are difficult to flush.

Patients of coeliac disease suffer from emaciation, weight loss, oedema over legs and feet. Abdomen is protuberant. Skin may bruise easily and bleed. Growth in children is stunted.

Diagnosis of the disease in children is easy especially if a correct detailed history is taken. History is quite helpful. Confirmation in adults is by barium meal study of gastrointestinal tract (dilatation of small intestines with loss of mucosal pattern, flocculation of barium and coin on end apperances of intestinal mucosa) and jejunal biopsy (villous atrophy and a flat mucosa).

Treatment of coeliae disease is by withdrawing of gluten from diet. Diet should be gluten-free but high in protein and low in fats. Anaemia is treated by use of iron, folic acid, vitamin B_{12} and fat-soluble vitamins.

Idiopathic steatorrhoea. It is adult form of coeliac disease characterized by passage of pale, watery, foul-smelling stools, dyspepsia, weight loss, anaemia osteomalacia, tetany and skin lesions.

Various aetiological factors like continuation of defect acquired in childhood, infection, defect in intestinal absorption, pancreatic deficiency and familial predisposition are considered.

Main defect in cases of idiopathic steatorrhoea is interference in absorption function of small intestines. Thus there is defect in absorption of various components of diet like fats, carbohydrates, sugar, calcium, iron folic acid and various other nutrients.

In addition to chronic diarrhoea patient shows wasting distended abdomen, anaemia (macrocytic, iron deficiency), tetany, dry scaly skin and clubbing of the fingers. Diagnosis of condition is made by biochemical investigations; glucose tolerance curve shows flat curve. Faecal fat excretion in 24 hours exceeds 10 gm (normal 5-7 gm). Barium meal study shows flocculation of barium (feathery appearance) and dilated mucosal folds of jejunum (Mulage sign).

Treatment is by low fat diet but with a high calcium and protein content. Anaemia is treated by folic acid, vitamin B_{12} and iron depending on the type of anaemia. In case of tetany, calcium and vitamin D is to be given.

Tropical sprue. It is a syndrome which occurs in people residing in tropics and is characterised by damage to the intestinal mucosa, malabsorption of two or more nutrients, chronic diarrhoea, loss of appetite, abdominal distension, pallor, weakness, sore tongue, oedema of the legs and even night blindness. The stools are watery to start with and become less liquid with the passage of time. Abdominal distension appears but there is no abdominal pain. As diarrhoea persists features of nutritional deficiency appear but in some remissions and relapses take place and diarrhoea tends to disappear.

People of all ages suffer from tropical sprue though adults are more prone to get it. Cases occur both sporadically and in epidemics.

Considerable controversy exists regarding cause of tropical sprue. Though exact cause is not known yet a number of factors ranging from bacterial and viral infections, protein malnutrition to altered immune response have been incriminated.

Characteristic clinical features include diarrhoea, abdominal discomfort, weight loss, anaemia, glossitis, burning feet, oedema and dysponea on exertion. Features of nutritional deficiency are more commonly seen and even night blindness in some due to vitamin A deficiency.

Investigations for malabsorption are abnormal in majority of patients. D-xylose test, fat balance studies are abnormal. Vitamin B_{12} malabsorption is assessed by Schilling test. Bone marrow examination shows megaloblastic bone marrow. Barium meal study of intestines shows dilatation of bowel loops, segmentation, flocculation and thickening of mucosal folds of intestines. Jejunal biopsy shows villous atrophy. Finger-like villi are replaced by flat mucosa, changes in epithelial cells and infiltration of lamina propria by chronic inflammatory cells.

Treatment. Natural remissions may occur in 50 per cent of cases. Specific therapy consists of oral tetracycline (1 gm) daily for 4-8 weeks along with oral folic acid 5 to 10 mg daily. In patients with vitamin B_{12} deficiency, this should be combined with 1000 µg of vitamin B_{12} given parenterally twice a week. In addition supportive measures in the form of electrolyte replacement, diet and symptomatic relief for diarrhoea may be employed. Majority of patients of tropical sprue do well with this line of therapy. Improvement is characterized by relief in abdominal symptoms though appetite and weight loss may take long time to improve. Some patients may get recurrence on cessation of therapy and may require intermittent courses.

Irritable bowel syndrome. Emotions control the intestinal movements to a large extent. Nervous diarrhoea occurs in highly strung individuals as a result of some situation producing emotional strain and is characterized by passage of loose stools after meals. It may be apparent or working subconsciously but is a great source of annoyance and suffering to the individual.

In this group is the disease called 'Irritable bowel syndrome' which affects not only the colon but also other systems and is aptly called a disease of civilization.

All races are known to be effected. It affects mostly adults especially in the age group of 30 and fifty years. It is more common in sedentary and professional workers but uncommon in manual workers.

Aetiology of the condition is poorly understood. Aetiological factors range from disordered motility of the intestines particularly large bowel, emotional factors, chronic infections like amoebiasis to hormonal imbalance. There can be no two views that emotional and psychological factors have a significant role to play in the aetiology of the irritable bowel. There is a definite close relationship between the onset and severity of symptoms of these patients corresponding to emotional upheavals. Heightened sigmoid contractions have been observed in people showing "coping" behaviour (expressed hostility), defensive attitude and feeling of self-sufficiency while there was diminution of sigmoid contractions with "giving up" behaviour (expressions of helplessness, depression, grief, guilt and feeling of personal inadequacy). Patients with irritable bowel have a specific type of personality. They react badly to physical stress and tend to be immature, dependent, rigid and conscientious with high standards of performance and behaviour. Some may show different behaviour patterns. Symptoms of generalized vasomotor instability like palpitation, sweating, flushing, headaches may also be seen. Often the patient is tense, apprehensive, meticulous, rigidly conscientious or deeply introspective.

Psychological stress to some degree is always present in such people and they are often worrying about multitude of small problems which could have been ignored usually. Psychosomatic factors vary from hysteria, anxiety, depression, obsessive compulsive neurosis to variable degree of stress. Very often an attack is triggered by acute stressful conditions.

Symptomatology. The symptomatology of a case of irritable bowel syndrome is as varied as its aetiology. The characteristic symptoms are pain in the abdomen, constipation or diarrhoea, abdominal distension, flatulance, fatigue, depression and feelings of anxiety.

Abnormal bowel habits are present in 75-90% of cases. It may be diarrhoea (either intermittent or constant) or constipation or alternating diarrhoea or constipation. Diarrhoea is steadily or intermittently present. Stools are semi-liquid or mushy in consistency often attended by great urgency or even tenesmus but are non-fatty and small in volume. Movements occur just before and after breakfast. They often contain conspicuous quantities of mucus and some appear to consist of mucus alone. Some patients suffer from episodes of explosive diarrhoea lasting hours or a day and this often leaves the patient exhausted and run down. Another group of patients may go to toilet several times a day, sometimes passing only a small amount of faeces and at other time pouring forth small volumes of liquid faeces.

Constipation when present is either a constant or intermittent symptom and the patient passes small dry hard stools in the form of pellets (Scybala or Rabbit or Sheep Pellets).

Pain is one of the cardinal symptoms and is present in the distribution of colon, lower abdomen or in left lower quadrant. Location of pain is variable and so its time of onset and duration. It may be dull discomfort, colicky, gripping or localized and sharp. The pain is often aggravated by eating or by drinking cold liquids. In more than 50 per cent of patients there is temporary relief of the pain when defaecation occurs and is considered an important point in the diagnosis since the link with defaecation should suggest the linking of abdominal pain to its being colonic in origin.

Increased abdominal distension related to meals and a sense of bloating is also commonly present. This symptom is often associated with inability to pass flatus. Some patients may massage their abdomen to relieve the gas and passage of flatus does afford some relief.

Since psychological factors play a major role in the aggravation of the symptoms, one would observe severely affected patients displaying signs of anxiety, aggression tension and often depression. These people have rather an obsessional compulsive character and have a tendency to worry over small matters easily.

Physical examination. On physical examination the general condition of the patient is good and the person looks well. But the patient often looks tense, is nervous and has cold clammy hands. Otherwise physical examination is non-contributory. There may be abdominal tenderness over part or whole of the colon but the abdominal tenderness is disproportionate to the symptoms complained of.

Diagnosis of irritable bowel syndrome is based mainly on clinical history and being aware of the condition. Often these patients have been suspected to be suffering from amoebic dysentery or colitis for which they have had received extensive treatment but without much significant relief.

Broadly speaking three-step approach to diagnosis of IBS is indicated. Firstly identify the symptom complex of the disease and its features which have been aptly described as follows (Manning Criteria).

1. Visible abdominal distension
2. Abdominal pain relieved by a bowel action
3. Looser stools with onset of pain
4. More frequent stools with onset of pain
5. Rectal passage of mucus and
6. A sensation of incomplete evacuation.

Majority of the patients of IBS shall satisfy more than one of Manning's criteria. Secondly recognition of the coincidence of periods of life stress and emotional disturbances with triggering of the disease. Thirdly search for any other disease process pertaining to the patient's symptoms and exclude any other organic disease.

Irritable bowel syndrome. Also labelled as mucous colitis, spastic colon, unhappy colon.

Three cardinal complaints

1. Abdominal pain
2. Disordered bowel function (constipation and/or diarrhoea)
3. Discomfort after meals. Often a feeling of bloatedness.

Diagnosis of irritable bowel syndrome is rather complex and it should be differentiated from ulcerative colitis, malignancy of gastrointestinal tract, thyrotoxicosis, etc. It is imperative that the clinical picture should be identified with the symptom complex and related to periods of stress in life and emotional tension.

Investigations include haemoglobin estimation, sedimentation rate, stools examination, sigmoidoscopy, rectal mucosal biopsy, barium enema and manometric studies.

The patient generally has got normal haemoglobin levels and ESR is also normal. If these figures are significantly abnormal, the diagnosis of irritable bowel should be suspected.

Repeated stools examination should be done to exclude parasitic infestations. Sigmoidoscopy is an important diagnostic aid since it helps in excluding organic diseases of the colon like ulcerative colitis or carcinoma.

In irritable bowel the mucosa is slightly hyperaemic with loss of clear vascular pattern but the flushed mucosa is not fragile and does not have any tendency to bleed. Excess mucus may be present. The colon may go into spasm when the instrument is manipulated and make the passage beyond rectosigmoid junction difficult. Insufflation of air into the colon may lead to reproduction of pain.

Aetiology

1. No specific cause known
2. Psychological basis important
3. Bowel infection predisposes to the condition
4. Regular intake of laxatives may be another causative factor
5. Obsessional personality. Tendency to worry easily over small matters.

Includes variety of colonic disturbances in the absence or organic disease.

Twice more common in women than in men; occurs principally in early adulthood and middle age.

Uncommon in patients aged less than 20 and above the age of 60 years.

Rectal biopsy shows basically a normal pattern. Barium enema not only helps in reaching a diagnosis but also excludes organic conditions like diverticulosis, ulcerative colitis and carcinoma, etc. Radiological studies show reduced size of colonic lumen, increased haustral markings (segmentation) and spasticity of the colon when barium is introduced into the colon.

Manometric studies of the lower colon shall show an active basal record with gross accentuation of activity, coinciding with the classical symptoms as seen after a meal or after an injection of prostigmine.

Management. For the management of a sufferer from irritable bowel syndrome, the patient should be treated as a whole rather than the individual symptoms. Irritable bowel syndrome has been an experimental ground for the trials of various regimens but there has not been much evidence to show that these various regimens are of much benefit. The treatment has varied from number of drugs ranging from anticholinergics to tranquillizers to high fibre diets but none has really proved efficaious. The approach has to be multipronged.

Diet is one factor that can be easily controlled so the aim of therapy should be to teach the patient how to live with his symptoms and how to manage them.

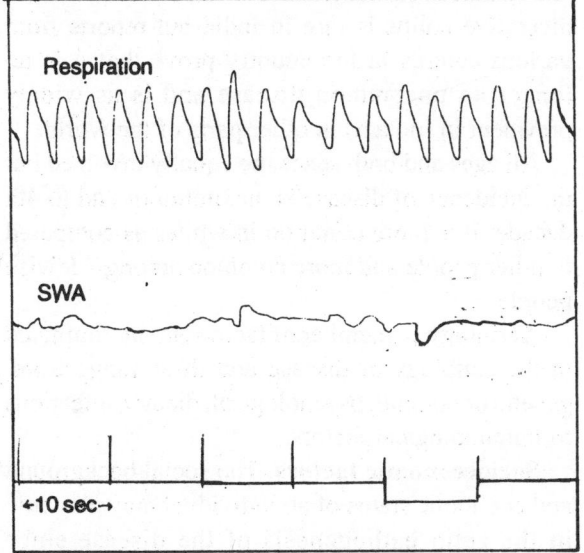

Fig. 2.24. Recordings of myoelectrical activity in a case of irritable bowel syndrome.

Physical examination. Patient looks well. Tense disposition.

Abdominal tenderness common over part or all of the line of colon:

Sigmoidoscopy	Essentially normal. Excess mucus present. Mucosa does not bleed readily.
Barium enema	Evidence of irritability, segmental spasm of the colon. Reduced size of colonic lumen
Rectal biopsy	Normal
Manometry	Increased colonic motility

For most patients a balanced, sensible and attractive diet should be prescribed. Those who suffer from constipation, high fibre diet should be advised. The patient can increase the amount of fibre by taking fruits and cooked vegetables in sufficient amounts. Those whose main complaint is diarrhoea,

food has to be soft and easily digestible. High fibre-containing foods have to be restricted initially but as the patient improves, gradually small amounts have to be added. Omission of cold liquids, soft and carbonated drinks, coffee, etc. also helps. Some patients do not tolerate certain foods like apples, tomatoes, salads etc. which should be avoided. A low lactase diet can also be helpful. Majority do not tolerate beer and alcohol. For those complaining of excessive flatus and bloating, legumes, onions and members of cabbage family be avoided.

There are no two opinions that that bulk producing substances like Isapghula husk, methyl cellulose, or bran should be prescribed and are really going to be beneficial. In most patients supporting therapy combined with symptomatic measures is sufficient to afford relief. Patient should be assured and be talked into opening discussion about his personal history, environment, home and work life so that tension factors in the patient's life be gone into. It has been rightly said that there can be nothing more devastating statement than to tell the patient that there is nothing organically wrong with him. Good results are achieved if the physician adopts a sympathetic approach and gives the patient opportunity to adjust to his environment and problems.

Placebos are of little benefit in such persons. A combination of tranquillizers with antidepressant effect, antispasmodics and antichlinergics are effective in the treatment of such patients.

For diarrhoea, symptomatic relief can be obtained by short-term use of lomotil (diphenoxylate monohydrate) 5 mg four times a day since it acts quickly. Loperamide 4 mg has same effect but fewer side effects. Codeine phosphate may also be used for same purpose but codeine should not be used in patients with spastic colon for it shall make the spasms worse. Similarly in patients of painless diarrhoea, anticholinergic drugs make the symptoms worse. The usefulness of sedatives and tranquillizers in the management of these patients cannot be ignored. A number of drugs ranging from phenobarbitone, diphenylhydantoin, meprobamate, trifluoperazine, to trimipramine have been employed with beneficial results. But these drugs cannot be recommended for long-term treatment.

Mebeverine, a phenyl ethylamine derivativie of reserpine, has a strong papaverine-like effect on smooth muscle of gut but with little or no atropine-like effect. It is a valuable drug since it has a direct smooth muscle relaxation effect and side effects are less. Dose is 100 mg tablet four times a day orally before meals. The treatment has to be continued for 4-6 weeks. Probanthine (propantheline bromide) 15 mg four times a day also gives relief though the side effects are there.

Majority of patients shall achieve relief with the combined therapy along with dietary control and psychological help but there are going to be still few where emotional factors arising from circumstances beyond their control shall make the problem a bit tricky. Though one has to bear in mind that psychological factors per se do not cause symptoms of irritable bowel syndrome. In some centres "Relaxation treatment" with aid of hypnosis has been employed and has been reported to be beneficial. Yoga and meditation shall also be other ways of looking at this problem. The ultimate prognosis in patients of irritable bowel syndrome is good. Patients may not be symptom-free for long periods though subjective relief may be there. Those in whom no psychological factors are apparently present, probably have worse prognosis and are difficult to manage.

Ulcerative colitis

An important but serious cause of chronic diarrhoea is ulcerative colitis.

It may be defined as a diffuse non-specific inflammatory disease of unknown aetiology which involves primarily the mucus membrane of part or whole of large intestines associated with ulceration. It is often called proctocolitis since rectum is invariably involved while a variable portion of the colon may or may not be involved. It may be acute, subacute or chronic following a variable course of relapse and remissions often going to severe form of disease with many local and systemic complications.

Incidence. Ulcerative colitis is universally prevalent throughout the world. Its incidence varies from country to country and from region to region. In varying proportions it occurs all over the world irrespective of environmental factors, and social difference. Generally it is in the range of 6.5 to 0.2 per 1,00,000 of the population in countries like England, Japan, USA, Norway, Spain, Austria, Iran and India. An earlier erroneous impression was that ulcerative colitis is rare in India but reports from various centres in the country prove that it is no longer an uncommon disease and is as widely prevalent in India as in other parts of the world.

All ages and both sexes are equally involved but the incidence of disease is maximum in 2nd to 4th decade. It is more common in whites as compared to other people and more common amongst Jewish people.

Aetiology. A member of factors are incriminated in the aetiology of disease and these range from, genetic or familial, psychological, dietary, infections to immunological factors.

Socioeconomic factors. The social background and economic status of an individual may play role in the aetio pathogenesis of the disease since repeated infection with bacteria or parasites is known to predispose to the ailment and people with poor social background fall easy prey to them.

Familial and genetic factors. The presence of ulcerative colitis in more than one member of the family is seen. It may be due either to genetic or environmental factor although not necessarily sex-linked. About 15-30% patients of ulcerative colitis have positive family history.

Persons with HLA (B5, DW35, BW35, BW40, AW24 and A2) are more prone to suffer from the disease. These genetic factors probably render the person more susceptible to the disease which may be precipitated by external agents like bacteria, viruses environmental pollutants, dietary agents and stress.

Psychosomatic factors. A particular type of personality has been described which is more prone to suffer from ulcerative colitis. These persons are generally timid, unable to express anger, with a tendency to nurse unexplained grievance; an abnormal dependence on some other person (often the mother) and an extreme sensitivity to strife or personal slight. Great importance has been attached to different behaviour patterns of patients with ulcerative colitis. Such people are often labelled as infantile, egocentric, hesitant and uncertain with few of there ideas being acted out into reality.

There is little doubt that emotional upsets like broken marital relations, loss of a family member, failure in exams, love relationship often initiates or precipitates an attack / relapse of ulcerative colitis. Though emotional factors play an important role in the aetiology of disease but often it has been doubted whether psychological factors are actually responsible for the initiation of the disease process though they are important for maintaining or prolonging an already existing disease. Feelings of anxiety, restlessness and even depression accompanying an attack of ulcerative colitis are important factors in modifying the course of the disease.

INFECTIOUS FACTORS

There is no clear cut evidence to implicate various infectious agents like bacteria, fungi or viruses. But it has been seen that frequency of cases of ulcerative colitis runs inversely parallel to that of infectious dysenteries. In susceptible individuals, the gut shows an altered reaction to a bacteria constituent or by combination of bacterial agents and their products, there is change in the relationship of bacteria with the bowel wall. Viral aetiology of the disease has been considered since there is clinical similarly between cases of ulcerative colitis and that of colitis due to viral aetiology. Often there is onset of ulcerative colitis after a viral illness. Then there is relationship between acute viral enteritis and flare up of a case of ulcerative colitis. Moreover there is no evidence of any seralogical abnormality in cases of ulcerative colitis.

Dietary factors. Some patients of ulcerative colitis are sensitive to food like milk, cornflakes and food deficient in fibre. Many patients remain well when milk is excluded from their diet but relapse soon after it is included. Two hypothesis have been put forward to explain this sensitivity that it is due

to an immunological reaction to milk proteins and that it is secondary to lactose intolerance. Though circulating antibodies to milk proteins are demonstrable in some normal subjects but there is an increased titre of these antibodies in patients of ulcerative colitis. Further early weaning from breast milk is twice as common in patients who later developed ulcerative colitis. The possibility of development of antibodies to cows milk perhaps during infancy may be the cause in these cases. But there is no concrete evidence to implicate dietary factors in cases of ulcerative colitis. High titres of milk antibodies found is more a consequence rather than cause of the disease.

Aetiological factors in ulcerative colitis

1. **Heredity and constitutinal factors:** 15-30% patients have positive family history. Persons with HLA (B5, DW35, BW40, AW24) more prone to suffer.
2. **Dietary factors:** Sensitivity to foods like milk. Circulating antibodies to milk proteins in patients with colitis.
3. **Psychosomatic factors:** Symptoms may be intiated by emotional upset. Particular personality type.
4. **Immunological factors:** Associated with immunologically mediated conditions. Presence of humoral antibodies to colon cells, bacerial antigiens.

Immunological factors. An immune mechanism has been involved to explain the pathogenesis of ulcerative colitis. This concept is based on the association of ulcerative colitis with immunologically mediated conditions such as iritis thrombocytopenic purpura, SLE etc. Moreover extra intestinal manifestations of ulcerative colitis such as arthritis, erythema nodosum, cutaneous vasculitis and autoimmune haemolytic anaemia represent autoimmune phenomenon. Patients with ulcerative colitis have humoral antibodies to colon cells, bacterial antigens, lipopolysoccharide and foreign proteins such as cow milk protein. Factors against auto immune theory include presence of ulcerative colitis in patients with IgA deficiency and agammaglobulinaemia. There is lack of increased frequency of immune complexes in patients of ulcerative colitis. But there are associated abnormalities of cell mediated immunity like cutaneous anergy, decreased responsiveness to various mitogenic stimuli and decrease in the number of peripheral T cells. There is depression of cell mediated response. However humoral antibodies are probably the consequences rather than a causative or precipitating factor in the disease.

Clinical presentation. The sufferer from the disease presents with loose stools containing blood and mucus. Diarrhoea consists in urgent passage of small quantities of blood stained discharge. The disease appears in adult and early middle age. Often the patient ascribes the start of illness to an emotional trauma or some alteration in life style.

The disease varies in its severity, the symptoms may range from the passage of small amounts of stools with rectal bleeding or there may be severe fulminant diarrhoea accompanied by considerable colonic bleeding, anaemia weight loss and toxaemia.

Mild form of colitis is the most common form of disease and is present in 80 per cent of the people. Neither colonic bleeding nor diarrhoea is severe in such cases. Generalized symptoms of toxaemia are either absent or present very minimally. There may be little bleeding in the absence of diarrhoea or short episodes of fatigue and lower abdominal discomfort. As the disease progresses the number of stools passed increases and these invariably contain blood. Mild low grade fever may appear.

Involvement of the whole or most of the colon leads to the passage of frequent liquid stools. Blood is usually mixed intimately with the stools and is often passed alone without faecal matter. Besides the liquid stools the patient is also troubled by urgency of defecation due to rectal inflammation.

Clinically ulcerative colitis may be classified into acute form often coming abruptly with fulminating course and a chronic insidious form which progresses slowly with periods of remissions and relapses.

Acute cases come with dysentery like picture with passage of blood and mucus. In chronic cases there may be abdominal pain and tenesmus.

Generally proximal part of colon is spared but the distal colon is severely diseased. The normal proximal bowel may become distended with mass of solid faeces leading to pain, distension and occasional passage of hard stools. Severe cramping abdominal pain indicates severe form of disease.

The degree of systemic upset varies widely. There may be toxaemia, high fever, dehydration, anorexia, malaise and rapid weight loss. Presence of abdominal pain, distension indicates severe form of disease.

Course of the disease is variable. It may be continuous though with slight variation in intensity of symptoms but no relief. Remissions and relapses are quite common. Often an acute attack is brought by an emotional disturbance or infection.

The duration of illness defines the shape of colon which is often dilated and thin walled, likely to tear easily. In long standing cases, the colon appears to be short, tube like and is thick walled.

When acuetly inflamed, the mucosa of colon is red, angry looking, swollen and there may be punctate erosions. The ulcers may be superficial or penetrate the whole thickness of mucosa and submucosa.

Physical findings. In mild cases there may be no physical findings except in acute cases, there are signs of toxaemia and dehydration. A chronic case shows nutritional deficiency signs. Abdomen may be distended and tenderness over the colon area may be elicited. Patient looks ill, anxious. There is tachycardia, and pulse rate is raised. Presence of anaemia, weight loss is evident.

Examination of stools is helpful in assessing the severity of disease. In mild cases patient passes blood and mucus alone and with formed stools. In more severe cases liquid stools mixed with blood are passed. A large volume of liquid blood stained faecal material indicates extensive involvement of colon.

Pathology. The disease is mainly confined to the rectosigmoid and distal colon but in some cases it extends to the proximal colon and in a small percentage of cases the whole colon is involved.

In acute stage the colonic mucosa is acutely inflamed, hyperemic, oedematous and is friable.

There are mucosal haemorrhages and formation of small ulcers. With the passage of time, as the disease progresses these ulcers coalese and form large irregular ulcers. These ulcers extend through the mucosa, submucosa and reach down to the muscularis wall. Joining of these ulcers literally denudes large parts of colon leaving mucosal bridge between adjacent ulcers. Reactive development of islands of mucosa results in oedema giving the mucosa a cobbles tone appearance.

Diagnosis: It is based on

a. Clinical presentation and by exclusion of other diseases like parasitic and infective causes. In acute cases leucocytosis is present and sedimentation rate is increased. Blood loss shall be evident by fall in haemoglobin levels. Sigmoidoscopy. It is essential for the diagnosis or exclusion of the disease. In milder cases, sigmoidoscopic finding may be the only abnormal findings. Normally the colonic mucosa is pale and mucosal blood vessels are seen ramifying through it. While looking at a diseased colon, one has to have an impression of the normal or abnormal mucosa, the presence or absence of normal vascular pattern, mucosal oedema and presence or absence of contact bleeding. Presence of contact bleeding and mucosal oedema are almost certain signs of patient having ulcerative colitis. Severity of ulcerative colitis is assessed on sigmordoscopic changes such as:

Mild changes:	Absent vessel pattern Little or no contact bleeding No free bleeding No mucus / Pus in lumen of colon
Moderate changes	Intermediate between mild to severe
Severe changes	Disappearance of normal vascular pattern Profuse contact bleeding Diffuse hyperemia with oedema of mucosal wall Free blood and pus in lumen Inflammatory polyps.

In acute cases ulcers may be seen and the mucosa is acutely inflamed which bleeds on little touch. With healing mucosa becomes granular.

b. Colonoscopy. It is done further to confirm the diagnosis and to assess the extent of involvement of the colon. Multiple biopsies, can be taken from various sites to confirm the diagnosis. Biopsy examination adds to the value of the sigmoidoscopic examination because in a few patients an apparently normal mucosa may be abnormal histologically while in some cases abnormal sigmoidoscopic changes may not be accompanied by histological change. Biopsy/cytological examination are important for excluding conditions such as amoebic colitis and Crohn's disease.

Radialogical investigations

A plain X-ray of the abdomen without preparation gives very important information. Patients of ulcerative colitis show empty colon with air while presence of faeces in the lumen indicates that the colon is normal. The absence of air in an empty part of the colon does not exclude the presence of deep ulcers in that part of intestines. However, a plain X-ray of the abdomen is an important help in making a diagnosis.

Barium enema. It is a classical method of diagnosing ulcerative colitis where both enema filled and post evacuation films are taken.

Mild form of colitis shows a thickened and slightly irregular mucosa. In more severe cases there are ulcers and projection of swollen mucosa into the lumen seen as polypoid projections. With advanced stage there are loss of haustrations with shortening of the bowel. In addition not only there is decreased length of the colon with decreased tone but also decrease in its distensibility and caliber. Colon assume pipe stem appearance.

Differential diagnosis. Cases of ulcerative colitis have to be differentiated from other conditions like amoebic colitis. Crohns disease and tuberculosis of the colon.

Complications. Ulcerative colitis produces both local and systemic complication. These include stricture formation, polyposis, perforation, toxic megacolon, haemorrhage and carcinoma. Anaemia is an important complication as a result of constant blood loss. An autoimmune haemolytic anaemia is occasionally seen in cases of ulcerative colitis.

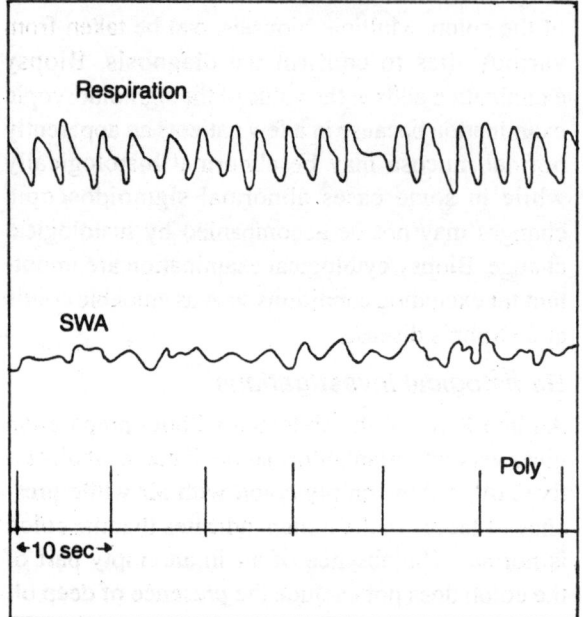

Fig. 2.25. Recording of myoelectrical activity in a normal subject

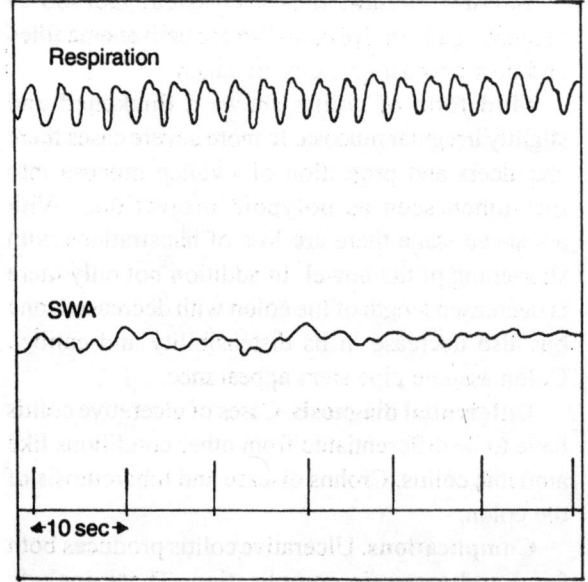

Fig. 2.26. Recording of myoelectrical obtained in a case of ulcerative colitis.

Two important skin lesions seen are erythema nodosum and pyoderma gangrenosum. Moniliasis and aphthous ulceration in the mouth are also commonly associated with the disease. Iritis, uveitis, episcleritis, arthritis and involvement of liver are other complications.

Management of ulcerative colitis. It depends on the severity and acuteness of the condition and may be grouped under two headings:

1. General measures
2. Specific therapy

General measures. Bed rest is advised only in acute cases while patients with milder and chronic form of the disease can continue with their occupation and daily chores.

Malnutrition is present in majority of cases due to insufficient food consumption, anorexia together with excessive nitrogen loss of blod, mucus and necrotic material. There is loss of large quantities of fluids, electrolytes and particularly potassium in the stools.

All patients to some extent have anaemia especially iron deficiency type. Blood loss combined with increased metabolism due to toxaemia increases the demand for nutrition. Diet in all patients oᶠ colitis should be soft, non-roughage, nutritious and well balanced. Milk and milk products are restricted and only given if patient tolerates.

Ulcerative colitis

Defined as a diffuse non-specific inflammatory disease of unknown aetiology affecting primarily mucous membrane of part or whole of large intestines associated with ulceration.

Almost always involves the rectum and extends variable distance to involve anything upto entire colon and even the terminal few inches of ileum.

Inflammation gererally is of an exudative and vascular type with unproductive granulation tissue or fibrosis.

On an average diet containing 2000 to 2500 calories per day containing at least 80-100 gms of protein per day is advised. Fats are permitted in small quantities while carbohydrates which shall form

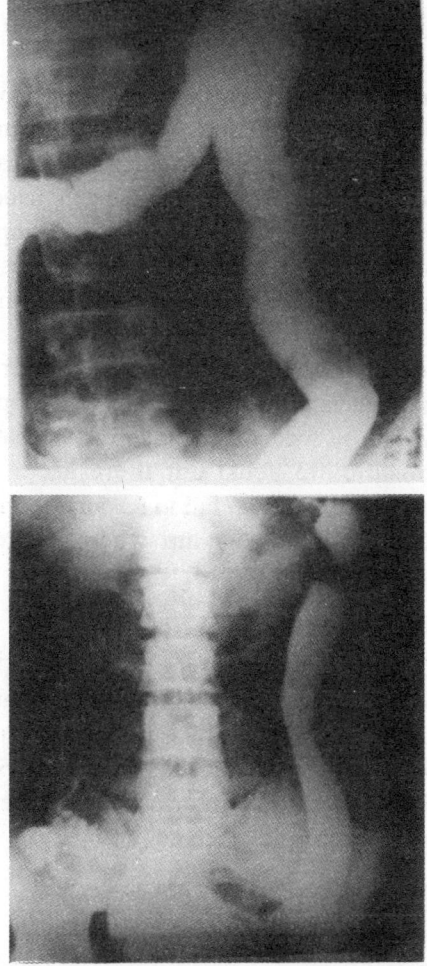

Fig. 2.27. Case of ulcerative colitis. Colon has got pipe stem appearance. Loss of haustrations.

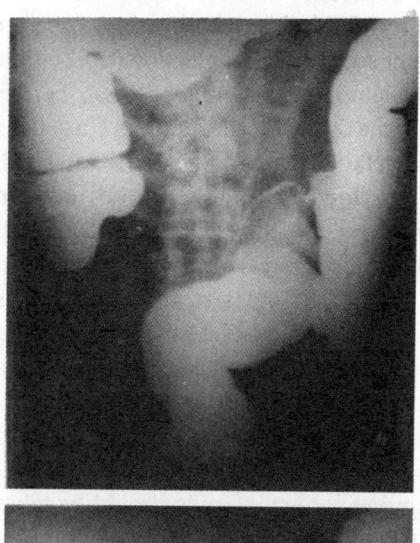

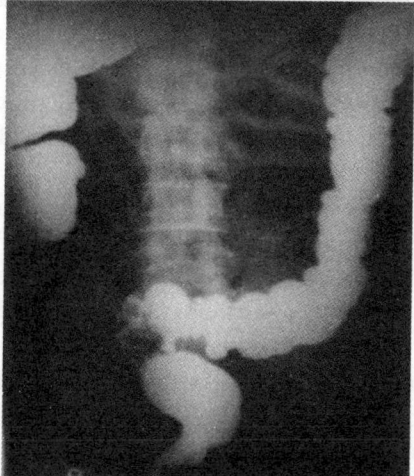

Fig. 2.28. Normal barium enema (a) shows dilated colon after barium enema. (b) normal haustrations after evacuation of barium

bulk of diet have to be given in sufficient quantity. Only easily assimilable food such as Sago, custard, rice, puddings etc. have to be given in acute stage. In cases of severe dehydration I/V fluids be given. Parenteral plasma or blood transfusion may have to be given when excessive blood loss is present.

Sodium loss is quite substantial in the faeces (approximately 100 meq/litre of stools) while potassium loss is even more (30 meq/litre of stools). Potassium loss may manifest in weakness, abdominal distension, asthenia and aches and pains

in body. Both electrolytes balance should be maintained by giving these salts either orally or parenterally in intravenous fluids.

Suitable mineral and vitamin supplements have to be given. Iron may not be tolerated orally and in severe form of iron deficiency, parenteral iron may be employed.

Specific therapy:

Corticosteroids. These form the main line of treatment. Dosage is Tablet Prednisolone 60 mg/

per day in divided doses. In acute cases or relapse Injection ACTH (20 units by slow intravenous 8 hourly) or ACTH depot injection (40-80 units once daily by intramuscular route) is very beneficial to tide over the crisis. Steroids produce a sense of well being with fall in temperature and toxaemia. Dosage is tapered slowly over a period of days and oral prednisolone substituted. Oral or injectable steroids have their side effects and it is desirable to have effect locally at the site of maximal disease. Hydrocortisone Hemisuccinate retention enemas is given. On an average patient requires at least one or two enemas daily with a total of 7-10 enemas. Retention enemas are contraindicated in toxic megacolon and impending perforation. Precautions while giving patient steroids should be taken since peptic ulceration, diabetes, pulmonary tuberculosis may be worsened. Side effects include moon shaped facies, cushings, muscular weakness, psychosis, hyperglycemia, hypertension, osteoporosis, delayed healing of wounds and Hirsutism.

Salazopyrin (sulfasalazine). An azo compound of salicylic acid and sulphapyridine is an effective drug and is poorly absorbed in the intestines. The drug is free from side effects of corticosteroids and is used on long term basis in chronic form of colitis.

Dosage is 1-2 gm (1 tablet 0.5 gm) 3-4 times daily for 3-4 weeks and afterwards patient is kept on maintenance dosage of 1.5-2 gm daily. Side effects include gastrointestinal symptoms (dyspepsia) haemolytic anaemia and skin rashes. To minimize dyspepsis and G.I. upset, the drug is preferably given after meals.

5-Aminosalicylic acid (mesacol). It is a metabolite of sulfasalazine, the drug which has been used to manage ulcerative colitis, 5-Aminosalicytic acid is the active moiety responsible for the beneficial effects attributed to sulphasalazine. The mode of action is topical rather than systemic and acts by diminishing inflammation by blocking cycloxygenase and inhibiting prostaglandin production in the colon.

The drug is safe and more effective than salazopyrin. Dose 3-6 tablets daily in divided doses (1 tablet 400 mg). Side effects include G.I. upset (loose stools, nausea, headache, fever, weakness and malaise). In addition to oral form, 5-aminosalicylic acid is also given in the form of enema in acute cases.

Immunosuppressive drugs. Based on the principle of ulcerative colitis being an auto immune disorder, immuno suppressive drugs in the treatment of severe form of colitis have been used and improvement has been seen. Commonly employed drug is 6-Mercaptopurine (Purinethol). Dosage is 50 mg tablet daily. Side effects include bone marrow depression and liver cell damage.

Success of medical treatment. Majority of patients of ulcerative colitis improve with supportive therapy and on medical regimen (corticosteroids, 5-aminosalicylic acid) but there are a small percentage of cases who fail to respond to medical treatment. It is this group where surgery is contemplated.

Main indications for surgery are:

1. Chronic continuous type of ulcerative colitis which does not respond to medical treatment.
2. Cases of colitis with complications such as perforation, stricture, carcinoma, persistent fistula, massive haemorrhage, toxic mega colon may require emergency surgery.

Two types of operations are advised:

1. Ileostomy with subtotal colectomy.
2. Colectomy.

Usual operation is ileostomy with colectomy and excision of the rectum performed either in one, two or three stages depending on the condition of the patient. An artificial passage for stools is created over abdomen. Risk of operation is 3% mortality and subsequent morbidity. Immediate relief aftersurgery is of toxaemia. Complications include fluid and electrolyte imbalance, dysfunction of ileostomy and severe skin excoriations.

Results of surgical treatment shall depend on the general condition of the patient especially the pre-operative condition. Long term results depend on the nature of the operation rather than severity of the disease.

Once colectomy is decided, a choice must be made between conservation of rectum and restoration of continuity by an ileo rectal anastomosis, total procto colectomy with formation of permanent ileostomy Or construction of an ileostomy with preservation of the rectum. An artificial anus is created over abdomen. An ileostomy drains into a bag supported by a belt and this fits well at waist level. Careful cleaning of the bag is required to prevent unpleasant odour as well as skin excoriations.

Management of chronic diarrhoea

Chronic diarrhoea constitutes a number of diseases of varied aetiology ranging from coeliac disease. Tropical sprue, irritable bowel syndrome, ulcerative colitis to uncommon diseases like Crohn's disease, diverticulitis, endocrinal disease (diabetes mellitus, thyrotoxicosis). Every case in itself shall have its clinical presentation and show varied picture on investigations. So we have to find out the cause of each case of chronic diarrhoea and manage the patient accordingly.

AMOEBIASIS

Amoebiasis is of worldwide distribution and in tropics it is widiely prevalent and one of the most commonly encountered diseases. The disease is caused by infection by protozoan parasite. Entamoeba histolytica gets lodged in the large intestine causing dysentery and may spread to liver and other organs. Infection of the intestines may become chronic and because of persistent ill-health E. histolytica may be harboured in the intestines for number of years without any symptoms.

Entamoeba histolytica exists in two forms—the protected cyst and the active trophozoites. Amoeba gain access to the body ordinarily in contaminated water or food. Flies may directly or indirectly convey the infection. Trophozoites are killed by the acids of the stomach while the cysts which resist adverse environment and are passed intact through the stomach and are carried to lower ileum where the cysts break open by the pancreatic juice. Released amoebae escape and multiply and invade the tissue of the colon wall. From there they may be carried by the circulatory system to the liver, lungs, brain and other organs of the body. The vegetative form (trophozoites) of amoeba are the invasive type, containing ingested erythrocytes within them and are actively motile. Trophozoites in the intestines may become cysts if the conditiions in bowel are not favourable for invasion and they are passed out in the faeces. Cysts-may be ingested again along with contaminated food or water and the life cycle is repeated.

Common source of transmission of cysts is water especially when it is contaminated by faecal matter, the sanitary conditions of water supply being defective. Discharge of sewage into water source is another important cause. Flies spread the infection by feeding upon either faecal matter or contaminated food. Autospread in a patient is equally important when cysts may get embedded underneath the nails and the person may get infection if the hands are not washed properly.

A person may go on passing cysts in the faeces and become a chronic carrier while in others trophozoites may develop from cysts and establish in the colon, multiplying by binary fission. These precystic amoeba are smaller, less actively motile and may persist for long periods without any symptoms, the person acting as a case of chronic amoebiasis or a carrier.

Pathology. Once the active form of amoeba, the trophozoites invade the large intestines, they ulcerate the mucous membrane causing toxic degeneration of the lining cells, necrosis and small abscesses which rupture producing superficial ulcers having undermined edges. As the amoeba further invades into submucosal layers of the colon, large bottlenecked ulcers filled with mucoid material, cell debris, degenerated blood and amoeba are produced. Basic lesion is a lytic necrosis of tissues with mononuclear and polymorphonuclear infiltration.

Maximum involvement of the colon is in caecum, ascending descending, sigmoid colon and rectum.

Descending and sigmoid colon may be considerably thickened and this is an important physical sign in cases of chronic amoebiasis patients. Ulcers in the colon are shallow with necrotic base covered with yellow or brown slough, with surrounding zones of hyperemia and normal healthy mucosa between the ulcers.

Ulceractive lesions generally are confined to the colon and rarely may spread beyond ileocaecal valve. Secondary bacterial infection may play a role in extensive ulcerative lesions. Rarely perforation may occur or when ulceration involves blood vessels, haemorrhage may take place.

Ulcer may heal sometimes of their own due to body's resistance. With repeated low grade infections, both bacterial as well as amoebic, there is scarring of the mucosa and thickening of the peritoneal surfaces, amoebic granuloma or amoeboma may develop. It is generally seen in caecum, sigmoid, and hepatic flexures of the colon.

Invasion of other organs in the body takes place via bloodstream. Liver is one of the commonest sites of involvement. Invasive amoebae reach the liver through mesenteric venules invading portal bloodstream and causing hepatitis as well as amoebic abscess. The same process involves other organs like brain, spleen, lung and other tissues where invasive amoebae produce necrosis and abscess. Cutaneous amoebiasis is a rare manifestation of amoebiasis and occurs in malnourished debilitated individuals by invasion of the skin by active vegetative form of amoebae.

Clinical manifestations. Amoebiasis is known to produce varied symptoms. These may range from symptomless carriers or cyst passers to mild symptomatic infection with gastrointestinal symptoms like chronic constipation, abdominal distension, chronic dyspeptic symptoms, attacks of pain in abdomen, nausea, flatulence, diarrhoea and chronic ill-health.

Incubation period of the disease is variable ranging from 3 weeks to 3 months. Onset is often insidious, patient coming with vague abdominal symptoms, diarrhoea and ill-health.

The two major presentations of amoebiasis are:

1. Amoebic dysentery
2. Amoebic hepatitis/abscess

Amoebic dysentery. It is generally of acute onset with patient passing 10-15 stools, containing blood and mucus with abdominal pain, often diffuse in nature. Constitutional symptoms are mild. When a patient has a fulminating course, the stools may become bulky and offensive, watery in nature, containing large amount of blood and mucus. Palpation of the abdomen may show diffuse tenderness.

As compared to acute amoebic dysentery, cases of chronic amoebiasis suffer from repeated attacks of diarrhoea, stools containing little blood and mucus. Often there is constipation. There is abdominal discomfort, flatulence and chronic ill health. Periods of symptom free intervals may last even for months and these may manifest at time of stress, dietetic indiscretion or any acute illness. Chronic cases of amoebiasis may show a thickened tender sigmoid colon or even an amoeboma which is felt as a sausage-shaped mass in the right iliac fossa, often mistaken for carcinoma of caecum or tubercular infection, or Crohn's disease. A tender hepatomegaly is often present in cases of chronic amoebiasis.

Diagnosis. Diagnosis of ameobiasis is made by the identification of Entamoeba histolytica in the stools in either the vegetative or cystic form. In the acute case mostly trophozoites are found.

For direct examination of amoeba, a portion of stool which might show blood and mucus is picked up and put in a triple mount of three preparations, one is in normal physiological saline, the other is in 2% iodine and the third is in 1% eosin.

The normal physiological saline preparation will serve to detect the vegetative forms of Entamoeba histolytica. Trophozoites are not found in formed stools but when diarrhoea or dysentery is present trophozoites may be identified.

Iodine stains the various vegetative forms and cysts and reveals details of the nuclei while the eosin preparation has a pink back ground and the E. histolytica cysts or vegetative form stand out against it.

Differential diagnosis of acute amoebic and Bacillary Dysentery		
Features	**Amoebic dysentery**	**Bacillary dysentery**
Incubation period	Prolonged weeks to months	Acute, generally less than a week.
Age	More in adults, less in children	All ages. Equally common in children
Onset	Gradual or insidious	Usually acute
Course	Chronic or subacute	Acute or fulminating
Toxaemia	Not common	Often severe
Fever	Uncommon	Present commonly
Bowel	Frequency of liquid stools with blood and mucus, Bulky, foul and offensive. Tenesmus may be present but not common	Frequency of stools with blood and mucus, faecal matter either little or absent. Stools are scanty but more frequent containing bright red blood. Tenesmus is invariably present and can be severe and distressing
Physical signs	Tenderness over the sigmoid descending and ascending colon.	Diffuse tenderness all over the abdomen.
Stool examination	Large number of red cells, degenerated polymorphonuclear cells, trophozoites (vegetative forms/and cysts of E. Histolytica present. Diamond shaped Charcot Leyden Crystals' may be present	Large number of macrophages, polymorphs and a few RBCs.
White cell count	Moderate leucocytosis	Marked leucocytosis in early stage of disease
Sigmoidoscopy	Numerous Flask shaped ulcers with surrounding hyperemia. Mucosa in between normal	No ulcers, mucous membrane inflamed, may bleed.

By stool concentration method, positive results may be obtained where routine smears are negative. Excretion of cysts in stools is cyclical and so at least 4 to 5 consecutive stool examinations must be done to detect cysts in stools. A fresh stool specimen should be preferred.

Sigmoidoscopy. In a patient with acute symptoms, rectal examination should precede sigmoidoscopy to exclude any local organic lesion.

Signoidoscope is inserted carefully with continuous observation of the intestinal mucosa. The typical picture is that of numerous small ulcers with surrounding hyperemia, interspersed with normal mucosa. The mucous membrane surrounding individual lesions is not itself inflamed. Large ulcers are rare. Scraping from amoebic ulcers and biopsies may provide valuable material for establishing the diagnosis.

Serological tests. These are of importance in diagnosing extraintestinal form of amoebiasis. Indirect haemagglutination test, amoebic flourescent antibody titre, countercurrent electrophoresis, indirect immunofluorescence and agar gel diffusion tests are the type of tests employed. Positivity of these tests is high in extraintestinal form of amoebaisis and low in asymptomatic cyst passers.

Complications. Complications in a mild form of amoebiasis are not common. It is generally a fulminating form of the disease which may result in perforation intestinal haemorrhage and retrocolic abscess. Rectal prolapse, colonic stricture, intussusception and peritonitis may develop rarely. Inflammation of appendix due to amoebiasis may occur in some. Amoebomas may develop in long-standing cases of amoebic infection in caecum or other parts of colon. Spread of amoebic infection to liver, lungs, brain, spleen, testicles, and skin may occur.

Differential diagnosis. Cases of acute amoebic dysentery have to be mainly differentiated from cases of bacillary dysentery. Cases of chronic amoebic infection may have to be differentiated from other causes of diarrhoea like ulcerative colitis, irritable bowel syndrome, tuberculosis of gastrointestinal tract. Amoeboma may have to be differentiated from malignancy of the caecum or colon depending on its site.

Treatment. Treatment of amoebiasis is by specific drugs. The ideal amoebicidal drug should kill the amoeba in the lumen of the intestine, in the wall of the intestines and in other tissues. Besides it should be active when given orally as well as parenterally and is safe, non-toxic. Despite availability of a number of antiamoebicidal drugs, the ideal is not there and every drug has its own plus and negative points.

Emetine. It is a powerful amoebiacide effective against trophozoites form but not against cysts of E. histolytica. It produces effective relief in acute amoebic dysentery but is of little use in chronic form of amoebiasis. Drug is effective when given parenterally. Dosage is 60 mg/day given intramuscularly or deep subcutaneously. Total dosage should not exceed 600 mg. Since it is a cumulative drug so patient must not be given the drug continuously. Initially give the drug for six days, give rest for 3 days and complete the course.

Side effects include local irritation at site of injection, tenderness, weakness of the muscles and rarely an abscess at the site. Most important side effects are on cadiovascular system in the form of tachycardia, hypotension, cardiac arrhythmia, myocarditis and pericarditis.

Electrocardiographic monitoring of the patient on emetine is essential. ECG changes in the form of ST segment depression. T wave inversion, prolongation of P-R interval and arrhythmias have to be considered. In view of its cardiotoxic effect, drug is contraindicated in elderly patients and those with pre-existing heart disease. To avoid cadiotoxicity patient must be confined to bed and avoid exertion of any kind. Sudden death while on the drug is known to occur.

Because of its side effects, Emetine is not used commonly except in special circumstances like amoebic liver abscess, brain abscess or where other drugs have failed.

The semi-synthetic form of emetine *dehydroemetine* is less toxic than emetine and is to be preferred. Dosage 60 mg/day I/M for 6 to 10 days.

Iodochlorohydroxy quinoline (Enterovioform, enteroquinol). It is an effective anti-ameobicide useful against cystic form of amoeba. It is not much absorbed from the gastrointestinal tract and its action is due to local effect.

Side effects are generally mild but in patients on prolonged use, a neurological syndrome consisting of peripheral neuritis and optic nerve involvement (subacute myelo optic neuropathy-SMON) has been seen. Because of its toxic effects the drug has been banned and is not recommended. Dosage is 250 mg tablet three times a day for seven days.

Diloxanide furoate (Furamide). It is a potent direct amoebiacidal drug effective in chronic intestinal amoebiasis in cyst passers and in cases with acute form. Its use in extraintestinal form of amoebiasis is of no value.

Dosage is 500 mg three times daily for 10 days. Side effects include gastrointestinal disturbances, nausea, flatulence and skin rashes.

Metronidazole (Metrogyl-flagyl). It is an effective antiamoebicide effective against both cysts and trophozoites. It is effective in most forms of amoebiasis and is almost completely absorbed from the small intestines. It is a valuable drug in the treatment of intestinal as well as extraintestinal amoebiasis. In severe and complicated cases the drug can be given intravenously (Injection Metrogyl 500 mg I/V 8 hurly). Dosage of the drug orally is 400-600 mg three times a day for 7-10 days.

Side effects include anorexia, nausea, metallic taste in the mouth, abdominal cramps, headache, giddiness, vertigo, and peripheral neuropathy.

Drug is contraindicated in neurological disorders, and first trimester of pregnancy.

Tinidazole. This analogue of metronidazole has got slower metabolism and its duration of action is longer. It has a longer half life and is better tolerated than metrogyl. Its spectrum of action is same as that of metroogyl.

Dosage 600 mg twice daily for 6-7 days.

Side effects include furred tongue, metallic taste, G.I. disturbances, dark urine, neuropathy and epileptic form seizures. Special precaution in pregnancy and when patient is on anticoagulants. Alcohol intake is to be avoided while taking the drug.

Secnidazole. It belongs to 5-Nitroimidazole group with longer half life. It is effective for both intestinal and extraintestinal amoebiasis. It is given orally in a single dose of 2 gms. Side effects include nausea, epigastric pain, glossitis, headache, loss of appetite, stomatitis, urticaria, rash, leucopenia.

Special precuations in CNS diseases, liver impairment. It is contraindicated during pregnancy and lactation. Use of alcohol while taking the drug is prohibited.

Management. Cases of acute amoebic dysentery are treated on general supportive measures, fluid and electrolyte imbalance correction. Diet generally is soft, liquid or semi liquid. Metrogyl (400 mg (2 tablets) three times a day for 5 to seven days or Tinidazole (600 mg) two times a day for 5 days is the preferred line of treatment. Relief is obtained within 24 hours. In very ill patients Injection Metrogyl 500 mg in 100 ml infusion is given 8 hourly. When superadded infection is suspected. Tablet Norfloxacin 400 mg twice a day forfour days is added.

Adjuvant therapy in the form of antispasmodics for relief of colic is added.

For cases of chronic intestinal amoebiasis, either metronidazole or tinidazole are the drugs of choice. A single dose of secnidazole (2 gm) may bring about relief in 80-90 per cent of cases. For complete eradication of parasite, repeated courses of anti-amoebicidal drugs may be required.

In addition to drugs, general sanitation, clean water supply and general hygienic principles of personal hygiene must be observed.

AMOEBIC HEPATITIS AND LIVER ABSCESS

Amoebic hepatitis and liver abscess are commonest complications of amoebiasis when amoebae are carried to the liver in the portal venous system causing hepatitis or abscesses. Amoebic dysentery may precede involvement of liver by months and in only 50 per cent of the cases of amoebic hepatitis history suggestive of intestinal involvement is available. Malnutrition, anaemia and alcoholism predispose to the liver involvement in cases of intestinal amoebiasis.

Amoeba after reaching the liver multiply and block small intrahepatic portal radicles, producing thrombosis and infarction resulting in necrosed areas surrounded by areas of congestion. The necrotic area consistsof degenerate liver cells, leucocytes, connective tissue strands and enmeshed in between entamoeba histolytica. Cytolytic enzyme liberated from amoebae destroy the liver parenchyma and fusion of these small necrosed areas results in abscess formation. An abscess generally is single but may be multiple. Its walls are lined by a shaggy necrotic zone in whose center there is thick reddish brown pus containing fragments of liver tissue, necrotic material and erythrocytes. The pus typically is called "Anchovy sauce" like and is sterile on culture.

Many factors govern the progression of hepatitis to abscess formation and these include virulence of the organism and resistance of the host. Most of the times an amoebic liver abscess is solitary involving mainly right lobe of the liver situated supero anteriorly. When a large amoebic abscess reaches the surface, adhesions may be formed with surrounding structures and even rupture may take place. A large abscess may produce compensatory hypertrophy of the other half of liver. In a small percentage of cases (20 per cent) secondary bacterial infection with Staphylococci, Streptococci, Pneumocoeci, Ps. Pyocyaneus and anerobic organisms may take place. The pus now instead of brown, or chocolate colour becomes yellow or greenish yellow and is foul swelling.

Clinical features. Onset of amoebic hepatitis is insidious and patient may come with irregular or intermittent fever. There is stretching sensation in the liver area. Gradually with the progression of disease, anorexia hepatic pain and epigastric discomfort appear. Examination shows a uniform enlargement of liver which is tender. There are signs of toxaemia. Jaundice is not very common.

When hepatitis progresses on to a liver abscess, pain in the liver area becomes a constant feature. Intermittent fever, loss of weight, lassitude, peculiar sallowness of skin, irritability, sleeplessness are common features. Depending on the site of abscess and its size, pain may initially be dull aching in liver area but subsequently may become sharp and stabbing. When abscess irritates the diaphragm, pain may be referred to the shoulders.

Physical examination shows an ill looking, toxic and emaciated individual with sallow skin. Liver is enlarged and tender. It may enlarge upwards in the chest, as well as downwards towards the epigastrium. There may be local oedema of chest or abdominal wall. Pain on firm pressure with finger tips in the lower inter costal spaces on right side is a valuable localising sign.

When abscess becomes very big, jaundice may appear. Presure over a major hepatic duct may produce features of obstructive jaundice. A large abscess may also bulge producing not only widening of inter costal spaces but also restricted movements ofthe chest wall.

An abscess in the left half of the liver is not very common but when present may produce swelling tenderness and rigidity in the epigastrium.

Investigations.

1. Total and differential white cell count show leucocytosis with rise in polymorphs (70-80%).
2. *Flouroscopy*. Right dome of diaphragm is raised with movements of diaphragm restricted on that side. A bulge or abscess may be seen. There may be obliteration of costrophrenic and cardiophrenic angle. Pleural effusion or basal pnemonia on right chest may be seen.
3. *Stools*. Both cysts and trophozoites form of E. Histolytica be looked for in stools. Invariably stools are negative but positive result favours the diagnosis.

4. *Sigmodoscopy*. It may be helpful when it shows shaggy and necrotic ulcers in the colon or healed scars may be seen.

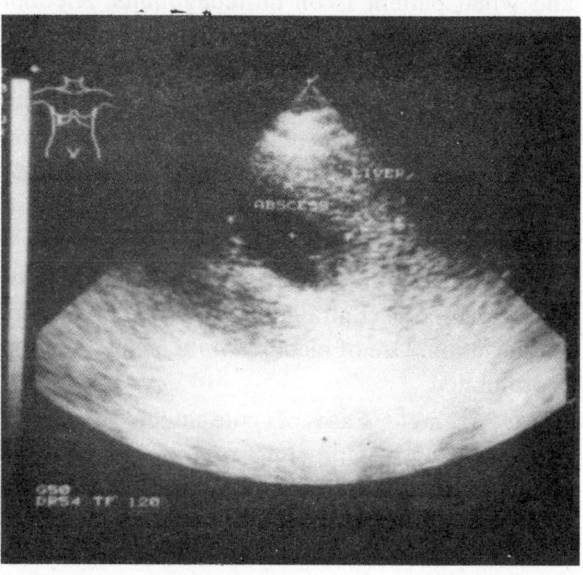

(1)

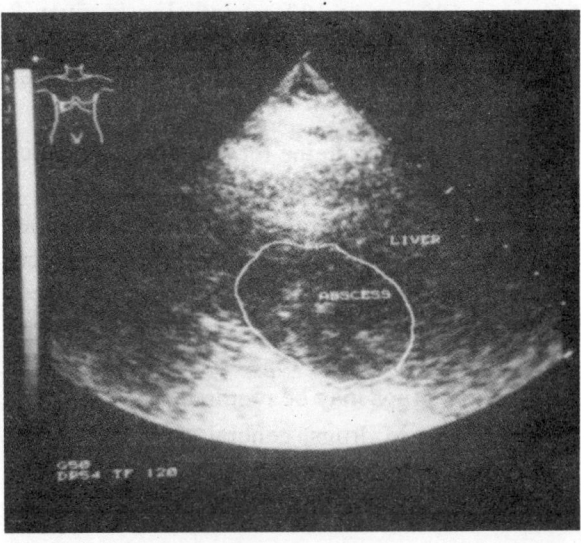

(2)

Fig. 2.29.1-2. Ultra-sound abdomen showing liver abscess.

5. Complement fixation test and amoebic fluroscent antibody titre is positive in 80-90%

of cases. Latex agglutination and haem agglutinations tests are also helpful in diagnosis.

6. *Ultrasonography*. It is an ideal non-invasive test which is helpful in detecting liver abscess.

7. Diagnostic aspiration. When abscess has been localised, diagnostic aspiration of the abscess is carried out. The pus may be whitish or greenish to start with and as the aspiration proceeds it becomes chocolate coloured or typical anchovy sauce type. Often the microscopic examination of the pus may reveal Entamoeba histolytica. Absence of anchovy pus does not rule out the diagnosis of amoebic liver abscess. After aspiration, air or radio-opaque material may be introduced into the abscess to demonstrate its boundaries.

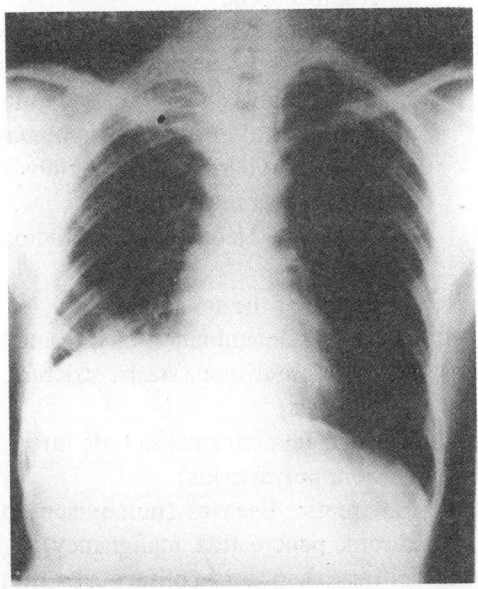

Fig. 2.30. Xray Chest (PA View) A case of amoebic liver abscess. Right dome of diaphragm is markedly elevated

Treatment. A combination of drugs is effective in the treatment of amoebic hepatitis. Metronidazole or tinidazole are the drugs of choice. Dosage of metrogyl (400 mg three times a day) or tinidazole (600 mg twice a day) for 7-10 days. In addition chloroquine diphosphate in the dose of 500 mg thrice daily for 11 days or thrice daily for 2 days followed by twice daily for 21 days. Chloroquine is completely absorbed from the gastrointestinal tract and is concentrated maximum in the liver. It is effective in the treatment of hepatic amoebiasis but has no action either on trophozoites or cysts of Entamoeba histolytica.

Cases of amoebic liver abscess be treated on Injection Dehydroemetine 60 mg I/M daily for 6 days along with Tablet Tinidazole 600 mg three times a day for 7 days and Tablet Chloroquine 500 mg three times a day for 11 days.

If liver abscess is large, is pointing outwards and there is danger of its rupture as well as failure of medical treatment, abscess should be aspirated and all fluid pus etc. be removed. Open drainage of pus may be undertaken if there is large amount of pus secondarily infected or if there are signs of pus but aspiration is negative. Depending on the patients response further aspiration of the abscess may be carried out.

Pulmonary amoebiasis. It is not common but abscess in lungs may occur due to extension from liver abscess or there may be empyema secondary to rupture of liver abscess. Very occasionally liver abscess may rupture through diaphragm into lungs and the content may be coughed up in the form of chocolate-coloured pus. It may leave behind a pneumonic lesion in the lungs. Treatment of pulmonary amoebiasis is on the same lines as in amoebic liver abscess.

Results of treatment. Cases of intestinal amoebiasis and amoebic hepatitis respond satisfactorily to the various amoebicidal drugs. Sometimes it may be difficult to eradicate amoebic infection completely since reinfection is quite common because of poor sanitary conditions, improper water supply and bad personal hygiene.

MALABSORPTION SYNDROME

It encompasses a number of conditions in which absorption of food and nutrients is defective. Absorption of substances takes place by different mechanisms. Thus passive diffusion is the mechanism of absorption of fat-soluble vitamins like A, D, E and K and of water-soluble vitamins including folic acid. Intestinal membrane acts an effective barrier to the diffusion of water-soluble substances. The mechanism of active transport means the movement of a metabolite across a membrane against an electrochemical gradient, and it is the mechanism for a number of substances such as glucose, galactose, amino acids, fatty acids, vitamin B_{12}, sodium and other electrolytes.

A substance is also absorbed by competitive inhibition against a concentration gradient meaning thereby that when some metabolites are not soluble in the membrane, they may combine with a receptor and cross the barrier as a soluble complex and are loaded inside the cell. The mechanism by which a receptor substance acts as a transporter is called facilitated diffusion.

In nutshell absorption of nutrients and other substances is facilitated by these three mechanisms acting on the mucosal surface and derangement of any of these mechanisms shall result in malabsorption.

The rate of absorption of nutrients and their rate of transit in the small intestines is equally important. The distribution of active transport mechanism is of importance since absorption of substances such as glucose, folic acid, iron or water-soluble vitamins takes place rapidly in jejunum while dietary fat escapes absorption proximally and passes on to be absorbed in ileum. The result is reabsorption of bile salts in terminal half of ileum and vitamin B_{12} throughout the ileum. In other words diseases involving the proximal and distal parts of small intestines have their own pattern of malabsorption depending on which segment of intestine is involved.

Causes of malabsorption:

1. Defects of gastric function as in partial and total gastrectomy. Here the total capacity of stomach is decreasd and there is rapid rate of gastric emptying with the result that upper part of small intestines gets food at a rapid rate that it can absorb. Further there is rapid intes-

tinal transit due to passage of food down to ileum from jejunum reslting in imperfect mixing. Role of impaired pancreatic and biliary flow as well upper intestinal infection is also there. The malabsorption following gastrectomy is usually mild unless complicated by chronic pancreatic exocrine insufficiency or a pre-existing gluten sensitive enteropathy or blind loop syndrome.

2. Intestinal malabsorption
   i. Congenital defects of intestinal mucosa
      a. Disaccharide malabsorption (lactase, sucrose, deficiency)
      b. Amino acid transport defects.(Hartnup disease, cystinuria)
   ii. Disorders of absorption
      a. Coeliac disease
      b. Tropical sprue
      c. Idiopathic steatorrhoea
      d. Infiltrative lesions (intestinal tuberculosis, Crohn's disease, scleroderma, reticulosis and intestinal lymphomas)
      e. Parasites (Giardia, strongyloidosis, D. latus or fish tapeworm).
      f. Drugs like Neomycin, Phenindione
      g. Irradiation
   iii. Resection of the small intestines
   iv. Bacterial contamination of the small intestines (blind loop, stasis, stricture, diverticulosis)
   v. Vascular (superior mesenteric artery occlusion, polyarteritis)
   vi. Pancreatic diseases (mucoviscoidosis, chronic pancreatitis, malignancy)
   vii. Biliary disorders (biliary obstruction when bile salts are not excreted in the bile through enterohepatic circulation and in their absence in jejunum fat digestion and absorption becomes defective).
   iix. Endocrine disorders: Addison's disease, thyrotoxicosis, diabetes mellitus, hypoparathyroidism. Zollinger-Ellison syndrome
   ix. Miscellaneous (hypogammaglobulinaemia, pernicious anaemia).

Clinical features. Depending on the underlying

cause, the clinical picture of a case of malabsorption shall vary. But there are few features which are common in almost all the cases.

Gastrointestinal. Bowel abnormality in the form of diarrhoea, abdominal distension, discomfort and excessive flatus are common features. Diarrhoea generally is of steatorrhoeic type with passage of loose, ill formed stools, pale frothy, foul smelling and difficult to flush.

General. Symptoms are as a result of malabsorption of major nutrients. There is anaemia, sore mouth, loss of weight, fatigue and lethargy. In advanced stage oedema on the dependent parts and skin changes are seen. A megaloblastic anaemia due to lack of folic acid or vitamin B_{12} is common. Bone pains may be due to hypocalcaemia and lack of vitamin D leading to rickets, osteomalacia and tetany. Low serum albumin, and hypoproteinaemia are responsible for oedema on dependent parts while skin shall show loss of elasticity, pellagra like features and tendency to bleed readily (vitamin K deficiency). Night blindness and other features of vitamin A deficiency are equally common. In addition patients of malabsorption may suffer from peripheral neuropathy, irritability and general lack of confidence.

Physical signs. *In a case of malabsorption look for:*

1. Evidence of anaemia, glossitis, stomatitis, peripheral oedema. Tongue may be red, angry-looking or bald.
2. Skin changes for pellagra, bleeding tendency.
3. Peripheral neuropathy—tender calves with diminished deep reflexes.

Investigations of a case of malabsorption:

1. Stools for ova, cysts to exclude parasitic infestation.
2. Blood examination. Haemoglobin for anaemia: Peripheral blood smear for type of anaemia. Generally macrocytic type of picture: Sometimes microcytic depending on type of deficiency. Bone marrow examination shows megaloblastic picture. Serum iron, folate, serum B_{12} and carotene levels are low. Pro-

thrombin time proglonged. Serum proteins are low. Calcium, phosphorus and alkaline phosphatase levels are deranged.

3. Tests of intestinal absorption

D-xylose excretion test. After an oral dose of 5 gm of xylose, its urinary excretion over next 5 hours is estimated. If excretion less than 1 gm in urine it indicates malabsorption.

Lactose absorption. In normal subjects, levels of glucose rise after oral administration. Cases of malabsorption show flat glucose tolerance curve.

Fat balance study. In normal person stool fat is below 6 gm per day on a diet which contains 50 g of fat per day for 3 days before the test. Fat in excess of this in stools indicates steatorrhoea. Faecal nitrogen in excess of 2.5 gm per day indicates malabsorption.

Vitamin B_{12} absorption (Schilling test). This is tested by giving radio activie labelled vitamin B_{12} (CO58-labelled vitamin B_{12}) by mouth and measuring urinary excretion. Normal subjects excrete more than 10 per cent of the oral dose, less than 7 per cent excretion indicates malabsorption.

Folic acid deficiency (Figlu test). Folate deficiency is detected by measuring urinary excretion of Figlu after a loading dose of histidine. Figlu is an intermediate in the histidine breakdown to glutamic acid and is excreted in the urine when further metabolism is blocked by folate deficiency. Normal excretion of Figlu is 17 mg or less in 8 hours.

Faecal fat excretion. Radioactive labelled fat (14C-trilein) is administered and when excreted in excess indicates fat malabsorption.

Breath tests. Administration of radio-labelled substances and their excretion in breath is estimated. These tests are useful in cases of steatorrhoea, lactose deficiency and bacterial overgrowth in the intestines.

Thus 14C-labelled trioleen with a lipid meal and estimation of $^{14}CO_2$ in breath in cases of steatorrhoea. 14C-Cholyglycine test in bacterial overgrowth in intestines and breath hydrogen levels in lactose deficiency are the tests employed and are helpful.

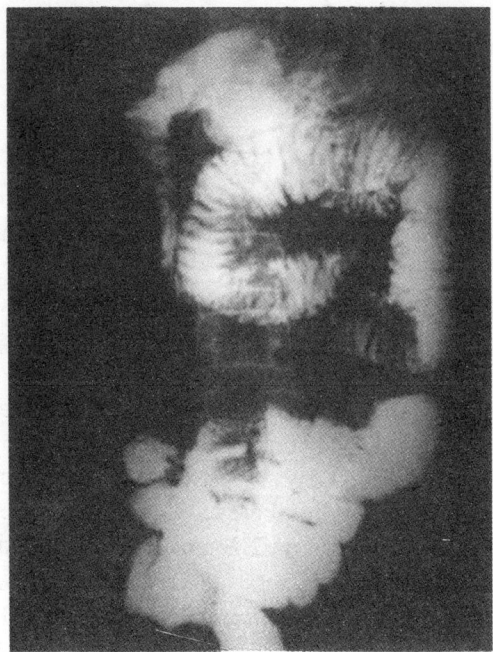

Fig. 2.31. Barium meal study G.I. Tract showing marked duodenal hypertrophy.

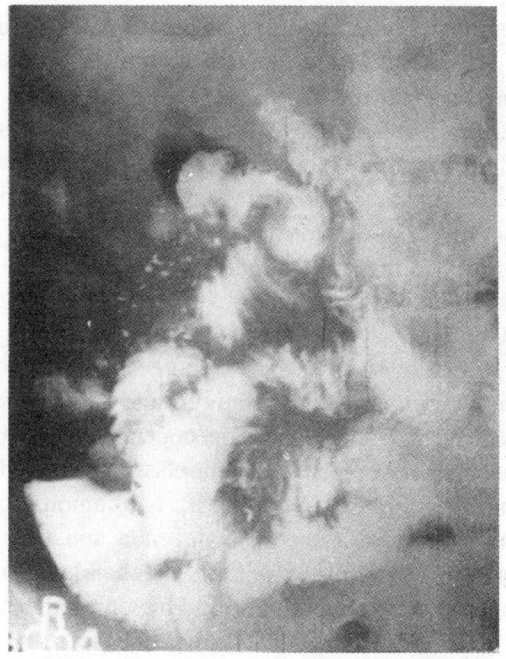

Fig. 2.33. Barium meal study showing coarsening (Hypertrophy) of jejunal mucosa.

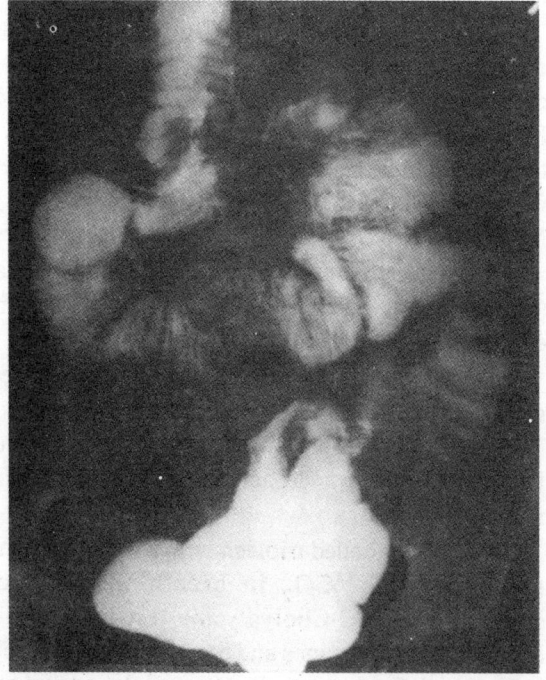

Fig. 2.32. Barium meal study showing jejunal mucosal hypertrophy also.

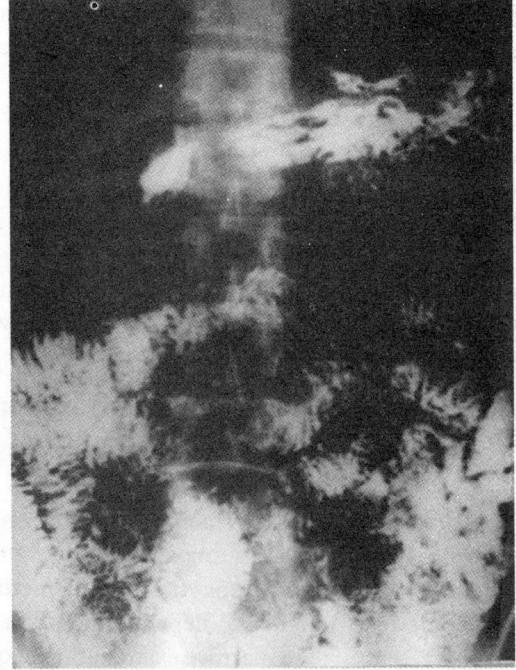

Fig. 2.34. Barium meal study shows moulage's sign flocculation and jejunal mucosal hypertrophy.

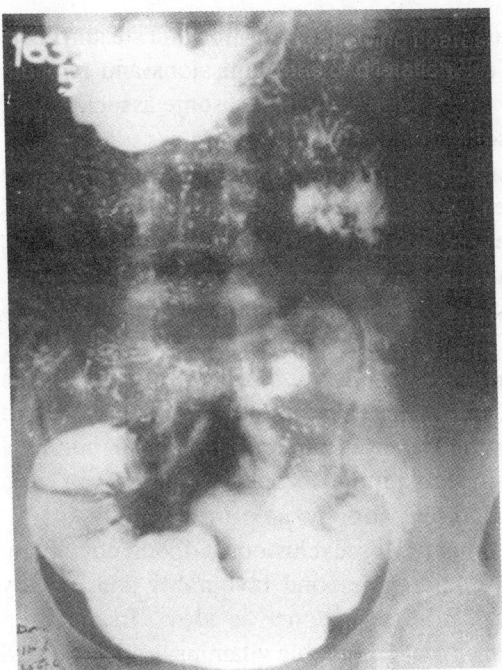

Fig. 2.35. Barium meal study showing flocculation.

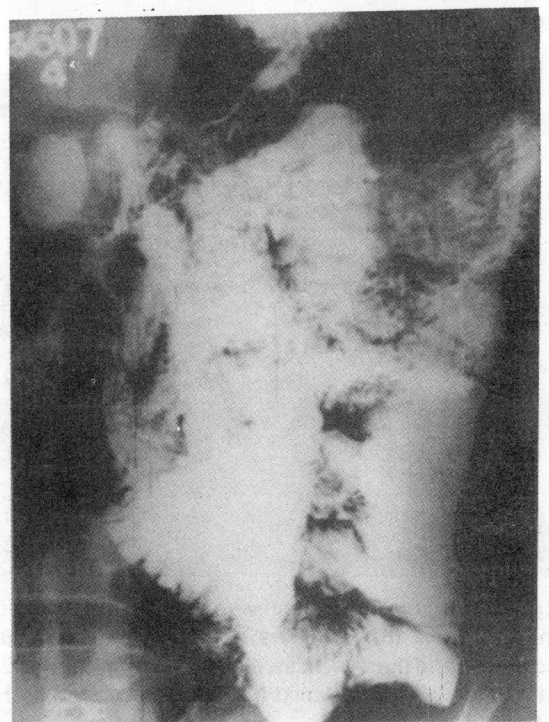

Fig. 2.36. Barium meal study showing coaresening of the jejunal mucosa with areas of dilatation.

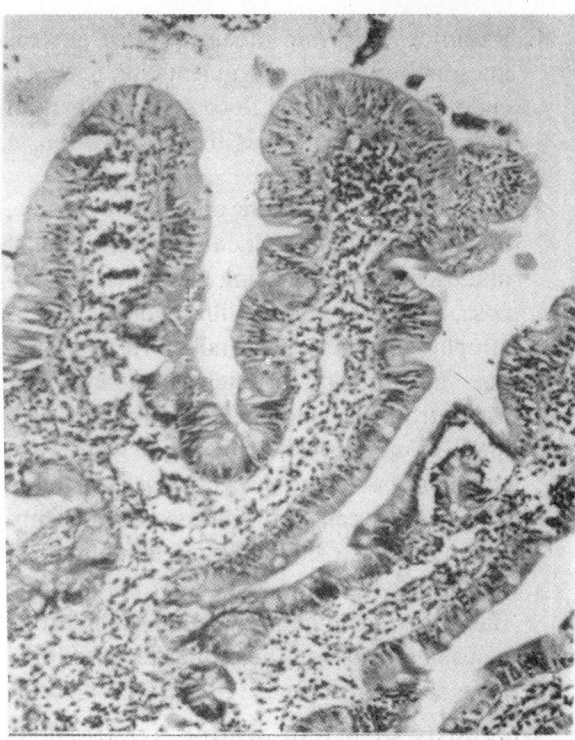

Fig. 2.37. Jejunal biopsy showing normal mucosa. The villi are tall and are covered by tall columnar epithelium. A normal sized crypt and a mild inflammatory infiltrate is seen in the lamina propria. H & E × 100.

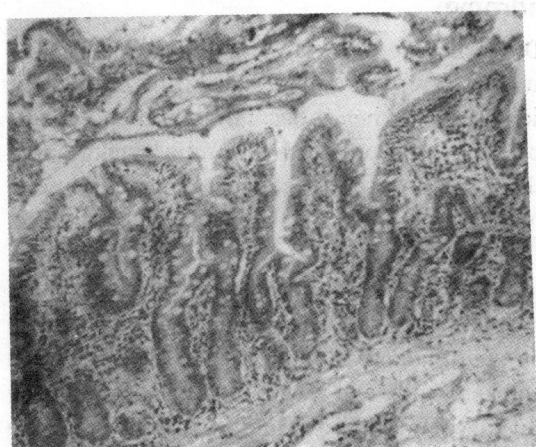

Fig. 2.38. Jejunal biopsy showing broadening and flattening of jejunal villi in a case of malabsorption syndrome.

4. Radiology. Barium meal study of gastrointestinal tract shows segmentation (coin on end appearances) and flocculation of barium in small intestines. It is the presentation in cases of malabsorption.

5. Jejunal biopsy. By means of a crosby capsule, jejunal biopsy is obtained. By conventional microscopy, most striking feature is flat mucosa, devoid of normal villi (subtotal villous atrophy). In others, intestinal villi show blunting, short, broad and thickened (partial villous atrophy). Under electronmicroscopy, there is a curious pattern of ridges, whorls and convolutions. There is severe disorganization of the surface cells of the mucosa. Histochemical studies also show marked diminution of many of the enzyme systems of the mucosa. Bacterial examination of the small intestine by using a capsule is helpful in cases of blind loop, stasis or a fistula.

Diagnosis of malabsorption syndrome is dependent on number of factors. To satisfy the rigid criteria out of three parameters (biochemical radiology and histology) patient must have two positive parameters to be labelled as a case of malabsorption syndrome.

Common diseases causing malabsorption syndrome:

Disaccharide deficiency. Deficiency of disaccharide enzyme leads to a picture of lactose deficiency and when it occurs in children appears to be congenital one with a familial background. Child suffers from chronic diarrhoea, and failure to thrive. In adults, the patient complains of flatulence, and abdominal discomfort. Flatulence and diarrhoea occur within one to 2 hours of taking milk. Diagnosis is suggested by a flat glucose curve after ingestion of 50 gm of lactose. Symptoms can be reproduced by intake of milk and its products. Treatment is by exclusion of milk and related lactose containing substances.

Coeliac disease. Often labelled as 'gluten sensitive entropathy' where the child is sensitive to gluten in the diet (wheat, rye and oats) and presents with failure to thrive, malnutrition and steatorrhoea. There may be periods of remissions and relapses over a period of time. There is some association of the disease with HLA system.

Adult coeliac disease may start in third and fourth decade. There are attacks of diarrhoea precipitated by intercurrent illnesses. In addition loss of weight, anaemia and features of malabsorption are seen. Family history may be available in small percentage of cases.

Diagnosis is by history, biochemical tests, barium study (loss of normal mucosal pattern, clumping of barium and increased transverse binding of intestinal mucosa) and jejunal biopsy (flat mucosa with subtotal villous atrophy).

Treatment is by exclusion of foods containing gluten. Children respond favourably and quickly while in adults response is slow. In addition supplements of fat-soluble vitamins, iron, folic acid and vitamin B_{12} are given. A few patients not responding to above regimen are to be treated with corticosteroids.

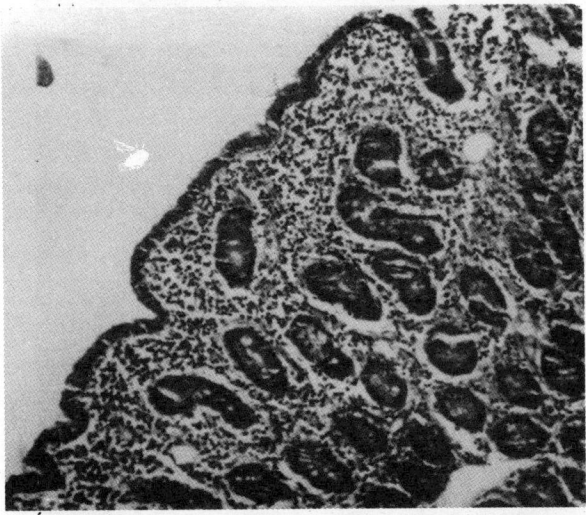

Fig. 2.39. Jejunal biopsy showing blunting and marked shortening of the villi. The depth of the crypts is increased and there is an increased inflammatory exudate in lamina propria-mild (partial) villous atrophy H & E × 100.

Tropical sprue. A disease prevalent in tropical and subtropical countries, is characterised often by a picture of acute diarrhoeal illness followed by steatorrhoea. Often the onset is gradual. Patient complains of anorexia, weakness, loss of weight, abdominal discomfort, flatulence and soreness of mouth. Cases of sprue suffer from a number of deficiencies and predominant picture is of a megaloblastic anaemia. Diagnosis is as per tests of malabsorption. Treatment of sprue is by rest,

correction of malnutrition and a nourishing diet. Oral Tetracycline 1 gm daily in divided doses for 6-8 weeks, results in improvement. In addition folic acid

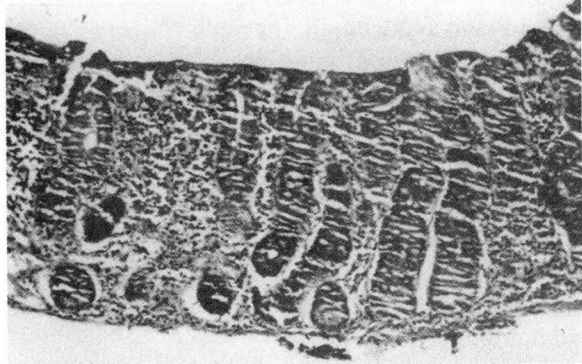

Fig. 2.40. Jejunal biopsy showing subtotal villous-atrophy. The mucosal surface is nonvilliform and the covering epithelium is flattened. There is a marked increase in depth of crypts. Dense inflammatory infiltrate is seen in lamina propria H & E × 100.

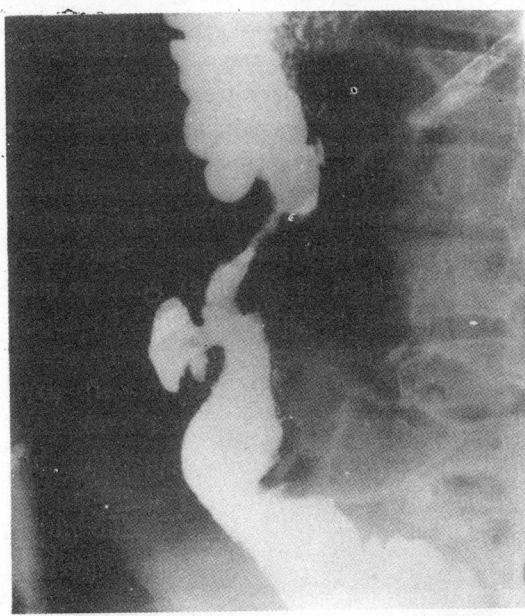

Fig. 2.42. Barium meal showing rat tail appearance in ileoceacal tuberculosis.

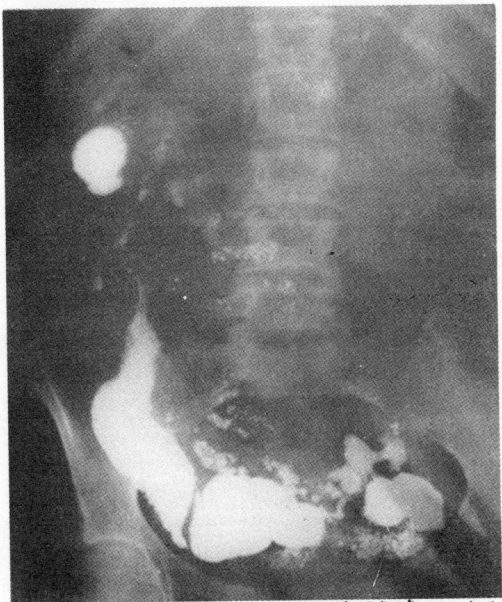

Fig. 2.41. Barium meal showing 'String Sign' in cases of ileoceacal tuberculosis.

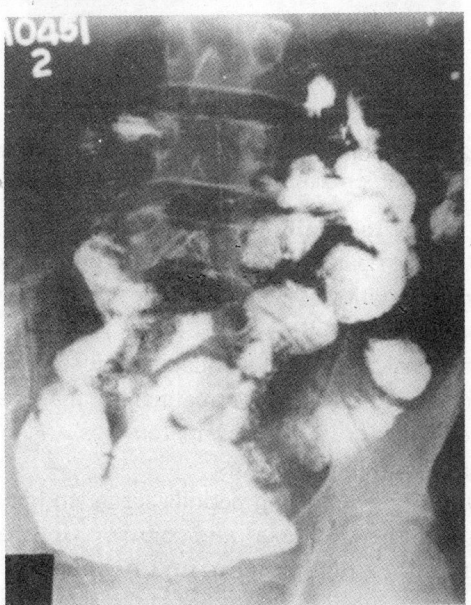

Fig. 2.44. Barium meal study showing flocculation and segmentation in cases of abdominal tuberculosis.

10 mg orally three times a day along with parenteral vitamin B$_{12}$ corrects the condition.

Infiltrative diseases of the small intestines. These include whipples disease (gradual onset of diarrhoea steatorrhoea and progressive weight loss. In addition skin changes, and lymphadenopathy). Amyloid disease (secondary to suppurative disease in lung, bones or primary which is very rare), reticulosis (lymphoma, leukaemia, hodgkin's disease) and collalgen disorders like scleroderma.

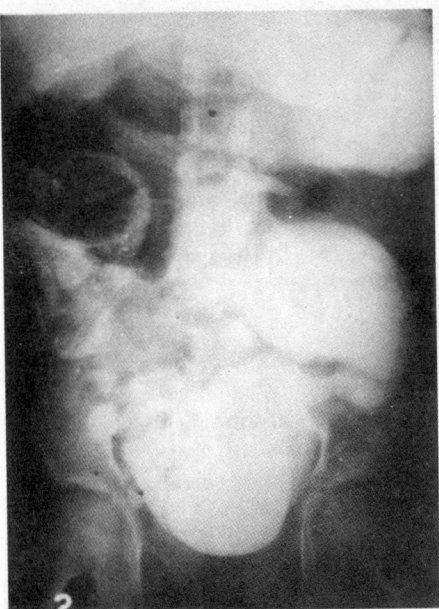

Fig. 2.44. Barium meal showing multiple structures in the ileum with proximal dilatation of small intestines.

Damage to small intestinal mucosa. This may result due to parasites like giardia, fish tape warm where infestation is heavy and they interfere with absorption.

Intestinal mucosa may be damaged by irradiation when applied to pelvis for treatment of malignancy of cervix, uterus, ovaries in females and other malignancies in both sexes.

Drugs taken for long periods are again liable to damage the mucosa and cause picture of steatorrhoea. Tubercular involvement of the intestines (enteritis, stricture, fistula, stagnation of intestinal contents) and Crohn's disease are important cause of malabsorption by inflammatory

damage to the intestinal mucosa and a blind loop situation.

Resection of the small intestines. Depending on the extent of resection and the part of intestines removed (proximal or distal) picture of malabsorption shall result. Resection of the proximal part of intetine has less adverse effects as compared to distal resection when B$_{12}$ absorption is interfered with.

Bacterial contamination of small intestines (blind loop syndrome). In people with anatomical lesions of the small intestines such as blind loop diverticulosis, stasis or fistula, there is proliferation of bacteria which mainly interfere with the absorption of fat and vitamin B$_{12}$ causing steatorrhoea and to some extent with glucose and folic acid absorption. Result is picture of malabsorption.

Treatment is by correction of anatomical abnormality (stricture, diverticulae, fistula, blind loop) by surgery. In addition broad spectrum antibiotics (tetracycline 1 gm in divided doses four times a day) low fat diet, fat soluble vitamins and vitamin B$_{12}$ be given.

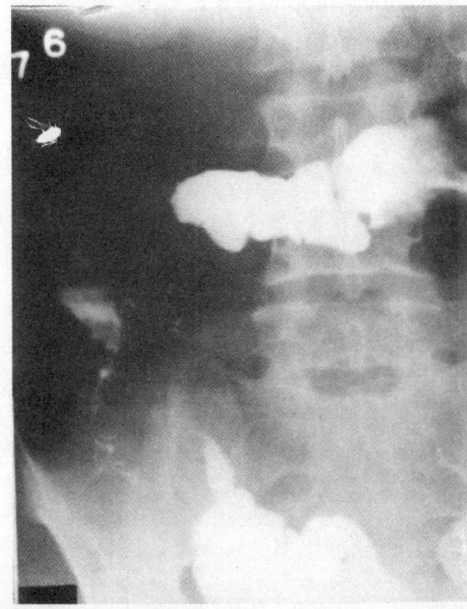

Fig. 2.45. Barium meal showing ceacal changes in intestinal tuberculosis.

Miscellaneous causes of malabsorption. A

number of varied causes though not very common are associated with causation of malabsorption. These include vascular lesions (chronic obstruction of the superior mesenteric artery). Endocrine disorders like Addison's disease, hypoparathyroidism, diabetes mellitus, Zollinger-Ellison syndrome and thyrotoxicosis. These are uncommon causes and often present with steatorrhoea and loss of weight. Diagnosis of these conditions shall depend not only on carrying tests of malabsorption but also of the underlying condition.

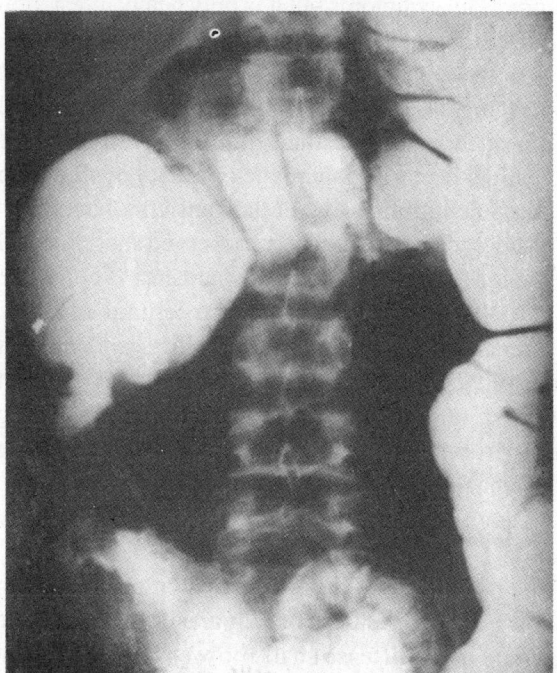

Fig. 2.46. Barium enema showing non-filling of caecum and shortening of ascending colon.

Management of malabsorption syndrome. Malabsorption syndrome encompases a number of conditions with varied aetiology. Treatment and management shall depend on the underlying condition and has to be individualized. But in addition care should be taken to manage general nutrition of the patient by means of adequate nutritional supplements in diet as well as adequate dose of fat soluble vitamins, folic acid and vitamin B_{12}.

Cases of coeliac disease have to be put on gluten free diet while cases of tropical sprue and blind loop syndrome shall require oxytetracycline for 4-6 weeks. Similarly in patients with lactose intolerance (disaccharide enzyme deficiency) treatment is by lactose restricted or free diet.

GIARDIASIS

For more than a century, Giardia lamblia intestinalis had been considered a harmless inhabitant of the small intestines especially the upper part, the duodenum, but its pathogenicity is now universally well recognised. The incidence of giardiasis infection is prevalent all over the world though it is known to be higher in the tropics.

The pear-shaped parasite inhabits the human intestine mainly duodenum and jejunum and often gets lodged in the bile ducts. By its suckers present on its concave surface it gets attached to the intestinal mucosa and multiplies by longitudinal fission. In its encysted form it may persist and passed in the faeces for a number of years but in its trophozoite (flagellate) form it is passed to the large bowel and when transit is rapid these are passed unchanged in the liquid stools and may perish rapidly. Healthy individuals who harbour the parasite may suffer from periodic attacks of diarrhoea when large number of flagellate form of giardia are passed.

Cysts of giardia are the ones which are infectious and transmitted to new hosts by faeco-oral route. Giardiasis is a disease of poor hygiene, bad sanitation and improper purification of water supply. Cysts persist in cold water for months together and even chlorination of water fails to eradicate the infection. It is an important cause of water-borne diarrhoea and inadequate filtration and purification of water supply remains the main culprit. Direct person to person infection also occurs especially amongst closed communities. Poor sanitation, improper disposal of sewerage and poor standards of personal hygiene shall contribute to a large extent in the spread of the disease.

Persons suffering from immune deficiency, protein caloric malnutrition, achlorhydria and deficiency of IgA are more prone to suffer from it.

Clinical presentation. The symptomatology of patients with giardiasis is very variable. It may range from no symptoms to multiple complex symptoms. Most of the individuals may have minor gastro-intestinal symptoms and are passing encysted form of giardia in the stools. Attacks of explosive watery diarrhoea with foul-smelling stools without any blood or mucus occur in some and stools of these patients contain large number of flagellar form of giardia.

Epigastric discomfort, ulcer-like features, abdominal distension, gas formation, flatulence, chronic diarrhoea, steatorrhoea, headache, dizziness are the other symptoms complained of. Loss of weight and failure to thrive are important features in children.

Diarrhoea-like features persist for a long time in many sufferers of diarrhoea due to giardiasis. Even after therapeutic cure these symptoms only disappear after a period of time and may take even one to two month to resolve.

The role of giardia in causing chronic intestinal malabsorption is controversial. Studies in children suffering from giardiasis tend to show that malabsorption can be caused due to parasite. On the contrary studies in adults have been controversial. Since there is susceptibility of patients with secretory IgA deficiency to symptomatic giardiasis it has been presumed that giardiasis may be solely resposible for diarrhoea disease. In children it is well accepted that giardiasis can cause malabsorption which is reversible with the eradication of the parasite. But in adults mal-absorption has been found only in a small proportion of cases and not in all. Many have doubted the presence of malabsorption solely due to giardiasis.

The question arises as to how giardia is capable of producing malabsorption. The possible factors which have been incriminated include (i) presence of large number of parasites in mucosal surface of the intestines so that the absorptive surface of the intestines is considerably reduced, (ii) increased motility of gut so that the time of exposure of nutrients to the absorptive surface is reduced,

(iii) bacterial overgrowth, (iv) invasion of pancreatic duct, (v) injury to mucosa possibly by the mucosal invasion by the parasite and lastly a barrier provided by the parasite to the active transport of various nutrients. There is no doubt that giardia is capable of causing steatorrhoea in adults but it produces malabsorption in insignificant number of cases though this may not hold true for children where giardiasis should be considered an important factor responsible for malabsorption.

Pathogenesis. Mild infection with giardia may produce no symptoms but it is only heavy infestation with the parasite which causes pathological features. Though the exact mechanism for this is not known but factors like mechanical blockage of the intestinal villi, changes in intestinal motility, overgrowth of intestinal bacteria, pancreatic or biliary dysfunction and competition for essential nutrients have been considered. It has also been observed that mucosal invasion of the intestine by the parasite may provoke a T cell-mediated insult to the jejunal mucosa. Patients with immunological defects and protein malnutrition are more prone to suffer from it suggesting some degree of immune response acting as a protective factor in adults not having these deficiencies.

Diagnosis. Diagnosis of giardia can be easily made by stool examination of fresh specimen. Patients who pass liquid form of stools are likely to show trophozoites form of the parasite while chronic carriers of the disease shall show cyst form. Repeat examination of three stools done daily shall contribute to the high positivity rate. Since giardia is a common habitat of small intestine, duodenal intubation can be done by means of String test and the organism can be seen in the duodenal aspirate. Rarely jejunal biopsy may be done to demonstrate the organism.

Elisa test. Immunodiagnostic tests are the other methods employed but in majority of patients simple stool examination shall clinch the diagnosis.

Treatment. Though giardia is a universally distributed parasite yet it has attracted little attention because of its being considered mostly non-pathogenic specially in adults. Whatever symptoms are seen and reported these are mostly seen in children. But if one carefully studies adults who come with vague abdominal discomfort, loss of appetite and chronic ill-health coupled with either chronic constipation or diarrhoea one finds that in quite a high percentage of them the cause is giardiasis and requires adequate treatment.

An important factor to be considered is to ensure a good personal hygiene and clean water supply. Similarly patient should be advised to take high protein diet since it itself is likely to cause the infection to die while high carbohydrate diet is likely to increase ten-fold daily faecal output of cysts.

Of the various drugs employed quinacrine (mepacrine) is a well-known old remedy and was found to be quite good as far as clinical cure was concerned but numerous side effects like yellow colouration of skin, psychosis, nausea vomiting, etc. has made the use of the drug rather undesirable. Dosage employed 100 mg thrice a day for 5 days. Cure rate varies from 60-70 per cent. Another drug employed is Erythromycin (Estolate or Stearate) either in a single dose (150 mg tablet 4 tablets at bed time) or two tablets twice a day for five days.

Further on these drugs gave place to antiamoebic drugs like Furazolidone, Metronidazole, Tinidazole and Secnidazole.

Furazolidone is an equally useful drug but efficacy ranges from 62-67 per cent. Dosage is 100 mg thrice a day for 7 days. Side effects include nausea, vomiting.

Metronidazole (200 mg thrice a day for five days) is equally effective giving a cure rate of 80-90 per cent. However this drug is not to be employed in pregnant women. Side effects include metallic taste, leucopenia, urticaria, dark urine, neuropathy, etc.

Tinidazole is a better substitute to Metrogyl. Dosage is 300 mg twice a day for six days. It has less side effects as compared to Metrogyl and cure rate is 80-90 per cent.

Secnidazole is another effective drug. It may be employed as single dose (2 g in adults, 30 mg/kg in children) or given in divided doses spread over a period of four days. Success rate with this drug is again upto 92 per cent.

Most of these drugs give substantial degree of cure in patients of giardiasis though the chances of reinfection always remain high. However when failure occurs, a combination of two drugs is always better. If required the drug may be repeated after three weeks. But in addition patient must be advised to have clean pure water supply, avoidances of potentially contaminated food and ensuring proper personal hygiene.

In pregnant women where giardiasis is causing distressing symptoms all the above drugs are contraindicated. Paromycin, a member of aminoglycoside family of antibiotics has been employed. It is an effective luminal amoebicide and also effective against giardiasis. Side effects include G.I. upset, diarrhoea.

Thus giardia can act an important pathogenic organism in some people and can produce a number of distressing symptoms. Patients without any symptoms and silent passer, of cysts of giardia may require no treatment. It is the symptomatic individuals who should be given the therapy along with advice to ensure clean sanitation, water supply and personal hygiene.

PAINFUL SWALLOWING

Swallowing is a normal physiological process and is governed by a number of factors.

Oesophagus connects the oropharynx to the stomach and it starts from the lower margin of the cricopharyngus muscle. It is composed of striated muscle and a coordinated action of the muscular layers of body of the oesophagus helps in the passage of the food boluses and liquid from the pharynx down to the stomach. A series of reflexes constitute the normal act of swallowing which is a painless process. The process of swallowing may be interfered with either due to functional or pathological conditions. There may be difficulty in swallowing because of the pain during the act and this is called Odynophagia. Painful swallowing is a condition which can not be ignored and a number of conditions may be responsible for it. These may range from chemicals, poisons. Infections, trauma following instrumentation, foreign body impaction oesophagitis, diverticula, webs to malignancy etc. Let us look at some of these conditions.

Trauma. It can be important cause of painful swallowing and often follows instrumentation of the upper G.I. tract like oesophagoscopy. At the same time a feeling of pain and rawness often persists after intubation. These symptoms are of short duration and persist only for a few days. Again one has seen patients suffering from asthma who had perforce swallowed small live fish and they complain of rawness in throat and difficulty in swallowing.

If a careful history is taken in all such patients it shall not be difficult to arrive at the underlying cause of painful swallowing.

Infection. Mild oesophagitis with substernal pain and painful swallowing may complicate infections of the upper respiratory tract. A number of inflammatory conditions effecting upper part of gastrointestinal tract may be important cause and these include stomatitis, ulcers of the tongue (traumatic, tubercular, gummatous, septic, malignant) tonsillitis, pharyngitis, quinsy and injuries by accidental swallowing of corrosives like strong alkalis or acids. Various inflammatory conditions of larynx, retropharyngeal abscess, diphtheria and malignancy of base of the tongue often present with painful swallowing more because of pain rather than any mechanical obstruction.

Acute oesophagitis alongwith painful swallowing is often seen in diabetic patients, patients on immunosuppressive drugs, broad spectrum antibiotics where candida and a number of viruses such as herpes simplex and cytomegalovirus invade the body. Patients with AIDS (acquired immune deficiency syndrome) are other likely victims and will show white patches of candidiasis any where in the oral cavity which are superimposed upon a hyperemic oesophagus and in severe cases on ulcerated oesophageal mucosa. Cases with Herpes simplex infection show confluent or discrete ulceration but the characteristic white patches of moniliasis, are not seen. Similarly monilial over growth leading to painful swallowing is a frequent occurrence in patients of cancer who are under treatment with a variety of antimitotic agents. Such patients are often debilitated, under nourished, wasted and immunocomprised. A careful analysis of the underlying condition with appropriate examination including endoscopy and microbiological help should be able to clinch the diagnosis. In majority of the cases the clinical picture is so classical that often microbiological examination is not necessary.

Chemical. The ingestion of strong alkaline or corrosive agents produces a form of oesophagitis which may range from mild to severe degree depending on the amount of chemical agent swallowed. This is going to produce a severe degree of oesophageal stenosis and painful swallowing. Very often this is either suicidal or accidental and there are tell tale signs. In an acute stage one may often see burns round about the oral cavity which shall tell the whole story about the true picture of the cause.

Foreign body. An impacted foreign body is an important cause and often produces severe degree of pain during the act of swallowing. All types of foroeign bodies are known to be impacted in the upper part of oesophagus especially in children but a fish bone swallowed during a meal is a common cause in adults and should be especially kept in mind in an apparently healthy individual.

Gastro-oesophageal reflux. The reflux of gastric contents into the oesophagus may produce not only heart burn but picture of oesophagitis. Oesophagitis not only produces a picture of substernal discomfort but difficulty in swallowing. Drugs like NSAID (Non-steroidal anti-inflammatory drugs) slow releasing potassium salts, steroids are known to produce ulceration in oesophagus. Prolonged and severe reflux may lead to stricture formation resulting in not only painful swallowing but also dysphagia.

Plummer-Vinson syndrome. Young females with iron deficiency anaemia glossitis and koilonychia may complain of food sticking in the throat and pain during the act of swallowing. Anaemia especially of iron deficiency type is common in such patients. A barium swallow may reveal a circoid web in the post cricoid region of such patients. These webs respond to treatment with iron and regress spontaneously. But these are also considered as premalignant.

Oesophageal spasm. It may be diffuse type of spasm resulting in painful swallowing. A number of conditions quite unrelated to gastrointestinal tract may be responsible for it and these range from functional, manifestation of aging, mucosal irritation, neuromuscular diseases such as myasthenia gravis, diabetic neuropathy, motor, neurone disease, scleroderma, connective tissue disorders and idiopathic group. Spasm when severe often produces pain, difficulty in swallowing and inability to push the food down.

Malignancy. Precancerous and malignant conditions especially in upper part of oesophagus should be seriously considered as causes of painful swallowing especially in persons after the age of fifty. Difficulty in swallowing solids is the patient's first complaint which may or may not be painful. The dysphagia which is initially intermittent progresses quickly over a period of weeks. There is pain either in the sternum, the back or in the neck. Swallowing is invariably painful. This is especially so on swallowing hot liquids and has often been ignored by the patient. Progressive weight loss with regurgitation of oesophageal contents often blood stained is common symptom. Diagnosis in such cases is not much of a problem if one keeps this condition in mind. Barium swallow shall shown an asymmetrical diffuse thickening of the oesophageal wall or stricture or protrusion of growth into the lumen. Further investigations shall be by oesophagoscopy and biopsy from the site to clinch the histological diagnosis. The tumour can be either fungating, infiltrative or ulcerative. Commonest is squamous celled carcinoma.

Extrinsic causes. These include conditions which put pressure on the oesophagus from outside and include aortic anaeurysm, growths including glands in the mediastinium (tubercular, Hodgkin's, Malignancy, Lymphoma etc) and retrosternal goiter and sometimes a large thymus.

Oesophageal diverticula. These are an important cause and often missed. These are small pouches present immediately above the upper oesophageal sphincter. The aetiology of these diverticula is not clear though factors like abnomal motility and incoordination of oesophageal sphincter have been incriminated. Commonly these diverticula are small but when they become large symptoms are produced and painful swallowing is one of them.

Diagnosis. The condition of painful swallowing should not be ignored in any patient since a number of benign as well as malignant conditions may be the underlying cause.

A thorough detailed history shall be helpful. Thus malignancy of oesophagus in elderly people, plummer Vinson Syndrome in young females suffering from anaemia, corrosive agents in accidental or suicidal cases and inflammatory causes should be looked into. Look for tell tale signs of Herpes and candidia.

Precipitating factors include swallowing of a foreign body especially in children or an emotional upset in an emotionally labile individual. Associated symptoms such as body wasting, anorexia shall favour a malignancy. Cough, dysponea and toxaemia shall suggest inflammatory pathology. A good clinical history with details of symptomatology and a thorough physical examination shall go a long way in clinching the diagnosis. Every case of a painful swallowing should be submitted to an X-ray examination including X-ray of the chest and barium swallow which is a must in every case. In addition oesophagoscopy and biopsies from any suspicious site in the oesophagus be carried out.

Further investigations shall depend on the aetiology of the condition like AIDS, diabetes, myasthenia gravis, candidiasis etc.

Management of a case of painful swallowing

shall depend on the underlying cause and appropriate treatment instituted. A foreign body can be removed under direct vision and similarly monilial infection be treated with drugs like Miconazole, ketoconazole or fluconazole. In a case of malignancy of oesophagus, appropriate surgical treatment has to be advised.

Prognosis of a case shall depend on how quickly the underlying condition is diagnosed and appropriate treatment instituted.

Diseases of Liver

Liver the largest organ in the body lies in the right upper quadrant and plays an important role in carbohydrate, protein, bile salt metabolism and detoxification of noxious substances. Liver inactivates certain hormones which include sex hormones, adrenal cortical hormones and possibly antidiuretic hormone of post pituitary. The Kupffer cells being hepatic sinusoids play important role in the production of immune bodies, in phagocytosis and in blood formation.

Liver is also involved in proteins concerned with blood coagulation such as prothrombin, fibrinogen factor 7 and enzymes.

Liver has great capacity for regeneration and the result is that people with extensive damage can survive with rudimentary parts of liver.

TESTS FOR LIVER FUNCTIONS

Biochemical tests play important role in the diagnosis of liver disease and multiple tests are required to reach accurate diagnosis.

Serum bilirubin. It consists of two fractions, the conjugated which gives a direct reaction and unconjugated the lipid soluble indirect fraction.

The normal total serum bilirubin concentration ranges form 0.4 to 1.0 mg/dl. Rise in conjugated levels indicates impairment of secretion into the bile while unconguated levels indicate impaired conjugation. Rise in non-conjugated levels occurs in conditions such as haemolytic anaemia and congenital hyperbilirubinaemias (Gilbert's or Crigler-Najjar syndrome).

Although measurements of both conjugated and unconjugated fractions will determine as to which form of bilirubinaemia is predominent yet this disinction is of limited significance, since in majority of cases with hepatobiliary disease, it is conjugated levels which rise.

Serum bilirubin rise occurs in acute hepatitis, hepatocellular and obstructive jaundice.

Serum alkaline phosphatase. Normal values are between 3-13 King Armstrong units (K.A.) or 1.5 to 4 bodansky units per 100 ml. Rise in alkaline phosphatase over 30 K.A. units occurs in obstructive jaundice while in hepatocellular jaundice levels are raised but usually less than 30 K.A. units. Rise in these levels is a good index in tumours of liver (primary or secondary) though normal values do not exclude metastasis. Elevated levels of alkaline phosphatase are also seen in diseases of bone.

Serum proteins (Albumin and globulin). Serum albumin levels normally are between 3.5-4.5 g while globulin levels range from 2.0 to 3.2 g. It is better to have electrophoretic estimation of the proteins.

Albumin levels decrease with elevation in gamma globulin in portal cirrhosis while in acute viral hepatitis, albumin levels are slightly decreased and there is rise in gamma globulin and beta globulin. In obstructive jaundice there is increase in alpha2, beta and gamma globulins.

Changes in protein levels are slow to develop and are of importance in chronic liver disease indicating derangement of protein metabolism.

Sero flocculation tests. These include thymol turbidity (0-4 units) thymol flocculation (0-1+) zinc sulphate turbidity (4-12 units) and cephalin-cholesterol flocculation (0 to 1+) tests. These tests reflect a delicate imbalance of the various protein fractions of the serum and are useful for assessing the severity of cirrhosis or hepatitis.

Brom sulphalein tests. This is a test for assessing liver dysfunction in cases of cirrhosis and for following its progress. But normal result does not exclude a compensated case of cirrhosis. This test is also useful in confirming complete recovery from viral hepatitis.

In this test sterile BSP in a dose of 5 mg/kg body weight is injected intravenously. Normal person should retain only 0-10 per cent of the dye in 30 minutes and less than 3 per cent in 45 minutes.

Serum enzymes. A number of enzymes are estimated and help in assessing hepatocellular damage. But rise in enzyme levels may be seen in diseases of heart, kidney, lung and musculoskeletal tissue.

Of the various enzymes, aspartate amino-transferase (AST/SGOT) and alanine aminotransferase (ALT/SGPT) are most important. Their normal values range upto 40 units. High levels are found in hepatic necrosis and diffuse and focal liver diseases.

Another enzyme 5-nucelotidase levels rise in hepatobiliary disease. Its principle importance is to confirm the hepatic origin of elevated alkaline phosphatase in conditions like bone disease coexisting with liver disease. However levels of 5-nucleotidase do not always parallel that of alkaline phosphatase in liver diseases.

Needle biopsy of the liver. When it is required to confirm and to study the extent of liver damage in cases of diffuse parenchymal disorders (cirrhosis, hepatitis) and disseminated focal liver disorders (granulomatous or tumour infiltrates) a needle biopsy of the liver is helpful in making a diagnosis.

In the method employed either a Vimsilverman or Meghini needle is employed, mainly through the ninth or tenth intercostal space and piece of liver obtained for histology.

Liver biopsy is not to be done in patients with jaundice, bleeding disorers, and low platelet count. Cases with massive ascites make biopsy procedure rather difficult.

Complications after biopsy include haemorrhage, biliary peritonitis, pleurisy, perihepatitis and sometimes puncture of other viscera.

Percutaneous trans-splenic portal veno-graphy. This technique is emplyed to measure intrasplenic pressure as well as demonstrating the patency of portal vein and pattern of splenic and portal veins and their radicals.

In this procedure, a needle is inserted into the spleen usually in 8th or 9th intercostal space in the mid axillary line, the intransplenic pressure is measured and a contrast injected through it. Serial films are taken and results analysed.

Deep jaundice, low prothrombin time and bleeding disorders are contraindications to this procedure. Complications include haemorrhage, infection and perisplenitis.

Normally the dye when injected reaches liver within a few seconds. Splenic and portal veins are filled. The intrahepatic branches of portal vein show branching and reduction in their caliber.

In case of portal hypertension, venogram may show filling of large number of collateral and gross distortion of intrahepatic branches of portal vein.

In case of extrahepatic portal obstruction, large number of vessels running from spleen and splenic vein to the diaphragm and other structures are filled while intrahepatic branches usually are not seen.

The procedure of portal venography is essential before portacaval anastomosis as well as postoperatively to demonstrate the patency of portacaval anastomosis.

Cholecystogram. This method is undertaken to visualize the functioning of gall bladder and presence of any gall stones. Oral tablets of contrast medium (telepaque) are taken night before and X-ray plates taken next day.

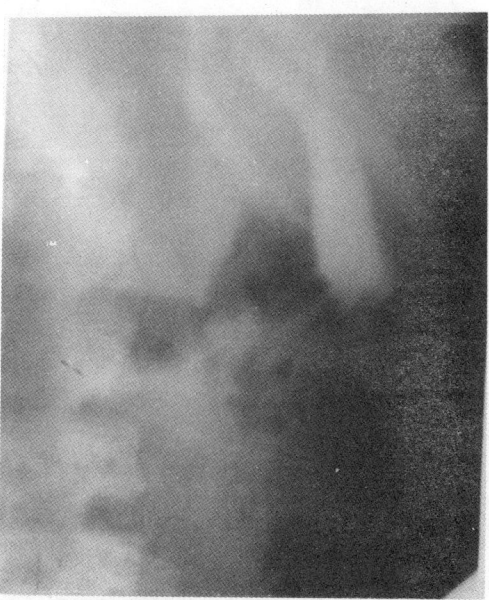

Fig. 3.2. Same case after fatty meal. Gall bladder has contracted indicating normal functioning of gall bladder.

Cholecystography is also of use in differentiating calcification or any mass in right hypochondrium.

Intravenous cholangiography. In this procedure biligrafin is injected intravenously and gall bladder, hepatic and common bile ducts are visualized. Generally it takes 20 minutes after injection to visualize the various structures.

This procedure is required after cholecystectomy to visualize the presence of any calculi or bile strictures after surgery on gall bladder.

Percutaneous transhepatic cholangiography (PTC). Here through a fine needle, contrast is injected into the liver to visualize the biliary tree. Its main use is to demonstrate extrahepatic biliary obstruction in patients of jaundice who have dilated intrahepatic bile ducts. By this procedure, site of obstruction can be demonstrated.

Contraindications to the procedure are low prothrombin time and platelet count. Complications include bleeding, cholangitis and biliary peritonitis. Rarely death may occur.

Ultrasound. It is an important non-invasive diagnostic aid in cases of liver disorders especially for visualizing size of liver, spleen and presence of any space occupying lesions. The gall bladder,

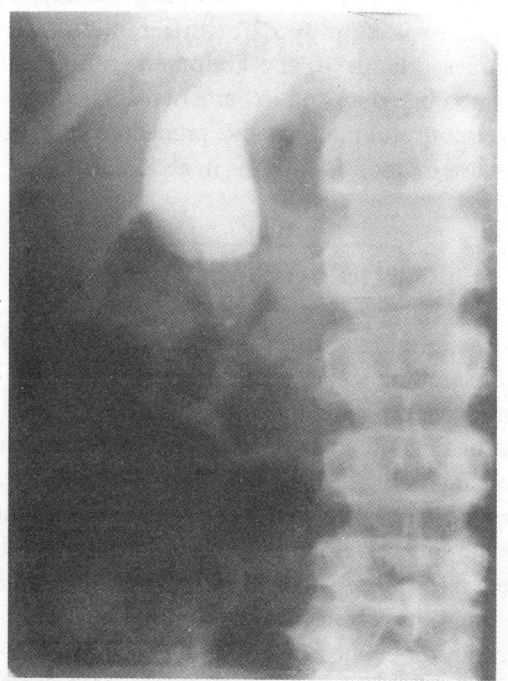

Fig. 3.1. Oral cholecystogram Observe normally filled gall bladder.

Normally gall bladder concentrates the contrast within 12 hours to show a shadow and presence of any filling defect (gall stones). A fatty meal is given and contraction of gall bladder observed. One to two hours after a fatty meal the gall bladder contracts to one half or less of its size.

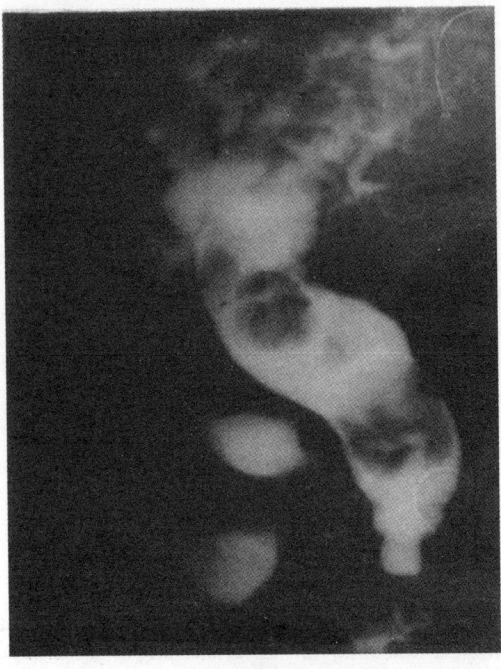

(3)

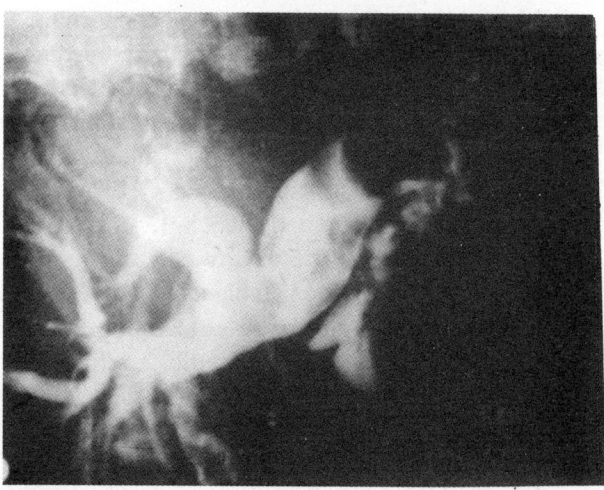

(4)

Fig. 3.3-4. Percutaneous tans hepatic cholangiography (PTC) both figures show filling defects at lower end of common bile duct (Gall stones), there is massive dilatation of intrahepatic ducts and common bile duct.

common bile duct, portal veins and pancreas can be visualized. Further distinction between intrahepatic and extrahepatic causes of jaundice can be made. Ultrasound has to a large extent replaced P.T. cholangiography.

Computed tomography (C.T). This is a very useful aid in all cases of hepatobiliary disorders. In this not only various structures are visualized but abnormalities in their size and shape are also detected.

Endoscopic retrograde cholangio pancreatography (ERCP). By means of an endoscope, ampulla in the second part of duodenum is cannulated and contrast is injected and both pancreas as well as gall bladder along with their ducts visualized.

ERCP is not only used as a diagnostic aid but also for therapeutic purpose like removal of stones from common bile duct.

Complications include pancreatitis, infection and cholangitis.

Magnetic resonance imaging (MRI). This procedure is employed for differentiating liver tumours, glands in the abdomen, round about common bile duct and in porta hepatis.

It is a useful non-invasive procedure and has its own use in doubtful masses in abdomen.

HEPATOMEGALY

Lying in the right upper quadrant of the abdomen and extending to the epigastrium and to some extent in the left upper quadrant, liver lies covered by ribs or costal cartilages, the upper border corresponding to the level of the 5th rib while the lower border crosses obliquely upwards from 9th right to the 8th left costal cartilage. It crosses the midline about midway between the base of the Xiphoid and the umbilius. The left lobe extends to the left of the sternum for about 5 cms.

Normally liver is not palpable except in cases where because of alterations in the position of the diaphragm it may be displaced or there is accessory or reidels lobe. A palpable liver does not mean hepatomegaly since liver may be displaced because of ptosis, a low lying diaphragm in cases of pleural effusion, pneumothorax and pulmonary emphysema. Liver enlargement (hepatomegaly) is always taken with reference to its palpability below the costal margin. It may be mild (viral hepatitis) moderate (cirrhosis, hepatitis) or gross reaching upto umblicus (leukaemia, Hodgkin's malignancy).

Causes of hepatomegaly.

Infections:

Viral hepatitis. Inflammation of liver due to viral hepatitis is a common cause of producing a tender hepatomegaly. There is moderate enlargement of liver which is smooth with consistency varying from soft to firm. History of loss of appetite, nausea and vomiting is available. Jaundice is present. There are features of low grade fever, toxaemia and pain in right hypochondrium. Serum bilirubin and enzymes (AST/ALT) levels are elevated.

Amoebic liver abscess. There is moderate to huge enlargement of liver depending on the size of liver abscess. In amoebic hepatitis enlargement is moderate. Liver is tender and there is tenderness on the lower costal cartilages on right side. Jaundice is uncommon though a massive liver abscess may produce it. Fever and toxaemia are present. Blood count shows luecocytosis with raised polymorph count. Movements of diaphragm on right side are restricted. Ultrasonography and diagnostic aspiration of liver absecess confirm the diagnosis.

Bacterial liver abscess. Multiple small pyogenic abscesses or a single large abscess as a result of generalized systemic pyaemia or infection in the gastrointestinal tract invloves the liver, mainly right lobe, producing an enlarged tender liver. Patient is toxic and wasted. There is dull aching pain in the liver area. Jaundice appears late. Skin over a large abscess is reddened and oedematous. A fluctuating mass inliver may be palpable. Diagnosis is based on history of fever coming with rigors and chills generally following acute infective process in the abdomen (appendicitis, cholecystitis). Total and differential white cell count shows polymorph leucocytosis. A plain X-ray abdomen may demonstrate fluid level in the abscess. Ultrasonography shall confirm the diagnosis. Aspiration of abscess with culture of pus is diagnostic.

Typhoid, malaria, kala-azar, tuberculosis. All these diseases invlove the liver in variousways. Malaria may produce moderate enlargement of liver with massive splenomegaly. There is history of fever coming with rigors and chills. In malignant form of malaria there is often mild jaundice, hepatomeglay and tenderness over the liver.

In kala-azar there is skin pigmentation and hepatosplenomegaly along with history of being resident in endemic area. Diagnosis is made by demonstration of Leishman Donovan bodies in bone marrow smear.

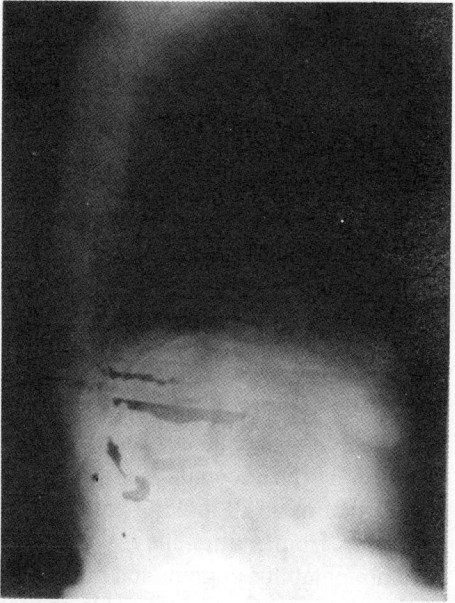

Fig. 3.5. Plain Xray abdomen showing calcified hydatid CYST in liver.

In typhoid, liver enlargement generally is mild, liver surface is smooth and there is no tenderness. There are features of toxaemia, jaundice is usually not present. Liver enlargement is present in varying degrees. Diagnosis of typhoid is based on widal test, blood/bone marrow culture Tuberculosis produces enlargement of liver primarily in miliary form of disease. Liver enlargement is smooth, and non-tender. In addition to other tests for tuberculosis, liver biopsy shall confirm the diagnosis of liver involvement where a caseous lesion along with acid fast bacilli can be demonstrated.

Hydatid disease. Hydatid cysts usually involve

the right lobe of liver involving its anterior or posterior inferior surfaces. Most of the times there are no symptoms and theonly complaint may be a dull ache in the right hypochondrium. Liver is palpable. In large hydatid cysts, hydatid thrill may be elicited. Diagnosis is based on positive complement fixation test and casoni test. Eosinophilia may be there. Calcification of cyst when seen on plain X-ray abdomen confirms the diagnosis. Further aid is obtained by ultrasonography.

Circulatory disturbances:

1. **Chronic venous congestion.** Congestive heart failure is an important cause of hepatomegaly moderate to massive. Liver is firm and tender. There are signs of underlying heart disease in the form of cardiomegaly, murmurs along with signs of congestive heart failure (raised jugular venous pressure, peripheral oedema, cyanosis). Constrictive pericarditis and pericardial effusion have massive hepatomegaly. Here patient has engorged neck veins, low pulse pressure and pulsus paradoxus. Heart sounds are feeble and apex beat is not visible.

2. **Hepatic vein occlusion (Budd-Chiari syndrome).** It is an uncommon condition and picture is that of an ill looking patient generally suffering from malignancy, polycythaemia, thrombophlebitus migrans and portal pyaemia. Patient has picture of intractable ascites with enlarged and tender liver. Mild jaundice is often present. Collaterals develop over the abdominal wall due to development of portal hypertension. In more chronic cases spleen may become palpable. Hepatic vein occlusion should be suspected when a patient with tendency to thrombosis or suffering from malignant disease develops an enlarged tender liver with resistant ascites.

Portal cirrhosis. There is mild to moderate enlargement of liver in cases of post necrotic cirrhosis. Liver has got a nodular surface. Jaundice may or may not be present. Splenomegaly and ascites appear in late stages. Patient has features of liver decompensation like spider naevi, clubbing, palmar erythema, gynaecomastia, testicular atrophy in men, dupuytren's contractures, loss of axillay and pubic hairs, white nails and peripheral oedema.

Diagnosis of cirrhosis is based on biochemical changes and liver biopsy.

Malignancy of liver. Involvement of liver leading to hepatomegly occurs in simple (primary) and malignant growths.

In primary growths of liver, it enlarges not only downwards but also upwards. A hard irregular lump may be felt in right upper quadrant. It is continuous with liver. In left lobe involvement mass is present in the epigastric region. Multiple masses may be felt but they are not tender. Jaundice is not constant. Ascites occurs in only small number of cases.

In secondary tumours of liver, size of liver is variable. Massive enlargement may be present. Tumour deposits give liver a hard nodular umbilicated feel. There are features of loss of weight, malaise and cachexia. Jaundice is only mild, deep jaundice appears when there is invasion of large bile ducts in the porta hepatis.

Diagnosis is based on biochemical tests (raised levels of AST/ALT and alkaline phosphatase). Diagnosis is confirmed by liver biopsy and peritonoscopy.

Reticuloendothelial diseases. These include leukaemia, hodgkin's disease, lymphomas and myeloproliferative disorders.

Liver is enlarged from mild to moderate degree depending on the underlying pathology. Thus liver is grossly enlarged in myeloid leukaemia and Hodgkins disease. Liver enlargement in lymphoid leukaemia is never massive.

Liver in all these condition is non-tender. Jaundice generally is not present but if present it is mild.

Patient generally has anaemia. Lymphadenopathy, splenomegaly and tendency to bleed. Diagnosis is based on peripheral blood examination, bone marrow, gland and liver biopsy.

Miscellaneous disorders. These include fatty liver in cases of severe anaemia, malunutrition and chronic alcoholics. Liver is moderately enlarged, smooth, non tender. There is no ascites or jaundice.

Features of anaemia and malnutrition are generally present.

Amyloidosis is one condition where liver is predominantly involved in secondary form. It commonly follows chronic diseases like pulmonary tuberculosis, pulmonary suppuration, ulcerative colitis and rheumatoid arthritis. Liver when involved is moderately enlarged, smooth, non-tender with a rubbery feel. There is evidence of amyloid involvement inother organs.

Diagnosis is based on demonstration of massive albuminuria and a positive congo red test. Confirmation is made by gum, kidney or liver biopsy.

In glycogen storage disease, liver is smooth, firm and markedly enlarged. There is no jaundice but features of physical retardation and failure of general health. Diagnosis is made by demonstration of low blood sugar levels and by liver biopsy.

Lipoid storage disorders (Gaucher's disease, Niemann picks disease) are characterised by pigmentation on exposed parts, massive splenomegaly and liver which is enlarged, smooth and firm. While Gaucher's disease may occur in adults, Niemann picks disease occurs only in infants. Diagnosis is made by bone marrow biopsy.

Diabetes of long standing produces hepatomegaly which is mild to moderate. Hepatic enlargement in young adults and children with uncontrolled diabetes is massive. Fatty infiltration of liver giving rise to mild enlargement of liver occurs in young diabetics and in women during pregnancy.

Haemochromatosis is characterised by an enlarged liver which is firm, non-tender. Left lobe may be more enlarged than right. When liver capsule distends due to intrahepatic iron deposits, pain in liver area appears which sometimes is very acute. Diagnosis is based on skin changes, presence of congestive failure, diabetes and secondary sexual changes. Diagnosis is confirmed by liver biopsy.

Haemolytic anaemias also produce mild to moderate enlargement of liver which is non-tender. Jaundice is usually mild. Splenomegaly, dark coloured urine and increased osmotic fragility of blood shall favour the diagnosis.

Causes of hepatomegaly

1. *Infections*
   a. Viral hepatitis
   b. Amoebic liver abscess
   c. Bacterial liver abscess
   d. Typhoid fever
   e. Malaria
   f. Kala-azar
   g. Tuberculosis
   h. Hydatid disease

2. *Circulatory distrubances*
   a. Congestive heart failure
   b. Constrictive pericarditis (pericardial effusion)
   c. Hepatic vein occlusion (Budd-Chiari syndrome)

3. *Portal cirrhosis*

4. *Tumours*
   a. Primary tumour (Hepatoma)
   b. Secondaries in liver

5. *Reticuloendothelial disorders*
   a. Leukaemia
   b. Hodgkin's disease
   c. Myeloproliferative disorders

6. *Miscellaneous causes*
   a. Diabetes mellitus
   b. Anaemia
   c. Chronic alcoholism
   d. Haemochromatosis
   e. Haemolytic anaemia
   f. Amyloidosis
   g. Lipoid storage diseases (Gaucher's disease and Niemann-Pick disease)

7. *Biliary cirrhosis*

Biliary cirrhosis. It is generally seen in a middle-aged female who is well nourished. Liver is markedly enlarged, smooth, firm and non-tender. Spleen is palpable and there is skin pigmentation along with jaundice. This has to be differentiated from extrahepatic biliary obstruction.

Patients of biliary cirrhosis have insidious onset, painless obstructive jaundice, no fever and a large liver with palpable spleen. Ascites usually is absent. Skin xanthomas develop frequently. Urine contains bile pigment and urobilin. Blood biochemistry shows raised bilirubin, alkaline phosphatase, normal serum albumin and slightly raised globulin levels. Electrophoresis shows an increase in alpha-2 and beta globulin levels.

ASCITES

Collection of fluid in the peritoneal cavity is called ascites and at least 1500 ml of fluid must collect in the peritoneal cavity before it is detected by physical examination. Causes of ascites shall include local as well as general causes.

Development of ascites depends on number of factors.

1. Plasma colloid osmotic pressure and the portal venous pressure. Plasma albumin level controls the colloid osmotic pressure and a lowered plasma albumin level is essential for the development of ascites. Factor of raised portal venous pressure and diminished plasma protein levels when present together shall produce ascites.

   Failure of liver to synthesize albumin because of poor hepatocellular function shall result in diminished albumin contributing further to a low plasma osmotic pressure. Intra hepatic portal venous obstruction compounding portal hypertension further increases amount of fluid in peritoneal cavity. Factors leading to sodium and water retention shall include stimulation of the adrenal cortex with increased production of aldosterone, and activation of renin angiotensin aldosterone system.

2. Fall of renal blood flow with lowered glomerular filtration rate shall be leading to sodium retention and fluids. This is further compounded by increased production of antidiuretic hormone with resultant water retention and its depressed excretion.

Thus production of ascites is dependant on number of factors ranging from plasma osmotic pressure to renal blood flow changes, aldosterone activity to antidiuretic hormonal activity.

Clinical picture. Cases of ascites present with adbominal distension developing over a period of weeks or it may develop quickly in a period of days.

Pathogenesis of Ascites

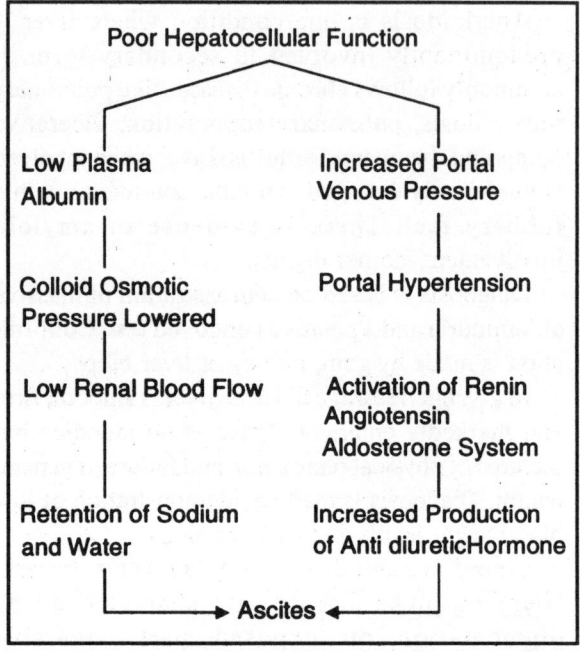

Presence of ascites is seen by bulging of abdomen, prominence being in the flanks. Confirmation of fluid is done by demostration of fluid thrill and shifting dullness. In cases of massive ascites, shifting dullness may not be demonstrable and in cases with small amount of fluid or localized ascites, fluid thrill may not be elicited.

Skin over the abdomen is stretched, umbilicus is everted and in line with the abdomen. Features of malnutrition are often present. Oedema over ankles and feet if present is due to hypoproteinaemia. Because of abdominal distension diaphragm may be pushed upwards and often there is respiratory distress. Pleural effusion on right side may be present due to leakage of peritoneal fluid through the diaphragmatic lymphatics into the pleural space. Urinary output is reduced.

Development of sudden abdominal pain with fever, toxaemia in a case of ascites should make one suspect spontaneous bacterial peritonitis.

Causes of ascites:

1. Diseases of peritoneum

Tuberculous peritonitis. Generally it is a young

undernourished individual. It may be primary or secondary to pulmonary tuberculosis. Ascites is moderate, never massive. Abdomen has a plastic or doughy feel with coils of gut matted with glands or omentum. Ascitic fluid is generally turbid or haemorrhagic. Specific gravity more than 1.015. Protein content more than 2.5 g%. Cell count of fluid shows predominant rise in lymphocytes. Confirmation of diagnosis by peritoneal biopsy. Culture of ascitic fluid for acid fast bacilli and guinea pig inoculation.

Causes of ascites on nature of fluid

Exudate

1. Tuberculous ascites
2. Malignant ascites
3. Chylous ascites
4. Pyogenic peritonitis

Transudate

1. Congestive heart failure
2. Constrictive preicarditis
3. Nephrotic syndrome
4. Portal cirrhosis
5. Anaemia, hypoproteinaemia
6. Meig's syndrome
7. Inferior venacaval obstruction
8. Beri-beri

Malignant peritonitis. In this amount of ascites is small. It is common in malignancy of gastrointestinal tract, secondaries in peritoneal cavity; occult malignancy and disseminated carcinoma from genitalia in females. Fluid generally is straw coloured, haemorrhagic or mucinous. Specific gravity more than 1.015. Protein content more than 2.5 g%. Cell count is variable. Further confirmation of diagnosis by peritoneal biopsy and cytology demonstrating malignant cells.

Evidence of primary disease in some organs may be seen. Patients with malignant ascites are markedly emaciated and show a down hill course.

2. Portal hypertension. This includes cirirhosis of liver, where there is splenomegaly, ascites which is disproportionate to the oedema over legs and feet. Ankle oedema is often preceded by abdominal distension. The liver may be enlarged or contracted

and impalpable. Rapid filling of ascites may take place after paracentesis pointing to poor hepatocellular function.

Causes of ascites

1. Diseases of peritoneum
   a. Tuberculous peritonitis
   b. Malignant peritonitis
2. Portal cirrhosis
3. Inferior venacaval obstruction
4. Meig's syndrome
5. Chylous ascites
6. Ascites associated with generalized anasarca
   a. Congestive heart failure
   b. Constrictive pericarditis
   c. Nephrotic syndrome
   d. Anaemia, hypoproteinaemia
   e. Beri-beri

Portal vein thrombosis is characterised by rapid development of ascites along with splenomegaly. Portal vein may be obstructed by either due to primary or secondary enlarged lymph glands. There is ascites and often mild jaundice.

3. Inferior vena caval obstruction. There is abdominal distension, ascites and prominent abdominal veins with reversal of blood flow. Often there is history of previous thrombosis in legs. Oedema is present over the dependent parts.

4. Meig's syndrome. In females triad of ascites, ovarian tumour and pleural effusion characterises this disease. Ascites often/is massive.

5. Chylous ascites. Ascites here has a turbid, milky and opalescent appearance. It is most often the rsult of lymphatic obstruction from tumour, trauma, tuberculosis or filariasis. Chylous ascites accumulates rapidly and has often to be differentiated from pseudochylous ascites which accumulates slowly. In chylous ascites, fat droplets are small and uniform with fat content high. Fat globules can be seen stained by Sudan staining. Ether extraction will lead to clearing of the turbidity if it is due to lipids. In contrast pseudochylous ascites has low fat content and cellular proteins which will dissolve by alkalinization and turbidity reduced.

6. Ascites associated with generalized anasarca. This will include cases of congestive heart failure, nephrotic syndrome, severe anaemia, hypo-proteinaemia, constrictive pericarditis, polyserositis and beri-beri.

Ascites associated with congestive heart failure has got oedema over legs and feet, engorged neck veins, enlarged and tender liver and evidence of cardiac disease.(Cardiomegaly, Murmurs)

Cases of nephrotic syndrome have puffy face, oedema maximum in early hours of morning and generalized anasarca. Urine shows massive albumi-nuria. Blood chemistry shows hypoalbumin-aemia and hyper cholesterolemia.

When ascities is due to anaemia with hypo-proteinaemia there is severe degree of anaemia and deficiency state. Ascites generally is moderate, oedema over feet is marked. Blood shows low serum proteins, albumin globulin ratio disturbed.

Constrictive pericarditis has got ascites, engorged neck veins. Pulsus paradoxus, enlarged liver and feeble heart sounds. Oedema over legs and feet is minimal. A picture of polyserositis may be seen where in addition to massive ascites, there is pleural and pericardial effusion. Oedema over the legs is not much.

Beri-beri though not very common is associated with vitamin B_1 deficiency. Patient has ascites, oedema, neuropathy and cardiomegaly.

Of the other causes, a case of ascites may still has to be differentiated from obesity. Pregnancy and an ovarian cyst where there is massive enlargement of abdomen. There may be fluid thrill but no shifting dullness. Upper border of cyst will be defined as convex whereas in ascites due to any cause it shall be horse show shaped with concavity above.

Diagnosis. Ascites is a symptom of a number of diseases and based on aetiology, the diagnosis of basic underlying disease is arrived at.

Most of the time cause of ascites may appear obvious. Thus an emaciated wasted individual with moderate amount of ascites shall favour either a tuberculous or malignant ascites. Presence of anaemia, hypoproteinaemia shall be suggestive of malnutrition while a history of haematemesis and melaena shall suggest cirrhosis and respiratory difficulty will be a pointer towards a cardiac lesion.

Similarly a case of nephrotic syndrome with massive anasarca will have history of decreased urinary output and swelling appearing over face on getting up in morning.

Investigations. Every case of ascites has to be investigated on individual lines depending on suspected aetiology but one test which is helpful in almost all cases is diagnostic paracentesis where ascitic fluid should be examined for its gross appearance, Protein content and cell count. In some cases cytologic examination, acid fast stain and culture including guinea pig inoculation are required.

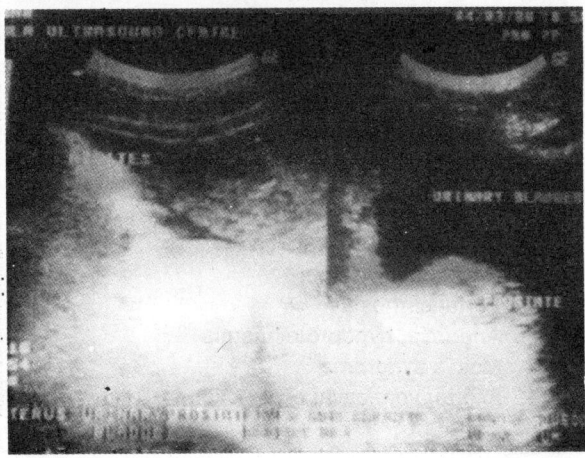

Fig. 3.6. Ultra-sound of abdomen showing ascites.

Differences between various types of ascitic fluids

	Trasudate	Exudate
Colour	Clear	Turbid haemorrhagic
Specific gravity	Between 1.000 and 1.015	Greater than 1.015
Protein content	Less than 2.5 g%	More than 2.5 g%
Cell count	Occasional cell mesothelial or mononuclear	Cell count more than 1000 cells. Predominant lymphocytes

When ascitic fluid is clear, with specific gravity between 1000-1.015, protein content less than

2.5 g%, few cells usually mesothelial or mononuclear, this is called transudate and is generally seen in congestive failure, nephrotic syndrome cirrhosis, hypoproteinaemia, constrictive pericarditis. Compared to transudate, ascites which is mainly inflammatory in nature, is turbid or haemorrhagic or chylous is called exudative form. Its specific gravity is more than 1.015, protein content more than 2.5g%, cell count more than 1000 with predominant polymorph leucocytes and lymphocytes (70%). Exudative ascites is seen in tuberculous peritonitis, malignant peritonitis, pyogenic peritonitis etc.

Further investigation shall depend on the suspected disease. A case of cirrhosis liver shall require liver function tests and liver biopsy. Constrictive pericaditis shall require cardiac imaging and cardiac catheterization while peritoneal biopsy will confirm the diagnosis in tuberculous peritonitis. Histologic examination along with ascitic fluid culture and animal inoculation will further substantiate the diagnosis. Cytological examination of ascitic fluid for malignant cells along with ultrasound, CT scan and MRI shall be helpful in further evaluating a case of suspected malignant ascites.

Management. It depends on the underlying pathology. For tuberculous aetiology, anti-tubercular therapy, for congestive failure, digitalis and diuretics, for malignancy chemotherapy. Heavy doses of vitamin B_1 for case of beri-beri, iron, folic acid and blood transfusion for anaemia and hypoproteinaemia. In every case of ascites:

1. Oral diuretics (frusemide, spirnolactone, either daily or on alternate day) are administered. Electrolytes have to be monitored since frusemide (dosage 40-80 mg) produces potassium loss while spirnolactone (dosage 25-100 mg) is a potassium-sparing diuretic. Both diuretics may be combined for better effect.
2. Restrict sodium intake. Diet low in sodium content (cucumber, peas, tomatoes, apple, dates, oranges, grapes, wheat, puffed rice, jelly, etc.) be prescribed. All foods with high sodium content be avoided.

3. In cases where ascites is massive, producing cardiorespiratory embarassment, abdominal paracentesis be done and fluid be drained slowly. Side effects include infection at the site of puncture, and peritonitis. Vaso vagal attack if fluid is withdrawn rapidly may occur. In a case of cirrhosis if too much fluid is drawn rapidly hepatic coma may be precipitated.

JAUNDICE

It is a condition where there is yellow pigmentation of the skin or sclera by excess of bilirubin in the blood. Normal levels of bilirubin in the blood range from 0.8 to 1.2 mg and most of this is unconjugated. When levels of bilirubin exceed 2 mg or above, clinical jaundice becomes apparent. Preponderance of unconjugated bilirubin indicates haemolytic jaundice while rise in conjugated occurs in either obstructive or hepato cellular jaundice.

Jaundice is a symptom complex and number of diseases are responsible for it. Broadly there are three forms of jaundice—haemolytic, obstructive and hepatocellular jaundice. In addition there is a group of cases where there are disturbances of bilirubin conjugation in the microsomes producing chronic non hemolytic jaundice.

Haemolytic jaundice. In this there is excessive breakdown of red blood cells in the reticulo-endothelial system, with the result that bilirubin is produced in excess from haemoglobin. Increased bilirubin is carried to liver for excretion, which raises levels of faecal stercobilinogen producing dark brown sools. Stercobilinogen is absorbed from the intestines in amounts greaterthan that can be reexcreted and result is that large quantities are passed out in the urine as urobilinogen.

Causes of haemolytic jaundice. *These shall include:*

1. Physiological jaundice, jaundice of prematurity
2. Defect in shape of erythrocytes
   a. Spherocytosis
   b. Sickle cell anaemia

3. Parasitic destruction of erythrocytes: Malaria in patients with glucose-6-phosphatase dehydrogenase deficiency
4. Toxic agents: These include metals like lead, poisons like snake venom, drugs like sulfonamides, nitrofurantoin and FAVA beans.
5. Bacterial toxins, septicaemia
6. Incompatible blood transfusions
7. ABO and Rh blood group Incompability
8. Extensive burns of the body.

Classification of jaundice:

1. Haemolytic

a. Physiological: Jaundice of prematurity
b. Congential: Spherocytosis, sickle cell anaemia
c. Parasitic destruction of erythrocytes: Malaria
d. Toxins: Heavy metals
e. Poisons: Snake venom
f. Drugs: Sulfonamides, nitrofurnatoin
g. Bacterial toxins: Septicaemia
h. Incompatible blood transfusions—ABO and Rh blood group incompatibility
i. Extensive burns

2. Obstructive

a. *Extrahepatic*
1. Obstruction within the bile ducts—gall stones, neoplasm, round worm.
2. Obstruction due to changes in the wall of the ducts: Congenital obstruction (biliary atresia), traumatic (following surgery), sclerosing cholangitis.
3. Pressure from without: Carcinoma of liver (primary/secondary) gumma, hydatid cyst, enlarged glands in porta hepatis (Hodgkin's, leukaemia, tuberculosis) carcinoma head of pancreas, cancer stomach.
b. *Intrahepatic (obstruction without mechanical cause)*
1. Drugs like chlorpromazine, antitubercular drugs, methyl testosterone, oral contraceptives.
2. Viral hepatitis with prolonged cholestasis.

3. Jaundice of pregnancy
4. Primary biliary cirrhosis

3. Hepatocellular

a. Virus hepatitis
b. Infectious monoucleosis
c. Yellow fever
d. Bacterial diseases with fever, typhoid
e. Malaria
f. Weil's disease
g. Chemicals like chloroform, halothane, trinitrotoluene, carbon tetrachloride
h. Post-necrotic cirrhosis
i. Alcoholic hepatitis
j. Haemochromatosis

4. Congenital hyperbilirubinaemia

a. Without liver pigment:
   1. Gilbert's disease
   2. Criggler-Najjar syndrome
b. With liver pigment:
   1. Dubin-Johnson syndrome
   2. Rotor syndrome

Obstructive jaundice. Here bilirubin conjugation takes place normally in the liver but it does not reach the intestines and goes into the blood stream, the result being rise of bilirubin levels. Since bile is unable to reach the intestines and the faeces, stools in absence of stercobilinogin are clay coloured. Urine contains bilirubin while urobilinogen is absent. Causes of obstructive jaundice include both extrahepatic and intrahepatic causes. Thus there may be obstruction in the bile ducts either within or pressure from outside.

Extra hepatic:

1. *Obstruction within the bile ducts.* Commonest cause is gall stones. Other causes shall be a neoplasm, or rarely a round worm blocking the duct after entering from the duodenum.
2. *Obstruction due to changes in the wall of the ducts.* Congenital obliteration of the duct in infants (biliary atresia) inflammation, stricture following injury during operation, sclerosing cholangitis.

Pressure from without. Pressure upon the bile ducts from without occurs in number of diseases. Carcinoma of the liver both primary or secondary is the commonest cause. Uncommon causes shall include gumma, abscess and a hydatid cyst of liver.

Enlarged glands in the porta hepatis due to any cause (Hodgkin's, leukaemia, tuberculosis). Carcinoma of head of the pancreas, cancer of stomach when the growth spreads to lesser omentum and presses on the common bile duct even invading its wall are the other causes.

Intrahepatic. In this there is no mechanical obstruction in the bile ducts andcauses include intake of drugs like chlorpromazine, antitubercular drugs, methyl testosterone, oral contraceptives. Alcoholic hepatitis, post necrotic cirrhosis, virus hepatitis with prolonged cholestatsis, primary biliary cirrhosis and uncommonly jandice of pregnancy developing in the last trimester.

Hepatocellular, toxic or infective jaundice. There is failure of liver cells to conjugate and excrete all the bile pigment. Because of poor functioning of liver cells, it is unable to re-excrete stercobilinogen which is removed by the kidneys and excreted into urine as urobilinogen which is present there in excess. Stools are paler but not acholic indicating less amount of stercobilinogen.

Causes:

1. Infections like virus hepatitis, yellow fever, infectious mononucleosis, septicaemia, malaria, typhoid, Weils disease.
2. Chemical poisons like chloroform, halothane, gold, trinitrotoluene, carbon tetrachloride.
3. Postnecrotic cirrhosis, alcoholic hepatitis, haemochromatosis.

Chronic non-hemolytic jaundice. This group comprises cases where there is decreased bilirubin conjugation and a deficiency of the enzyme glucuronyl transferase. Gilbert's disease is the commonest variety, with a familial incidence and inherited as dominant. It generally manifests with mild form of jaundice starting in childhood. Liver histology is normal and the disease carries good prognosis. Compared to this there is more severe form of unconjugated hyperbilirubinaemia (Crigler-Najjar syndrome). Bilirubin levels are very high and there is kernicterus. Most of these infants die usually within first year of life. Those who survive are left behind with neurological defects.

Another variety of chronic non-hemolytic jaundice are cases of idiopathic conjugated hyperbilirubinaemia (Dubin-Johnson and Rotor syndromes) where levels of conjugated bilirubin are increased in blood and bilirubin appears in urine. Both are familial and carry good prognosis.

Symptoms. Symptoms of a case of jaundice shall vary with the type of jaundice the patient is suffering from and the underlying condition. Commonest form of jaundice is due to hepatitis where the patient may start with malaise, low grade fever, vomiting and loss of appetite. The person may take his/her morning breakfast normally and as the day passes, appetite for food almost disappears. In smokers, urge to smoke is the earliest to go. Yellowness appears first in the conjunctiva and then the mucous membrane of the lips and palate became pale. Urine is high coloured while in earlystage, the stools may remain of normal colour.

When a person has got features of obstructive jaundice, colour of conjunctiva is yellowish green. Stools become clay coloured and there is severe degree of itching. Pulse becomes slow. There are tell tale signs of itching in the form of scratching. Patient may suffer from bruises and bleeding from mucous surfaces due to lack of fat soluble vitamin K.

If jaundice remains for prolonged periods as in case of malignancy patient suffers from marked asthenia and wasting.

Investigation of a case of jaundice:

Age and sex. Transient jaundice appearing in infants few days after birth is called 'Physiological jaundice' and disappears in a few days. It may have a slightly prolonged course in premature infants. A progressive jaundice, obstructive in nature developing within a week or so of birth is suggestive of congenital obliteration of bile ducts (biliary atresia). Jaundice appearing in young adults is commonly due to infective hepatitis while in females (fat, forty) gall stones become a common cause. In last trimester of pregnancy uncommonly mild jaundice with pruritis develops in some women. It is called cholestatic type of jaundice, disappears after delivery but recurs during subsequent pregnancies.

Persistent jaundice in persons above the age of 40 should make one suspect carcinoma (cancer of bile ducts, hepatic metastasis—primary or secondary, carcinoma head of pancreas etc.).

Occupation of the patient. Weil's disease in sewer workers or fish handlers is common.

Family history. History of chronic cholecystitis or gall stones in the family. Familial incidence of congental hyperbilirubinaemia (Gilbert's disease, Crigler-Najjar syndrome, Dubin Johnson and Rotor syndromes).

Personal history of contact where viral hepatitis is endemic. History of receiving any injection, blood transfusion during the preceding six months. Appearance of jaundice shall favour serum hepatitis. History of intake of drugs like gold, sulfonamides, chlorpromazine, antitubercular drugs, oral contraceptives, methyl testosterone or any other hepato-toxic agent since these are known to produce jaundice.

Previous history of fatty dyspepsia, biliary colic shall favour chronic cholecystitis and gall stones. Nausea, anorexia and malaise preceding jaundice is suggestive of infective hepatitis while epigastric pain with progressive jaundice will point towards carcinoma pancreas.

Jaundice which follows surgery of the biliary tract may suggest a residual calculus, stricture of the bile duct or sclerosing cholangitis.

History of excessive alcohol intake in cases of alcoholic hepatitis. Pruritis favours obstructive jaundice. Painless jaundice with loss of weight, and wasting suggests malignancy.

Colour. Jaundice of toxic and infective hepatitis is bright yellow or orange coloured. In haemolytic jaundice it is lemon yellow and in obstructive jaundice it is greenish yellow.

Colour of stools and urine. In obstructive jaundice stools are clay coloured (acholic) in hepatocellular or infective jaundice they are usually of normal brown colour while in haemolytic jaundice stools have dark brown colour.

Urobilinogen is absent in urine in obstructive jaundice while bilirubin is present. In hepatocellular jaundice and haemolytic jaundice, urobilinogen is present in excess while biliirubin is absent in haemolytic jaundice though present in hepatocellular form of jaundice.

Course of the disease. Patient of infective hepatitis over a period of time show improvement in general condition and jaundice. In obstructive jaundice, levels of bilirubin progressively rise and if obstruction is complete further rise shall occur suggestive of malignancy.

Physical examination. Patient may show signs of anaemia, malnutrition suggestive of malignancy or cirrhosis. In cirrhotics look for spider naevi, white nails, enlargement of parotid glands, testicular atrophy, palmar erythema, gynaecomastia, oedema over legs and feet, and ascites.

There may be scratch marks on skin suggestive of cholestasis due to obstructive jaundice, Bruising and Petechial spots indicating prothrombin deficiency in alcoholic or Laennec's cirrhosis may be observed.

Liver may be palpable, smooth and tender in infective hepatitis, hard and nodular in malignancy.

Gall bladder becomes palpable when obstruction at the level of common bile duct is incomplete (courvoisier's law). A hard, small nodular gall bladder may be palpated in carcinoma. In chronic cholecystitis, gall bladder may be palapable and tender (Murphy's sign). In addition to looking for signs of disease in general examination, look specifically in abdomen for ascites, liver, spleen and any lymphadenopathy. Rectal examaination may be carried out for any primary growth in rectum.

Biochemical tests

1. Serum bilirubin estimation to assess the level of jaundice. Flocculation tests (zinc sulphate and thymol turbidity) are positive in hepatocellular jaundice but negative in obstructive and haemolytic jaundice. *Alkaline phosphatase* levels are normal to less than three times normal levels in haemolytic and hepatocellular jaundice while levels four times

Differential diagnosis of main varieties of jaundice

	Obstructive jaundice	Hepatocellular jaundice	Haemolytic jaundice
Age	Middle aged or elderly	Young adults	Infants, young adults
Previous history	History of dyspepsia attacks of pain	Exposure to contacts, serum transfusion. Intake of drugs	History of exposure to infections/toxins Acquired or congenital haemolytic anaemia
Pain	Constant or colicky pain	Dragging pain over liver	None
Rate of development of jaundice	Slow but may rise rapidly in malignancy	Slow	Slow but rapid in haemolytic crisis
Pruritis	Present	Present in cholestatic phase only	Absent
Type of jaundice	Greenish yellow	Orange yellow	Lemon yellow
General symptoms	Weight loss, asthenia, wasting, Bruises,scratch marks	Average health except malaise. In cirrhosis, palmar erythema, ascites, oedema	Apparently in good health
Liver	Enlarged	Enlarged and tender	Moderately enlarged
Spleen	Absent	Often enlarged especially in cirrhosis	Splenomegaly common
Faeces	Clay coloured	Clay coloured for few days	Dark brown
Urine	Urobilinogen absent.Bilirubin present	Urobilinogen in excess. Bilirubin present	Urobilinogen in excess. Bilirubin absent
S.alkaline phosphatase KA units	Greater than 30.	Less than 30	Less than 30.
Flocculation tests	Negative	Usually positive	Negative
Prothrombin time	Prolonged. Response to vitamin K satisfactory	Prolonged. Response to vitamin K poor	Normal
Serum albumin/globulin	Normal	Slightly depressed. Rise in globulin levels	Normal
Radiology	Plain *X-ray* abdomen shows gall stones. Barium meal shows widening and displacement of duodenum in carcinoma head of pancreas	Oesophageal varices in portal hypertension	Not significant
Ultraeonography	Helpful	Not of much use	Not of much use

than normal indicate obstructive jaundice and often malignancy.

Serum albumin levels are low and globulins levels are high in chronic hepatocellulr jaundice.

Electrophoretic pattern suggests predominence of alpha and beta globulin levels in obstructive jaundice while gamma globulin elevation suggests hepatocellular jaundice.

Transaminases (AST/ALT) are raised in infective/toxic hepatitis. Prothrombin time is prolonged in obstructive jaundice and hepatocellular failure as in cirrhosis.

Haematology. A raised while cell count with polymorph leucocytosis indicates severe infective hepatitis or cholangitis. In haemolytic jaundice, blood film shows immature cells and spherocytosis. Erythrocyte fragility is increased. Coomb's test is positive.

Other tests include Australian Antigen (Hb S AG) Viral studies for hepatitis A, B, non-A, non-B, autoimmune antibodies for primary biliary cirrhosis, alpha fetoprotein for liver malignancy.

Radiology. Plain X-ray picture of abdomen may show raised dome of diaphragm in a malignant liver. Gall stones may be seen.

Barium meal study of oesophagse for oesophageal varices in cases of cirrhosis. Widening or displacement of duodenum in carcinoma head of pancreas. Intravenous cholecystogoraphy may show poor functioning of gall bladder in chronic cholecystitis.

An ultrasound may show primary or secondary tumour of liver, pancreas, size of bile ducts and level of obstruction as well as presence of tumour or glands. Ultrasonography is a useful non-invasive test.

Aspiration needle biopsy of liver. It has to be done with caution in the presence of jaundice. Prothrombin time must be normal before undertaking the test. Instead of Vim Silverman's needle, Meghini needle is employed. It is safe and less traumatic. The histological appearances of three types of jaundice (obstructive, hepatocellular and hemolytic) are distinctive.

Other tests include percutaneous transhepatic cholangiography (PTC), endoscopic retrograde cholangiopanceratography (ERCP) which are employed in reaching aetiological diagnosis peritonescopy is a very useful method to study various abdominal structures and reach a diagnosis. But there shall be still a small percentage of cases who will require a lapratomy to confirm the diagnosis.

Treatment. Jaundice is a symptom complex and treatment is to be directed towards the underlying cause. In general supportive measures, patient should be given small frequent feeds of fat free, low protein and high carbohydrate diet which can be easily assimilated. In addition vitamin B complex, vitamin C orally be given in high doses. In obstructive jaundice, vitamin K should be given daily (10 mg) parenterally. Sedatives should preferably be not given in a case of jaundice since they are likely to precipitate hepatic coma.

VIRAL HEPATITIS

Viral hepatitis is a clinical entity where systemic infection causes inflammation and hepatic cell necrosis producing typical clinical, biochemical, immunological and morphological features. A number of viruses may cause hepatitis like picture but five viruses specific for liver have been identified. They are hepatitis A virus (HAV). Hepatitis B virus (HBV), two types of non-A, non-B hepatitis virus (NANB) and hepatitis delta virus. All these viruses produce almost similar clinical picture though the viruses can be differentiated by their antigens characteristics.

Epidemiology. Viral hepatitis is of worldwide distribution and infection is transmitted by three main routes, faecal oral route, direct person to person and by parenteral route.

Hepatitis A virus (HAV) is excreted in faeces and the spread is mainly through faecal contamination of water supply and most cases occur in epidemic form while sporadic cases follow person to person contact. A case of viral hepatitis excretes the virus for about two weeks before the start of illness and for a few days afterwards. This is the most infectious period in a case of hepatitis. Epidemics of viral hepatitis (HAV) are reported worldwide and often result from contamination of water supply.

Hepatitis B virus (HBV) is mainly spread by parenteral route i.e. by transfusion of infective blood and blood products or by use of contaminated instruments, syringes, needles, tattooing, acupuncture. This is particularly important in case of drug addicts. Vertical transmission from mother to child is another route of infection.

Epidemics of hepatitis B have also been seen. Any procedure involving intravenous, intramuscular, subcutaneous injection, transfusion of blood, plasma and its products and dental procedures all carry the risk. The virus is mainly spread by parenteral route and is present in the blood during its long incubation period though faeces of a patient of serum hepatitis are not infective.

Delta virus hepatitis (HDV) also is of worldwide distribution and is spread by parenteral route mainly by blood and its products. It mainly occurs in association with hepatitis B infection especially in drug addicts or in those who are already infected by HBV infection.

Non-A, non-B hepatitis. It mainly consists of two type of viruses. Hepatitis C virus which is spread by blood transfusion, parenteral route especially in intravenous drug abusers, in dialysis units. Haemophilics and transplant recipients. Other form of non-A, non-B hepatitis is termed hepatitis E virus (HEV). Its spread is mainly through contaminated water supply.

Clinical profile. Clinical features in all patients of hepatitis are almost the same except slight variations. These may range from mild form of disease to serious form like fulminant hepatitis. In general type A, type B and non-A and non-B hepatitis run the same clinical course but HBV hepatitis tends to be more severe and may be associated with a serum sickness like syndrome.

The mildest attack of hepatitis may be without symptoms and is marked only by rise in transaminase levels. The patient may be anicteric but suffers gastrointestinal and influenza-like symptoms.

Cases of hepatitis may pass through three phases:

1. Preicteric or prodromal phase
2. Icteric phase
3. Post icteric phase.

Preicteric phase. Often referred to as prodromal phase it lasts for three to seven days or even longer before the appearance of jaundice. Patient in this period feels unwell, suffers digestive symptoms (anorexia, nausea) has headache, general malaise and may have mild pyrexia. Rigors are unusual. Anorexia is marked and patient may not stand the site of food. Loss of desire to smoke or take alochol is present. A small pain develops in the right hypochondrium and may be increased by movement. Liver is palpable and tender. Malaise almost invariably is severe and gives the patient a wretched feeling.

Cases of serum hepatitis may show rashes (maculo papular, urticarial or erythematous) transient migrating arthralgia and arteritis. These are uncommon manifestation present only in small percentage of cases and disappear with the appearance of jaundice.

Icteric phase. The prodromal phase is followed by the appearance of jaundice which develops rapidly. There is darkening of the urine and stools become pale. Symptoms tend to decrease. Temperature returns to normal. Appetite improves and nausea, vomiting subside. Pruritis may be seen transiently for a few days. Liver is enlarged, smooth, tender and palpable in seventy to seventy five per cent of cases while spleen is palpable only in 20 per cent of cases. Patient may loose weight. Jaundice which initially may be severe, gradually subsides in a period of one to four weeks the average patient usually makes an uneventful recovery. The stools regain their colour, urine becomes normal. Appetite becomes good.

After apparent recovery, lassitude and fatigue persist for some weeks. Clinical and biochemical recovery takes longer time and usually takes upto six months after the onset of illness.

Posticteric phase. After recovery from jaundice, patient may experience a sense of fatigue and general lassitude. Posticteric phase usually is between two to six weeks. Appetite in this phase is good, stools and urine regain their normal colour and a sense of well-being develops gradually though complete clinical and biochemical recovery may take longer time.

Pathology. The liver changes in all types of virus A, B, non-A, non-B infection are similar and essential lesion is acute inflammation of the whole liver. There is diffuse liver cell injury with hepatic cell necrosis associated with leucocytic and histiocytic reaction and infiltration. There is centrilobular necrosis and portal tracts show great cellularity. The sinusoids show hyperplasia of Kupffer cells and inflammatory changes. Fatty change is absent.

Focal spotty necrosis may be seen. The reticulum frame work is well preserved even in the midst of extreme disorganisation, the necrotic cells appear to have dropped out. If reticulum frame work is intact, liver cells regenerate from without inwards and recovery is usually complete. Inflammatory cells disappear gradually from the portal tracts and some new connective tissue can be formed. During recovery phase, reticuloendothelial activity increases.

In severe forms of hepatitis, massive fulminant necrosis involving the whole lobule is seen. There may be bridging or subacute or confluent necrosis when large areas of liver cells drop out with collapse of reticulum frame work. Bridging necrosis may be followed by the development of fibrous septa, nodules and a subacute course leading to scar formation (post necrotic scarring) and subsequent post necrotic cirrhosis.

Macroscopically the liver is reduced in size, flaccid and shrunken. Nodular regeneration may be seen in those where the course is prolonged. Liver shows a nut meg appearance with red areas of haemorrhage alternating with yellow patches of necrosis.

Continuation of inflammatory activity and fibrosis in the portal zones with preservation of liver architecture constitutes picture of chronic persistent hepatitis which is benign self limiting condition. In some cases portal tracts may enlarge and become irregular with inflammatory cells reaction. Liver cell necrosis is seen at the junction of the portal zone and there is collapse of reticulum frame work. There is progressive replacement of bridging necrosis with fibrosis. This is chronic active hepatitis where there is progressive distribution of hepatocytes over number of years eventually leading to developmrnt of cirrhosis. It is significant that histological changes in liver are found even before the development of jaundice.

Laboratory investigations:

Urine. Bilirubin appears in the urine before jaundice appears (preicteric phase) and its urinary threshold varies in hepatitis. It is found when the serum levels of bilirubin are raised, later it disappears although serum levels of bilirubin remain elevated.

Urinary urobilinogen appears in the late preicteric phase and with the onset of obstructive features it disappears from the urine to reappear in recovery phase. Complete disappearance from urine indicates complete functional recovery of liver cells.

Stools. With the start of jaundice, stools become light coloured while in obstructive phase they are clay coloured and with recovoery colour of stools changes to light brown.

Haematology. Blood shows leucopenia with relative lymphocytosis. This reverts to normal with onset of jaundice. ESR is raised in pre icteric phase, again returning to normal with onset of jaundice and rises again when jaundice subsides. With complete recovery it returns to normal. A persistent raised ESR indicates activity of disease process.

Biochemistry. Biochemical tests reveal the degree of liver impairment. An increase in the serum bilirubin level may be earliest indication of hepatitis though clinical jaundice is not seen till bilirubin levels in blood exceed 2 mg% (normal 0.8 to 1.2 mg%)

In the prodromal stage, serum bilirubin may be normal while urinary bilirubin precedes it and is useful in making a diagnosis. Bilirubin levels both conjugated and unconjugated continue to rise in the initial period and may take 3 to 4 weeks to return to normal.

Serum enzyme levels (SGOT/SGPT) rise before or one to two days before the appearance of jaundice. Very high levels (above 1000 units) indicate the extent of damage and are not a good sign. In a case of hepatitis the usual levels are between 300-500 IU. With recovery the levels return to normal though in some cases raised levels may persist for a few months after clinical recovery.

Serum alkaline phosphatase levels are slightly raised but are below 30 KA units. Levels above this occur in obstructive jaundice and is an important differentiating parameter between obstructive and hepatocellular jaundice. Prothrombin time is prolonged in severe cases of jaundice and indicates hepatocellular damage. Other tests like serum proteins estimation, flocculation tests are not of much value except that these tests may be positive in early stage of disease.

Serological tests. In HAV infection, IgM antibodies rise occurs early in acute phase (anti-HAV IgM). It disappears in 4-5 weeks.

In hepatitis B infection, hepatitis B surface antigen (HbSAg) and hepatitis B surface antibody (anti-HbS) are looked for and their presence indicates that either the person has acute infection or incubating it. It generally appears in the blood from 6 weeks to 3 months after an acute infection. The persistence of HbSAg in the serum and hepatitis B core antigen (HbCAg) in the liver cells following an attack of acute hepatitis B is associated with the development of chronic active or chronic persistent hepatitis.

Diagnosis of hepatitis D is by finding IgM anti-HD at the same time as IgG Hbc. While hepatitis E diagnosis rests on Elisa test for IgG and IgM anti-HEV and hepatitis C is diagnosed by detection of anti-HCV Antibodies (Elisa Technique).

Liver biopsy. It is rarely required since majority of cases of hepatitis can be diagnosed by clinical presentation and biochemical tests. Its main indication is in cases of cirrhosis presenting with post-hepatitis picture.

Radiology. Plain X-ray abdomen is done to exclude the presence of stone in bile duct. Further help is sought by doing an ultrasound of abdomen which shall exclude any biliary tract obstruction.

Differential diagnosis. This shall vary depending on the phase in which a case of infective hepatitis is seen. A case of hepatitis in preicteric stage has to be differentiated from viral fever, typhoid, gastroenteritis and malaria. In the presence of jaundice, all other causes of jaundice like drug-induced hepatitis, biliary tract obstruction, malignancy, amoebic hepatitis, portal hypertension, etc. have to be differentiated.

Patterns of hepatitis:

Hepatitis A. This is the commonest type of hepatitis and its spread is almost exclusively by the faeco-oral route. Its incubation period is short-ranging from 15 to 45 days. It generally involves children and young adults and has a benign, self-limiting course. Rarely it causes fulminating hepatitis.

The virus is small 27 nm, single-stranded RNA enterovirus. It is stable at 4°C for weeks to several months but is inactivated by heating to 100°C for 5 minutes. Its shedding in the stools begins 2 weeks before onset of symptoms and continues for a few days afterwards.

The spread of disease is dependent on state of hygiene and water supply. There is no sex difference in susceptibility. There is no chronic viremia or faecal carrier state; infection spreads from infected individuals in acute state. Most of the time infection is by oral route, is water- or food-borne and rarely by parenteral route. Virus is present in blood three days before onset in acute phase. Serum antibody (anti-HAV) appears as the stools become negative for virus, and reaches maximum in several months. Chronic carriers have not been identified. Hepatitis A virus may be shown in liver biopsies of patients of hepatitis by immunofluorescence.

Hepatitis B. Type B hepatitis spreads by blood and its products and is mainly by parenteral route. Use of unsterilized instruments, needles, acupuncture, tattooing, drug abuse are common modes of spread of disease. Blood and body fluids of infected individuals (saliva, tears, seminal fluid, breast milk, gastric juice) act as important reservoirs of infection and spread occurs through intimate personal contact. Homosexuals are at higher risk of contracting hepatitis B. Accidental transmission may also occur in healthcare personnel (laboratory workers, doctors, nurses) especially in transfusion services, and renal dialysis units. Hepatitis B occurs at any age, has an insidious onset, its incubation period ranging from 6 weeks to 6 months.

Clinical Features of Hepatitis B

1. Loss of appetite, Fatigue, Fever, weight loss, nausea vomiting.
2. Transmission through Parenteral route. (Pin Prick blood transfusion). Sexual exposure, shared razors, tattooing, mother to new born (Perinatal).
3. Incubation period 6 weeks–6 months.
4. Abnormal LFTs (Raised SGOT/SGPT). Presence of HbsAg. If HbeAg present it indicates continued infection stage or acute or chronic HBV infection.

The virus itself is a sphere about 42 nm in diameter composed of a central 27 nm core formed by the liver cell nucleus and an outer surface coat (HbSAg). This is called Dane particle. The inner core contains double-stranded DNA polymerase and the core antigen (HBcAg) and the e antigen (HBeAg). These three particles including surface antigen HBsAg (Australian antigen) constitute complete hepatitis B virus (HBV). During the presymptomatic stage of hepatitis B, the principal serum markers are first HBsAg and then HBeAg and as the disease progresses and the patient becomes symptomatic, antibodies to core antigen (HBcAg) become detectable.

Presence of HBsAg indicates either a current or chronic infection or carrier state. HBcAg may appear early and is related with severity of the disease process. Clinical features of hepatitis B resemble those of hepatitis A except that it follows a more serious course. Sometimes immune complex-like mediated picture in the form of polyarthritis or even nephritis may be seen.

Non-A, non-B hepatitis. The elimination of hepatitis A and hepatitis B from transfused blood did not eliminate post-transfusion hepatitis. This led to the identification of another virus termed non-A, non-B (hepatitis C). Other viruses in this group include Hepatitis D virus (an incomplete virus with an RNA genome) and Hepatitis E virus which has a 7600 nucleotide RNA genome.

Hepatitis C. It is a single stranded RNA virus 50-60 nm in size, belonging to flavivirus group. Six major strains of HCV have been identified (genotypes 1-6). The mode of transmission is by parenteral route though it is not the sole mode of transmission. Transfusions of contaminated blood and blood products (plasma, factor VIII, immunoglobins) accounts for 75% of cases of hepatitis C. Other methods of transmission include intranvenous drug abuse, sexual transmission (Homosexual and heterosexual). Vertical transmission (Mother to infant) is extremely low unless mother is coinfected with HIV. Hepatitis C is not transmitted through kissing, sneezing etc where there is no blood to blood contact. Parenteral exposure may occur in families through sharing of razors or tooth brushes. There are also risks of transmission through tattooing, ear piercing and acupuncture However, there may be small percentage of cases (10-20%) where possible source of infection is not identifiable. Incubation period of the disease ranges from 6-12 weeks and is shortened when viral load is heavy. The infection is primarily cytopathic but there may be immunological mediated liver injury.

Clinical Features of Hepatitis C

1. Parental route transmission, Blood and blood products, transfusion. Intravenous drug abuse.
2. Transmission through tattooing, ear, piercing etc. sexual spread uncommon.
3. Incubation period 6–12 weeks.
4. Acute Hepatitis–asymptomatic (75%) chronic hepatitis (60–70%).

Clinically disease presents both in acute and chronic form. Acute disease is generally asymptomatic in more than 90% of cases. Jaundice is present in about 10% of cases. Common symptoms are easy fatiguability, malaise, nausea and vomiting. Fever, arthralgia and skin rash are uncommon features. Although HCV accounts for 20% of acute cases of hepatitis but 70% of cases develop chronic hepatitis. Symptoms of chronic hepatitis include mild to severe fatigue, malaise, weight loss, weakness, irritability, feeling of malaise and pain in right side of upper abdomen. In 80% of cases of chronic HCV infection, there is smouldering infection for more than 6 months and 20 to 30% go on to develop cirrhosis of liver after 10-30 years while 15% of these develop carcinoma of liver.

Extra hepatic manifestations like lichen planus, autoimmune disorders (Hepatitis, thyroiditis, poly-arteritis nodosa), membranous glomerulo-nephritis, neuropathy, arthralgia, alpastic anaemia and mixed cryoglobulinaemia etc develop in 1-2% of cases.

Diagnosis of HCV is made from estimation of enzymes like AST and ALT which are usually elevated and by detection of anti-HCV antibodies by ELISA technique. HCV RNA is detected by polymerase chain reaction (PCR). It indicates active viraemia and is detectable for more than 6 months after exposure. Liver biopsy is important to assess the degree of liver involvement as well as progression of the disease. It generally shows inflammatory reaction with predominatly lymphocytic or plasma cell infiltration, piece meal necrosis and spread of fibrous tissues from portal tracts into lobules with associated degenerative changes.

Management of acute from of hepatitis C is symptomatic and on non-specific lines. Patients with normal enzyme levels and minimal or no changes in biopsy may require no treatment though these patients are still infectious.

In patients with raised enzyme levels (AST/ALT), abnormal liver biopsy and active disease. Interferon alpha is administered subcutaneously (3 million units) three times per week for 24 weeks. Long term remission occurs in 25% as patients are assessed by improved ALT levels and undetectable HCV RNA.

Relapse occurs in 50% of patients on stopping the drug.

National institute for clinical excellence (NICE) has recommended the use of combination therapy in such cases. Here interferon in dose (3 Mu units three times per week) with ribavirin (1000-1200 mg daily) is given for 24 weeks. In patients infected with HCV genotype 1 and a high viral load, further 24 weeks of combination therapy is given. Favourable response to combination therapy occurs in young females (below 40 years of age) genotype 2 or 3, low viral load and minimal fibrosis on biopsy.

Side effects of therapy include fever, rigors, chills, anorexia arthralgia, asthenia, alopecia, depression, increased sweating, taste alteration, insomnia, thyroid dysfunction, hypotension and depression.

Regular blood counts (total and differential white blood count, platelets) and AST/ALT levels be done periodically. Contraindications to interferon alpha treatment include decompensated cirrhosis, auto-immune liver disease, depression and neutropenia while ribavirin is contraindicated in end stage renal disease, coronary heart disease and decompensated cirrhosis.

Natural history of infection with HCV	
Acute hepatitis	– Chronic hepatitis (60-70%)
Chronic hepatitis	– Cirrhosis (20-30%)
Cirrhosis	– Hepatic decompensation (4-5%)
	– Hepatic carcinoma (15%)

In patient where response to treatment is poor and they pass on to end stage chronic liver disease, liver transplantation is the answer.

Delta hepatitis. It is caused by hepatitis D virus (HDV) which is a defective RNA virus requiring HbsAg for its replication. It is a small circular single stranded RNA virus and causes acute hepatitis only in the presence of HBV infection or in chronic carriers of hepatitis B.

Delta hepatitis is transmitted by parenteral route in drug addicts and after blood transfusion. It should be suspected when there is double peak in AST/ALT levels in a case of hepatitis B infection or a picture of acute hepatitis is observed in a chronic carrier of HbsAg.

Clinical Features of Hepatitis D

1. Asymptomatic in majority.
2. Delta Hepatitis occurs generally in persons having chronic HBV infection (Delta-super infection).
3. Transmission by parenteral route after blood transfusion and in drug addicts.
4. Clinical presentation variable.
5. Complete recovery in 80–90% of patients.
6. Chronic Hepatitis. Fulminant Hepatitis and cirrhosis in those already having HBV infection.

Delta hepatitis produces morbidity in chronic carriers of HBV in the form of fulminant hepatic failure (5%) and chronic viral hepatitis (75%). Diagnosis is made by demonstration of anti HDV 1 g M antibodies. If there are high levels of HbsAg and Ig M anti Hb C it indicates coinfection.

Treatment of delta hepatitis is unsatisfactory. Response to interferon alpha therapy is not encouraging.

Hepatitis E (HEV). Hepatitis E is an RNA virus which is primarily transmitted by oral route. The virus occurs in two forms namely epidemic and sporadic; the epidemic form is seen in outbreaks and is related to contamination of water while endemic form is common in endemic regions. The virus mainly involves young adults producing a picture of acute hepatitis but carries high degree of morbidity and mortality in pregnant women.

Clinical Features of Hepatitis E

1. Faecal-oral transmission through contaminated water.
2. Mainly two forms – Epidemic and sporadic.
3. No transmission through parental route.
4. Incubation period 2–10 weeks.
5. Transplacental transmission possible (Mother to new born).
6. Mortality low.

Clinically picture resembles that of asymptomatic to acute and fulminant hepatitis. It is self limiting and does not lead to chronic carrier state or chronic hepatitis. Diagnosis of HEV infection is made by detection of HEV antibodies. Presence of 1g M antibodies against HEV indicates a recent infection.

No specific treatment is available against hepatitis E. It is mainly symptomatic in the form of bed rest, high carbohydrate diet, vitamin C and B complex.

Course of acute hepatitis. A case of acute hepatitis may follow one or the other of following courses.

i. Complete recovery occurs in majority of cases (90% of cases).

ii. A small percentage of cases go to subacute hepatic necrosis progressing to chronic hepatitis which leads to cirrhosis either compensated or a progressive liver failure.

iii. Fulminant hepatitis in 1 per cent of cases and may lead to death.

iv. Chronic carrier state in 5-10 per cent of patients with hepatitis B.

v. Post-hepatitis syndrome in small percentage followed by complete recovery.

Complications. A small percentage of cases develop complications though majority of patients of hepatitis make an uneventful recovery.

Subacute hepatitis. Some patients do not recover completely and continue to have low grade pyrexia and varying levels of jaundice. Liver is enlarged and tender and spleen is palpable. It has a slow downhill course and patient may pass on to hepatocellular failure with high degree of morbidity and mortality.

Relapsing or recurrent hepatitis. A small percentage of cases especially of hepatitis A may get relapse weeks to months after clinical recovery. There is recurrence of symptoms with rise in enzyme levels. Relapse is probably precipitated by premature activity or alcohol consumption during period of convalescence. Relapsing or recurrent hepatitis has a mild course and patient recovers completely.

Cholestatic hepatitis. Occasionally cases of hepatitis A may develop a prolonged course with cholestatic features characterized by deepening jaundice and marked degree of pruritis. It starts acutely and may last for few weeks after which the

Diseases of Liver 149

patient starts feeling better. There are no physical signs except marks of itching and hepatomegaly. This type of picture in a case of hepatitis may have to be differentiated from biliary duct obstruction or drug induced hepatitis.

Post-hepatitis cirrhosis. Cases of hepatitis may pass on to a subacute stage which shows features of liver cell failure. Some may die during this phase while others may apparently recover and come back after a number of years with fullfledged picture of portal hypertension and patient now has picture of splenomegaly, liver which may be shrunken and ascites.

Fulminant hepatic failure. It is not a common complication of hepatitis A but generally develops in patients of hepatitis B, non-A, non-B hepatitis and delta hepatitis. It is a very serious complication, often life threatening and develops very rapidly. Patient shows features of hepatic encephalopathy (delirium, violent behaviour, coma, flapping tremors, fetor hepaticus). Cerebral oedema, respiratory failure, renal failure and bleeding from various sources may develop. Hepatic failure carries very high degree of mortality (80-90%).

Chronic persistent and active hepatitis. This is a late complication of hepatitis B where there is persistence of symptoms of hepatitis like anorexia, malaise and weight loss. It generally resolves within six months being benign and self-limiting. This is then known as chronic persistent hepatitis. If it persists for six months or more it is called chronic active hepatitis where symptoms persist and may progress onto cirrhosis. Chronic active hepatitis is seen not only in hepatitis B but also in those with superinfection with Delta virus and non-A, non-B hepatitis following transfusion.

Chronic asymptomatic carriers. Cases of hepatitis B infection may become carriers though this occurs only in small percentage (5-10%). Though carriers may remain asymptomatic but carry the risk of infecting others. Carriers with HBeAG antigen may develop chronic hepatitis and cirrhosis. Persistence of this state for 25 years or more may predispose the patient to develop hepatocellular carcinoma.

Post-hepatitis syndrome. Some patients especially medical personnel (doctors, nurses) who are familiar with the course of hepatitis may harbour anxiety or fear about developing some major complication. These people have ill-health, fatigue, malaise, anorexia and failure to gain weight. There is discomfort in the right hypochondrium. Liver may be just palpable and slightly tender. All biochemical tests including liver biopsy are generally normal except liver histology shows mild portal zone cellularity and fatty change.

Patients of post hepatitis syndrome require no treatment except assurance. Most recover completely within a few months.

Treatment. There is no specific treatment for a case of hepatitis and only supportive measures are employed.

Bed rest. Rest in bed is advised since it helps in speeding up recovery. It is preferable to advise bed rest till jaundice has cleared up and enzymes levels have returned to normal. Inadequate rest or early resumption of activity may lead to development of complications.

Diet. Traditionally high carbohydrate, low fat is preferred since it is palatable. Plenty of carbohydrates like sweetened fruit juices, honey, glucose water, sweet biscuits, corn flakes, sago etc. are given. Dietary proteins should be given in normal daily requirements (1 g/kg). In ill patients with very high levels of bilirubin and transaminase levels, proteins in diet may have to be restricted. As far as possible, a normal diet which can be easily digested is to be given. When there is severe degree of anorexia and nausea, one may have to give parenteral glucose. Alcohol is to be avoided during acute attack and six months after recoveory.

Drugs. Vitamin supplements in the form of vitamin B complex and vitamin C in heavy doses are beneficial. All hepatoxic drugs like paracetamol, anti-tubercular, oral antidiabetics, tetracyclines, sulfonamides, oral contraceptives, anti epileptic etc. should be avoided. No sedatives or tranquilizers since these may precipitate hepatic coma. For severe vomiting, metoclopramide may be given parenterally along with intravenous fluids.

Electrolytes must be monitored and adequate control maintained. If patient has got persistent fever and either secondary infection or liver cell necrosis is suspected Ampicillin upto 2-4 g may be given orally since it shall be useful for sterilization of the gut.

For cholestasis when severe pruritis is problem, steroids (Tab. prednisolone 40-60 mg per day in divided doses) be given. Role of steroids otherwise in hepatitis is controversial. In severely ill ptients use of steroids is advocated since steroids may not effect the underlying process but give a sense of well being, improve the appetite and buy time for the liver to regenerate.

Complications of hepatitis. Mainly are subacute hepatitis, portal cirrhosis and fulminant hepatitis failure. These should be treated on appropriate lines.

Prophylaxis. HAV infection can be prevented by meticulous personal hygiene, disposal of excreta and avoiding contacts with infected person. Water should be taken boiled since boiling shall kill the virus.

In persons who are exposed to risk with HAV infection, and travellers to areas where prevalence of hepatitis A is high, contacts of infected persons, homosexuals, abusers of injectable drugs, haemophilics, persons with multiple sexual partners or in places where there is higher incidence of disease, hepatitis A vaccine (HAVRIX) offers confirmed protective efficacy and is highly immunogenic. Dosage in adults is 1 ml by intramuscular route and second dose (1 ml) after two weeks. A booster dose is recommended any time between six and 12 months after the initiation of the primary course in order to ensure long-term antibody titres.

Hepatitis B. Prevention against hepatitis B means avoidance of professional donors blood, screening of blood and its related products for surface antigen (HbSAg). All laboratory personnel should avoid unnecessary pricks punctures and contact with infected fluids.

Passive immunization may be required in those who do not have antibodies against HBsAg. Hepatitis B immune globulin (HBIG) may afford passive protection if given within two days of exposure like pin pricks, sexual partners of patients with acute hepatitis B. Dose is 0.05 to 0.07 mg/kg body weight (500 Iu HBIG) given intramuscularly. A second dose is given after 3-4 weeks. Efficacy of passive immunization has not been established. It only reduces the frequency of clinical illness but does not prevent infection. Hepatitis B vaccine prepared from circulating HbSAg of symptomless carriers is immunogenic, and effective. Patients with hepatitis B may act as carriers of hepatitis B virus (HBV). All these patients of chronic HBV infection are at risk of developing chronic liver disease (chronic hepatitis, cirrhosis and hepatocellular carcinoma).

Treatment of carrier state is by administration of Interferon (3 million units) at weekly intervals be 16–24 weeks. Sero conversion is achieved in 30–50 percent of patients.

Hepatitis B vaccine gives effective immunization against hepatis B virus infection and is safe. It should be given to all persons at risk from hepatitis B, persons coming in contact with blood or body fluids of patients, sexual contacts of HbSAG carriers. Three injections of vaccine at 0, 1, and 6 months (1 ml contains 20 mcg of hepatitis B surface antigen protein) to be given intramuscularly in deltoid region are recommended. Hepatitis B vaccine gives immunity in more than 95 per cent of people. For more rapid immunization third dose can be given two months after the initial dose with a booster at 12 months. Vaccination is not recommended to pregnant women.

Delta hepatitis. There is no separate vaccine against delta hepatitis though infection by this virus can be prevented by giving hepatitis B vaccine in susceptible individuals.

Hepatitis C: Except for preventive measures like screening of blood and blood products for the virus antibodies, no vaccine is available.

Prognosis. Prognosis in a large majority of patients of viral hepatitis is good since it is a benign, self limiting disease and patient makes uneventful recovery. In a small minority, patient does develop fulminant hepatitis which carries poor prognosis.

In patients with serious underlying medical disease (anaemia, congestive heart failure, diabetes) and elderly people, the course of the disease is prolonged and may be more serious and severe. Hepatitis B as compared to hepatitis A has a more serious profile and the incidence of complications is also high. Similarly superinfection with Delta virus in a patient with hepatitis B, chances of developing fulminant hepatitis are increased and with it the degree of morbidity and mortality.

In any case of hepatitis bad prognostic signs (clinical and laboratory) shall be severe anaemia, rapidly developing fulminant hepatits, bleeding tendencies, delirium, signs of hepatocellular failure, very high bilirubin and transaminase levels, low blood sugar, prolonged prothrombin time and a low serum albumin.

Chronic active hepatitis

It is an important cause of chronic liver disease, cirrhosis and hepatocellular carcinoma. Of the known hepatitis viruses, the three that can cause persistant infection and chronic hepatitis, the hepatitis B virus, (HBV) the hepatitis C virus (HCV) and the hepatitis delta (Hepatitis D) viruses are important cause. Of the other two viruses hepatitis A and hepatitis E they cause only acute self limiting disease.

In addition to viral artiology other causes include auto immune and administration of drugs like methyldopa, Isoniazid and nitrofurantoin. Alpha-1 antitrypsin deficiency has also been incriminated as one of the aetiological factors.

Chronic active hepatitis is characterized by continuous hepatic necrosis, active inflammation and fibrosis which ultimately lead to cirrhosis / liver failure. The cause of this continued liver damage is not known but it is considered to be associated with defective immunological responses though there is no association between auto immune or any particular genetic markers.

Clinical picture. It has an insidious course. Many patients remain asymptomatic for a variable period ranging from weeks to months when they may present as an acute case of hepatitis. Features suggestive of chronic active hepatitis develop in a period of 1-2 years. These include fatigue, persistent or recurrent jaundice, malaise, low grade fever and loss of appetite. Subsequently some patients develop features of cirrhosis. In addition to features suggestive of liver disease other features include arthralgia, skin eruptions, erythema nodosum, pleurisy pericarditis etc.

Laboratory investigation. There is elevation of serum bilirubin levels along with alkaline phosphatase AST and ALT levels. Hyper gammoglobulinemia is common and there is presence of circulating antibodies against DNA, IgG, smooth muscle and mitochondria. Hb S Ag is found positive in 30% of patients. Sero diagnosis is made using ELISA and various other markers.

Diagnosis. Besides clinical features, laboratory investigation, liver biopsy is the only way to establish the diagnosis of chronic active hepatitis. Typically it will show piece meal necrosis along with distortion of lobular structure and fibrosis. Bridging hepatic necrosis may be seen in advanced form of the liver disease.

Treatment. In cases of chronic active hepatitis not associated with hepatitis B or non-A, non-B virus, glucocorticoids are the drug of choice and give good clinical response. In patient with chronic hepatitis B, antiviral agent interferon alfa is employed. A course of four to six months duration induces a long term remission in 25 to 40 per cent of patients. The recommended regimen of interferon alfa is either 5 million units daily or 10 million units thrice weekly given subcutaneously for four months. The effects of therapy are maintained by measuring aminotransferase levels at two to five weeks interval along with serologic assays for Hb S Ag Hb e Ag and Hb V DNA.

Adverse effects of interferon include flu like illness with fever chills and myalgia which appear six to eight hours after the first dose. Other side effects include changes in mood, alopecia and unmasking of depression.

When therapy is stopped patient should be followed up to document whether HBV DNA, HB e Ag and Hb sAg have disappeared. A beneficial response can be said to have occurred if the patient is negative for both HBV DNA and HBeAg and has normal or nearly normal aminotransferase values six months after therapy is stopped.

Prognosis. If the patient responds to therapy the prognosis is good but once cirrhosis develops, prognosis becomes poor. Development of carcinoma is another poor marker.

HEPATIC CIRRHOSIS

A widely prevalent disease not only in India but all over the world is characterised by diffuse involvement of the liver in the form of necrosis of liver cells, collapse of hepatic lobules, reticulin framework followed by difuse fibrosis and formation of structurally abnormal nodules. This interferes not only with the liver blood flow but also its functions. This results in the clinical picture of cirrhosis which is due to inadequacy of liver cells and portal hypertension. Cirrhosis may be present in compensated or decompensated forms where clinical signs of the disease become apparent.

Aetiology. *Commonest causes of cirrhosis are:*

1. *Post-necrotic cirrhosis following infective hepatitis.* In only a small percentage of people history of hepatitis may be available and absence of history shall not exclude previous hepatitis since in these people the hepatitis may have been mild. Further it is seen that there is increased chance of patients with hepatitis B, non-A, non-B hepatitis, hepatitis D to develop cirrhosis.

2. *Alcoholic cirrhosis.* Chronic alcoholism over a number of years results in repeated injury to liver cells which initially results in fatty liver followed by hepatitis, ultimately leading to cirrhosis. The amount of alcohol and duration of its consumption in addition to poor food intake with malnutrition act as complement to each other though poor nutrition per se may not cause cirrhosis. Alcohol injury of liver is reversible till hepatitis stage and when cirrhosis has developed, the whole process becomes irreversible. There is destruction of liver cells, fragmentation, and formation of fibrous septa, dividing the liver into small nodules. In final

stages the liver shrinks and full fledged picture of cirrhosis results.

Classification of portal cirrhosis

Clinical

a. Post-necrotic cirrhosis
b. Cryptogenic cirrhosis
c. Miscellaneous causes. Malaria, haemochromatosis, alpha-1-antitrypsin, deficiency, autoimmune chronic active hepatitis, Wilson's disease, schistosomiasis, venoocclusive disease, hepatic venous congestion.

Pathological

a. Micronodular cirrhosis
b. Macronodular cirrhosis
c. Mixed type

---

3. Cryptogenic cirrhosis. There are quite a few cases where no known cause of cirrhosis is operative. There is no history of excessive alcoholic intake or suggestion of viral hepatitis in the past or other numerous causes of cirrhosis. Such cases come under the group of cryptogenic (unknown) cirrhosis.

4. Miscellaneous causes. In addition to the common causes a number of other aetiological factors may cause cirrhosis. These range from haemochromatosis, alpha-1-anti-trypsin deficiency, autoimmune chronic active hepatitis, Wilson's disease, malaria, schistosomiasis venoocclusive disease, hepatic venous congestion to drugs like methyl dopa, methotrexate, arsenic and oral contraceptives.

Pathology. There is wide spread necrosis of liver cells, disorganization of hepatic lobules and formation of diffuse fibrous septa with collapse of reticulin frame work. Subsequent to the damage of reticulin frame work, there is formation of abnormal nodules which give the liver its nodular appearance. Depending on the size of nodules, histologically cirrhosis has been classified into miconodular, macronodular and mixed picture.

In micronodular cirrhosis the nodules are less than three mm in size involving almost the whole of liver. The nodules are surrounded by fibrous bands, while in macronodular type, the nodules are of coarse type, irregular and give the liver a grossly distorted surface. Mixed type has got features of both. Micronodular type picture of liver generally is seen in alcoholic cirrhosis while macronodular type is seen in postnecrotic cirrhosis.

Clinical features. A case of cirrhosis may present either in compensated or decompensated forms.

A compensated case of cirrhosis has features of dyspepsia in the form of morning anorexia, nausea, vomiting and vague ill health. This is more so when it is early stage of alcoholic cirrhosis. There is palmar erythema, spider naevi, splenomegaly and hepatomegaly with a non-tender liver. There is loss of weight, ill health and oedema of the ankles. There may be no firm signs of cirrhosis and diagnosis is made on clinical suspicion to be confirmed by biochemical investigations and liver biopsy.

This stage of compensated form of cirrhosis may continue for a variable period of time ranging from months to years and bleed from oesophageal varices may draw attention to the disease or some precipitating cause like severe bacteraemia may produce hepatocellular decompensation.

A decompensated cirrhosis is characterised by a downhill course, abdominal distension, ascites, weight loss, oedema over the dependent parts, cirrhotic facies (sunken eyes, hollow cheeks, pinched nose) skin dry and sallow. Jaundice may appear indicating progressive liver cell destruction. Liver may be palpable with irregular surface or it may not be palpable when it is shrunken. Splenomegaly is present in 80 per cent of patients. Nails are white and clubbed. Endocrinal changes in the form of spider naevi, palmar erythema, gynaecomastia, loss of axillary and pubic hair, and testicular atrophy are seen. There may be bleeding spots or bruising due to prothrombin deficiency. Ascites may be massive and is disproportionate to the oedema of feet.

Hepatocellular failure may supervene as liver cell necrosis proceeds. Breath becomes foul smelling often giving a mousy smell (Fetor hepaticus). Flapping tremors and encephalopathy appear (delirium, restlessness, irritability, coma). Appearance of jaundice, rapid accumulation of ascites and development of hepatic encephalopathy are poor signs in cirrhosis.

Clinical signs in hepatocellular failure
1. Spider naevi
2. Palmar erythema
3. Gynaecomastia
4. Testicular atrophy
5. Changes in the distribution of body hair
6. Dupuytren's contracture
7. Ascites
8. Easy bruising, pupuric spots
9. Flapping tremors

The above picture is seen in almost all cases of hepatic cirrhosis irrespective of aetiology. But there are a few distinctive features in cases of alcoholic cirrhosis.

In early stage when picture is of alcoholic hepatitis, symptoms are often mild in the form of anorexia, nausea, vomiting, weight loss, tender hepatomegaly, splenomegaly (30-40%) and spider naevi. But as the disease progresses ascites and oedema over ankles develops. Alcoholic cirrhosis as such may also remain silent for a number of years, progressing insidiously with only symptoms of anorexia, wasting and weight loss.

Features which may distinguish alcoholic cirrhosis are. A middle aged person between 35-45 years, presenting with jaundice, ascites, anaemia, wasting, peripheral neuropathy, parotid gland enlargement and in men features of feminization and in women features of masculinization. Patient has low grade pyrexia, with a palpable liver which is often large while spleen is palpable only in small percentage of cases.

Diagnosis. In a classical presentation of ascites, oedema over the ankles, splenomegaly, hepatomegaly with a history of progressive weight loss, anorexia, abdominal distension, vague abdominal pain and features of hepatocellular decompensation like spider naevi, palmar erythema, parotid enlargement, gynaecomastia and testicular atrophy favour diagnosis of portal cirrhosis. If history of viral hepatitis is available it shall favour a post necrotic cirrhosis, while in alcoholic cirrhosis, there is always history of intake of alcohol spread over number of years. The diagnosis of cryptogenic cirrhosis is considered when no apparent aetiological cause can be incriminated.

Often a case of cirrhosis has to be differentiated from tubercular or malignant peritonitis or constrictive pericarditis.

Confirmation of diagnosis is made by carrying out the investigations.

Investigation:

1. *Haematology.* Anaemia which may be macrocytic or normocytic. But when there has been gastrointestinal bleed, it may be microcytic. Bone marrow shows macronormoblastic reaction. Prothrombin time is prolonged. Platelet count is low.

2. *Biochemistry.* In early stages of cirrhosis, biochemistry may be normal. But in advanced cases, there is rise in bilirubin levels, serum transaminases, alkaline phosphatase levels in varying degrees. Serum albumin levels are low while globulin levels are raised. Flocculation tests (thymol turbidity, zinc sulphate) are abnormal.

   Electrophoretic analysis of serum shall show a rise in alpha and to less extent in beta globulins. **Ascitic fluid** is transudate with protein content less than 2 g%.

   Serum electrolytes for serum sodium and potassium. Increased urinary loss of potassium may occur due to hyperaldosteronism. Blood ammonia levels are raised in the presence of hepatic encephalopathy. Viral markers (hepatitis B antigen HbsAg) and smooth muscle mitochondrial and nuclear antibodies are done to demonstrate the aetiology.

3. *Barium swallow for oesophageal varices.* Ultrasound of abdomen shall demonstrate the size and shape of liver which is shrunken in post necrotic cirrhosis. Presence of any malignancy can also be detected. Hepatic scan is also helpful in some cases.

4. *Gastroendoscopy* to demonstrate varices which appear as bunch of grapes in the oesophagus.

5. *Liver biopsy.* Sometimes in a case of cirrhosis with massive ascites. It is difficult to perform liver biopsy. But a liver biopsy is often necessary to confirm the degree of liver damage and to assess its prognosis. Histologically there shall be irregular random areas of massive fibrosis alternating with other areas of scarring producing nodularity. The broad scars are interposed between islands of disorderly regenerating liver cells or areas of normal liver and where extensive necrosis has taken place, two or more portal triads may be seen within the scars.

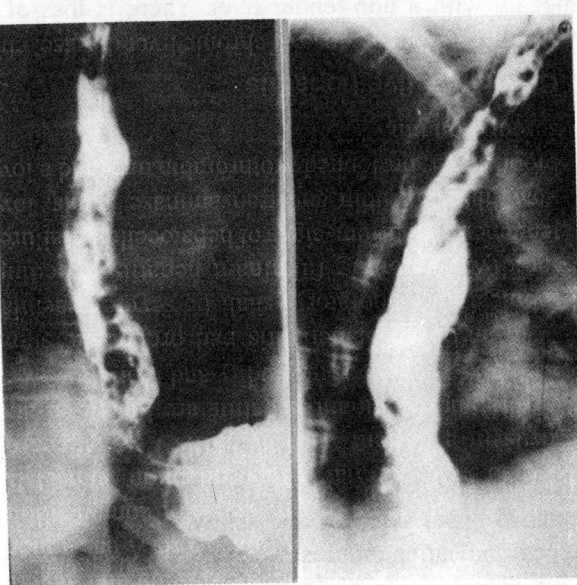

Fig. 3.7-8. Showing oesophageal varices in a case of portal cirrhosis.

Complications. A case of cirrhosis may suffer number of complications:

1. Development of intercurrent infection especially gram-negative septicaemia leading to peritonitis.

2. Tuberculosis of the abdomen coexisting with cirrhosis.

3. Malignancy of liver, especially in those with hepatitis B, non-A, non-B hepatitis as aetiological factor. Serum alpha fetoproteins shall be a useful test for detection of hepatoma.

4. Haemorrhage from oesophageal varices.

5. Development of hepatocellular failure which generally is a terminal feature.

Course of the disease. It is extremely variable depending on number of factors:

1. Presence of anaemia, malnutrition, jaundice, rapid accumulation of ascites, repeated bouts of haemorrhage from oesphageal varices, bleeding from mucous surfaces, failure to respond to therapy, progression to hepatocellular failure carry poor prognosis.

2. Aetiologically alcoholic cirrhosis carries better prognosis as compared to post-necrotic cirrhosis especially in early stages when abstinence from alcohol may reverse the process to some extent.

3. A large liver indicates that regeneration has taken place while shrunken liver tells the story of hepatic necrosis. Abnormal biochemical tests including electrolyte abnormalities and hypoprothrombinaemia of severe degree carry poor prognosis. Once a case of hepatic cirrhosis has gone into decompensation stage, a great majority of patients follow a downhill course and do not survive for more than 3-4 years.

Sequelae of cirrhosis. A case of portal cirrhosis develops a number of sequelae in the course of disease and *these are:*

1. Portal hypertension.
2. Gastrointestinal haemorrhage
3. Hepatic encephalopathy.
4. Ascites
5. Hepatorenal syndrome
6. Hepatocellular carcinoma
7. Spontaneous bacterial peritonitis.

PORTAL HYPERTENSION

Normal portal pressure in portal vein formed by the union of superior mesentric and splenic veins is between 5-7 mm Hg. Normally the portal blood passes through sinusoids and is drained with a small gradient across the liver to the hepatic veins and then to inferior vena cava. Portal hypertension (por-

tal veins pressure > 12 mmHg) results from increased resistance to portal blod flow and it may occur at three levels, Intrahepatic, suprahepatic and extrahepatic levels. Intrahepatic causes shall include all type of cirrhosis, non-cirrhotic portal hypertension while extrahepatic portal hypertension may occur due to portal venous obstruction or thrombosis of speenic vein by localised pressure of adjacent structures or spread from umbilical vein.

Suprahepatic portal hypertension results due to obstruction of the main hepatic veins (Budd-Chiari syndrome) or obstruction of small radicles of hepatic veins (veno-occlusive disease) or secondary to general rise in systemic venous pressure (congestive heart failure, constrictive pericarditis). Of all the causes of portal hypertension, cirrhosis is the commonest followed by portal vein obstruction.

Clinically a patient of portal hypertension has acites, splenomegaly, dilated abdominal wall veins (caput medusae) palmar erythema, spider naevi, anaemia and history of bleed from oesophageal varices.

There is development of portal systemic collateral channels and these are commonly at lower end of oesophagus (gastric veins communicating with oesophageal veins) rectum (inferior mesenteric and haemorrhoidal veins) abdominal wall and hepatic veins communicating with diaphragmatic veins in the falciform ligament of the liver.

Diagnosis of portal hypertension is based on clinical features. Demonstration of oesophageal varices by barium swallow and endoscopy. Portal venous pressure may be measured directly by percutaneous transhepatic catheterization when both occluded or wedge presssure or free hepatic pressure are measured or by measuring intrasplenic pressure since it bears a close relationship to portal venous pressure.

Percutaneous trans-splenic portal venography is helpful where radio-opaque dye is injected into the spleen when splenic and portal veins and their collaterals are visualized. In portal cirrhosis, there is filling of large number of collateral vessels as well as distortion of their intrahepatic pattern. In extrahepatic portal hypertension there is filling of large number of vessels running from spleen to diaphragm and abdominal wall. There may be block in portal vein. Intrahepatic branches are generally not visualized. Splenoportovenography helps in visualization of spleno portal circulation and is also essential before undertaking portacaval anastomosis. Major side effect of carrying out this procedure is haemorrhage which sometimes may be massive.

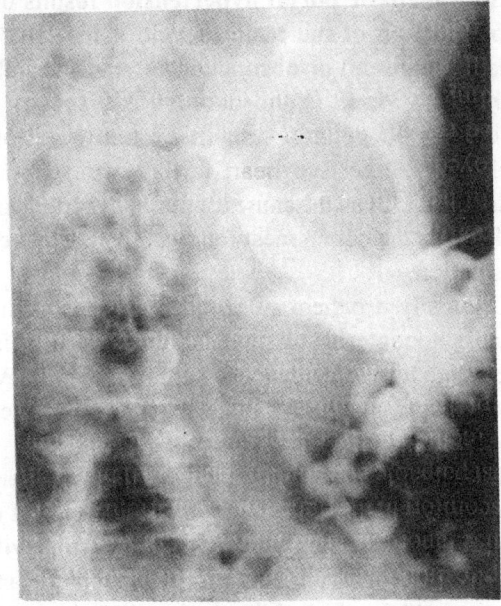

Fig. 3.9. Splenoportovenogram in a case of portal hypertesion showing collaterals.

Gastrointestinal haemorrhage. Bleeding from oesophageal varices is the commonest cause of gastrointestinal haemorrhage in cases of cirrhosis. It may be slow, the patient presenting with malaena or when massive patient presents with haematemesis. Bleeding from varices occurs when portal pressure is high and there is severe liver disease. Bleed from varices has injurious effect on liver cells and is likely to precipitate hepatic failure because of increased absorption of nitrogenous products from the intestines. Diagnosis of gastrointestinal bleed is not difficult. An emergency endoscopy shall locate the site of bleed.

Ascites. There is accumulation of excess fluid in the peritoneal cavity. Ascites in cirrhosis is generally massiveand is disproportionate to the peripheral oedema. Factors of portal hypertension, hypoalbuminaemia and reduced plasma osmotic pressure, sodium retention, increased plasma renin activity and aldosterone secretion play their role in causation of ascites. Ascites is not demonstrable clinically unless 500 ml of fluid in abdominal cavity collects. Excessive accumulation of fluid may cause cardio respiratory embarrasment.

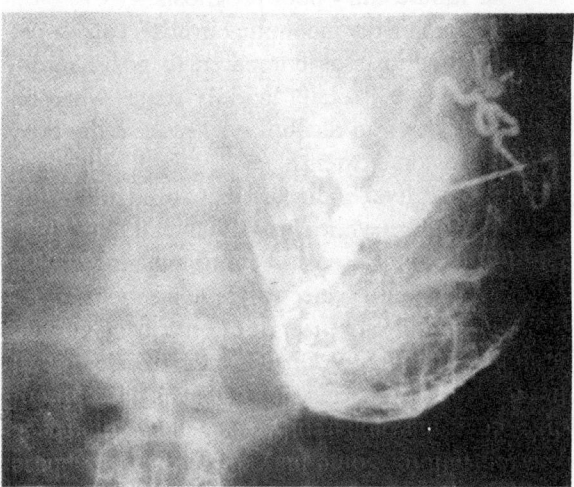

Fig. 3.10. Splenoportovenogram showing perisplenic collaterals.

Hepatic encelphalopathy. Progressive failure of liver cells may produce a picture of encephalopathy characterised by delirium, alterations in consciousness, behaviour disturbances, flapping tremors progressing ultimately to coma. Hepatic encephalopathy is a very grave complication or sequlae of cirrhosis and carries very serious prognosis. Common precipitating factors include gastrointestinal bleed Electrolyte disturbances (hypokalemia, alkolosis) infection, use of drugs like morphine, sedatives, tranquilizers. Intense diuresis which produces hypokalemia and hyponatremia, minor and major surgery including porto systemic shunt surgery and high intake of dietary protein in a case with advanced liver disease.

Diagnosis of hepatic encephalopathy in a case of cirrhosis is not difficult on clinical examination. Further confirmation may be obtained by estimating blood ammonia levels and by an electroencephalogram which shows slowing of normal alpha waves (8-13 Hz) to delta waves (1.5-3 Hz).

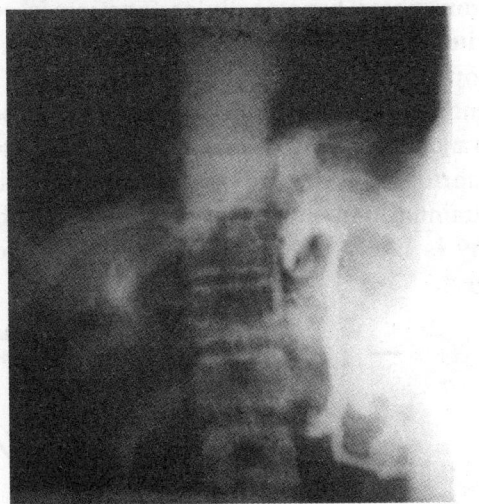

Fig. 3.11. Splenoportovenogram. Splenic vein is well seen. There is obstruction of portal vein.

Hepatorenal syndrome. It is a serious complication and is characterized by worsening renal failure with sodium retention, oliguria, low sodium excretion and features of renal failure. There is no identifiable cause of renal dysfunction but probably arterial renal haemodynamics play part in the causation of this complication.

Spontaneous bacterial peritonitis. It is an uncommon but serious complication. There is development of acute bacterial peritonitis without an obvious primary source of infection. There is sudden onset of fever, chills and abdominal pain. Ascitic fluid shows a leucocyte count of more than 500 cells per cubic millimeter with predominant polymorphs.

Hepatocellular carcinoma. Cirrhosis may predispose to the development of hepatocellular carcinoma which may be suggested by progressive deterioration of health, weight loss, rapid enlargement of liver or resistant ascites.

Treatment of hepatic cirrhosis. Management of hepatic cirrhosis shall be mainly of the basic disease, prevention of factors which may lead to progressive hepatocellular failure and treatment of various sequlae/complication.

A well compensated case of cirrhosis requires a good high caloric diet (2500-3500 calories) with a high content of first class proteins. If underlying cause like alcohol is there the cause should be removed and complete abstinence from alcohol enforced.

If there is anaemia it should be corrected. Sometimes blood transfusion may have to be given. Avoid use of hepatotoxic drugs, sedatives and tranquilizers. Infection should be treated at the earliest. Any acute illness should make the patient take bed rest and adequate treatment.

Attempt should be made to detect complications in a decompensated form. Patients with compensated cirrhosis can lead as normal life as possible.

Use of vitamin B complex and vitamin C is helpful.

Ascites. *Management of ascites requires:*

1. High carbohydrate and protein diet with adequate calories.
2. Low salt diet preferably limit the consumption of salt to minimum.
3. Diuretics orally twice a week. Frusemide 40 mg orally or in resistant cases by parenteral route. Diuretics cause loss of sodium and potassium. Oral potassium supplements be given on the day diuretics are given. Combination of potasium sparing diuretics like Spironolactone (200 mg) or Amiloride (10 mg) is effective as diuretic agents. With these diuretics potassium intake in diet should be restricted.
4. When ascites is massive and causing respiratory difficulty paracentesis of abdomen is carried out and upto 2-3 litres can be removed. Drainage of ascites should be done slowly and only minimal amount of fluid removed slowly. Rapid drainage of fluid may precipitate hepatic coma. Other complications include shock, infection. In resistant cases of ascites not responding to diuretics and paracentesis intravenous infusion of albumin and dextran may be helpful.

Gastrointestinal bleed. Bleeding from oesophageal varices is a serious emergency and requires urgent management.

1. Correct shock by rapid blood transfusion plasma. Maintain fluid and electrolyte balance.
2. Oesophageal compression by Sengstaken tube where constant pressure is maintained by inflating the balloon and keeping it in place for 24 hours. Constant gastric aspiration is done. Tube is only removed when there is no blood in gastric aspirate. In between pressure is eased to see whether bleed is there or not. Prolonged use of tube may cause ulceration. As a rule not more than 3 days intubation is maintained.

Where there is failure of bleed to stop, emergency endoscopy is done and a sclerosing agent is injected into varices to control bleeding by producing thrombosis.

In addition vasoconstrictor agents are also employed to control bleed. Vasopressin infusion of 25 units per hour or Octreotide, a Somatostatin analogue (250 µg bolus followed by infusion every hour) are helpful drugs in lowering portal venous pressure and causing splanchnic vasoconstriction.

Beta-adrenergic blocking agents (Propranolol) may sometimes play role in acute variceal bleed.

When drugs, ballooning and sclerotherapy fail to control variceal bleed, emergency surgery like oesophageal resection and ligation of the bleeding varices or porto systemic shunt surgery has been employed. Surgical procedures carry high degree of mortality.

Portal hypertension. A decompensated case of cirrhosis with raised portal pressure should be watched carefully for any episode of variceal bleed.

Prophylactic sclerotherapy may have to be undertaken and repeated at appropriate intervals.

Oral propranolol (40 mg per day) should be given to reduce portal pressure and be continued as prophylactic measure. Adequacy of dosage can be assessed by watching the pulse rate which should reduce by 25 per cent of the resting rate.

Surgery in portal hypertension is undertaken in select number of patients where there is:

i. Recurrent history of bleed/haemorrhage from gastro-oesophageal varices.
ii. Raised portal pressure.

An ideal patient for surgery is generally a young person where hepatocellular function is good. Ascites is not present. Spleen is usually large, oesophageal varices are demonstrated, and splenoportovenography has shown a patent portal vein and hepatocellular functions are good. Presence of mildest form of encephalopathy is a contraindication since post operative encephalopathy is likely to complicate following portal surgery.

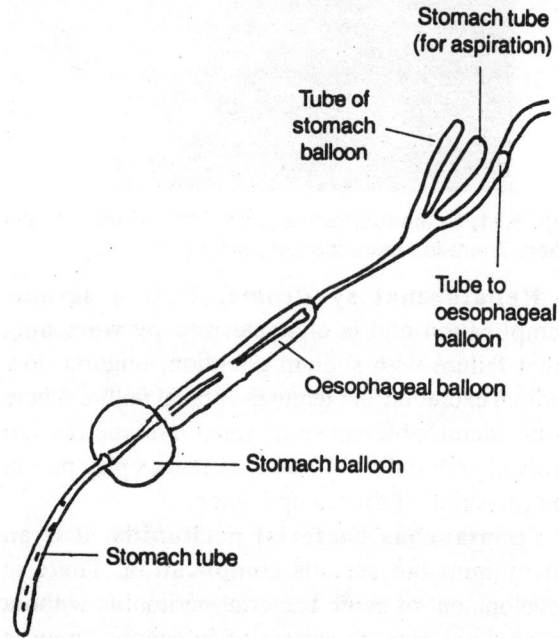

Fig. 3.12. Blakemore-sengstaken tube. (After Sherlock)

Two types of surgeries are advocated.

Portocaval anastomoses or spleno renal shunt. Porto caval anastomosis means end to end or side to side shunt. Portal vein is joined to inferior vena cava either end to side with ligation of the portal vein or side to side maintaining its continuity. End to side shunt gives a greater fall in portal pressure than side to side procedure.

Shunt closure is often due to operating on a partially thrombosed, thickened or calcified portal vein and often results in development of acute or chronic neuropsychiatric complications. Hepatic failure is the usual cause of death.

In splenorenal shunt aim is to divide veins feeding the oesophagogastric collaterals while allowing drainage of portal blood through short gastric and splenic veins through a spleno renal shunt to inferior vena cava. In this procedure an adequately functioning right kidney must be there since anastomosis is usually end to side with preservation of left kidney and splenectomy while in the other splenectomy with left nephrectomy is done.

It is difficult, time-consuming operation and is mainly advised for extrahepatic portal hypertension.

HEPATIC ENCEPHALOPATHY

It refers to the deterioration in the mental state of a patient with liver disease. It may occur in a case of acute liver failure or with chronic liver disease. The neuropsychiatric syndrome seen in patients of cirrhosis and portal systemic shunting is known as portal-systemic encephalopathy. Acute encephalopathy can occur in patients of acute hepatic failure. The pathogenesis of hepatic encephalopathy is not clear but a number of factors are known to play part. These include elevated inhibitory neurotransmitter activity (gamma aminobutyric acid: endogenous benzodiazipene) and accumulation of false neurotransmitters. Many toxic substances including ammonia, free fatty acids and mercaptans have been incriminated as causative factors. While increased levels of aromatic amino acids and reduced branch chain amino acids occur, elevated levels of blood ammonia play an important role.

Clinical features. The classical features of hepato cellular failure are invariably present and these include general deterioration of the condition, fever, anorexia, nausea with or without vomiting. Jaundice to a variable degree is present. While in cases of acute failure it runs parallel to the extent of liver damage but it is not so in cases of chronic liver disease since liver in such cases has been able to achieve a balance between hepatic damage and regeneration. Patient has features of hyperkinetic circulation as shown by flushed extremities, bounding pulse and increased capillary pulsation. There is a sweetish, feotid smell coming out of breath. It is very typical of a case of hepatocellular failure and is called fetor hepaticus. Neurological features develop due to over whelming cerebral oedema. These include disorders of sleep intellectual deterioration. Personality changes, a slow and slurred speech along with characteristic neurological abnormally cailed 'Flapping tremors' (Demonstrated by extending the arms with hyper extension of the wrist when patient shows flapping of the wrist and fingers like that of a bird). Gradually confusion and delirium supervens, patient showing bizarre behaviour.

The encephalopathic features have been graded as follows:

Grade I Altered sensorium, drowsiness inappropriate behaviour.

Grade II Stupor, Personality changes with neurological abnormality. Inarticulate speech.

Grade III Advanced confusion, disorientation. Coma but response to painful stimuli.

Grade IV Deep coma. No response to painful stimuli.

Most of the time the neuropsychiatric features are fluctuating ranging from mood alterations, sleep disturbances, a slurred speech to disorientation.

Depending on the aetiological causes the physical signs shall very. The liver span is generally shortened and liver dullness is obliterated. Ascites may be present. There may be bleeding spots in the skin.

Aetiology. Commonst causes are hepatitis and portal cirrhosis. The acute onset of the disease is precipitated by a number of factors such as:

1. Gastrointestinal bleeding
2. Increased intake of dietary proteins in a case of liver dysfunction leading to increased production of nitrogenous substances in the colon.
3. Fluid and electrolyte disturbances due to diuretic therapy.
4. Paracentesis of ascites with resultant hypovalaemia.
5. Acute infections.

6. Drugs like hypnotics, sedatives.
7. Portosystemic shunt operations.

Diagnosis. It is based on clinical history, physical examination and varied neuro psychiatric disturbances in a case of hepatocellular diseases. Liver biochemistry shows abnormal tests. There are raised levels of bilirubin, AST/ALT and blood ammonia.

EEG shows symmetrical high voltage waves with synchronous slow wave bursts (2.5 /sec).

Management. It is general and specific. In general measures, maintain fluid and electrolyte balance. Measure urinary output. Care of oral hygiene. Prevent bed sores by turning the patient from side to side. If patient is deeply comatose, endotracheal intubation may be required.

Specific measures

1. Start with 20% glucose intravenously so as to meet energy requirements. If patient is vomiting then nothing orally, otherwise a Ryle's tube be passed and patient given glucose through it. Eliminate proteins from the diet.
2. Oral neomycin 1 G 6 hrly.
3. Lactulose 20-30 ml three times daily. It is a semi-synthetic diasaccharide of fructose and lactose and is not digested or absorbed in the small intestines. It shall enhance bowel movements as well as reduce blood ammonia levels. It is broken down in the colon by bacteria to osomotically more active products.
4. Bowel wash twice a day to wash away the nitrogenous products from the bowels.
5. Treat infection vigorously. Injection amoxycillin 1 g I/v 8 hourly.
6. No sedative / tranquilizer, If patient is restless injection phenergan 25 mg I/M may be given.
7. Injection vitamin B complex: Heavy doses of vit. C.
8. Role of steroids is controversial but has been employed in seriously ill cases.
9. In patients who are deeply comatose, levodopa in the dose of 2 gm to start with followed by 1 gm in the evening and further so in the next 24 hrs through the ryles tube is given. Its role is mainly to improve the level of consciousness without any specific effect on the hepatic failure and its prognosis.

Above is the standard procedure to be adopted in a case of hepatic encephalopathy. As the patient improves protein in the diet is added (20 gm/day). Patient is advised to avoid constipation. Lactulose 10-30 ml thrice a day is continued. All factors which could precipitate hepatic failure are to be avoided. Patient should not take alcohol for at least 6-12 month after recovery.

Despite all the necessary measures, cases of hepatic failure carry poor prognosis. Many measure like exchange blood transfusion, plasma exchange, cross circulation, Colon by pass, total body wash out, extra corporeal liver perfusion to liver transplant have been employed but mortality still ranger from 80-90%.

LIVER TRANSPLANTATION

During the last few decades advances have been made in the transplantation of liver. Patients with end stage or irreversible liver disease are being considered for liver transplantation. It is of two forms. 'Heterotopic' where an extra liver is implanted at an ectopic site without the removal of diseased liver while in 'Orthotopic' liver transplantation the homogroft is transplanted in place of diseased liver after its total removal. The results with heterotopic transplantation are not encouraging.

Potential candidates for liver transplantation are children and adults who suffer from severe irreversible liver disease for which alternative medical or surgical treatments have been exhausted.

Commonest indication for transplant in children is biliary atresia where there is progressive distortion of intra hepatic ducts leading to cirrhosis of liver and liver failure. Metabolic disorders which are genetically transmitted and are associated with progressive liver failure both in children and young adults, are another field which requires a liver transplant.

In adults main indications are non-alcoholic cirrhosis. Primary biliary cirrhosis, sclerosing cholangitis and hepatic vein thrombosis. Transplantation in these condition is considered when the condition of patient has deteriorated and end stage has reached. Transplantation in cases of carcinoma of liver is generally not under taken as the chances of recurrence of malignancy are high.

Selection of patients. It is very important to select the right patient for liver transplantation. Patients with life threatening systemic diseases, infections, pre-existing respiratory or cardiac diseases and malignancies are not good candidates for liver transplant. Even in patients with alcohol related liver disease, results of transplant are rather disappointing. Though transplant has been done in patients with chronic viral Hepatitis B with variable results but patients of delta hepatitis are poor risks. A successful liver transplant programme requires team work consisting of physician surgeon, blood bank, primary care and excellent anesthesia services.

Course and management. Transplant may be total or partial. In the post operative period most patients succumb to infections. Immuno suppression therapy (Cyclosporine) has to be given and may be continued life long. Rejection of graft occurs in majority of patients one to six weeks after surgery. Chronic rejection of liver transplant is relatively rare.

Prognosis in all cases of liver transplant is guarded. Children fare slightly better than adults. Children who survive initial three post operative months, one year survival rates are 96 percent as compared to 89 per cent in adults. Five year survival is seen in more than 50 per cent of cases. Quality of life after surgery is not bad and one has to guard against possible chances of infection etc. Some women who underwent transplantation and received immuno suppressive therapy have also conceived and carried the pregnancy to full term without any demonstrable ill effects to the child.

CHAPTER 4

Diseases of the Cardiovascular System

1. Diagnostic approach in cardiology
2. Rheumatic fever
3. Valvular heart disease
4. Infective endocarditis
5. Congenital heart disease
6. Congestive heart failure
7. Hypertension
8. Coronary heart disease
9. Refractory heart failure
10. Disorders of heart beat (cardiac arrhythmias)

DIAGNOSTIC APPROACH IN CARDIOLOGY

An important basis of diagnosing cardiac dysfunction is a good clinical history (history of palpitation, dyspnoea, pain in chest, nocturnal dyspnoea and dyspnoea on effort) and physical examination including pulse, its character, rate, rhythm, volume, blood pressure—high or low, Oedema over dependent parts, ascites. Jugular venous pressure, hepatomegaly, apex beat, its position and character, cardiac impulse, heart sounds and abnormal heart sounds, murmurs, pericardial rub etc. are of significance since in every cardiac patient an abnormal physical sign may help in diagnosing the underlying condition. But in addition a number of diagnostic methods (invasive and non-invasive) are employed to confirm the dignosis.

X-ray of the heart. Size and shape of the heart is assessed by radiograph of the chest. Normally the cardiothoracic ratio is less than 50 per cent as measured by the ratio of transverse diameter of the heart to the internal diameter of the chest at a point above the level of the diaphragm. A number of conditions ranging from hypertension, ischaemic heart disease, cardiomyopathy to valvular heart disease produce cardiac enlargement. Left ventricular enlargement often causes convexity of the left cardiac border and the cardiac apex is displaced downwards producing a 'Boot shaped heart' characteristic of left ventricular disease commonly seen in aortic valve pathology.

Right ventricular enlargement has no representation in the frontal plane and causes an upward displacement or tipping up of the cardiac apex.

An enlarged left atrium in cases of mitral valve disease may produce a 'double shadow' in the center of the cardiac shadow. There is prominence of left atrial appendage on left border of heart. Further confirmation of left atrial enlargement is done by right anterior oblique views when a barium filled oesophagus is displaced backwards by an enlarged left atrium.

X-ray of heart may show characteristic configuration in different cardiac disorders.

1. A pericardial effusion produces a globular shadow where configurations of heart assume a straight line. Money bag appearance of heart is characteristic of pericordial effusion (tuberculous, rheumatic).

2. Uraemic lung. Butterfly shadows round about Hilum.

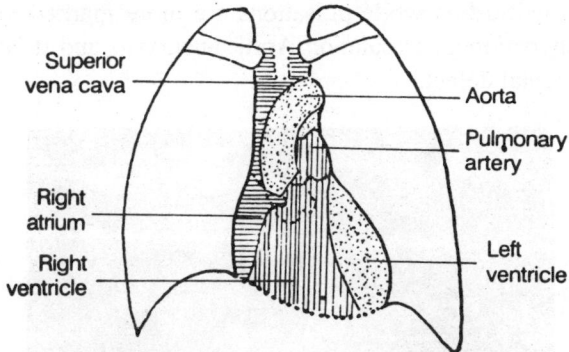

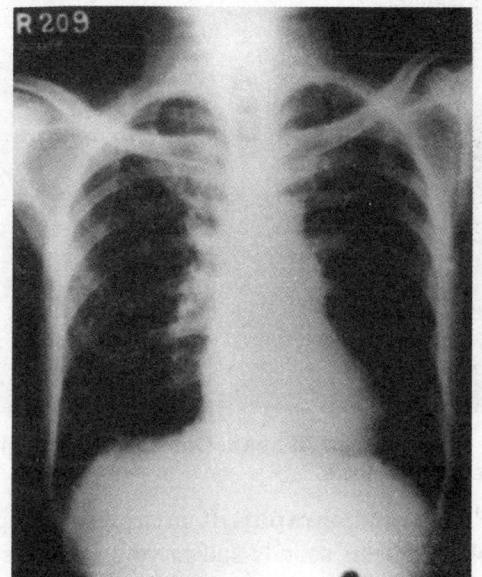

Fig. 4.1. Radiological anatomy of heart (Anterior view)

3. Pulmonary congestion or oedema occurs in congestive heart failure.

Chronic interstitial pulmonary oedema is seen as haziness round the vascular shadows. In severe cases thickening of the interlobular septa shows up as horizontal lines (Kelley's B lines) extending inwards for a few centimeters from the periphery at the base of lungs just above the diaphragm.

Pulmonary plethora is characterised by increase in vascularity of lung fields as in left to right shunts (Atrial or septal defects).

Pulmonary oligaemia manifests by reduced pulmonary blood flow and vascular markings and occurs chracteristically in Fallot's tetralogy, pulmonary stenosis, pulmonary embolism.

Pulmonary infarction shows up as a triangular shadow in the lungs or even as a patch of consolidation.

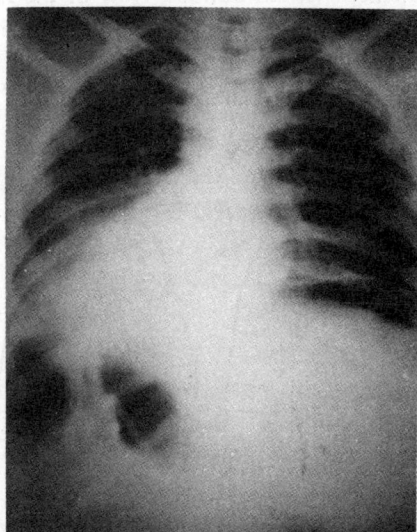

Fig. 4.2. X-ray heart (PA view) heart is present on right side as compared to its normal position on left side of chest. This is called Dextrocardia and is a congenital anomaly.

4. Notching of lower border of ribs is seen in coarctation of aorta. Mediastinal enlargement is characteristically seen in aortic anerusym which is further confirmed by fluoroscopy when a pulsatile mass is seen. Similarly fluor-

oscopy is helpful in pericardial effusion or constrictive pericarditis where cardiac pulsations are poor.

5. Calcification sometimes seen in X-ray film is also of great help. Pericardial calcification is seen in pericarditis commonly tubercular in aetiology. It is in the form of a plaque like opacity over the heart shadow.

Mitral valve calcification is seen in a thick rigid mitral valve due to stenosis whereas calcification in aortic valve or knuckle occurs due to atherosclerosis and is usually seen in persons above the age of 40 years. Syphilitic aortitis may produce calcification in the ascending oarta while descending aorta is involved due to atherosclerosis.

Coronary artery stenosis is rarely seen and indicates atherosclerosis of the vessels.

Right anterior oblique view (RAO). It is the best method to demonstrate the left atrial enlargement when an oblique view of the heart is taken after giving barium to the patient. Barium filled oesophagus is displaced backwards by an enlarged left atrium characteristic in case of mitral stenosis.

upwards and forwards while an enlarged left ventricle projects downwards and backwards, its posterior aspect normally clearing the spine with the patient rotated to an angle of 60° or less in relation to plane of the film. But when the left ventricle is enlarged it overlaps the spine when the patient is rotated 60° or more. Similarly in patients with marked right ventricle enlargement, posterior displacement of ventricle occurs. An enlarged right atrium may also cause a bulge in the upper anterior cardiac segment.

Fluoroscopy is helpful in certain cardiac conditions, when one looks for cardiac pulsations. Cardiac pulsations are poor in pericarditis, pericardial effusion. Constrictive pericarditis and myocarditis while pulsations are more marked in hyperkinetic circulation, Aortic aneurysm, and atrial septal defect.

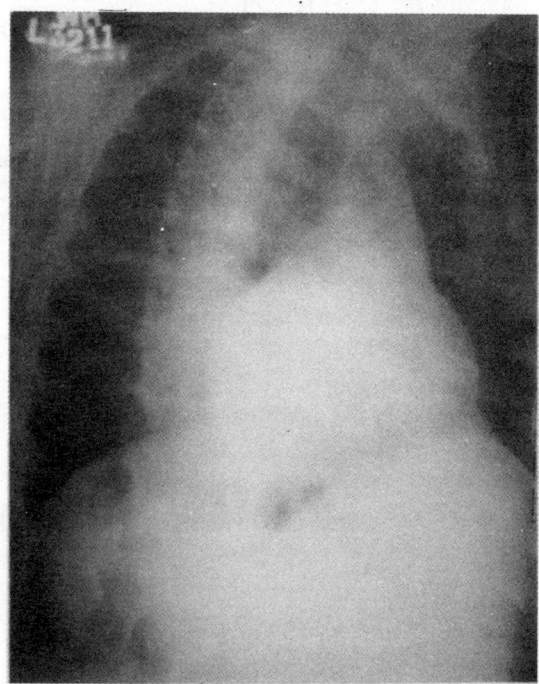

Fig. 4.5. LAO view of heart. Observe shadow of enlarged left ventricle.

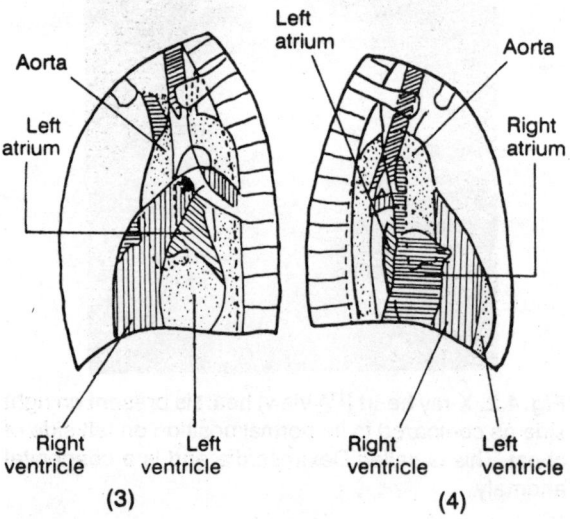

Fig. 4.3-4. Radiological anatomy of normal heart. Left oblique view and right oblique view.

Left anterior oblique view (LAO). It shows enlargement of the inflow tract of right ventricle in best form. An enlarged right ventricle projects

Phonocardiography. It provides a graphic display of heart sounds and murmurs. Filters are employed to allow selective passage of low and high frequency sounds. Usually cardiac, carotid or

PLATE IX

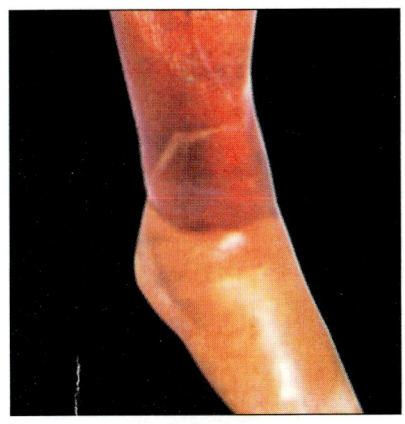

Congestive heart failure

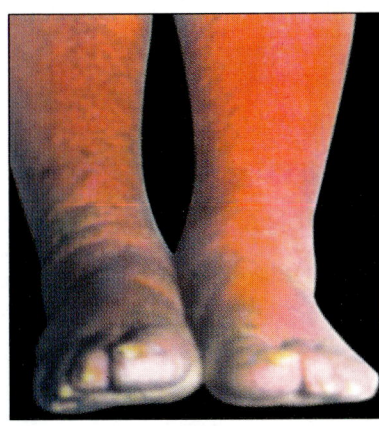

Chronic lymphedema

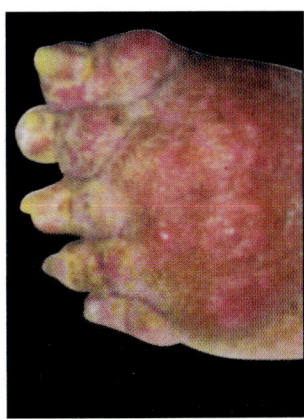

Chronic oedema

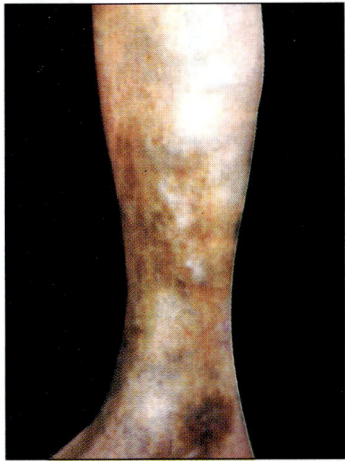

Varicose veins

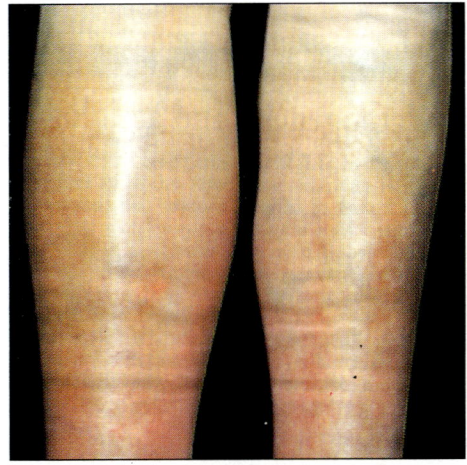

Deep vein thrombosis

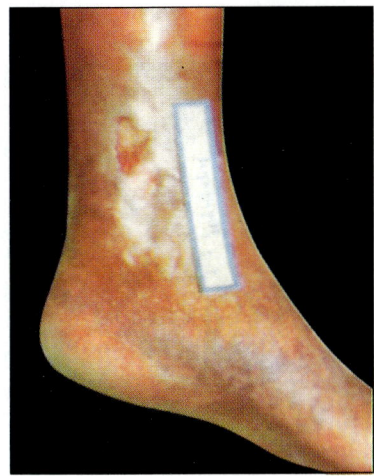

Venous leg ulcer

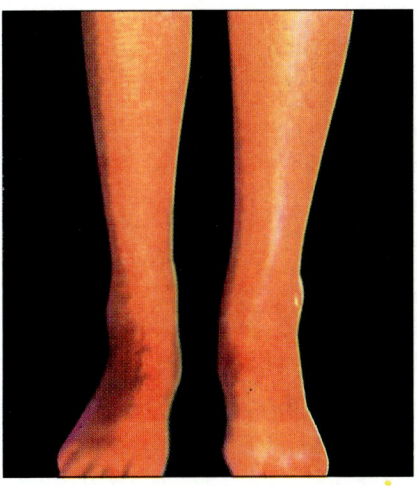

Deep vein thrombosis

PLATE X

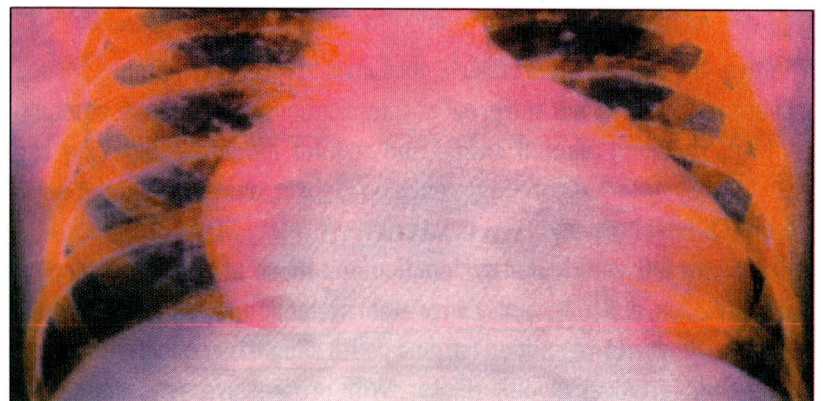

Ventricular dilatation in dialated cardiomyopathy

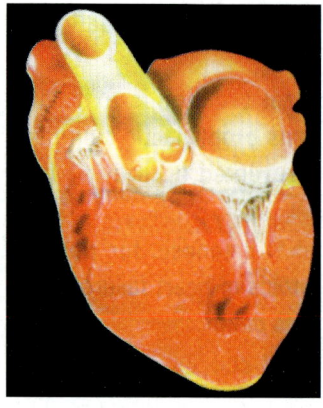

Heart in a case of hypertrophic cardiomyopathy

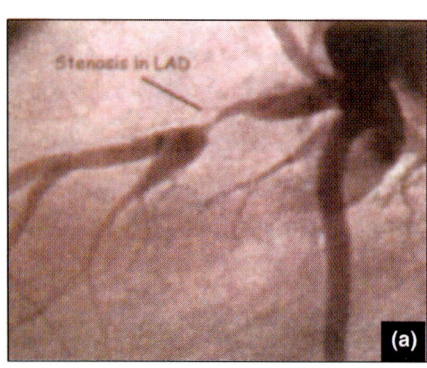

Stenosis in LAD

(a)

(b)

Angiography in a case of IHD: (a) narrowed LAD artery disease and (b) after angioplasty

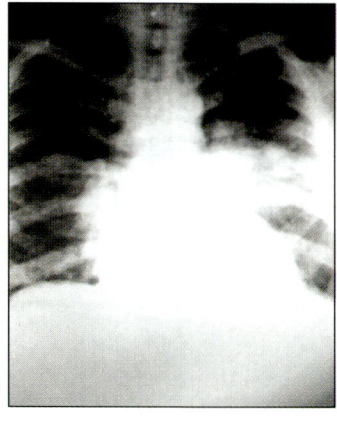

X-ray heart (PA view) in a case of pulmonary oedema

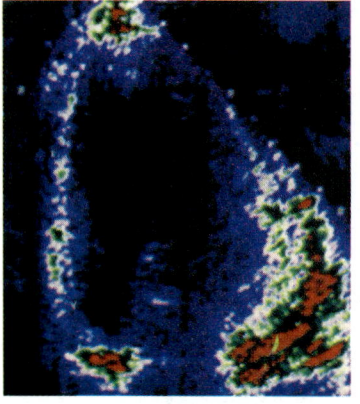

Echocardiogram of a case of left ventricular hypertrophy

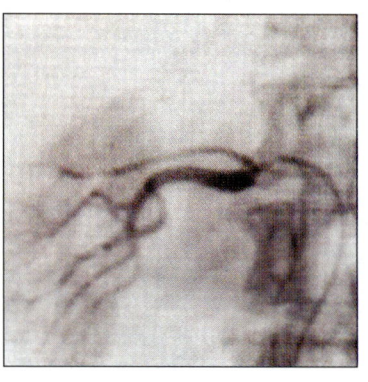

Arteriogram in a case of hypertension showing renal artery stenosis

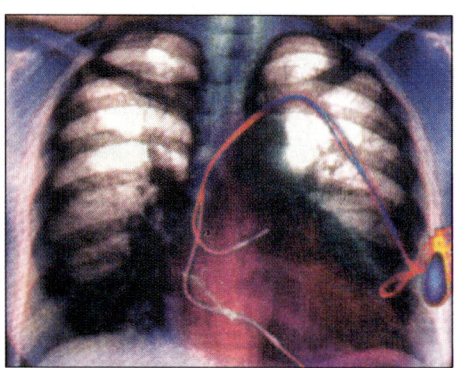

Cardiac pacing

jugular recordings are done at the same time. Phonocardiography is now mainly used for research purposes.

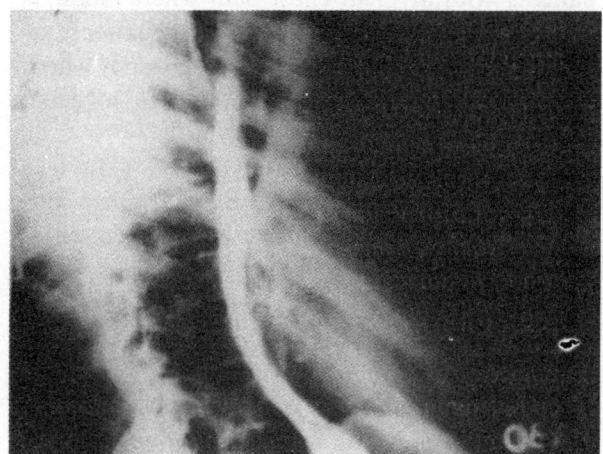

Fig. 4.6. RAO view of heart, Note barium filled oesophagus.

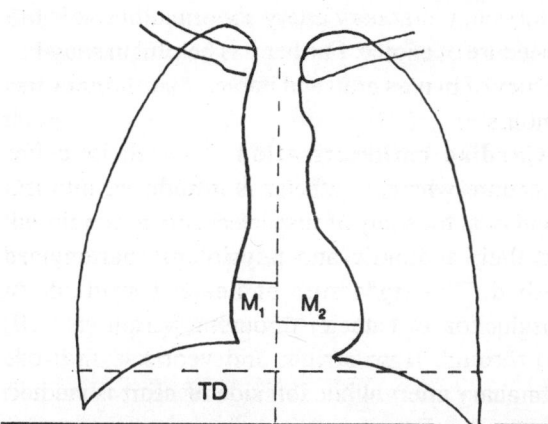

Fig. 4.7. Showing diameters of normal heart. Diameter of normal heart M1 + M2 < 50% TD.

Echocardiography. It implies the recording of pulsed ultrasound waves from the various parts of the heart and for studying the detailed images of the heart. A transducer is used to reflect both transmission of sound and as receiver of reflected waves. Three types of studies are performed. M-mode, two-dimensional and Doppler echo-cardiography.

In M-mode a single transducer is used to record from the parasternal position, motion patterns of

aorta, aortic valve, mitral valve, left and right ventricles to left atrium while two-dimensional echocardiography helps in evaluating valve orifice area, congenital heart lesions, left ventricular functions as well as delineating the structures seen on M-mode.

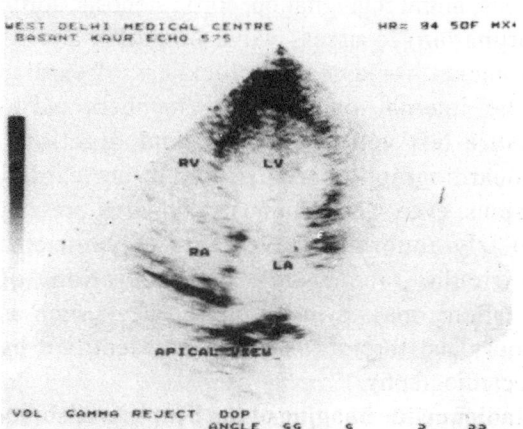

Fig. 4.8. Normal Echocardiogram. Shows various cardiac chambers. Cardiac valves are structurally normal.

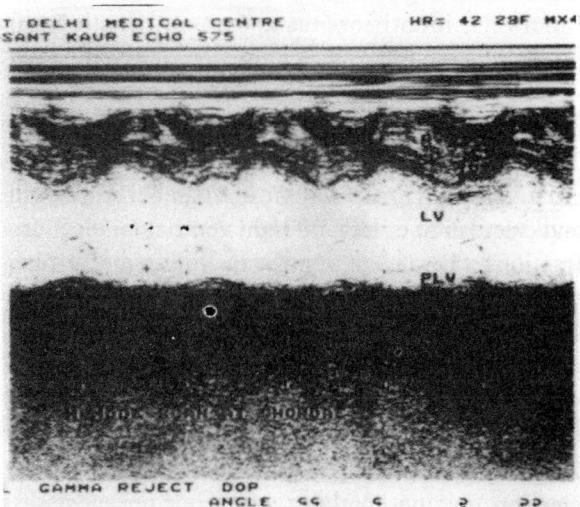

Fig. 4.9. 2-D study to show the motion of ventricular chambers. In this echocardiogram apical portion of intraventricular septum and adjoining wall of left ventricle shows hypokinetic motion.

Doppler echocardiography helps in assessing abnormal flow of blood, its velocity and turbulence. It is useful in spatial localization of flow disturbances in valvular stenosis, regurgitation and septal defects as well as localization of vegetations > 2 mm in cases of infective endocarditis.

Echocardiography is a useful non-invasive technique in diagnosing a number of cardiac conditions.

Its main uses are in valvular heart disease (mitral stenosis, mitral regurgitation, aortic stenosis, aortic regurgitation) to assess valve thickness and its movements, for assessing thickness of cardiac muscle, internal dimension of chambers and to measure left ventricular size and functions. Echocardiography can also detect pericardial effusions, even when minimal amount is present. Similarly abnormal movements of ventricles (ventricular aneurysm) demonstration of vegetations, masses involving the heart such as tumours and thrombi can also be identified by echocardiography.

Radionuclide imaging of the heart. Availability of radionucleides such as technetium 99 m and thallium 201 has helped in isotopic studies for assessment of systolic and diastolic ventricular functions, identification and quantification of intracardiac shunts as well as myocardial perfusion.

Flow studies. Dynamic flow studies are performed by using technetium 99 m compounds. These help in (1) delineating heart chambers and great vessels, (2) estimation of chamber volumes, and calculation of left and right ventricular ejection fractions, (3) rates of ventricular filling and stroke volume ratios and demonstration of akinetic segments of the ventricular wall following myocardial infarction. A low resting ejection fraction in a case of acute myocardial infarction has been related with increased incidence of morbidity and mortality in such cases. Similarly a reduced resting ejection fraction corelates with poor prognosis in patients with mitral or aortic regurgitation.

Myocardial scanning. Thallium 201 which is a potassium analogue is used to study its uptake by myocardium where its uptake depends on myocardial blood flow. Its concentration in the myocardium indicates the health of its cells and thus areas of myocardial necrosis, fibrosis or ischaemia show diminished perfusion and these are called 'cold

areas'. Thallium 201 scan is commonly used to detect stress induced myocardial ischaemia. It is also useful for detecting ischaemia during pacing, in patients with atypical chest pain where exercise electrocardiogram is not helpful, in patients of bundle branch block, ventricular hypertrophy where conventional methods are unable to localize ischaemia.

Fast computed tomography (CINE-CT). It is useful in the evaluation of hypertrophic and congestive cardiomyopathies, pericardial disease, pericardial and intracardiac masses. Coronary artery bypass graft patency. Further it is of use in assessing complications following myocardial infarction as well as analysing ventricular functions.

Magnetic resonance imaging (MRI). It is a secondary method of investigation where primarily disease has been demonstrated by conventional methods including echocardiography. In anatomical anomalies of the heart such as coarctation of aorta, aneurysm, pulmonary artery abnormalities, it is the procedure of choice. Further it is helpful in showing patency of bypass graft and intracardiac thrombi and tumours.

Cardiac catheterization. It is an invasive procedure where a catheter is introduced into the circulation for study of suspected cardiac conditions and their anatomic and physiologic parameters studied. The right side of heart is studied by introduction of catheter through a peripheral vein and through right atrium and ventricle into the pulmonary artery while left side of heart is studied by introduction of catheter through a peripheral artery. The pressure in different chambers of the heart can be recorded during catheterization both by direct method as well as indirectly by wedge pressure through pulmonary artery. Pressure measurements are used to identify anatomical abnormalities. Blood samples can also be collected from different locations and thus estimate oxygen concentration and gauge left to right or right to left shunts.

Main indications for cardiac catheterization are:

a. Patients with acquired valvular heart disease in which haemodynamic assessment and angiocardiographic studies are required to assess nature and severity of a valvular defect rendering it amenable to surgical treatment.

b. In congenital heart disease to assess the primary cardiac lesion and presence of any associated lesion.

c. To study haemodynamic characterization in cases of dilated cardiomyopathy and valvular heart disease.

d. To measure cardiac output, cardiac index and pulmonary wedge pressure (reflecting left atrial pressure). Pressure tracing of the ventricles enables assessment of inflow and outflow obstruction as well as any septal defect.

e. To calculate systolic ejection time.

f. To assess patency as well as success of bypass surgery in patients of coronary heart disease.

Complications during cardiac catheterization include start of cardiac arrhythmias (premature beats, supraventricular tachycardia, atrial fibrillation and ventricular tachycardia) air embolism, perforation of the heart, haemorrhage, hypotension, stroke, myocardial infarction and sudden death.

Cardiac angiography. It involves injection of a radio-opaque substance via cardiac catheter into either cardiac chambers or a vessel.

Selective angiocardiography is used for imaging of cardiac chambers and flow of dye during various phases of cardiac cycle. By this method anatomical and functional abnormalities of the heart are assessed.

Coronary angiography. It is the commonest procedure involving injection of contrast material into the right and left coronary arteries through a catheter. Each coronary artery is assessed for severity of atherosclerosis, stenosis or any abnormal anomaly of artery. This procedure is must before embarking on coronary bypass surgery.

Coronary angiography is performed by selective injection of 5 to 10 ml of contrast medium directly into each coronary artery orifice by means of specially designed catheters.

Side effects of coronary angiography include cardiac arrhythmias, infection, embolism, cerebral thrombosis, haemorrhage and rarely death.

Electrocardiography. It is a commonly used non-invasive method of diagnosing cardiac disorders and is of special use in cases of myocardial infarction, cardiac arrhythmias, pericarditis, systemic diseases which affect the heart (Myxoedema, diphtheria: typhoid) Electrolyte abnormalities (Hyperkalemia, hypokalemia, hypocalcemia) and effect of drugs (Digitalis, Quinidine). An electrocardiogram is a graphic recording of electrical activity of the heart which is generated by individual cardiac cells.

An electrocardiogram consists usually of 12 leads—three standard leads (LI, LII, LIII), three augmented unipolar limb leads (aVR, aVL, aVF) and six precordial leads (V1 to V6).

Lead I (LI) is the difference of potential between the left arm and the right arm (LA-RA). Lead II between left leg and right arm (LL-RA) and lead III between left leg and left arm (LL-LA).

The relation between the three leads is expressed by Einthoven's equation

Lead II = Lead I + Lead III

Events affecting the anterior surface of the heart are best seen in lead I and those involving the inferior surface in leads II and III.

In augmented unipolar limb leads (aVR, aVL, aVF) the voltage of unipolar limb leads is augmented as much as by 50 per cent.

Unipolar chest leads. A single exploring electrode is used to record cardiac activity from various sites on the chest wall. Conventionally recordings are taken from six chest positions on the precordium (V1-V6).

V1 – Fourth intercortal space at right sternal border.

V2 – Fourth intercostal space at left sternal border.

V3 – Equidistance between V2-V4.

V4 – Fifth intercostal space in left mid clavicular line.

V5 – Fifth intercostal space in anterior axillalry line.

V6 – Fifth intercostal space in mid axillary line.

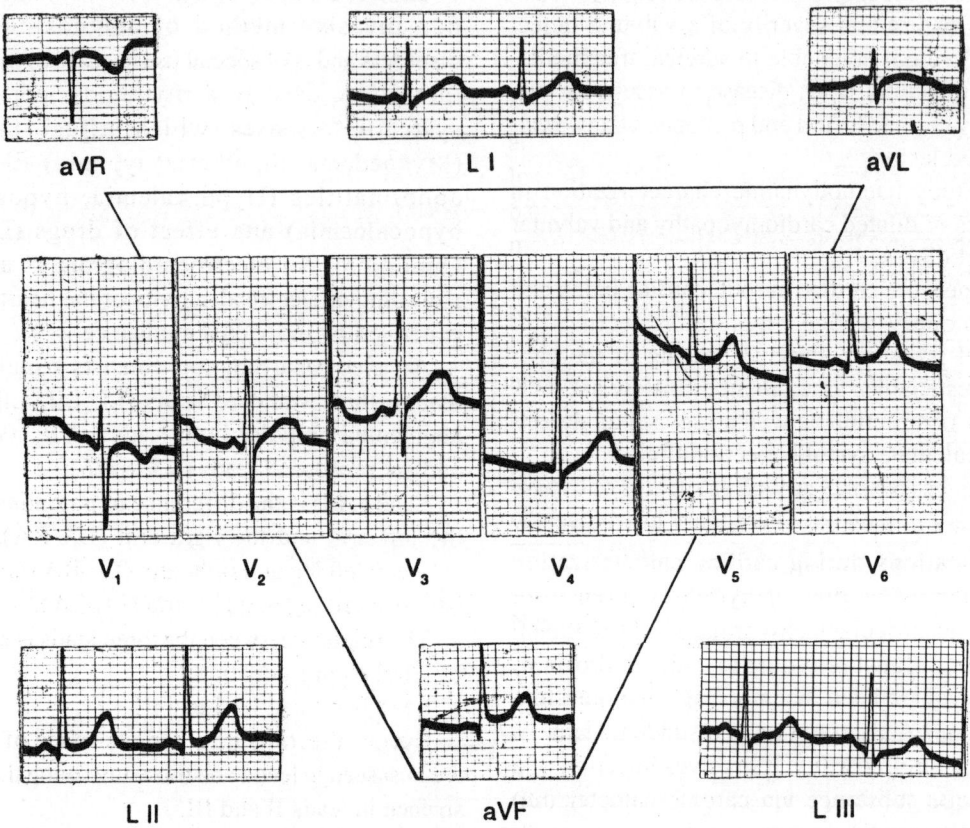

Fig. 4.10. Normal Electrocardiogram

Sometimes to explore further the inferior surface of the heart two further leads are recorded. V7 in posterior axillary line, V8 in posterior scapular line in 5th intercostal space.

Right precordial leads are taken in cases of chronic cor pulmonale or diseases affecting right ventricle where it is required to demonstrate right ventricular hypertrophy. V3R-V4R are taken on the right side of the chest in the same location as the left sided leads. Right precordial leads taken one space above V3R-V4R are labelled 3V3R-3V4. while recordings taken over the ensiform cartilage is labelled VE.

Oesophageal leads are taken from within the oesophagus and its nomeclature is derived from the distance in centimeters from the tip of the nares to the electrode. Thus generally recording's are from a distance of 50 cms from the nares (E40-E50) E15-25 (Atrial area) E25-E35 (region of atrioventricular groove).

Oesophageal leads are useful for recording and defining atrial complexes in cases of tachycardias and for exploring the posterior surface of the heart in suspected myocardial infarction where conventional precordial leads are not helpful.

Normal electrocardiogram. Electrocardiograms are recorded routinely on the graph paper which runs at speed of 25 mm/s. Each small square is 1 mm apart (0.04 seconds) and one large square equals 0.20 seconds. Voltage calibration is upwards and is measured along vertical lines. Expressed as mm calibration is 1 mV = 10 mm. Capitals letters (Q, R, S) refer to relatively large waves (over 5 mm) while small letters (q, r, s) refer to relatively small waves (under 5 mm).

Heart rate is calculated by counting number of

small squares between two R waves, provided the heart rate is regular and dividing 1500 by this.

A normal ECG recording consists of P-wave which is the initial wave of activity during cardiac cycle and results from atrial depolarization.

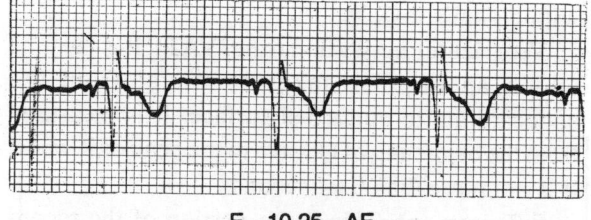

E   10-25   AE

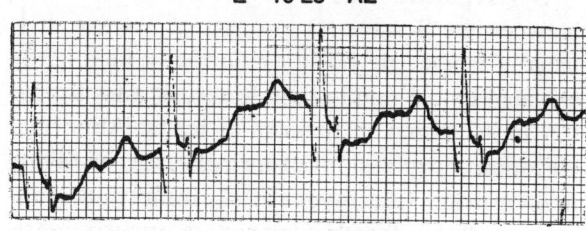

E   25-35   AVE

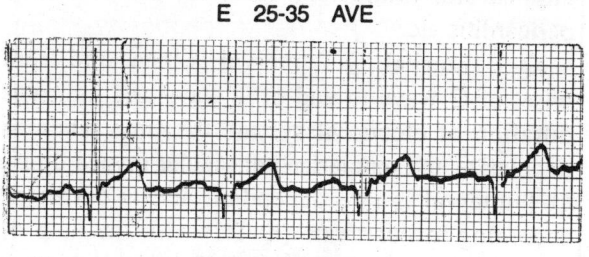

VE   40-50

Fig. 4.11. Normal Oesophageal leads.

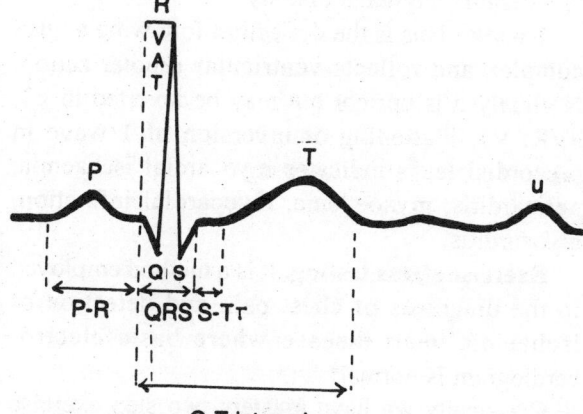

Fig. 4.12. Normal electrocardiographic complex.

A Q-wave is an initial negative wave, an R wave a positive wave following Q-wave and S-wave again

a negative deflection. QRS represents ventricular depolarization and T-wave its repolarization. T-wave is sometimes followed by a small positive deflection, u wave which is considered to represent repolarization of papillary muscle.

The interval between end of QRS complex and beginning of T wave is called ST segment, and is the period of time between depolarization of ventricles and its rapid repolarization. ST segment is very important in cardiac disorders especially myocardial ischaemia where its shape, configuration, elevation or depression have to be considered.

P-wave. It results from atrial depolarization and since the spread of impulse from SA node to A-V node is from head to foot direction, P is normally upright in leads I,II, avF and V3-V6. It is normally inverted in aVR and occasionally in V1 and may be upright, diphasic, flat or inverted in LIII and aVL. Best leads to study it are LII, aVR and aVL. Normally P wave is not over 0.11 seconds in duration and over 2.5 mm in height.

P-wave height more than 2.5 mm and it assuming tall, spiky shape (P pulmonale) indicates right atrial hypertrophy and commonly seen in chronic cor pulmonale.

When P-wave becomes widened and assumes a bifid shape (duration more than 0.11 seconds) it indicates left atrial hypertrophy P mitrale and is found in mitral stenosis. Biphasie P wave indicates bilateral atrial hypertrophy. Absent P waves are seen in atrial fibrillation (replaced by fibrillary waves) complete heart block. S.A. block while inversion of P wave, is seen in atrial premature beats, sick sinus syndrome and A-V nodal rhythm.

P-R interval. It is the time taken for atrial depolarization and repolarization plus the normal time taken for excitation in the A-V node. It is measured from the beginning of the P wave to the onset of the QRS complex. It varies normally between 0.12 to 0.20 seconds and is usually shorter at faster heart rates. Slower the heart the longer the P-R interval. Prolongation of P-R interval indicates delay in conduction at the A-V node and is seen in cases of first degree heart block (myocarditis, coronary heart disease, digitalis intoxication). A shortened P-R interval is seen in W.P.W. syndrome.

QRS complex. This is the measurement of ventricular depolarization and is measured from the onset of Q-wave (or R-wave if no Q is present) to the termination of S wave.

Q describes an initial negative deflection, an R an initial positive deflection and S a subsequent negative deflection. A secondary R wave is usually termed R and a totally negative deflection is termed QS. The QRS complex may start with a Q-wave which should normally be less than 0.04 seconds in duration and 25 per cent or less of the amplitude of the complex.

A QS deflection is present normally in aVR and also in V1 and V2. This is because these leads resemble a right ventricular cavity lead. The duration of QRS complex is 0.10 seconds and its prolongation indicates bundle branch block (right or left, partial or incomplete or complete). Slight prolongation of QRS interval (between 0.10 and 0.11 seconds) is termed partial or incomplete bundle branch block and prolongation beyond 0.12 seconds is termed complete bundle branch block. Right bundle branch block (RsR', rSR' complex in V1-V2. Wide S wave in V5-V6. VAT 0.06 seconds or more in V1-V2, QRS interval 0.12 seconds or more) may be seen in any type of organic heart disease including coronary heart disease, diseases which produce right ventricular hypertrophy i.e. chronic cor pulmonale. Pulmonary valve disease, congenital heart disease involving the septum-atrial septal defect.

A right bundle branch block may also be found in normal individuals especially in elderly people. Left bundle branch block is best diagnosed by looking at precordial leads. There are wide, slurred R waves or rSR' or RSR' complexes in left precordial leads (V4-V6), QRS complex more than 0.12 seconds, VAT more than 0.09 seconds in V4-V6, ST segment depression and T wave inversion in V4-V6. Extremity leads show pattern similar to V4-V6 in aVL (if heart is horizontal, in aVF if heart is vertical). Standard leads shall reflect the same pattern as in extremity leads.

Left bundle branch block (LBBB) presence alway signifies serious cardiac ailment like ischaemic heart disease, hypertension and aortic valve disease. A transient LBBB may occur in cases of acute myocardial infarction, acute myocarditis or in cases with digitalis toxicity.

Ventricular activation time (VAT). It is the time which an impulse takes to travel from the endocardium to epicardial surface. It is measured from the beginning of Q wave to the peak of R wave. It is not more than 0.04 seconds.

S-T segment. This is the portion of the record between the S wave (J) to onset of T wave. It is usually isoelectric but may normally be slightly elevated upto 1 mm in limb leads and vary from − 0.5 to +2.0 mm in precordial leads. Abnormal elevation or depression occurs in diseases involving myocardium like myocardial, infarction, sub-endocardial infarction, coronary insufficiency pericarditis etc.

Q-T interval. Q-T interval is measured from onset of Q wave to end of T wave and indicates duration of electrical systole the time taken to depolarize and repolarize ventricular myocardium. Q-T interval is rate dependent and is corrected according to heart rate (Q-TC) with the help of nomogram. Normal Q-Tc is 0.42 seconds in men and 0.43 seconds in women. It is altered in myocarditis, digitalis toxicity.

T-wave. This is the deflection following a QRS complex and reflects ventricular repolarization. Normally it is upright but may be inverted in L3, aVR, V1. Flattening or inversion of T wave in precordial leads indicates myocardial ischaemia, pericarditis, myxoedema, myocardial infarction, myocarditis.

Exercise stress testing. It is a method employed in the diagnosis of chest pain and detection of ischaemic heart disease where basic electrocardiogram is normal.

Classically we have masters two step exercise test where two steps each nine inches high eight to 10 inches deep and 18 to 27 inches wide are used and the patient is instructed to walk up anddown the steps for a definite number of trips in one and a half minute. Criteria for a positive test include ST segment depression of more than 0.5 mm, change from an upright T to a flat or inverted T in any lead except LIII and appearance of cardiac arrhythmias. In patients where exercise test is normal, double two step test is performed where patient performs double the number of trips of single test in three minutes. Criteria for diagnosing positively of test remain the same.

Treadmill stress test (TMT). Tread mill test is an important test and is done to evaluate cardiac function in a patient who is suffering from angina and his/her ECG is normal. It is not to be done in cases of unstable angina, uncompensated heart failure fresh myocardial infarction, uncontrolled malignant hypertension, seriously ill patients and those with serious cardiac arrhythmias.

Stress testing is performed by walking on a treadmill with continuous monitoring of pulse, BP, ECG, heart rate and patients symptoms like chest pain, breathlessness recorded. The exercise in this test is graded and the speed is gradually increased. If a patient can do more than nine minutes of exercise without any problem he is said to have good tolerance. Two common types of machines employed for stress testing are a bicycle ergometer or motor driven treadmill.

Stress testing tells us whether the coronary circulation is capable of increasing the oxygen supply to the heart in response to increased demands. Patients who are labelled as high risk due to strongly positive test (greater displacement of ST segment and its longer persistence before recovery, development of disorders of conduction, sustained fall in blood pressure) have better prognosis with surgical treatment while those with mildly positive test respond well to medical treatment. A strongly positiveTMT showing triple vessel disease requires further testing by coronary angiography and is a fit case for bypass surgery.

Holter. It is an important test for recording transient changes such as brief periods of arrhythmias which often go undetected as well as transient cardiac ischaemia.

It is a small fully computerised machine carried by the patient on the waist belt with electrodes applied to the chest. The recordings are made on an audiocassette which after 24 hours is put in a special computer analyser and useful information about premature beats, any cardiac irregularity and periods of cardiac ischaemia are recorded and evaluated.

Holter monitoring is a useful test to assess the health of the heart, to detect potentially dangerous arrhythmias which often go undetected and the response of the heart to various day to day activities.

RHEUMATIC FEVER

It is an inflammatory disease which follows as a delayed sequel to pharyngeal infection with group A haemolytic streptococci and is thought to develop as an autoimmune reaction to the infecting organism. It virtually manifests in involvement of heart, joints, skin, subcutaneous tissues and central nervous system. Clinical features in acute stage are migrating joint pains, fever, toxaemia and involvement of heart in the form of carditis. Rheumatic chorea, subcutaneous nodules and erythema marginatum are other signs.

Incidence. Although it may occur at any age yet it is a disease of children and young adults and commonly appears between the ages of 5 and 15 years. It is disease of poor and developing countries and factors such as overcrowding, poor sanitation, dampness, economics and factors related to the high incidence of streptococcal infection predispose to it. It is more common in countries with poor health services and economy such as Asia, Africa and Eastern Europe but rare in developed countries of the west.

Etiology. There is enough evidence to demonstrate close association between group A streptococcal infection and rheumatic fever. There are increased titres of antibodies to streptococcal antigens in acute stage of rheumatic fever. Prompt treatment of streptococcal infection with antibiotics in acute stage prevents the development of rheumatic fever.

Though there is association between

streptococcal infection and rheumatic fever yet precise mechanism by which it occurs is not known. Most likely it is an autoimmune reaction since cases of rheumatic carditis may have circulating antibodies.

Pathology. There is a widespread involvement of the various tissues in the body (heart, connective tissues, skin, central nervous system) and all the three layers of the heart (myocardium, pericardium and endocardium). Synovial membranes and tendons are effected by inflammation with oedema, hyperemia and leucocyte infiltration. Characteristic lesion of rheumatic inflammation is an Aschoff nodule which is considered pathognomic of the disease. These may persist in patients of chronic rheumatic inflammation and rheumatic heart disease for a long time after subsidence of acute rheumatic fever. Involvement of valves especially mitral and to a lesser extent aortic with pin head warty vegetations may take place. In some aggressive forms of rheumatic fever, valve tissue may rapidly be destroyed and its subsequent scarring leads to valve changes of chronic rheumatic heart disease. Rheumatic endocarditis and pericarditis may occur in acute stage. Involvement of joints, synovial membranes and subcutaneous nodules also occur. Pulmonary (pneumonia) and pleural (pleurisy) lesions are not very common though chorea as a late manifestations is quite common.

Clinical features. The presenting features of a case of rheumatic fever are fleeting and migratory joint pains with features of toxaemia, fever and malaise. Almost all joints are involved and several large joints may be involved at the same time.

Heart is involved in the form of carditis. There is tachycardia and involvement of the heart may be either an inapparent inflammation to severe form of pancarditis. In majority of cases carditis in acute stage of rheumatic fever is not diagnosed and only at a later stage when rheumatic heart disease is diagnosed, an old history of rheumatic fever is considered.

When cardiac involvement is suspect, diminished intensity of first heart sound or the development of systolic murmur in mitral area are the early signs. A transient mitral diastolic murmur (Carrey Coomb's) may be heard. It is due to mitral valvulitis. Aortic regurgitation may occur later on. Myocarditis pericarditis or endocarditis presence is suggested by tachycardia, cardiac enlargement, features of congestive heart failure and development of cardiac arrhythmias (prolonged P-R interval, extrasystoles, other arrhythmias). Pericarditis is characterised by retrosternal pain and pericardial rub.

Clinical features of rheumatic fever

1. Fever, malaise
2. Fleeting and migratory joint pains
3. Carditis, myocarditis, pericarditis, endocarditis
4. Erythema marginatum
5. Chorea
6. Subcutaneous nodules

Extracardiac features *include subcutaneous nodules* (small pea sized swellings, painless in character present over, bony prominences like scapula, scalp elbows). Erythema marginatum (transient pink rash with clear centre and slightly raised round margins). The rash may rapidly enlarge to form irregular patches and is mostly seen on trunk and extremities) and chorea where patient develops sudden purposeless, irregular movements of limbs exaggerated by effort or excitement. Chorea often appears as a delayed reaction of rheumatic fever and at that time other features like polyarthritis are not present. Carditis may be detected at this time. Patient with chorea may develop marked choreiform movements and even find difficult to do normal chores like walking talking or sit up and holding of objects.

Laboratory investigations:

1. Blood sedimentation rate (ESR) and C-reactive proteins. Raised levels indicate activity of the rheumatic process.
2. Throat swab for group A streptococcus; a quarter of patients may show a positive culture.
3. ASO titres (antistreptolysin O) of 300 Todd units or above suggests recent streptococcal infection.
4. Chest radiograph for cardiac enlargement.

5. Electrocardiogram for evidence of prolongation of P-R interval, abnormalities of ST segment, and T wave, Cardiac arrhythmias.
6. Echocardiography for confirmation of ventricular dilatation or evidence of pericardial effusion.

Diagnosis. Diagnosis of rheumatic fever is based on criteria evolved by Duckett-Jones where a patient of rheumatic fever must have either two or more major criteria or one major and two or more minor criteria.

Major Criteria:

1. Carditis
2. Polyarthritis
3. Chorea
4. Erythema marginatum
5. Subcutaneous nodules

Minor criteria:

1. Fever
2. Arthralgia
3. Previous rheumatic fever or rheumatic heart disease
4. Raised ESR/C reactive proteins
5. Prolonged P-R interval on ECG
6. Leucocytosis

In addition there should be supporting evidence of preceding streptococcal infection (positive throat culture for group A streptococcus, raised ASO titres (more than 300 units).

Treatment:

1. Bed rest till acute symptoms and fever subside. With rest and improvement in disease. Pulse rate, ESR, haemoglobin and white cell counts levels return to normal. Prolonged rest may be necessary where disease process remains active.
2. Injection Penicillin (5-10 lac units I/M 6 hourly) for 7 to 10 days in every patient to kill any remaining haemolytic streptococci in throat. Where patient is allergic to penicillin, erythromycin 2-4 gm in divided doses in 24 hours be given.
3. Aspirin is effective in combating pain and fever. Daily dose is 15-20 mg/kg in children and 50 mg per kg body weight divided into four hourly doses (average 6-8 gm in adults perday). Of the various salicylate preparations, aspirin is the cheapest and most effective. Gastric intolerance can be diminished by administering aspirin after meals or by giving antacids. Dosage of aspirin can be increased to the level of tolerance (development of Tinnitus) or until the clinical effect is achieved. Side effects of aspirin include nausea, dizziness, headache. Tinnitus and deafness in early stage followed by vomiting, hyperventilation and confusion. Aspirin relieves symptoms but has no effect either on course of the disease or development of carditis.
4. Prednisolone 60-80 mg per day in divided doses has been found effective in acute stage. Dosage is to be gradually tapered off in 2 weeks. Role of steroids in prevention of development of cardiac lesion is doubtful.
5. Treatment of other manifestations of rheumatic fever like Erythema marginatum, carditis is the same. Patients of chorea require sedatives and tranquilizers, Diazepam (2-5 mg) or Phenobarbitone (30-60 mg) twice a day is useful.

Duckett-Jones criteria for rheumatic fever

Major criteria

a. Carditis
b. Polyarthritis
c. Chorea
d. Erythema marginatum
e. Subcutaneous nodules

Minor criteria

a. Fever
b. Arthralgia
c. Raised ESR/C-reactive proteins
d. Leucocytosis
e. Prolonged P-R interval on ECG
f. Previous rheumatic fever or rheumatic heart disease

Prevention of recurrence. The frequency of recurrence is dependent on severity of streptococcal infection and presence or absence of rheumatic heart disease. If a patient has not developed carditis or any significant cardiac lesion prevention of recurrence carries excellent prognosis.

A fortnightly injection of Benzathine Penicilline (Penidura-LA) 1-2 mega units intermuscularly is to be given fortnightly till the patient reaches the age of 21 years. Patient who had carditis or one with rheumatic heart disease or recurent sore throat deserve maximum protection and care.

VALVULAR HEART DISEASE

It is one of the commonest cardiac ailment in young adults and follows rheumatic fever in more than 50 per cent of cases. Principal world wide cause of symptomatic valvular heart disease is rheumatic but other causes include congenital, infectious and degenerative disorders.

Chronic rheumatic disease most commonly affects the mitral valve, (Mitral stenosis and incompetence) aortic valve the next (aortic stenosis or insufficiency) tricuspid valve occasionally and very rarely the pulmonary valve. Combined mitral and aortic valve involvement also occurs and constitutes about 40 per cent of the cases.

Mitral stenosis. Commonest cause of mitral stenosis is rheumatic fever and a history of one or more attacks of rheumatic fever or chorea can be elicited from more than 50 per cent of cases of adult rheumatic disease. Pure mitral stenosis is the commonest lesion and is almost alway due to rheumatic endocarditis. Other causes include congenital (Lutembacher's syndrome, congenital mitral atresia), Functonal obstruction of valvular orifice by bacterial vegetations or thrombosis.

Causes of mitral stenosis

1. Rheumatic (commonest)
2. Congenital
   a. Lutembacher's syndrome combination of an acquired mitral stenosis with atrial septal defect
   b. Congenital mitral atresia
3. Functional obstruction of mitral orifice by bacterial vegetations or thrombi.

The disease process may take number of years to develop after an attack of rheumatic fever and many patients may have subclinical episodes of the disease. On an average it takes about 7-10 years after the initial episode of rheumatic fever but in India because of the severe form of disease, a classical picture of mitral stenosis may develop rapidly in young children and adults (Juvenile mitral stenosis).

Pathology. Normal mitral valve orifice is 5 cm^2 (square cm). Because of the disease process the cusps become thickened, rigid and fibrosed. Commissures of the valve become adherent and the chordae are often short and deformed. Mitral valve becomes distorted and narrowed with subsequent calcification of the mitral valve in long standing cases. There is progressive immobility of the mitral valve leaflets. Size of orifice of about 2.5 cm^2 indicates mild form of stenosis but when mitral valve orifice is reduced to 1 square centimeter or less, severe mitral stenosis results.

Since adequate cardiac output has to be maintained, and there is resistance offered by a narrowed mitral valve, increase in left atrial pressure Pulmonary venous and pulmonary capillary pressures occurs. Maintenance of blood flow through the narrowed mitral orifice is governed by excess of left atrial over left ventricular pressure in diastole. This difference is termed mitral gradient and this in mitral stenosis is usually between 5-30 mm Hg at rest and indicates severity of disease process.

Rise in left atrial pressure results in left atrial dilatation, with blood flowing into left ventricle and diminished left ventricular stroke output. Cardiac output can be maintained only by a rise in left atrial, pulmonary venous and pulmonary capillary pressure leading to pulmonary hypertension. This leads to right ventricular hypertrophy and dilatation. A sudden increase in pulmonary venous pressure may precipitate. Pulmonary oedema while left atrial dilatation may be accompanied by atrial fibrillation. All cases of mitral valve disease develop pulmonary hypertension as a result of increase in pulmonary venous pressure leading to rise in pulmonary arterial pressure as well as structural changes in the pulmonary vascular bed putting an exra strain on right ventricle which subsequently enlarges producing right ventricular hypertrophy and dilatation. Patients with mitral stenosis with a large left atrium are at risk from left atrial thrombus and subsequent systemic thromboembolism especially in presence of atrial fibrillation.

Mitral stenosis may be isolated or associated with mitral regurgitation or tricuspid regurgitation or aortic valve disease.

Clinical features. Cases with mild to moderate degree of mitral stenosis may have no symptoms and those cases who remain well compensated may live a normal life. It is only cases with severe degree of mitral stenosis who become symptomatic.

Shortness of breath induced by exertion is the commonest symptom. The gradual reduction in the size of mitral orifice results in the development of symptoms which may take long time to develop but once a patient of mitral stenosis becomes symptomatic, continuous progression of the disease takes place.

The extra demands put on the heart by severe exertion, infection, pregnancy bring about impairement of cardiac function and this along with tachycardia or atrial fibrillation may precipitate a deterioration and bring on breathlessness, even at rest. Precordial distress and palpitation are early symptoms and are as frequent as dysponea.

Pulmonary congestion causes cough which is worse at night. Haemoptysis may occur in 10 per cent of cases and results from rupture of pulmonary, bronchial venous connections. It may also occur due to pulmonary embolization and infarction. Haemoptysis may also occur with moderate pulmonary engorgement and tends to subside as pulmonary hypertension develops. Further development of pulmonary vascular resistance and right ventricular failure leads to fatigue, weakness, hepatic congestion and ankle oedema. Gross enlargement of left atrium predisposes to development of atrial fibrillation with symptoms of palpitation. It may further produce both systemic and pulmonary emobilization.

Physical signs:

1. Patients with mitral stenosis especially fair skinned have malar flush on the face (dusky pink discoloration present over the cheeks bilaterally).
2. Pulse is low volume. If atrial fibrillation is present then it is irregularly irregular.
3. Signs of right heart failure may be present depending on the stage at which patient presents. These are engorged neck veins (jugular venous pressure raised) tender hepatomegaly, ankle oedema.
4. Heart shows a right ventricular hypertrophy impulse which is tapping in character. A diastolic thrill over the apex may be palpated. If pulmonary hypertension is present, a parasternal heave along the left border and pulmonary second sound may be felt in the second left intercostal space.

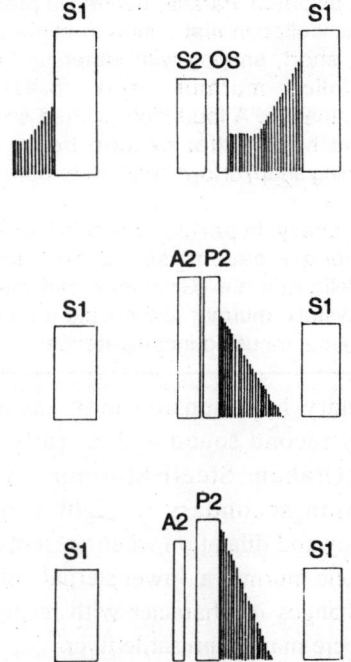

Fig. 4.13. Graphic representation of Heart sounds and murmurs in valvular heart disease. a. Mitral stenosis. Opening snap. Mid-diastolic murmur with presystolic accentuation. b. Aortic incompetence. Early diastolic (Decrescendo) murmur with soft second sound. c. Pulmonary incompetence. Early decrescendo distolic murmur. Pulmonary second sound loud.

On auscultation first sound in mitral area is loud, short snappy and there is either mid disastolic or late diastolic murmur with presystolic accentuation. Opening snap of the mitral valve, a high pitched sound is audible in expiration at or just medial to the apex. The intensity of first heart sound and opening snap correlates with the mobility of the anterior mitral leaflet and decreases in valves with fibrosis and calcification.

Presystolic accentuation of the diastolic murmur disappears with the appearance of atrial fibrillation.

Physical signs in mitral stenosis

1. Malar flush on face in fair-skinned people.
2. Low volume pulse. If atrial fibrillation, then irregularly irregular pulse.
3. If right heart failure is present, engorged neck veins. Prominent 'a' waves in neck. Tender hepatomegaly. Ankle oedema.
4. A tapping apex beat. Diastolic thrill over the apex palpated. Parasternal heave present.
5. On auscultation first sound in mitral area is loud, short, snappy with either mid or late diastolic murmur and presystolic accentuation. A loud high pitched snapping sound heard after second heart sound (opening snap) at lower end of sternum medial to apex.
6. Pulmonary hypertension produces loud pulmonary second sound and an early diastolic murmur (Graham steell murmur), Pansystolic murmur in tricuspid area due to functional tricuspid incompetence.

Pulmonary hypertension may cause a loud pulmonary second sound and an early diastolic murmur (Graham Steell Murmur). Tricuspid regurgitation secondary to right ventricular. Hypertrophy and dilatation when present produces a pan systolic murmur at lower sternal border. This murmur changes its character with respiration. In addition there may be pulsatile liver.

Investigations:

1. *X-ray heart* shows typically a mitralised heart which consists of cardiac enlargement. Prominent pulmonary conus. Hypoplastic aorta and enlarged left atrium often seen as double shadow. Occasionally calcification of mitral valve may be seen. RAO view of heart demonstrates an enlarged left atrium causing a backward displacement of barium filled oesophagus.

2. *Electrocardiogram* shows a bifid broad P wave P mitrale best seen in leads II and V_{2-5}. There is evidence of right ventricular hypertrophy.

3. *Echocardiography.* It allows estimation of severity, rigidity and state of calcification of mitral valve cusps as well as size of left atrium and state of ventricular functioning. Doppler may be employed to study mitral valve gradient as well as size of mitral valve orifice.

4. *Cardiac catheterization.* It is done to assess the severity of mitral stenosis, presence of mitral in competence and to measure pressure gradient across the valve.

Complications of mitral stenosis. *The various complications are:*

1. Congestive heart failure.
2. Atrial fibrillation
3. Subacute bacterial endocarditis.
4. Systemic and pulmonary embolisation.
5. Ball-valve thrombus causing sudden death.
6. Hoarseness due to left recurrent laryngeal nerve paralysis as a result of compression of nerve between dilated left pulmonary artery and aorta.
7. Dysphagia due to pressure of dilated left atrium on oesophagus.
8. Chest infections
9. Palmonary hypertension

Treatment:

1. A mild or asymptomatic case of mitral stenosis requires no treatment. Prophylactic measures against any infection by use of adequate antibiotics must be taken promptly.

2. When patient has signs of congestive heart failure in the form of dysponea, ankle oedema, hepatomegaly treatment is by salt restricted diet Digitalis and Diuretics. (Tab Digoxin 0.25 mg twice a day, Dosage may be adjusted according to heart rate. in addition Frusemide 40 mg tablet twice a week)

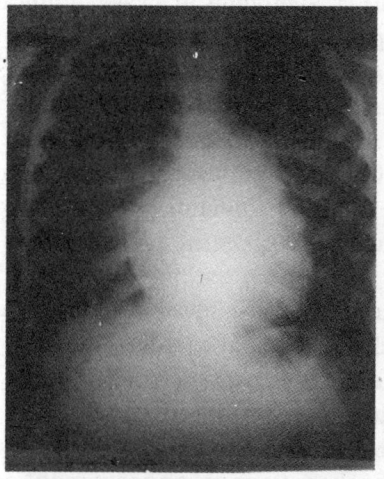 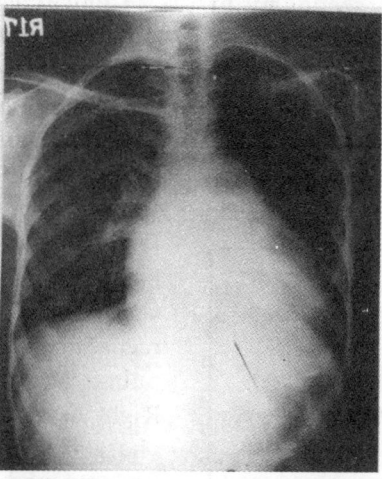 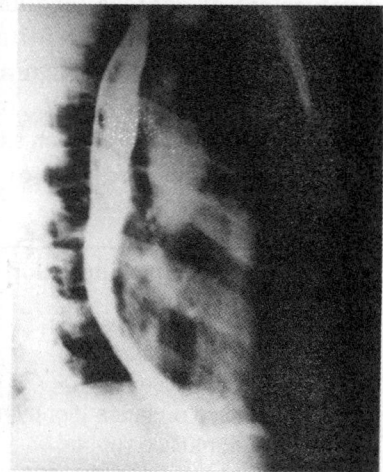

Fig. 4.14 and Fig. 4.15. X-ray Heart (PA view). Mitralised heart. Shadow of enlarged left atrium is seen. Pulmonary conus is prominent.

Fig. 4.16. RAO View in a case of mitral heart Barium filled oesophagus is displaced backwards by an enlarged left atrium.

3. Development of atrial fibrillation requires treatment with Digitalis and anticoagulation to prevent systemic or pulmonary embolization.
4. Surgery is the definitive treatment in all cases of mitral stenosis with a grossly narrowed mitral orifice.

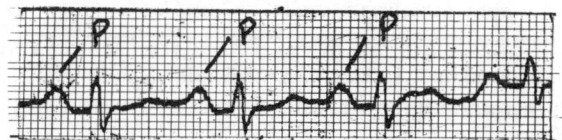

Fig. 4.17. P mitrale. P wave is notched and broad. Best seen in L-II, avF, V2-V5. Indicates left atrial hypertrophy.

Mitral valvotomy (closed or open) is the surgical treatment of choice in cases with pure mitral stenosis without evidence of mitral regurgitation and a thin mobile and non-calcific mitral valve.

Often open valvotomy is done to safeguard against development of traumatic mitral regurgitation.

In cases of gross damage of mitral valve or mitral incompetence coexisting, valve replacement is undertaken.

Success with surgery depends on the stage of disease, presence of any complication and expertise of surgeon. Generally after surgery relief may be obtained for 5-15 years. Restenosis of valve may occur in some cases.

Mitral regurgitation. A number of diseases which cause left ventricular dilatation are known to cause mitral regurgitation but rheumatic heart disease is responsible for more than one third of cases of mitral insufficiency.

Other causes are:

1. Bacterial endocarditis.
2. Aortic valve disease.
3. Rupture of papillary muscle in a case of coronary heart disease.
4. Hypertensive heart disease.
5. Congenital mitral insufficiency due to perforation in the valve leaflet or a congenital cleft (endocardial cushion defect).
6. Connective tissue or degenerative collagen disorders.
7. Hypertrophic cardiomyopathy.
8. Traumatic mitral insufficiency as a result of surgery in cases of mitral stenosis.

In sum total mitral insufficiency is seen in patients with massive left ventricular dilatation as seen in cases of hypertensive heart disease, aortic regurgitation, rupture of papillary muscles, involvement of chordae tendinae, secondary to bacterial endocarditis or following an acute myocardial infarction. It can also result from dilatation of the mitral valve ring with diseases involving the myocardium such as rheumatic fever, diphtheria, myocarditis or hypertrophic cardiomyopathy.

Causes of mitral regurgitation

1. Rheumatic heart disease
2. Bacterial endocarditis
3. Aortic valve disease
4. Mitral valve prolapse (floppy mitral valve)
5. Papillary muscle rupture
6. Hypertensive heart disease
7. Hypertrophic cardiomyopathy
8. Congenital (endocardial cushion defect)
9. Connective tissue/or collagen disorders
10. Traumatic (following surgery in mitral stenosis)

Mitral valve prolapse syndrome is a congenital condition where mitral cusps prolapse into the left atrium during systole and mitral regurgitation is present.

Chronic rheumatic heart disease commonly has coexisting mitral stenosis or aortic valve disease along with mitral regurgitation depending on the degree of damage of the mitral orifice. Fusion and calcification of the anterior mitral valve leaflets produces predominant mitral stenosis while shortening of chordae tendinae, loss of substance of posterior leaflets and of valve shall have mitral regurgitation over shadowing stenosis.

Pathophysiology. There is regurgitation of blood into the left atrium because of inability of mitral valve to close during systole and this results in increased left atrial pressure. The enlarged output of the left atrium increase the left ventricular and diastolic volume and as the regurgitation increases left ventricular function deteriorates. There is left ventricular dilatation and hypertrophy. As left ventricle dilates further dilatation of mitral valve ring also occurs. With further deterioration left ventricular failure occurs followed by right ventricular failure and finally biventricular failure supervenes.

Clinical features. Symptoms in a case of mitral regurgitation depend on the degree of severity of incompetence and as to how suddenly it has developed. Many patient with mild form of incompetence remain asymptomatic for a long time. With progress of the disease dysponea on exertion and later on even at rest, palpitation, weakness and fatiguability are the prominent symptoms. Fatiguability is due to low cardiac output. Left ventricular failure develops in severe form of mitral regurgitation and a patient may present as a case of pulmonary oedema and marked breathlessness. Right heart failure though late in developing is characterised by hepatomegaly ascites, ankle oedema and marked venous engorgement is associated with severe degree of pulmonary hypertension. Subsequently patient goes into a full picture of congestive heart failure.

Physical signs in mitral regurgitation

1. Peripheral/radial pulse is good in volume.
2. Apex beat is displaced downwards and outwards. It is diffuse, forceful and thrusting. A systolic thrill often conducted to axilla palpable at apex.
3. On auscultation first heart sound is soft and feeble. A pansystolic (holosystolic) murmur at apex radiating to axilla.

Second heard sound at apex is faint and inaudible. Pulmonary second sound is accentuated and split.

Physical signs. Peripheral or radial pulse is good in volume and often described as pseudocollapsing. There is cardiac enlargement with apex beat displaced down and out. Apex beat is diffuse, forcible and thrusting type with a palpable systolic thrill often conducted to the axilla. There is a pansystolic murmur which is loud and prolonged often replacing the first heart sound which is soft and feeble. The murmur may start immediately after first sound and occupies most of systole (Holosystolic) radiating to the axilla. High pitched musical murmurs may be seen in mitral regurgitation with ruptured chordae tendinae or papillary muscle dysfunction. The second sound at apex is generally inaudible or faint. Pulmonary second sound may be accentuated and split.

A third heart sound is heard at the apex but there is no opening snap.

Complications. A case of mitral regurgitation may develop certain complications depending on the severity of disease process.

1. Acute left heart failure
2. Pulmonary oedema
3. Congestive heart failure
4. Subacute bacterial endocarditis: More common in mitral insufficiency as compared to pure mitral stenosis
5. Cardiac arrhythmias, atrial fibrillation, atrial flutter or flutter-fibrillation.

Investigations:

Electrocardiogram. A mild case of mitral regurgitation shows a normal ECG. In cases with significant mitral insufficiency there is evidence of left ventricular hypertrophy (SV1 + RV5 or RV6 > 35 mm).

X-ray chest. Heart is enlarged with left ventricle extending outward and downward and may be rounded. Posterior enlargement of left ventricle is better seen in left anterior oblique view.

Echocardiography. Flow and doppler echocardiography are helpful in the assessment of mitral insufficiency and the flow of regurgitant jet. Vegetations, enlargement of left atrium, and rupture of chordae tendinae are identified.

Cardiac catheterization. It is helpful for assessing severity of mitral regurgitation and by injecting contrast into left ventricle, assessment of haemodynamic abnormalities and pressure in left atrial as well as pulmonary wedge pressure are measured.

Treatment. In a case of mitral incompetence, treatment is directed to the basic myocardial disease.

A patient presenting with symptoms of palpitation breathlessness shall be treated with Digoxin and Diuretics.

Similarly case with acute pulmonary oedema or congestive heart failure are to be treated with O_2, digoxin, diuretics.

But in cases with severe mitral incompetence who are not responsive to medical therapy. Mitral valve replacement or even repair of the damaged valve (mitral valvuloplasty) are the surgical procedures adopted. Before undertaking surgery, infective endocarditis (if present) and congestive failure must be treated. Thromboembolism and late valve failure are important complication following surgery.

AORTIC VALVE DISEASE

Aortic valve may be involved in the form of either aortic stenosis or regurgitation in rheumatic involvement where the aortic valve cusps become thickened, fused and narrowed resulting in a bicuspId valve which may ultimately show degenerative changes and even calcification.

Aortic stenosis. Aortic stenosis due to rheumatic fever in isolated form is not very common and is often associated either with mitral stenosis or aortic regurgitation.

In addition to rheumatic being a cause of aortic stenosis other causes include:

1. Congenital bicuspid or unicuspid aortic valve stenosis.
2. Atherosclerotic
3. Degenerative calcified aortic valve in elderly people.

Aortic stenosis produces left ventricular outflow tract obstruction and besides it other lesions in the heart may produce this picture. This comprises of:

1. Supravalvular stenosis produced by congenital narrowing of either ascending aorta or of diaphragm above aortic valve.
2. Subvalvular stenosis in which there is a membranous diaphragm or fibrous ring below the aortic valve.
3. Subaortic obstruction where hypertrophy of interventricular septum produces obstruction.

Causes of aortic stenosis

1. Rheumatic
2. Congenital
3. Atherosclerotic
4. Degenerative

Classic example is cases of hypertrophic cardiomyopathy.

Pathophysiology. The normal circumferance of aortic valve is 7.5 cm. The degree of narrowing is variable but significant haemodynamic disturbances are produced only when the aortic circumference is reduced to 2 cm or less. Basic abnormality is obstruction to left ventricular outflow leading to increased left ventricular pressure. Result is left ventricular dilatation and hypertrophy. The resting cardiac output is usually within normal limits in majority of the patients but in cases with severe aortic stenosis it is diminished and does not increase with exercise. Result is relative ischaemia of myocardium and interference with coronary artery blood flow.

Clinical features. Mild cases of aorotic stenosis may have no symptoms and even cases with moderate severity may remain asymptomatic for a long time.

Main features are syncope from a decrease in cardiac output, dysponea on exertion, angina prctoris and features of left heart failure (orthoponea, paroxysmal nocturnal dysponea, and pulmonary oedema in advanced stage of disease).

Fatigue is often the earliest symptom. Other features include palpitation, cardiac pain, dizziness or faintness and cardiac arrhythmias. Sudden death may occur in a case of aortic stenosis due to coronary artery occlusion, heart block or ventricular fibrillation.

Physical signs include a low volume, slow rising pulse (Anacrotic). Apex beat is forceful, a sustained and thrusting type, may be displaced inferiorly and laterally in the presence of left ventricular hypertrophy. A systolic thrill is palpable at the base of heart in the second intercostal space along the right sternal border (aortic area) and in jugular notch and along the carotid vessels.

Auscultation reveals a loud pitched, rough rasping mid systolic ejection murmur which starts shortly after first heart sound, raches peak towards the middle and stops short of second heart sound. This murmur is best heard over the aortic area or basal areas, with patient in sitting position and bending forward it radiates to the neck vessels.

Aortic second sound may be inaudible or becomes soft when the aortic valves become immobile. An ejection click is heard in valvular form of aortic stenosis.

Physical signs in aortic stenosis

1. Low volume pulse or slow rising (anacrotic).
2. Apex beat is displaced downwards and outwards. Forceful, sustained and thrusting type. A systolic thrill is palpable in the aortic area.

   Auscultation reveals a loud pitched, ejection systolic murmur over the aortic area, radiating to the neck vessels. Second heart sound is soft.

Investigations. *X-ray of the chest* shows little or no cardiac enlargement when there is no or slight left ventricular hypertrophy. But later on as left ventricular hypertrophy takes place, there is blunt rounding of the lower left cardiac border.

There may be dilatation of the ascending aorta with post stenotic dilatation. There may be calcification in the aortic valve in cases of severe aortic stenosis. In late stage when left ventricular hypertrophy and dilatation takes place, heart size is enlarged and there is pulmonary congestion.

Electrocardiogram. It shows left atrial and left ventricular hypertrophy. Abnormalities of T wave in the form of inversions and ST segment depression in left ventricular leads are seen.

Conduction disturbances like left bundle branch block, intraventricular conduction defects, partial and complete heart block may be seen.

Echocardiogram. It demonstrates left ventricular hypertrophy and the nature of aortic valve and severity of stenosis. It is particularly useful for demonstrating other valvular abnormalities such as mitral stenosis and aortic regurgitation which may be present in association with aortic stenosis as well as measuring pressure gradient across the valve.

Cardiac catheterization. It is used to determine the gradient across the aortic valve which together with measurement of cardiac output can be used to calculate the size of aortic valve orifice and the degree of aortic valve obstruction.

PLATE XI

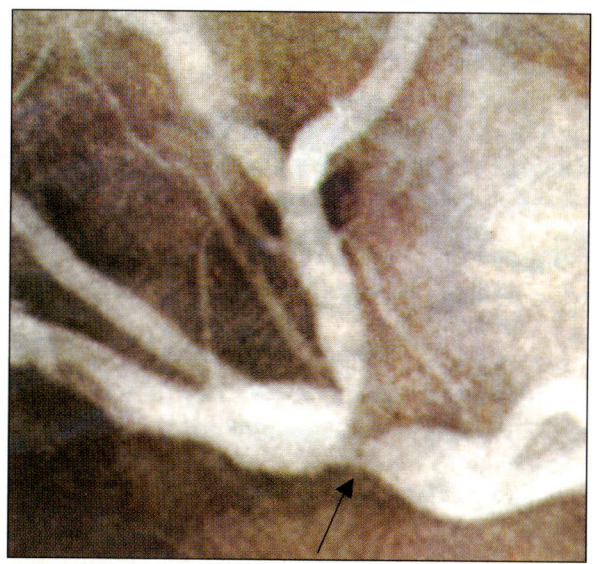

Angiogram in a case of CAD showing narrowing
of coronary artery (↑)

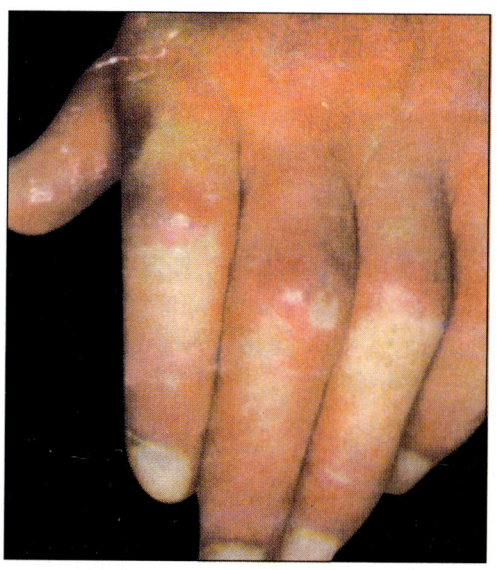

Raynaud's disease: Blisters on hand

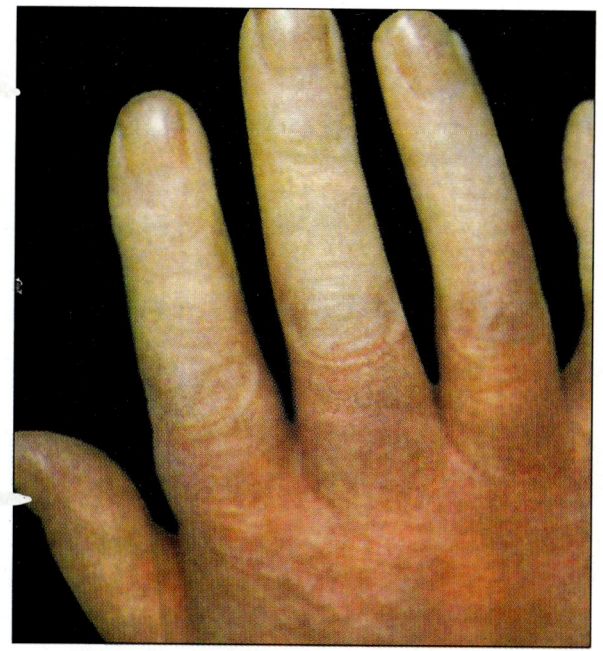

Raynaud's disease: Skin is white due to ischaemia

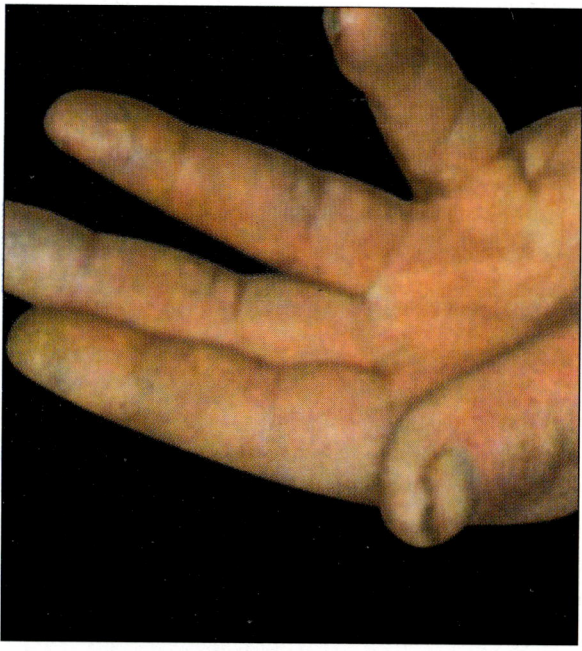

Raynaud's disease: Blue appearance due to venous stasis

PLATE XII

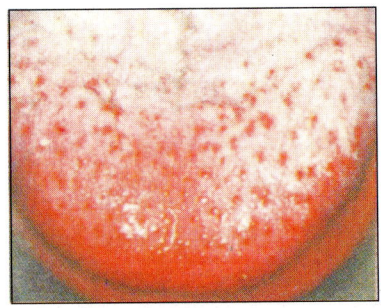

Strawberry tongue

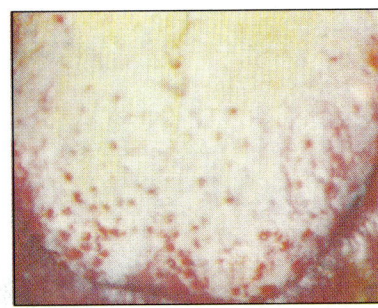

Candida infection of tongue

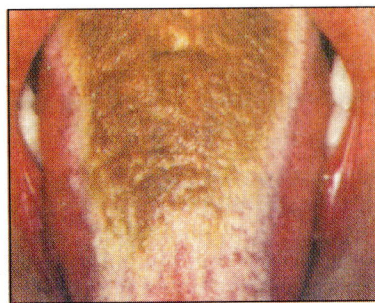

Black hairy tongue

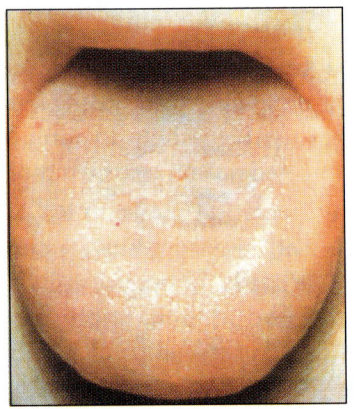

Pernicious anaemia

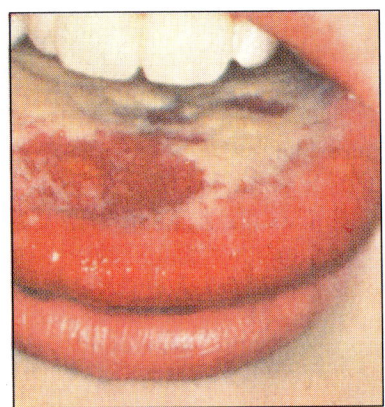

Aphthous ulcer

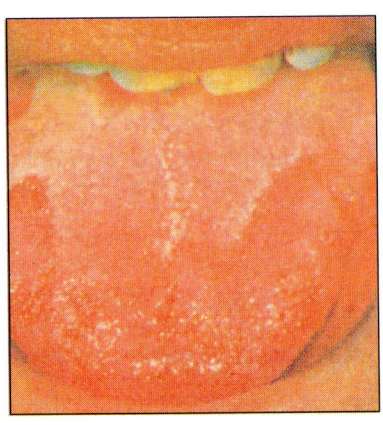

Geographical tongue

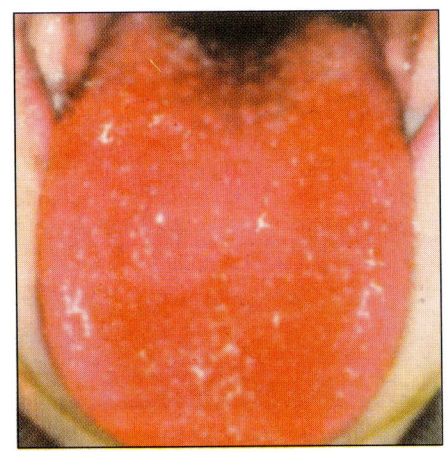

Scarlet fever

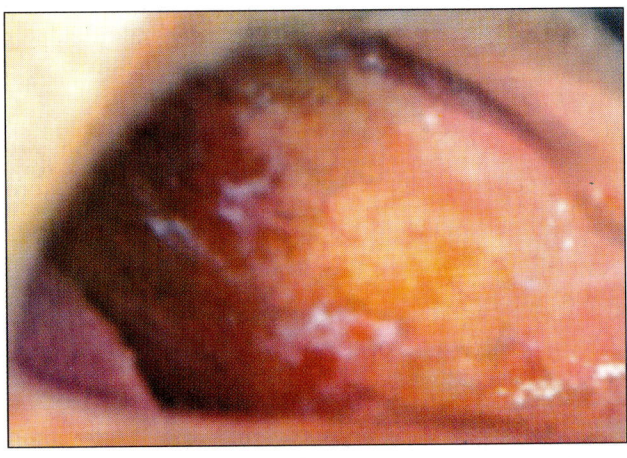

Lichen planus

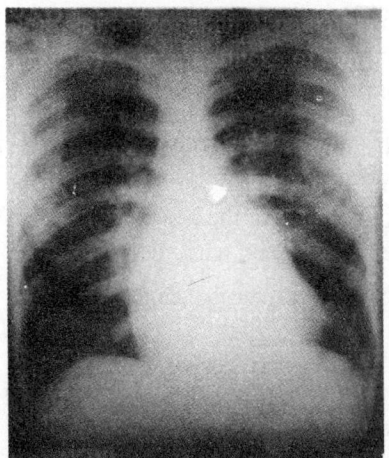

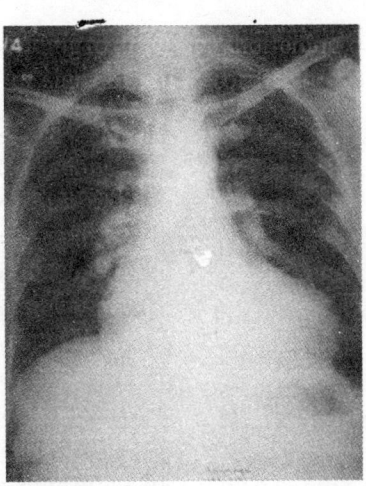

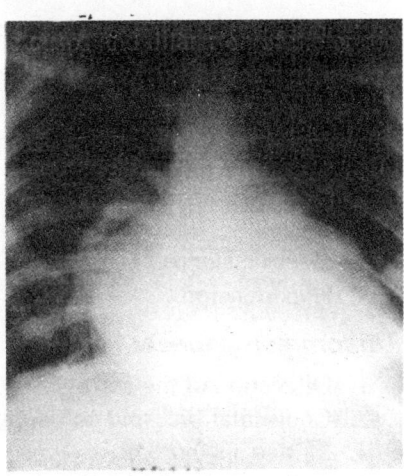

Fig. 4.18. X-ray heart (PA view). Mitralised heart.

Fig. 4.19. X-ray heart (PA view). A case of valvular heart disease (aortic) with left ventricular enlargement (boot-shaped heart).

Fig. 4.20. X-ray heart in a case with mitral and aortic valve disease. Note huge cardiomegaly.

Angiographic studies are helpful for delineating the size of left ventricular cavity, degree or aortic valve deformity and its mobility as well as for demonstrating obstruction in coronary arteries.

Complications of aortic stenosis. Left heart failure followed by congestive heart failure is important complication. Once it supervenes prognosis becomes poor.

Bacterial endocarditis is uncommon in pure aortic stenosis and patients who develop it have associated aortic regurgitation.

Angina pectoris, myocardial infarction, sudden death may occur. Syncopal and Adams-Stokes attacks may occasionally prove fatal.

Treatment. Mild cases of aortic stenosis may remain asymptomatic for a long time and require no treatment. Patients with aortic stenosis should be advised not to do undue physical activity. Development of left heart or congestive failure requires treatment with digitalis and diuretics. Anginal pain may be relieved by Nitrates or Beta blockers.

Surgical treatment is the treatment of choice. When patient of severe aortic stenosis starts complaining of anginal pain not responding to drugs or gets recurrent attacks of syncope or signs of left ventricular decompensation start appearing, surgery is definately indicated.

Aortic valvotomy or replacement of aortic valve under cardiopulmonary bypass either with a prosthetic or heterograft valve are the type of surgical procedures undertaken. In young children and in elderly patients with severe calcific aortic stenosis, percutaneous balloon aortic valvuloplasty is another alternative procedure.

Results with surgery are good and overall survival after surgery is upto 10 years.

Complications during surgery include ventricular fibrillation, haemorrhage, cerebral and pulmonary embolism and heart block.

Aortic regurgitation. Aortic regurgitation or insufficiency is produced by a number of diseases but majority of cases are due to acute rheumatic carditis often associated with other valve involvement and infective endocarditis. Unlike rheumatic where aortic valves are involved, syphilis, an important cause of aortic insufficiency hardly attacks the aortic valve cusps directly but mainly involves the aortic valve commissures (valvulitis) and produces widening of the commissures, shortening of the cusps and dilatation of the aortic orifice.

Causes of aortic insufficiency:

Common causes:

1. Acute rheumatic carditis
2. Infective endocarditis
3. Syphilis
4. Traumatic (direct trauma or following surgery in aortic stenosis)
5. Hypertension

Uncommon causes:

1. Dissection of the aorta
2. Congenital bicuspid aortic valve
3. Marfan's syndrome
4. Ankylosing spondylitis

In rheumatic heart disease occasionally pure aortic insufficiency may be seen but commonly both mitral and aortic valves are involved.

Causes of aortic regurgitation

1. Acute rheumatic carditis
2. Infective endocarditis
3. Syphilis (syphilitic aortitis)
4. Traumatic
5. Hypertension
6. Dissection of aorta
7. Congenital bicuspid aortic valve
8. Ankylosing spondylitis
9. Marfan's syndrome

Pathophysiology. There is significant regurgitation of blood from the aorta to the left ventricle and the amount of reflux depends on the degree and size of the leak. The cardiac output is usually normal or slightly reduced at rest but fails to rise normally during exertion. The left ventricle receives blood from the left atrium and aorta during diastole leading to rise in diastolic filling and left ventricular end diastolic pressure. In order to maintain cardiac output, blood pumped into the aorta increases, due to a more forceful contraction of the left ventricle. Result is dilatation and hypertrophy of the left ventricle. Because of large size of left ventricle due to dilatation, myocardial oxygen demands are not met and in some myocardial ischaemia may develop.

Clinical features. In the absence of any complication cases of aortic regurgitation remain asymptomatic for a long time and lead a normal life. But once cardiac decompensation takes place they follow a downhill course and prognosis becomes poor. Earliest symptoms which a patient complains of are palpitation, pounding of the heart, distressing throbbing, dizziness associated with sudden change of position, exertional dysponea and attacks of chest pain due to myocardial ischaemia. As the disease progresses patient goes into acute left heart failure and subsequently into congestive heart failure. Very often due to association of other valvular lesions, the clinical picture may be modified.

Physical signs. Peripheral pulse is of good volume bounding or collapsing (water hammer type). There is wide pulse pressure. Apical impulse is forceful and apex beat is displaced downwards to the left and laterally. A diastolic thrill is often palpable along the left sternal border.

On auscultation there is an early high pitched diastolic murmur heard best in the third left intercostal space. In early cases where the murmur is soft it is best heard by asking the patient to lean forward and holding the breath in expiration and by using bell piece of the stethoscope.

Murmur of the aortic regurgitation starts immediately after the second heart sound, and radiates widely down to the left lower sternal edge. Diastolic murmur of rheumatic origin is best heard along the left border of sternum while that of syphilitic origin is better heard in the second right interspace.

Murmur may assume a 'cooing' or musical character due to eversion or retroversion of the right anterior aortic cusp vibrating in the regurgitant stream.

An apical systolic murmur may also be present due to left ventricular dilatation producing relative mitral insufficiency.

In severe form of aortic regurgitation, soft rumbling (late or mid diastolic) murmur called Austin-Flint, heard over apex.

Peripheral signs of aortic incompetence include in addition to a water hammer pulse, prominent capillary pulsations in the nail bed as well as in retina and pistol shot sounds over the femoral arteries. There is low diastolic and wide pulse pressure. Instead of normal 30 to 50 mmHg the pulse pressure usually exceeds 80 mmHg or more. Auscultation over the vessels while applying presure reveal systolic murmur above the site of compression and diastolic murmur below that (Durozier's sign).

Physical signs in aortic regurgitation

1. Good volume bounding or collapsing pulse (water-hammer pulse).
2. Capillary pulsations in nail bed and retina.
3. Pistol shot sound heard over the femoral artery.
4. Auscultation over the femoral artery after applying pressure shows systolic murmur above the site of compression and diastolic murmur below that (Durozier's sign).
5. Head nodding with each heart beat.
6. Apex beat is displaced downwards to the left and laterally. Apical impulse is forceful and thrusting.
7. A diastolic thrill may be palpable along left sternal border.
8. On auscultation there is an early high pitched diastolic murmur present in the third left intercostal space. It is best heard by asking the patient to lean forward and hold breath in expiration.

Often in cases of aortic regurgitation, a low pitched, soft rumbling late or mid-diastolic or presystolic apical murmur is heard. It is called Austin Flint murmur and is probably produced by the displacement of the anterior mitral valve leaflat by the regurgitant aortic stream. This murmur has to be distinguished from a diastolic murmur of mitral stenosis where first heart sound is loud and snappy often with an opening snap.

Investigations. Blood serology (STS, VDRL, Kahn: Test) to exclude luetic aetiology.

X-ray heart shows enlargement of heart. The lower left cardiac contour which represents the left ventricle becomes elongated and enlarges downwards and to the left. This shape of heart seen in anterior posterior view of X-ray is called a 'Boot shaped heart', the rounded apex of the heart corresponds to the toe of the shoe.

Electrocardiogram. There is evidence of left ventricular hypertrophy and strain, the R wave in left ventricular leads of strikingly high voltage.(R in V5/V6 >25 mm)

Echocardiogram. It is helpful in demonstrating a dilated hyperdynamic left ventricle and rapid fluttering of the anterior mitral leaflet as a result of impact of a regurgitant jet from aorta in severe form of aortic regurgitation.

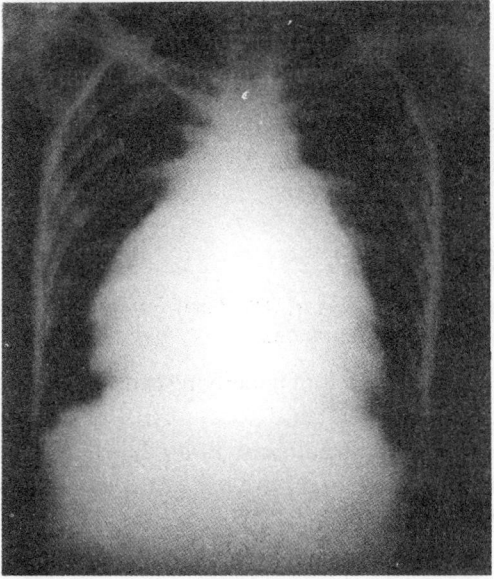

Fig. 4.21. X-ray heart (PA view). A case of biventricular enlargement of heart. This shadow gives the appearance of 'Money Bag' which is characteristically seen in pericarditis with effusion.

Colour doppler flow and doppler echocardiography are useful for the detection of aetiology of aortic regurgitation and its severity.

Cardiac catheterization and angiography are useful for measurement of magnitude of regurgitation, haemodynamic disturbances and assessment for surgery.

Complications. Common complications include congestive heart failure, acute left heart failure or pulmonary oedema, subacute bacterial endocarditis. In aortic incompetence due to syphilis there is always narrowing of coronary ostia and result is anginal pain and often sudden death.

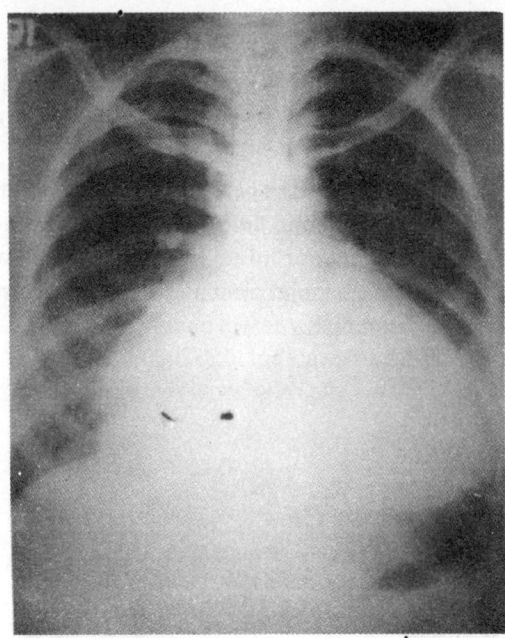

Fig. 4.22. X-ray Heart (PA View) Percardial effusion. Money bag appearances.

Treatment. It is of underlying causes when aortic regurgitation is due to syphilis or infective endocarditis, treatment is by heavy doses of penicillin and it may have to be to given for at least six weeks.

For all patients with symptoms of left heart failure treatment is by digitalis, diuretics and ACE inhibitors. Cases of aortic incompetence shall require valve replacement. Surgical treatment is undertaken before significant symptoms appear and timings of surgery is based on relevant investigations (haemodynamic echocardiographic and angiographic).

Damaged aortic valve is replaced by a mechanical or a tissue valve prostheses. Surgical repair is successful if undertaken early since after surgery a damaged myocardium does not recover fully. Antibiotic prophylaxis should be given before and after surgery as prevention against infective endocarditis.

Tricuspid stenosis. It is an uncommon valvular lesion and is usually seen in association with mitral or aortic valve disease.

Commonest cause of tricuspid stenosis is rheumatic fever. Rarely it may be congenital or a big thrombus or vegetation or a tumour projecting into the atrium may cause picture of tricuspid stenosis.

Pathophysiology. Rheumatic inflammation causes fusion and adhesion of the tricuspid cusps to each other with the result that a single fused cylindrical rigid aperture is produced. Normal circumference of tricuspid valve is 11 to 13 cm but with severe stenosis the tricuspid valve area falls below 1 square cm.

The right atrium is dilated and hypertrophied while the right ventricle is small. The flow of blood from right atrium to right ventricle is obstructed. There is pronounced rise in right atrial pressure and abnormal pressure gradient between right atrial mean pressure and diastolic pressure in right ventricle. Cardiac output falls and there is systemic venous congestion leading to right sided failure.

Clinical features. Since isolated tricuspid stenosis is uncommon and usually there is either mitral or aortic valve disease so the symptoms are often variable. As a result of low cardiac output there is easy fatiguability, dysponea on exertion and pain in right upper abdomen. Because of chronic venous congestion symptoms of anorexia, nausea, pain abdomen and generalized weakness are seen.

Physical findings. There is low volume pulse, jugular veins are engorged and there is prominent 'a' wave. There is a rumbling mid diastlic murmur best heard at the lower sternal border and it increases in intensity during inspiration. First heart sound is often split. An opening snap may occasionally be heard. Signs of right heart failure like hepatic enlargement, ascites, oedema over peripheral parts, effusions in pleural cavities (hydrothorax) may be present.

Investigations:

X-ray of heart shows cardiac enlargement with prominent right atrial bulge.

ECG. A tall atrial P wave with features of right ventricular hypertrophy.

Echocardiography shows a thickened tricuspid

valve. Further delineation is done by cardiac catheterization and angiocardiography when an enlarged right atrium is demonstrated.

Physical signs in tricuspid stenosis

1. Low volume pulse
2. Neck veins engorged and there is prominent 'a' wave, slow 'y' descent.
3. A rumbling mid diastolic murmur best heard at lower end of sternum. Increases in intensity during inspiration. An opening snap may occasionally be heard.
4. Signs of right heart failure—oedema over dependent parts. Tender hepatomegaly, ascites.

Treatment. In the presence of venous congestion, diuretics, and digitalis are indicated. Since tricuspid stenosis often coexists with mitral stenosis, tricuspid valvotomy or commissurotomy is done at the same time as mitral valvotomy.

Tricuspid regurgitation. It may be either functional or organic. Organic tricuspid insufficiency is invariably caused by rheumatic carditis or infective endocarditis while uncommon causes include Ebsteins anomaly and endocardial cushion defects. Functional tricuspid insufficiency results in conditions associated with failure and dilatation of right ventricle. Most common cause are pulmonary hypertension and chronic cor pulmonale.

Tricuspid regurgitation is recognised by an incompetent tricuspid valve when blood from right ventricle regurgitates into right atrium during systole. The right atrial pressure is markedly elevated along with that of right ventricle both in systole and diastole. This is reflected in the elevation of systemic venous pressure with features of venous hypertension and right heart failure.

Clinical features. Patients of tricuspid incompetence suffer from fatiguability and dysponea in exertion. Physical signs include peripheral oedema, ascites, hepatomegaly marked elevation of jugular venous pressure with prominent 'V' waves and 'y' descent. Liver may be pulsatile. On palpation, there is right ventricular impulse along

left parasternal region and at lower end of sternum, a palpable systolic thrill. On auscultation there is a pansystolic blowing high pitched murmur which increases in intensity during inspiration and decreases during expiration. Atrial fibrillation is commonly present and may change pulsations in neck vessels when prominent 'V' wave may be replaced by small fibrillary waves.

Physical signs in tricuspid regurgitation

1. Jugular venous pressure raised, prominent 'v' waves in neck and a rapid 'y' descent.
2. Right ventricular impulse along left parasternal border can be palpated and a pan systolic thrill at lower end of sternum.
3. On auscultation there is high pitched blowing pan systolic murmur at lower left sternal edge. It changes its charcter with respiration.
4. Pulsatile liver
5. Peripheral oedema, ascites and hepatomegaly.

Investigations:

X-ray of heart shows right atrial enlargement as well as that of right ventricle. Electrocardiogram may show evidence of right atrial and right ventricular hypertrophy.

Echocardiography is helpful in demonstrating an incompetent tricuspid valve as well as right ventricular dilatation.

Treatment. Since functional tricuspid incompetence follows or accompanies severe form of right ventricular hypertrophy, treatment is to be directed towards treating right heart failure.

In cases where tricuspid valve is damaged extensively and medical treatment is of not much help, surgical repair of valve is to be undertaken (annuloplasty or narrowing of annulus). Where severe regurgitation is present. Valve replacement is considered.

Pulmonary stenosis. This condition is almost always congenital and is often associated with other congenital lesions of the heart.

Acquired pulmonary stenosis is extremely rare and its causes include rheumatic valvulitis, bacterial endocarditis, trauma and rarely due to carcinoid syndrome.

Pathology. The main disturbance is increased pressure in right ventricle with normal and diminished pressure in pulmonary artery. Pulmonary stenosis produces right ventricular hypertrophy and dilatation. Normal cardiac output is maintained initially despite the obstruction. With progressive failure of right ventricle, right atrium also gets dilated and hypertropied. Cardiac output falls. Left chambers of heart remain normal unless there is associated disease. The valve itself becomes dome like with a very narrowed orifice. The pulmonary artery is usually dilated beyond the stenosis.

Clinical features. Most cases of pulmonary stenosis remain asymptomatic for a long time. As cardiac output falls, patient complains of easy fatiguability, tiredness and breathlessness on exertion. Occasionally there is chest pain on effort or syncope.

Physical signs include features of right ventricular hypertrophy producing a parasternal heave. There is a loud rough ejection systolic murmur in the second or third left intercostal space. The pulmonary second sound is either weak or absent. A thrill may be palpated.

Investigations:

X-ray heart. There is evidence of right ventricular enlargement with prominent pulnonary artery in cases of post stenotic dilatation (Coeur en Sabot).

Electrocardiogram. Prominent p wave, Right atrial and right ventricular hypertrophy.

Echocardiogram. It shows normal pulmonary valve without flow tract obstruction. There are features of right ventricular hypertrophy and dilatation. Further confirmation by colour doppler echocardiography and cardiac catheterization.

Treatment. In cases with severe degree of pulmonary stenosis with a high resting gradient treatment is by surgery (valvotomy or balloon valvuloplasty).

Pulmonary regurgitation. Organic pulmonary insufficiency is very rare. In majority of the cases the insufficiency is functional secondary to other cardiac lesions like mitral stenosis, pulmonary hypertension or dilatation of the pulmonary artery.

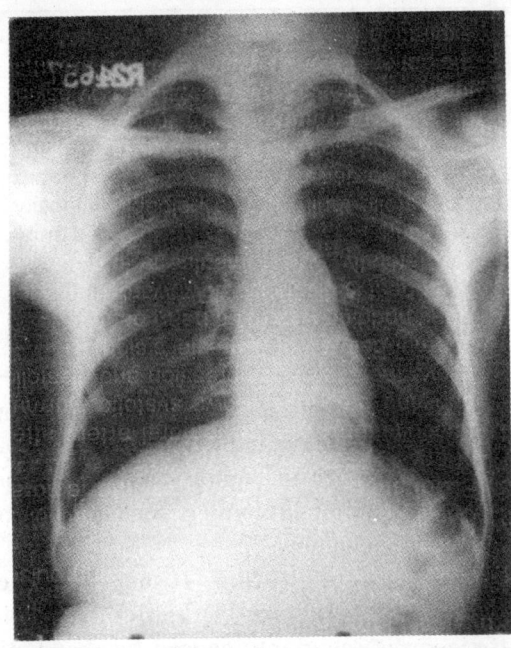

Fig. 4.23. Pulmonary Stenosis. A case of pulmonary stenosis with post-stenotic dilatation. Lung fields are oligaemic.

Heart in cases of pulmonary insufficiency shows right ventricular hypertrophy and considerable dilatation of pulmonary artery.

Clinically patients of pulmonary insufficiency have symptoms of underlying disease. There is cough, breathlessness on exertion, cyanosis and haemoptysis.

Physical examination shows dullness in pulmonary area on percussion. Often pulsations are present at site of pulmonary area. On auscultation there is a soft or loud blowing early diastolic murmur in second or third left intercostal space. When there is associated mitral stenosis it is called a Graham, Steell murmur. An associated systolic murmur due to dilated pulmonary artery may be heard. Second pulmonary sound may be accentuated.

Investigations:

X-ray heart. Evidence of right ventricular hypertrophy with dilatation of pulmonary artery. On fluoroscopy there are increased pulsations in pulmonary artery. Hilar shadows are prominent.

Electrocardiogram. Right ventricular hypertrophy.

Diagnosis of pulmonary incompetence is made on characteristic clinical findings and X-ray appearance.

Treatment. Since pulmonary incompetence is generally secondary to other diseases, treatment is directed towards the underlying condition.

INFECTIVE ENDOCARDITIS

Infective endocarditis may be defined as inflammation of the endocardium by bacteria resulting into exudative and inflammatory lesions. It may be acute, or subacute. Acute, the fulminating type of endocarditis often called ulcerative type is a serious ailment which generally proves fatal.

Commonest form of endocarditis is subacute form (subacute bacterial endocarditis) which is less serious as compared to ulcerative variety and runs an insidious course.

Etiology. Generally organisms attack an already damaged heart such as congenital heart disease (ventricular septal defect: Patent ductus arteriosus Fallots Tetralogy and coarctation of the aorta) and rheumatic heart disease. Occasionally a normal heart may be involved by virulent organisms especially when the person is immunologically compromised. The development of subacute bacterial endocarditis is dependent on the entry of microorganisms into the blood stream when they colonize on the endocardium, valves or already damaged parts of the heart and are implanted there by way of general blood stream. Localization and implantation of bacteria are determined mainly be haemodynamic alterations when bacteria settle and multiply at places where they are sprayed. Combined valvular lesions are more often the seat of involvement as compared to pure valvular lesions. Regurgitant mitral and aortic valves are commonest to be effected. In addition to rheumatic and congenital heart lesions, syphilitic aortic valve disease,

biscuspid aortic valves, arteriovenous fistulas, prosthetic valves, grafts and surgical procedures on heart like introduction of pace makers may be seat of starting subacute endocarditis. Intravenous drug users may get endocarditis, the microorganism from their skin may start the process.

Organisms. Although a number of organisms are known to be responsible for causing subacute bacterial endocarditis yet commonest are *Streptococcus viridans*, *Streptococcus faecalis* and *Staphylococcus aureus* or *albus* which account for more than 90 per cent of cases. Less common organisms include *Strep. pneumoniae*, haemolytic streptococci (Lancfield group A), *Neisseria gonorrhoae*, *E. coli*, Staphylococci, *Salmonella*, *Brucella*, Meningococci, *H. influenzae*, *B. proteus*, *Psuedomonas*, Friedlander's bacillus, Listeria, etc. Very rarely spirochetes, rickettsiae, candida and aspergillus may cause endocariditis.

Most of the organisms are inhabitants of the human body and may be found in upper respiratory tract, oral cavity, genitalia and urinary passages. It has been observed that subacute bacterial endocardilitis develops following a dental extraction, dental surgery, tonsillectomy, operative procedures of genitourinary tract such as, prostatectomy, cystoscopy, and catheterization. Urinary instrumentation, abortion or medical termination of pregnancy cause transient bacteremia and invade blood stream involving the damaged cardiac tissue and produce subacute bactrial endocarditis.

Of the various organisms, streptococcus viridans since it inhabits upper respiratory passages, is the one likely to be the causative organism in operative procedures in this region while streptococcus faecalis infection follows commonly procedures of the genitourinary tract. Staphylococcus aureus is a normal commensal of skin and causes endocarditis in great percentage of drug abusers or where procedures like cardiac pacing is done.

Pathology. Circulating organisms get implanted on a damaged site in the heart and proliferate. These get over laid by fibrin and erythrocyte coating. Further growth results in the formation of friable structures called vegetations which primarily consist of infecting organisms, platelets and fibrin. The vegetations form at areas of trauma to the endothelium, areas of turbulence where blood flow and changes in pressure dynamics are induced by valvular stenosis or insufficiencies or at cardiovascular shunts.

Microorganism responsible for subacute bacterial endocarditis

Common organisms:
1. Streptococcus viridans
2. Streptococcus faecalis
3. Staphylococcus aureus/Staphylococcus albus

Uncommon organisms:
1. Strep. pneumoniae
2. Haemolytic streptococci (Lancfield group A)
3. E. coli
4. Neisseria gonorrhoeae
5. Staphylococci
6. Salmonella typhi
7. Brucella melitensis
8. Meningococci
9. H. influenzae
10. B. proteus
11. Friedlander's bacillus
12. Rickettsia
13. Candida
14. Aspergillus

Endocarditis tends to occur in high pressure areas on the left side of the heart and is unusual at sites with small pressure gradient (atrial septal defect). The vegetations have a broad base of altered degenerated valvular substance with blood, platelets thrombi, and bacteria over laid by fibrin which may serve to protect them from the defence mechanism of the host. The agglutinating antibodies by clumping together of bacteria increase the chance of bacteria laden vegetations.

Vegetations may increase in size and get implanted at various sites. Involvement of chordae tendineae and papillary muscles may lead to rupture, ulceration and severe degree of valvular incompetence.

Manifestations of bacterial endocarditis

1. **General.** Low grade fever, Anaemia, clubbing of fingers, splenomegaly. Loss of appetite, malaise.
2. **Embolic.** Osler nodes (painful tender pea-sized nodules on fingers and toes) splinter haemorrhages under the nail bed. Janeway lesions (painful flat raised erythematous lesions on palms and soles).
   Splenic and pulmonary infarction, involvement of peripheral vessels leading to claudication and gangrene. Cerebral embolisation producing hemiplegia, visual loss. Retinal artery involvement leading to retinitis, roths spots.
   Renal infarction, hematuria (frank and microscopic) glomerulonephritis.
3. **Heart.** Changing murmurs, conduction defects, rupture of chordae tendinae.

Embolism from the vegetations may take place and involve major organs in the body. Kidney gets involved with focal embolic glomerulonephritis, diffuse glomerulonephritis and renal infarcts (cause of hematuria). Other common sites are splenic infarcts, pulmonary infarction and mycotic aneurysms in the brain which may rupture, leading to cerebral, intraventricular or subarachnoid haemorrhage.

Repeated infection with microorganisms may produce circulating antibodies and immune complexes which are thought to be responsible for production of glomerulonephritis, myocarditis, arteritis and cutaneous manifestaiton of vasculitis.

Cases of endocarditis not treated properly ultimately die as a result of massive embolism, rupture of mycotic aneurysms, Renal failure etc.

Clinical features. Onset of the condition is generally insidious. A patient with a known cardiac ailment (rheumatic/congenital) may start complaining of vague ill health, fatigue, weakness and a low grade fever. Fever often is like a viral infection with marked aches and pains all over the body. But fever is the most constant symptom. It may be continuous, remittent or intermittent. Many patients have unexplained anaemia not responding to treatment and giving a muddy discoloration of skin.

Signs in a case of subacute bacterial endocarditis may be divided into:

1. **General or systemic.** Low grade fever or fever coming with rigors and chills. Anaemia, clubbing of the fingers and toes. Splenomegaly, spleen may be painful and if a splenic infarct, splenic rub is palpable. Haematuria due to renal infarct. Microscopic hematuria may be an important sign.
2. **Embolic lesions.** Embolization takes place in various organs. Oslers nodes may be present as tender pea sized nodules on fingers and toes pads. There are splinter haemorrhages under the nail beds. Painful, flat raised erythematous lesions on palms and soles (Janeway lesions). Splenic infarcts produce a painful spleen with palpable rub. Peripheral vessels may be involved leading to claudication and even gangrene. Cerebral embolisation may produce hemiplegia, visual loss, and cerebellar disturbances. Pulmonary embolism result in infarction in lungs, pleurisy. Retinal artery involvement leads to retinitis and white spots in retina (Roths spots). Renal infarction presents either as microscopic or frank haematuria.
3. **Cardiac signs.** These are essentially those of underlying cardiac lesion. But murmurs in subacute bacterial endocarditis change their character and sites and new murmurs may appear during observation. Changing murmurs is characteristic of the disease. Rupture of chordae tendineae or papillary muscles may produce rough rasping murmurs.

Complications. A number of complcations may occur in cases of endocordits

1. Renal insufficiency following repeated infarcts or glomeruconephritis
2. Congestive cardiac failure
3. Rupture of mycotic aneurysms in the brain leading to encephalopathies, hemiplegia, cerebral haemorrhage.
4. Sudden death due to rupture of aneurysm of the splenic artery or rupture of the splenic abscess into peritoneal cavity.
5. Pulmonary embolisation

6. Sudden blindness from embolism of central retinal artery, optic neuritis, retinitis.
7. Gangrene of peripheral limbs.

Investigations:

1. Haemoglobin and peripheral blood film shows anaemia generally of hypochromic normochromic type. Total and differential cell count show polymorphonuclear leucocytosis. ESR is raised—as well as C-reactive proteins.
2. Blood culture is important. Repeated blood cultures especially at height of fever are required. At least 5-6 blood ocultures must be done before finalising the diagnosis. Blood cultures are generally positive in 90 per cent of cases. In patients who had already received antibiotics, blood culture may be negative. Bone marrow culture may be done in such cases.
3. There is elevation of blood proteins due to increase in the serum gamma globulin fraction. Serum immunoglobulins are elevated.
4. Urine shows albuminuria and microscopic hematuria.
5. Echocardiogram is usefull for detecting vegetations as well as valvular dysfunction.
6. X-ray heart and electrocardiogram for state of heart and presence of any arrhythmias.

Diagnosis. It is dependent on clinical profile of a patient with valvular heart disease or congenital heart disease who has poor health, low grade or high fever along with classical features of clubbing, oslers nodes, changing murmurs in heart, embolic phenomenon and positive blood culture. Repeat culture have to be done since with treatment, microbial flora may change. It is equally important to have drug sensitivity of the organisms grown on cultures.

Treatment. Basic line of treatment is antibiotics which should be given early in adequate disease and for long periods depending on the sensitivity of the organism.

Since commonest organism causing endocarditis is streptococcus viridans the drug of choice is penicillin. High doses of crystalline penicillin (10-20 lac units) I/M six hourly where disease appears to be fulminating. Penicillin is also given I/V in drip form. Injection Gentamicin (1 mg/kg body weight) or Injection Streptomycin (1 gm) eight hourly may be combined in the initial period. Penicillin must be continued for minimum of six weeks.

For other organisms producing endocarditis appropriate antibiotics depending on culture and sensitivity have to be administered. Oral Amoxycillin (6-8 gm daily) in divided doses may be substituted for penicillin after the acute stage subsides and continued for 4-6 weeks.

Any source of infection in the body like dental abscess must be treated under cover of antibiotics. In cases where cardiac valve has been damaged extensively leading to progressive failure or there is infection of prosthetic valve surgical intervention may be done.

Prophylaxis. In every patient with a valvular heart disease or congenital heart disease, before surgery is contemplated, prophylactic antibiotics must be given before and after surgical procedure. Similarly cardiac patients susceptible to infective endocarditis should be cautioned about the absolute necessity of taking special care of teeth (Dental extraction, apical abscess) and have antibiotic cover for dental procedures. Usual procedure is to give amoxycillin 3 g orally one hour before opration and continued 0.5 g 6 hourly for next 1 week.

Infective endocarditis is a preventable disease and taking adequate precautions in cardiac cases can save lot of morbidity and mortality.

CONGENITAL HEART DISEASE

These form important part of cardiac ailments and are the abnormalities of the heart and great vessels due to defective development in the prenatal period. According to most reports, major congenital cardiac anomalies are found in not more than 1% of total live births.

Though there are no specific sex differences yet males are effected more than females. The exact aetiology is not known but a number of factors ranging from genetic to environmental factors play their role. Genetic abnormalities and chromosomal aberrations as well as single gene mutation have an important role to play. Normal development of the heart is effected by diseases involving fetal envelopes, amniotic fluid or its environment. This is further corrobrated by the fact that 15-23 per cent of extracardiac anomalies accompany significant cardiac defects.

Factors which play their role in the causation of congenital cardiac lesions include:

1. **Heredity.** Factors in favour include presence of associated anomalies which are considered of heredity nature e.g. polydactylism, clubbed foot etc. History of congenital heart disease in families, identical twins, association of genetic as well as chromosomal abnormalities (Down's syndrome, Turners syndrome) with cases of congenital heart disease.

2. **Maternal Infection.** Rubella (German measles) in the early months of pregnancy is an important factor. Since entire development of heart and great vessels is completed in first two months of pregnancy, infection at this time produces not only cardiac but also other anomalies. In addition maternal infections with cytomegalovirus, use of drugs in the early months of pregnancy, exposure of pregnant woman to radiation and alcohol abuse also play an important role in the aetiology of congenital heart disease.

Nutritional status of the mother, presence of chronic diseases like diabetes are also known to play their role.

Classification of congenital heart disease. Broadly congenital heart disease is classified into two major subgroups:

1. Cyanotic
2. Acyanotic

Common cyanotic congenital heart lesions.

1. Fallot's tetralogy
2. Transposition of great vessels.
3. Tricuspid atresia
4. Persistent truncus

5. Pulmonary stenosis with reversed interatrial shunt
6. Pulmonary atresia.

Acyanotic congenital heart lesions:

1. Atrial septal defect
2. Ventricular septal defect
3. Congenital aortic stenosis (valvular, supravalvular, subvalvular)
4. Coarctation of aorta
5. Patent ductus arteriosus
6. Pulmonary stenosis (valvular, infundibular, supravalvular)
7. Tricusid stenosis

Common signs and symptoms in congenital heart lesions. Cases of cyanotic heart disease have right to left shunts where mixing of venous with arterial blood is taking place. In cases with left to right shunts (VSD, ASD, patent ductus arteriosus) as a result of development of pulmonary hypertension reversal of shunt takes place and subsequently these patients present with cyanosis (Eisenmanger's syndrome).

Most of the children present with poor growth, difficulty in feeding, syncopal attacks and recurrent respiratory infections. Blue baby is a classic example of a cyanotic heart disease. Cyanosis may appear in such children on crying. Breathlessness on exertion is a striking feature and may appear in paroxysms.

Forms of atrial septal defect

1. Ostium secundum
2. Ostium primum
3. Sinus venosus type

Squatting after exercise is common in Fallot's tetralogy and is the posture adopted by such children. Excessive weakness and persistent cough, cold extremities and numbness of limbs are other features. Cerebral symptoms include faintness, dizziness, syncope and convulsions and these are due to cerebral hypoxia.

The most common physical signs include cyanosis which in some is present since birth (Fallot's tetralogy) or appears later in life with reversal of

shunt from left to right to right to left (Eisenmanger's complex). Cases with prolonged and persistent cyanosis have clubbing of the fingers and toes.

Complications. Common complications include congestive heart failure, subacute bacterial endocarditis. Paradoxical embolism, pulmonary tuberculosis and cerebral abscess.

Prognosis in a case of congenital heart disease depends on the underlying cardiac lesion, how early detected and whether it is amenable to surgery.

Atrial septal defect. It is the commonest form of congenital heart disease and is more common in females as compared to men. It may occur in isolation or in association with other anomalies like VSD, pulmonary stenosis, or mitral stenosis. Depending on the developmental defects, three types of defects are known.

1. Ostium secundum, commonest type of defect and is present in the region of fossa ovalis.
2. Ostium primum, a defect in the lower part of interatrial septum.
3. Sinus venosus type, a defect in the upper part of interatrial septum.

In an uncomplicated case of atrial septal defect, the shunt is from left to right due to increased left atrial pressure. Because of increased flow of blood from the right atrium to right ventricle, the chamber becomes large and hypertrophied. As a result of diastolic over load of right ventricle, pulmonary blood flow increases. Rise in pulmonary arteriolar resistance determines the magnitude of shunt and increased pulmonary blood flow.

Clinical features. A large number of cases of ASD remain asymptomatic for a long time but when symptoms appear the most common are breathlessness on exertion, palpitation, easy fatiguability and recurrent respiratory infections.

Children with the anomaly may show retarded growth and prone to recurrent chest infections. Adults generally in third or fourth decade may because of increased pulmonary hypertension and bidirectional flow in shunt develop features of congestive heart failure. Paroxysmal atrial tachycardia and atrial fibrillation may develop. Subacute bacterial endocarditis is uncommon.

Features of atrial septal defect

1. Most cases remain asymptomatic
2. Children with ASD have retarded growth and prone to recurrent chest infections.
3. Palpitation, easy fatiguability and breathlessness on exertion.
4. Atrial arrhytmias may develop.
5. Pulse is of good volume. Heart may be enlarged, right ventricular heave, systolic thrill palpable in the second or third interspace along the left border.
6. On auscultation, second pulmonary sound is accentuated with wide fixed splitting. An ejection systolic murmur in second left interspace. An apical diastolic flow murmur at tricuspid valve.

Clinically there may be cardiac enlargement. A systolic thrill is palpable in the second or third interspace near the left border of sternum. On Auscultation second pulmonary sound is acentuated with wide fixed splitting and a loud mid systolic ejection murmur. It is due to increased blood flow through the pulmonary valve. An apical diastolic murmur of functional tricuspid stenosis may be heard because of increased blood flow through the tricuspid orifice. In advcanced cases a pulmonary diastolic murmur of pulmonary insufficiency is present.

Investigations:

X-ray heart. There is gross dilatation and conspicous pulsation (Hilar dance) of the pulmonary artery and its branches. There is peripheral pulmonary plethora, hypoplasia of aorta and enlargement of right ventricle and right atrium.

Electrocardiogram. Right axis deviation a typical rSR pattern. Incomplete or partial or complete right bundle branch block.

Cardiac catheterization, echocardiogram and colour doppler. These will help in confirming and visualization of the defect as well as in measuring the flow velocities.

Treatment. Surgical repair of the defect (Atrioseptopaxy) at young age between three to six years under direct vision using cardiopulmonary bypass or hypothermia is the treatment of choice.

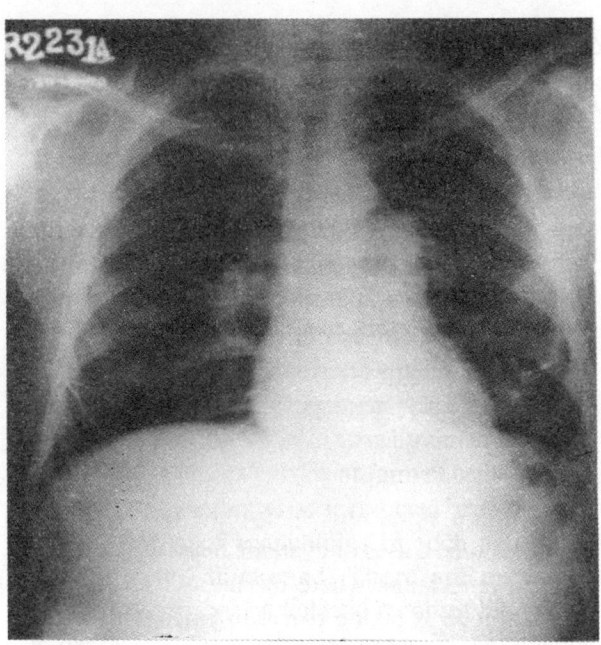

Fig. 4.24. X-ray Heart of a patient with an atrial septal defect. Notice the prominent pulmonary artery and the plethoric lung fields.

Results are good if surgery is carried before the development of pulmonary hypertension since cases with irreversible pulmonary hypertension with right to left shunt are not suitable for surgery.

Course and prognosis. A case with a very small defect and a left to right shunt may not require any surgery and be managed conservatively. Prompt treatment of respiratory infection, be given and prophylacticaly antibiotics be administered before any dental or surgical procedure to prevent development of subacute bacterial endocarditis.

In patients where surgery has not been carried out or the defect is haemodynanically significant. Pulmonary hypertension develops with reversal of shunt (right to left). This leads to development of cyanosis and progressive enlargement of right sided chambers (Eisenmenger syndrome). Course now is downhill. Congestive failure develops. Treatment at this stage is of congestive failure and other complications like arrhythmias (Supraventricular tachycardia, atrial fibrillation).

Ventricular septal defect. Ventricular septal defect is one of the commonest congenital cardiac defect in younger age group. It may be present in isolation or in combination with other cardiac anomalies (Fallot's tetralogy: Eisenmenger complex: Transposition of great vessels). A small ventricular defect may remain asymptomatic for a long time and functional cardiac disturbances are dependent on the size of the defect, blood flow and state of pulmonary vascular bed.

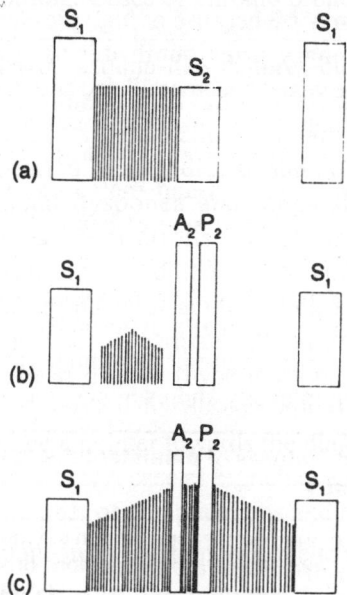

Fig. 4.25. Graphic representation of murmurs in congenital heart disease. a. Ventricular septal defect. Pansystolic (Roger's) loud murmur heard along parasternal line. b. Atrial septal defect. Ejection systolic murmur over pulmonary area. Wide and fixed splitting of second sound c. Patent ductus arteriosus. Continuous (Machinery) murmur.

In majority of patients the defect is situated in the anterior part of the membranous septum either anterior or posterior to crista supraventriculous while only in a small percentage it is found in the muscular part of the septum.

The flow of blood through the interventricular opening is from left to right ventricle because of the higher pressure on the left side. In small defects since the shunt is small, pulmonary blood flow may be only slightly more than systemic but with large defects the pulmonary blood flow increases, high pulmonary vascular resistance develops and

pulmonary hypertension with reversal of shunt (Eisenmenger's syndrome) occurs. The heart may be slightly enlarged, mainly involving right ventricle but with large defects left ventricle also gets dilated.

Clinical features. Mild and small septal defects remain asymptomatic carrying good prognosis and almost a normal life span. Cases with large defects and shunts suffers from stunted growth, recurrent respiratory infections and breathlessness on exertion leading on to congestive heart failure.

Clinical features of ventricular septal defect

1. Small septal defects remain asymptomatic.
2. Cases with large shunts suffer from stunted growth, recurrent respiratory infection and congestive failure.
3. Heart size normal in small defects, cardiac enlargement in large defects, apex beat forceful, parasternal heave may be present.
4. Systolic thrill in the third and fourth intercostal space, transmitted over precordium and back. Pansystolic murmur in third and fourth intercostal space. (Roger's murmur). Accentuated pulmonary second sound and a diastolic murmur in cases with pulmonary hypertension. Apical diastolic murmur due to increased blood flow across mitral valve.

Physical signs include a harsh pansystolic murmur associated with thrill best heard in the left 3rd and fourth inter costal spaces near the sternum (Roger's murmur). This is transmitted over the precordium and often to the back in the inter scapular or subscapular region. In a small VSD heart size is within normal limits but with large VSD cardiac enlargement takes place Apex beat is forceful, an apical diastolic murmur may be heard suggestive of increased blood flow across the mitral valve. Presence of pulmonary hypertension is suggested by an accentuated second pulmonary sound anda pulmonary diastolic murmur.

Complications. A large VSD is likely to develop number of complications ranging from congestive heart failure, Eisenmanger's syndrome, infective endocarditis and complete heart block often producing Adams-Stokes attack.

Investigations:

X-ray of heart in small defects is within normal limits. In large defects, heart is enlarged (both ventricles are enlarged but mainly left ventricle). Pulmonary artery is prominent and dilated. Aortic knuckle is small and less prominent.

Electrocardiogram shows incomplete right bundle branch block in small defects. With large defects initially there is left ventricular dominence with right ventricular hypertrophy pattern which as disease progresses shows both left and right ventricular hypertrophy patterns.

Echocardiogram. Two dimensional echocardiography will define and locate the defect as well as other cardiac anomalies.

Further confirmation can be done by cardiac catheterization and angiocardiography. These are helpful in defining the degree of shunt and status of pulmonary vascular bed.

Treatment. A small VSD which is generally asymptomatic does not require any surgical treatment except to take precautions during any surgical or dental procedures by prophylactic use of antibiotics. Operative correction is to be undertaken in moderate to large septal defects and a left to right shunt and where pulmonary hypertension is of mild to moderate degree. Surgical closure of the defect may be done either by closed method or under direct vision. Development of Eisenmengers syndrome is contraindication to surgery. Very small VSD's may close spontaneously by the age of 5-10 years and carry excellent prognosis.

Patent ductus arteriosus. It is one of the significant congenital cardiac anomaly seen in children which is completely curable by surgical management.

Ductus arteriosus arises from the bifurcation of the pulmonary artery connecting it with the descending arch of aorta below the left subclavian artery. In foetal life blood from right ventricle passes into pulmonary artery and through wide patent ductus arteriosus to descending aorta bypassing the lungs which are non-functioning. Blood supply to the lungs increases gradually until a fair pulmonary circulation is established. But immediately after birth lungs assume their function and large quantity of blood now passes from the pulmonary artery to pulmonary circulation and less through ductus arteriosus. Functional closure of the ductus occurs in 24 hours and anatomical closure usually by 3rd week. Sometimes it may take 2-3 months for closure to take place.

In cases where ductus arteriosus remains patent, blood from aorta because of high pressure flows to the pulmonary artery both during systole and diastole the vessel becomes dilated and its pulsations may be exaggerated. Because of increased flow of blood from high pressure to low pressure area (aorta to pulmonary artery) and increasesd pulmonary venous return, to left side of heart, dilatation and hypertrophy of left ventricle takes place. When pulmonary hypertension develops the shunt is reversed (Eisenmanger's syndrome). Patient may show differential cyanosis. Continuous murmur may decrease in intensity and even become inaudible.

Clinical features of persistent ductus arteriosus

1. Large number of cases remain asymptomatic.
2. Early symptoms are palpitation, breathlessness on exertion and easy fatiguability. Cyanosis when reversal of shunt.
3. Collapsing pulse, wide pulse pressure. Radial pulses on both sides are unequal.
4. Heart may be enlarged, left ventricular type.
5. Continuous machinery type murmur occupying both systole and diastole in second, third left interspace. A thrill may be palpable.

Second pulmonary sound is accentuated and split. An apical diastolic murmur may be audible.

Clinical features. A great number of cases remain asymptomatic till late in age. Earliest symptoms are palpitation, breathlessness on exertion and easy fatiguability. A case of PDA may present with infective endocarditis or when the shunt becomes large, heart failure may develop sooner or later. Cyanosis may appear with reversal of shunt due to pulmonary hypertension.

Physical signs include a collapsing or water

Hammer type of pulse. Because of large shunt, peripheral signs of wide pulse pressure are seen. Radial pulses on both sides are unequal and blood pressure is higher in the right arm than in the left. Heart may be enlarged andthere is left ventricular type of cardiac impulse. A continuous machinery type of murmur occupying both systole and diastole is audible in the second, third left intercostal space near the sternal border. A thrill may also be palpable.

Second pulmonary sound is accentuated and may be split because of pulmonary hypertension. An apical diastolic murmur may be heard because of excess blood flow.

Investigations:

X-ray heart. In a small shunt the heart size is normal but in cases with large shunts there is enlargement of left ventricle. Pulmonary artery is prominent and its pulsations may be exaggerated. Pulmonary plethora if shunt is large. Electrocardiogram shows left atrial and left ventricular hypertrophy.

Cardiac catheterization and echocardiography are helpful in delineating the ductus by measuring the pressure gradient, blood flow and oxygen content of the blood across the shunt.

Treatment. Premature infants with patent ductus may be treated with prostaglandin inhibitor (Indomethacin). Most of the cases of patent ductus remain asymptomatic. But ideal treatment is surgical closure ofthe ductus preferably between the ages of three to 5 years. Patients who develop infective endocarditis, surgery may have to be postponed and also delayed for several months after successful treatment of endocarditis.

Prompt surgical intervention in any case of PDA is indicaated where there is evidence of a large shunt, cardiac enlargement, signs of poor cardiac reserve and heart failure.

Prognosis is very good in majority of cases of PDA provided surgery is carried out at appropriate time before irrversible damage takens place.

Coarctation of the aorta. It means a stricture or contraction of the aorta at or below the insertion of the ductus but distal to the origin of left subclavian artery. Coarctation is often associated with other cardiac anomalies like bicuspid aortic valve, subaortic stenosis, mitral stenosis, and a septal defect. It is only in small percentage (20%) of cases when coarctation exists as the only anomaly. Depending on the site of constriction it may be classified as:

1. Pre-subclavian
2. Pre-ductal
3. Isthmus
4. Lower distal or subphrenic which comprises a very small group where stricutre is in the descending part of aorta well below the usual site above or below the renal artries. Nature of coarctation may be in the fom of an abrupt, elongated or imperforate lesion.

Clinical features. Majority of cases of coarctation remain asymptomatic till adolescence and often present with some complication like cardiac failure. Rupture of aorta or cerebral vessel takes place. Because of hypertension, there are complaints of headache, dizziness, tinnitus and epistaxis. Due to diminished blood supply to the lower half patient gives history of weakness, cold feet, easy fatiguability, cramps in the legs and intermittent claudication. As disease progresses features of progressive dysponea and congestive failure develop. Physical features include prominent pulsations in the supraclavicular region, dilated tortuous collateral vessels either visible or palpable over the back of chest, inner borders of scapula, in the axilla and sometimes in front of the chest. There is hypertension in upper limbs and wide differences in blood pressure levels in both upper and lower limbs. Femoral pulses are very weak, feeble and delayed. Heart is often enlarged. Apex beat is down and out, heaving in nature. There is a loud systolic murmur over the precordium and also heard at the back. Continuous murmur may be heard at the site of coarctation or over the collaterals. Often because of associated aortic valve lesion, there is an ejection systolic murmur over the right sternal border.

Investigations:

Electrocardiogram demonstrates left ventricular hypertrophy.

X-ray heart. Heart is slightly enlarged. Aorta is dilated. There may be indentation or concavity at the site of constriction with dilatation along the left para mediastinal shadow. Notching of the ribs on their under surface due to erosion by the dilated collateral vessels is an important sign.

Aortography will show the nature and site of defect while *echocardiography* helps in localising other associated cardiac anomalies.

MRI is important for visualizing the length and severity of the obstruction.

Complications. Common complications include congestive heart failure, bacterial endocarditis, rupture of aorta, cerebral haemorrhage.

Diagnosis. Diagnosis of coarctation of aorta is suspected in any young hypertensive who has got feeble or absent femoral pulsations and presence of collaterals over the chest wall. Confirmation is by the investigations like X-ray chest, electrocardiogram, aortography, MRI etc.

Treatment. When a person is diagnosed to be suffering from coarctation of aorta, surgical treatment is indicated which includes resection of the stenosed part and end to end anastomosis. If the narrowing is extensive, a graft may be needed.

Cases of coarctation who present with complications like congestive failure, endocarditis, appropriate treatment be instituted. Where surgery has been unusually delayed, hypertension may not reverse because of secondary damage to the kidneys. Ideal age for surgery is below the age of 15 years. Successful correction of coarctation carries good prognosis.

Tetralogy of fallot. It is the commonest cyanotic congenital cardiac anomaly in children and is associated with cyanosis and clubbing. It comprises of four components i.e. pulmonary stenosis, ventricular septal defect, over riding of the aorta and right ventricular hypertrophy.

Continous murmur may be heard at site of coarctation or over the collaterals.

The essential lesion is obstruction to right ventricular outflow tract either at supravalvular, subvalvular or valvular level associated with ventricular septal defect with resultant right ventricular hypertrophy. Depending on whether the obstruction is mild or severe, there is reduction in pulmonary blood flow, arterial desaturation, and large volume of venous blood is shunted from right to left across the septal defect into the over riding aorta. Result is deficiency in arterial oxygenation and production of cyanosis and polycythaemia.

Manifestations of coarctation of aorta

1. Cases often remain asymptomatic. Present with hypertension, congestive failure, rupture of aorta or cerebral vessels.
2. Symptoms of headache, dizziness, tinnitus, epistaxis, cold feet, easy fatiguability and intermittent claudication.
3. Physical signs include raised blood pressure in upper limbs. Difference in blood pressure level in upper and lower limbs. Prominent pulsations in supraclavicualr region dilated tortuous vessels over back of chest, inner borders of scapula, axilla. Femoral pulses are weak and feeble.
4. Heart is enlarged. Apex beat down and out. Loud systolic murmur over precordium and also heard at the back.

Clinical features. Main symptom is cyanosis which is present from infancy but the age at which it appears depends upon the severity of right ventricular outflow tract obstruction (RVOT). Cyanotic spells usually appear after the age of six months. There is breathlessness, fatigue, syncopal attacks and increasing degree of cyanosis. Child may adopt a squatting position to get relief. Paroxysmal attacks of dysponea may occur after exertion and there is often intensification of cyanosis. Clubbing of the fingers is present and may develop even after months or years after appearance of cyanosis. Eyeballs may be suffused because of polycythaemia. In late stages, dizziness and syncopal attacks and sometimes death may occur during one of such episodes.

Physical signs include central cyanosis (blue baby) clubbing. Heart size is within normal limits. A parasternal heave and a systolic thrill are palpable in the left upper sternal border in second intercostal space. On auscultation there is an ejection systolic murmur in the second space. Second sound is single and pulmonary component is weak or inaudible. There is no diastolic murmur.

Manifestations of tetralogy of Fallot

1. Cyanosis present since infancy. Cyanotic spells, breathlessness, fatigue, syncopal attacks. Child may adopt a squatting position to get relief. Growth of child stunted.
2. Clubbing of fingers suffused eyeballs. In late stage dizziness and syncopal attack.
3. Physical signs include central cyanosis, clubbing parasternal heave and a systolic thrill palpable in second left intercostal space. An ejection systolic murmur in pulmonary area. Second sound is single and pulmonary component is weak or unaudible.

Investigations:

Electrocardiogram shows evidence of right ventricular hypertrophy.

X-ray heart shows a hypertrophied and rotated right ventricle but cardiac enlargement is not marked. There is absence of pulmonary artery curve. No pulmonary congestion.

In adults heart shadow assumes a typical appearance called Coeur en sabot (like wooden shoe) where apex is elevated and blunted resembling a sheep's nose with prominence of right ventricle.

Echocardiography helps in assessing the defect while cardiac catheterization and selective angiocardiography evaluate the right ventricular outflow tract obstruction as well as pressure measurements and oxygen concentration in the right ventricle.

Course and prognosis. An untreated patient of fallots tetralogy runs risk of developing various complications which include congestive heart failure. Bacterial endocarditis, recurrent pulmonary infections, paradoxical embolism, cerebral abscess and coagulation defects.

Most of these complications develop in early period of life before adolescence. Rarely a mild case may reach adult life and lead a near normal life.

Treatment. Treatment mainly is surgical. Ideal time for surgery is between the ages of three and twelve but depending on the severity of the lesion, surgical correction can be done even during infancy.

Main aim of surgery is to increase the pulmonary blood flow by anastomosing left subclavian artery to pulmonary artery (Blalock-Taussig operation) thus increasing not only the blood supply but also oxygenation of blood.

Results of successful operation are dramatic and clinical improvement is significant (reduction of anoxemia, breathlessness and syncopal spells). Total correction of anomalies (closure of VSD, valvotomy of pulmonary valve and relief of RVOT obstruction) is also undertaken by aid of hypothermia, heart lung machine by open heart surgery. Results after surgery are good. Patients with cyanotic spells may get temporary relief by use of a beta blocker (Propranolol 40 mg twice a day/metoprolol 50 mg BD/Atenolol 50 mg once a day). These drugs relax the right ventricular (RVOT) obstruction and give relief.

CONGESTIVE HEART FAILURE

Congestive heart failure is one of the commonest condition of the heart in clinical practice. It may be defined as failure of the heart to meet the body demands of adequate circulation for its metabolising tissues. Cardiac failure may be described as acute or chronic, high output or low output or left sided or right sided and biventricular failure.

Acute form of heart failure develops suddenly following an acute myocardial infarction, rupture of chordae tendinae. hypertensive crisis or rapid transfusion of fluids in a compromised heart while chronic form develops slowly over period of time in patients with various chronic diseases as in ischaemic heart disease, rheumatic valvular disease, cardiomyopathy, hypertension etc.

Low output failure occurs when cardiac output is depressed secondary to diseases like ischaemic heart disease, hypertension, valvular heart disease, cardiomyopathy, congenital heart disease while high output failure occurs in cases where heart failure is primarily due to non-cardiac causes like hyper-

---

Forms of congestive heart failure

1. Acute form, chronic form
2. Low output failure, hight output failure
3. Left heart failure, right heart failure, biventri-cular failure
4. Compensated, decompensated

Causes of low output failure

1. Ischaemic heart disease
2. Hypertension
3. Valvular heart disease
4. Cardiomyopathy
5. Congenital heart disease

Causes of high output failure

1. Severe anaemia
2. Thyrotoxicosis
3. Chronic cor pulmonale
4. Beri-beri
5. Paget's disease
6. Pregnancy

---

7. Hypertension especially rapidly developing severe grades of hypertension.
8. Arrhythmias developing in case of compen-sated heart failure.
9. Massive acute myocardial infarction.
10. Rapid and excessive fluid load/blood transfu-sion.
11. Physical and emotional stress.
12. Thyrotoxicosis

Factors precipitating heart failure

1. Infections especially pulmonary
2. Severe anaemia
3. Pulmonary embolism
4. Pregnancy in a woman with preexisting heart disease
5. Bacterial endocarditis
6. Rapidly developing hypertension
7. Cardiac arrhythmias
8. Massive acute myocardial infarction
9. Cardiac overload (rapid transfusion of fluids including blood)
10. Thyrotoxicosis
11. Physical and emotional stress.

---

thyroidism, anaemia, pagets disease, chronic cor pulmonale, pregnancy and beri-beri. Patients with high output failure may have cardiac output either at normal level or slightly on the higher side but for that patients body requirements it is still less so that patient has all features of congestive failure. Again congestive failure may result due to inability of the heart to pump out a large volume of incoming blood i.e. there is increase in preload (atrial septal defect, aortic regurgitation) or there may be failure of heart to pump adequate amount of blood against increased resistance i.e. increase in after load (systemic hypertension). The very fact that a patient has got a compromised heart assumes significance since a number of factors are known to precipitate heart failure in such individuals and these factors range from.

1. Infections especially pulmonary are known to precipitate heart failure putting extra load on the heart.
2. Severe anaemia.
3. Pulmonary embolism.
4. Pregnancy in a woman with already existing valvular heart disease.
5. Myocarditis.
6. Bacterial endocarditis (acute/subacute).

Basically heart failure is the result of myocardial failure when there is defect in myocardial contractility either due to primary disease or secondary to ischaemia as in cases of ischaemic heart disease, Myocarditis, cardiomyopathy while in other group though the myocardium is healthy yet its functions may be strained beyond its capacity because of impairment of filling of ventricles due to mechanical factors or defects in its valves as in cases of rheumatic or congenital heart disease.

Causes of cardiac failure:

1. Myocardial causes where there is myocardial dysfunction leading to reduced contractile force of the heart. Causes include infections (rheumatic, typhoid, viral), toxins (diphtheria), nutritional (beri-beri), coronary heart disease, hypertension, cardiomyopathy, infiltrative lesions (amyloidosis), and degenerative diseases involving the heart.
2. Mechanical lesions of the heart. There is volume overload as in valvular heart disease

(aortic and mitral disease) syphilitic heart disease and congenital lesions (ASD, VSD, PDA).

3. Diseases interfering with diastolic filling of the heart i.e. constrictive pericarditis, pericardial effusion restrictive cardiomyopathy.
4. Rhythm disturbances especially in a compromised heart since they reduce the end diastolic volume due to reduction in diastolic interval. These range from atrial tachycardias, atrial flutter, atrial fibrillation to heart block.
5. Increased demands on a diseased heart either due to high fever, pregnancy or thyrotoxicosis shall be an important cause to look for.

Pathyophysiology. Normal functioning of the heart depends on its functional capacity as well as the load against which it has to work. When heart is diseased it tries to overcome it by compensatory mechanism like dilatation and hypertrophy of its chambers. Heart failure is the result of the failing heart to compensate the extra circulatory strain.

When the heart is failing, one or other ventricle fails to discharge its contents, the end diastolic volume of the ventricle rises, venous pressure gets elevated and there is more venous congestion behind the failing heart. It is called "Backward Failure" while due to "forward failure" theory there is inadequate discharge of blood due to fall in cardiac output and this coupled with salt and water retention through renin-angiotensin-aldosterone mechanism results in congestive failure. But basically in almost every case of congestive failure both factors of forward and backward failure operate to some extent.

Thus heart failure development depends on myocardial contractility, cardiac output, salt and water retention, elevated venous pressure, renin-angiotensin-aldosterone system and release of antidiuretic hormone (ADH) its excess activity leading to salt and water retention. Broadly speaking we have two forms of heart failure. Left heart failure and right heart failure and in later stages we have biventricular failure.

Left heart failure. *Common causes are:*

1. Hypertension
2. Ischaemic heart disease
3. Aortic valve disease
4. Mitral incompetence
5. Cardiomyopathy.

Clinical features of left heart failure

1. Progressive breathlessness more marked on exertion
2. Attacks of paroxysmal nocturnal dysponea
3. Features of low cardiac output—weakness, fatigue, palpitation and pain in chest.
4. In early case gallop rhythm, basal crepts.
5. Acute left heart failure charactrised by tachycardia, cold extremities, facial pallor, raised levels of blood pressure if hypertensive, pulsus alternans, Cheyne-Stokes breathing, gallop rhythm.

Basal crepitations in early case. Coarse and bubbling crepitations all over the chest more marked at bases in acute case.

Clinical features. Earliest symptom may be cough with progressive breathlessness more marked on exertion followed by orthoponea, attacks of paroxysmal nocturnal dysponea (cardiac asthma) with or without pulmonary oedema. Because of low cardiac output, weakness, fatigue, palpitation and pain, chest are important features.

Attacks of paroxysmal nocturnal dysponea often referred to as cardiac asthma may sometimes bring to light left heart failure. These attacks generally occur at night or in the early hours of morning when patient is sleeping comfortably in bed. Patient suddenly gets up feeling markedly breathless and a sense of choking sensation. He/she often goes to the window to get more fresh air. Face is pale, the extremities are cold and there are violent paroxysms of cough with little or no sputum though later on frothy sputum occasionally tinged with blood appears. Cardiac asthma has to be differentiated from bronchial asthma especially in middle-aged persons who have invariably a long history of bronchial asthma.

Cheyne-Stokes respiration may be another feature of left heart failure. It is characterised by waning and waxing periods of respiration and in between there are phases of slower breathing and recurring periods of apnea.

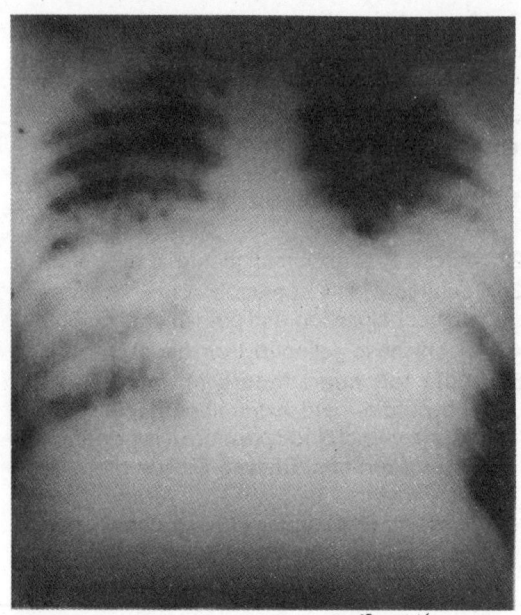

Fig. 4.26. Congestive Failure: X ray Heart (PA View). There are bilateral shadows in middle zones of lungs. Heart is enlarged. It is picture of pulmonary oedema.

Pulmonary oedema may accompany or complicate cardiac asthma. A cardiac case may suddenly go into pulmonary oedema as in acute myocardial infarction, hypertension or following I/V transfusion. Patient is acutely breathless unable to lie in bed, there is cough with rapid breathing accompanied by wheezing sounds or rattles. Patient often brings out frothy sputum tinged with blood. There is profuse sweating, air hunger and cyanosis. Unless treated promptly as an emergency. Pulmonary oedema may prove fatal.

Physical signs. In an early case of left heart failure there are no physical signs. But in acute attack, skin is cold and sweaty. Central cyanosis is present. There is tachycardia. Pulsus alternans is present. Blood pressure may be raised if hypertensive. Cardiac enlargement may be seen. A gallop rhythm may be heard at the lower end of sternum near the apex. Evidence of underlying heart disease may be seen (pansystolic murmur in mitral area in mitral incompetence, rupture of chordae tendinae: aortic diastolic/systolic murmur in aortic valve disease). Pulmonary signs include fine crepts at bases in early cases while in advanced cases there

are coarse and bubbling rales: present all over the lungs but more marked at bases. There may be rhonchi suggesting bronchospasm.

Investigations. X-ray heart shows cardiomegaly with pulmonary congestion (interstitial oedema and pleural effusion). Pulmonary oedema is characteristically seen in acute stage (BAT wing appearance).

Electrocardiogram. Left ventricular hypertrophy with or without strain.

Course and prognosis. It depends on the underlying heart disease. Acute pulmonary oedema following acute myocardial infarction, malignant hypertension carries poor prognosis. Patients of aortic valve disease once they go into left heart failure follow a rapid downhill course.

Right heart failure. This commonly follows left heart failure. Left heart failure with its associated pulmonary hypertension and pulmonary congestion is the commonest cause of right heart failure. Other causes include:

1. ***Primary disease of the lungs.*** Pulmonary vessels or pulmonary valve which cause strain on right side of heart and produce a picture of right heart failure (chronic cor pulmonale). Cor pulmonale may be acute due to massive pulmonary embolism while causes of chronic cor pulmonale shall be:

   (a) *Diseases of lungs.* Chronic bonchitis with or without emphysema, bronchiectasis, pulmonary tuberculosis, bronchial asthma, silicosis, pneumocentesis.

   (b) *Diseases of bony cage.* Kyphoscoliosis, massive resection of ribs.

   (c) Vascular disorders. Primary pulmonary hypertension

   (d) Valve defect. Pulmonary stenosis

2. Conditions which impair the function of the myocardium but produce predominant. Right sided heart failure as in myocarditis (rheumatic, toxic, diphtheria) severe anaemia, beri-beri.

3. Congenital heart disease such as pulmonary stenosis atrial and ventricular septal defect with left to right shunt.

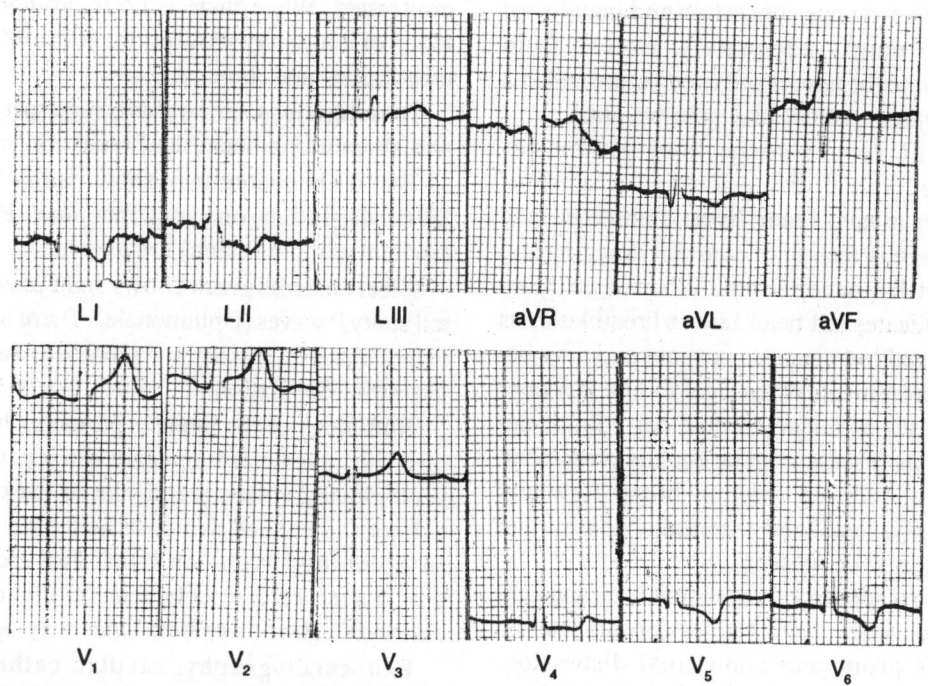

Fig. 4.27. ECG showing left ventricular Hypertrophy with strain. Deep S wave V₁ + RV₅ > 35 mm I wave inversion in left ventricular leads (V₅. V₆) indicates left ventricular strain.

4. *Valvular heart disease.* Tricuspid stenosis, mitral valve disease
5. Obstruction to inflow of blood into right atrium i.e. constrictive pericarditis.

Causes of right heart failure

1. Primary diseases of lungs (chronic bronchitis, bronchiectasis, pulmonary tuberculosis, bronchial asthma, pneumoconiosis, silicosis.
2. Diseases of bony cage. Kyphoscoliosis, massive resection of ribs.
3. Vascular disorders. Primary pulmonary hypertension, pulmonary valve stenosis.
4. Conditions impairing the function of myocardium. Myocarditis (anaemia, beri-beri rheumatic, toxic, bacterial).
5. Valvular heart disease, mitral stenosis, tricuspid stenosis.
6. Congenital heart disease: Pulmonary stenosis, atrial and ventricular septal defect.
7. Constrictive pericariditis
8. Secondary to left heart failure

Clinical picture. Since a case of right heart failure may accompany left heart failure it is a mixed picture of breathlessness on exertion and all features of left heart failure shall be present.

Clinical features of right heart failure

1. Generalized weakness and fatigue—Cough, breathlessness, anorexia, abdominal distension, pain and dragging sensation in right hypochondrium.
2. Headache, insomnia, restlessness, gain in weight, swelling of legs and feet, oliguria and nocturia.
3. Physical signs include cyanosis, warm extremities, engorged neck veins, jugular venous pressure elevated, hepatojugular reflux present, oedema over legs and feet, ascites, enlarged tender liver.
4. Cardiac size within normal limits. Pulmonary diastolic murmur due to pulmonary hypertension. Chest emphysematous, liver and cardiac dullness may be obliterated. Breath sounds vesicular with prolonged expiration, bilateral crepts and rhonchi. Signs of pleural effusion especially on right side may by present.

Generally there is weakness and fatigue. As a

result of passive venous congestion and inability of the heart to empty adequately, excess fluid accumulates into the tissues and even before oedema becomes apparent patient may gain weight.

Because of venous congestion, patient has anorexia, abdominal distension and a sense of fullness after meals. Since liver is enlarged and congested there is feeling of constant dragging and pain in right hypochondrium. When right heart failure complicates left heart failure breathlessness may be relieved but cyanosis appears and may become more prominent. When right failure is secondary to diseases of lungs (chronic cor pulmonale) features of lung disease shall be equally prominent.

Because of reduced cerebral blood flow and oxygen supply, headache insomnia, apathy and sluggishness may be present.

Oedema first appears on dependent parts and later on it becomes generalized. Ascites appears later on and there is prominent abdominal distension. Oliguria and nocturia occur frequently and diminution in urinary output indicates the severity of heart failure.

Physical signs. Patient generally is cyanosed. Clubbing may be present. Neck veins are engorged and pulsations are prominent. Jugular venous pressure is elevated. Hepatojugular reflux is present. There is oedema over the legs and feet. Ascites is present which sometimes is more prominent than oedema over legs (constrictive pericarditis). Liver is enlarged and tender. Occasionally in advanced cases of right heart failure jaundice may appear.

Heart generally is not enlarged until right heart failure is complicated by left heart failure. Signs of underlying lung or heart disease may be present. Because of predominant right ventricular failure there is parasternal heave. Pulmonary second sound may be loud and accentuated. Pulmonary diastolic murmur indicates pulmonary hypertension. Dilatation of the right ventricle may produce tricuspid incompetence and a functional pansystolic murmur may be heard. Lungs show pleural effusion most commonly on right side but in extensive disease there is bilateral hydrothorax. Chest may be emphysematous and cardiac dullness may be obliterated. When there is no hydrothorax auscultation of lungs may show prolonged respiration with crepitations and rhonchi.

Investigations. Urine shows high specific gravity and albuminuria because of renal congestion.

Blood chemistry may show rise in blood urea levels depending on renal functions. Electrolytes (sodium and potassium) are altered.

Electrocardiogram shows right axis deviation, tall spiky P waves (P pulmonale). There may be right ventricular hypertrophy and presence of arrhythmias like atrial fibrillation.

Radiology of the heart in pure right heart failure does not reveal cardiomegaly since enlarged right ventricle and atrium are displaced backwards. But oblique views shall demonstrate their enlargement. In combined right and left failure, there is pronounced cardiac enlargement. Pleural effusion either on right side or both sides may be seen.

Echocardiography, cardiac catheterization and radionuclide imaging as well as angiography are tests which may help in delineating the pathology.

Classification of heart failure. American heart association has classified the status of a cardiac case depending on the degree of heart failure. This classification is helpful in assessing functional status of the heart and so the prognosis in any case.

Grade I: Patient with heart disease but with no limitation of physical activity.

Grade II: Patients with slight limitation of physical activity. They are comfortable at rest and experience discomfort with more serious forms of physical activity.

Grade III: Patients with marked limitation of physical activity i.e. even milder form of physical activity produces discomfort.

Grade IV: Patients with inability to carry on any physical activity without discomfort. Thus patients with grade I group of congestive failure carry good prognosis as compared to those in grade IV.

Complications of congestive heart failure. These are the one associated with underlying heart

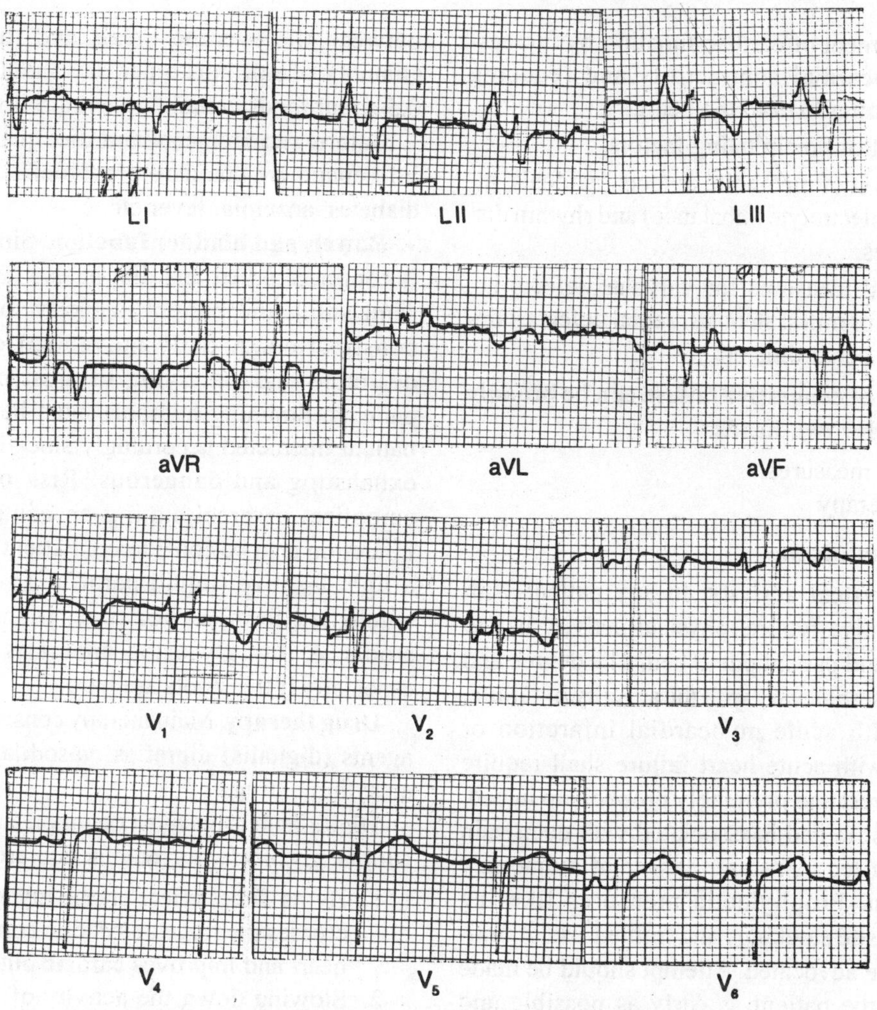

Fig. 4.28. ECG showing right ventricular hypertrophy. This is recorded in a case of chronic cor-pulmonale. P pulmonale in L II, L III, aVF. QR complex in aVR, V_1, R wave of greater voltage than S wave in V_1 (R:S > 10).

disease, congestion of various organs and with the therapeutic measures employed.

Complications of congestive heart failure

1. Pulmonary embolism
2. Cardiac arrhythmias
3. Pulmonary infections
4. Electrolyte disturbances
5. Renal insufficiency
6. Bacterial endocarditis
7. Systemic embolisation
8. Cardiac cirirhosis
9. Cardiac cachexia (weight loss and emaciation)

Pulmonary embolism is a common complication in those confined to bed because of thrombosis in the leg veins.

In patients with rhythm disturbances, systemic, embolisation may occur. Pulmonary infection, electrolyte disturbances, renal insufficiency, bacterial endocarditis, cardiac cirrhosis are other complication. In cases with long standing congestive failure, weight loss and emaciation may develop as a result of poor intake of food and wasting of tissues (cardiac cachexia).

Treatment of heart failure. *Main principles of treating a case of congestive heart failure are:*

1. Improvement of cardiac function by increasing myocardial contractility and reducing preload/after load of the heart.
2. Removal of precipitating factors.
3. Correction of metabolic defects (acidosis, alkalosis, electrolyte imbalance) and rhythm disturbances.
4. Remedial measures for valvular defects i.e. surgery for mitral stenosis, septal defects, constrictive percarditis etc.

Treatment of congestive failure can be broadly discussed under two heads.

a. General measures
b. Drug therapy

General measures:

Rest and physical activity. In any patient with severe congestive failure, physical activity has to be restricted and patient put to bed. The degree and duration of rest shall vary with the severity of failure. A patient with acute myocardial infarction or myocarditis with acute heart failure shall require absolute bed rest and preferably propped up in bed. Prolonged rest in bed is associated with deep vein thrombosis in leg veins and danger of pulmonary embolization. Prophylactic measures like leg exercises, elastic stockings and limited use of anticoagulants are advocated. Attempt should be made to ambulate the patient as early as possible and gradually activity introduced.

In addition to physical rest, mental rest be also ensured. A restful sleep at night is very essential. Diazepam (5 mg) at bed time be prescribed especially in acute stage.

Enforcement of physical and mental rest results in reduction in arterial pressure, and load on the myocardium. It minimizes the oxygen demands and thus reduces body's demands of increased cardiac output.

Diet. A nutritious, well balanced, soft palatable diet with low caloric and low salt intake should be basic principle of diet in congestive failure. Frequent small feeds be given. Over feeding and over loading of stomach at any time be avoided. Evening meals should be light and adequate interval should elapse between the evening meals and time of sleep. Quantity of salt intake per day should not exceed 0.5 g and foods containing extra salt be avoided.

Caloric requirements and diet quantity shall be influenced by coexisting problems like obesity, diabetes, anaemia, fever etc.

Bowels and bladder function. Since the patient is confined to bed and diet is also either liquid or semi solid, the patient is likely to suffer from constipation. A daily movement of bowels is desirable and satisfying to most of the Indian patients. Straining at stools must be avoided and patient instructed accordingly since it can be both exhausting and dangerous. Risk of pulmonary embolism or precipitating an acute myocardial infarction is to be considered. Patient may be given a light laxative (liquid paraffin 15-30 ml/day in emulsified form) at bed time. It shall soften the stools. A low glycerine enema is also helpful especially if the stools are hard.

Drug therapy. Main therapy consists of inotropic agents (digitalis) diuretics, vasodilators and antiarrhythmic drugs.

Digitalis. It is the most common and widely used cardiac glycoside. Its main action are:

1. By its direct effect on the myocardium, it increases the force of systolic contraction of the heart and improves cardiac output.
2. Slowing down the activity of SA mode and thus reduction of heart rate.
3. Depression of A-V conduction system with reduction of ventricular response. This is a result of vagal action and direct action of digitalis on the heart.

Dosages. In mild to moderate case of congestive failure start with Digoxin (0.25 mg tablet) twice a day. About 60% of the drug is absorbed. Absorption is effected by antacids, metaclopromide, antidiarrhoeals and neomycin. It is a cumulative drug and after oral administration the effect starts taking place in 30-45 minutes. Excretion of the drug is dependent on renal function. Special precaution should be taken when giving the drug in elderly people, patients with severe renal or hepatic disease. Once the therapeutic benefits have been achieved, dosage of the drug be monitored by clinical assessment, Electrocardiogram and plasma digoxn assay.

Rapid digitilization. In patients with severe congestive heart failure, acute left heart failure, failure with rapid heart rate, pulmonary oedema, injection Digoxin 0.5-0.75 mg is initially given intravenously slowly over a period of 5-10 minutes under electrocardiographic control. This may be repeated every 6-8 hourly (0.25 mg) depending on the clinical condition of the patient. The effect of intravenous dosage starts within minutes and maximum is reached in 2-3 hours.

Before administering drug intravenously, it must be ensured that the patient is not currently on digoxin and if not, the patient should not have had the drug during the preceding two weeks. If despite this, the drug is administered intravenously it may produce cardiac arrest.

Digoxin is contraindicated in early period of acute myocardial infarction, acute myocarditis, partial or unstable heart block, ventricular tachycardia and peripheral circulatory failure. Side effects of the drug include anorexia, nausea, vomiting, headache, visual disturbances, drowsiness, ventricular ectopics, PAT with 2:1 A-V block, ventricular tachycardia and fibrillation. Changes in Twave and ST segments of ECG (depression or scooping of ST segment and inversion of first portion of T-wave) are the earliest to appear. Hypokalemia from any cause enhances digitalis toxicity.

When signs of digitalis toxicity appear, stop the drug as well as diuretics. Estimate serum potasium levels. Administer potassium chloride (5-7.5 g) orally in divided doses. In severe cases, a solution containing 1-1.5 g of potasium chloride (40 meq of the drug) in 500 ml of 5% glucose can be administered intravenously over 2-4 hours with ECG monitoring and potassium levels as guide. Potassium is contraindicated in the presence of A-V block hyperkalemia or severe renal insufficiency. For frequent ectopics PAT with block oral or I/V propranolol or phenytoin are employed. Digitalis antibodies are specific antidote but are not available in our country. In every patient on digitalis: daily monitoring of pulse and heart rate be done and recorded. When rate is about 64/mt, be careful and if it falls below 60/mt, the drug has to be stopped. ECG monitoring should be done frequently to detect arrhythmias.

Diuretics. Next to digitalis, diuretics form the major mode of therapy in congestive failure and are indicated in all form of congestive failure. Commonly used diuretics are:

Frusemide. It is a potent diuretic and its effect starts within an hour after oral dosage (40-80 mg) and is complete by 4-6 hours while intravenous dose (40-100 mg) produces effect within 20 minutes lasting upto 2-3 hours. The drug acts along the entire nephron including loop of henle with the exception of distal site. It enhances potassium excretion. Hypokalemia is a serious side effect. Patient complains of weakness, fatigue, dizziness and cramps. Long term use may produce hyperuricaemia and hyperglycemia. Rapid diuresis in elderly patient may precipitate acute urinary retention. Cardiac arrest follows rapid intravenous, administration of frusemide. Frusemide can be safely given in the presence of renal disease but then the effective dose has to be higher.

For hypokalemia, patient be advised to take fruit juices or soup since they are rich source of potassium. Otherwise potassium supplements be given orally (pot. chloride 500 mg in 5 ml sorbitol) two to three times a day preferably after meals (10-15 ml).

Spironolactone (Aldactone). It is a potassium sparing diuretic and an aldosterone antagonist. It acts on the distal part of the nephron and prevents sodium reabsorption and potassium excretion. It is given orally in dosage of 25-100 mg either singly or in divided doses. It is a weak diuretic when given alone but when combined with other diuretics like Thiazide, frusemide, its action is potentiated as well as potassium is conserved. The diuretic response is observed only after a few days of therapy.

Side effects include headache, drowsiness, mental confusion rash etc. It is contraindicated in the presence of renal failure, addison's disease and anuria.

Triamterene. It resembles aldosteron antagonist spironolactone and when given orally increases excretion of water, sodium and chloride while depressing excretion of potasium.

It is a weak diuretic and is not used alone but in combination with other diuretics.

Dosage is 100-200 mg per day. After oral administration peak effect is reached in about 2 hours and lasts for 10-12 hours. Side effects include nausea, diarrhoea, cramps, skin rash, rise in blood urea levels. Care should be taken while using it in renal failure.

Amiloride. It again is a weak diuretic and has action similar to trimetrene, though more potent than it Dosage is 10-20 mg/day usually in combination with other diuretics.

Thiazide diuretics. These as a group constitute number of diuretics which have the same mode of action and differ from each other only in that minimal effective doses and duration of their action. Commonly used diuretics in this group include hydrochlorthiazide (Esidrex) chlorothiazide, chlorthalidone (hythalton, hygroton), bendrofluazide and metolazone (zaroxylin). Thiazide diuretics are effective when given orally and of use in patients with mild to moderate congestive failure. They act on the first half of the distal convoluted tubule and a portion of the ascending limb of loop of Henle preventing reabsorption of sodium and chloride. Because of their inhibitory action on sodium reabsorption, a large exchange of potassium with sodium takes place. This causes increased potassium loss (hypokalemia) and excessive renal loss of sodium (hyponataemia) and chloride (hypochloremia). Thiazide diuretics are to be administered once daily (esidrex 50 mg tablet hythalton 100 mg, Metolazone 5 mg). Because of prolonged use side effects like reduction in excretion of uric acid, hyperglycemia, skin rashes and thrombocytopenia may result. Hypokalemia is a serious side effect and produces marked weakness, lethargy and even precipitates digitalis toxicity. Oral supplementation of potassium chloride must be given on the day the diuretic is taken. Further potassium loss can be prevented by combining the drug with potassium sparing diuretics like spironolactone or triametrene.

Effect of thiazide starts within one hour of administration and lasts between 12-18 hours.

Importance of diuretic therapy. Diuretic therapy forms the first line of treatment for all stages of heart failure and especially so in mild and moderate stages. They relieve fluid overload by promoting renal excretion of sodium and water as well as blocking the reabsorption of sodium and chloride. Resulting fluid loss reduces cardiac over load and improves cardiac output. Dosage of diuretics has to be adjusted individually depending on the grade of congestive failure. Thus a patient with acute left heart failure, pulmonary oedema shall require intravenous administration of the diuretic. Over zealous use of diuretics may lead to excessive loss of salt and water, and a hypovolemic state. Hypokalemia may develop by use of thiazide diuretics. This has to be corrected. Occasionally patients may develop resistance to diuretics. This is corrected by change of diuretic and careful monitoring of electrolytes.

Vasodilators. In cases with severe and chronic congestive heart failure not responding to digitalis and diuretics, because of reduced cardiac output the neurohomoral mechanism are activated which constrict the peripheral vascular bed and increase peripheral vascular resistance and thus venous return. Such vasoconstriction of arterioles causes obstruction to the left ventricular ejection (after load) further increasing the work load of the heart while increased venous return raises the end diastolic ventricular pressure (preload). Both these mechanisms increase the work of the heart. Vasodilator therapy aims to reduce the after load by causing peripheral arteriolar dilatation and preload by vasodilatation. This is of therapeutic value especially in resistant cases of heart failure.

Of the vasodilators acting on the arteriolar system hydralazine (50-75 mg 6 hourly) is a smooth muscle relaxant while Prazosin (5 mg 8 hourly) an alpha adrenergic blocker are potent vasodilators. By reducing after load on the heart, they increase cardiac output.

Nitrates (Isosorbide dinitrite 20-40 mg orally or 5-10 mg sublingually 6 hourly) act on the venous side of the circulation and act primarily to reduce the preload on the heart. But there are balanced vasodilators which act both on arteriolar and venous system, thus reducing both preload and afterload on the heart producing beneficial effects on the failing heart. The drug of choice in this group are ACE inhibitors. ACE inhibitors are beneficial clinically and haemodynamically and are safe on long term use. It is always advisable to start therapy with small doses (Captopril 6.25 mg, enalapril 5 mg, Lisinopril 5 mg) as initial dose in order to avoid hypotension. Patients have to be kept on maintainence (Captopril 25 mg. enalapril 10 mg, Lisinopril 10 mg daily).

In acute heart failure, infusion of sodium nitroprusside is advocated but its use requires careful monitoring of the pressure and ECG control. The effect is short lived and lasts as long as infusion is given. This type of therapy is to be given only in a intestive care unit.

For all cases of chronic congestive failure, ACE inhibitors are the drug of choice because of their easy administration and improvement in cardiac output, survival and reduction in mortality.

Other therapy. In addition to digitalis, diuetics patient should be propped up in bed especially in acute stage. A back rest be given. If there is infection, approprirate antibiotics given. Most of the patients with congestive failure are anxious and apprehensive. For alleviation of these symptoms and for a restful sleep Tablet Alprazolam (0.25-0.5 mg twice a day) or Tablet Diazepam (5 mg twice a day) are advised.

Acute pulmonary oedema. It is a serious and life threatening emergency. Most common causes of pulmonary oedema are hypertension. Acute myocardial infarction, mitral incompetence and aortic valve disease.

Treatment of pulmonary oedema must be started immediately and basic line of approach shall be:

1. Put the patient in bed. Preferably hospitalize. Back rest be provided as the sitting position tends to reduce venous return.

2. O_2 inhalation.
3. Injection Morphine 15 mg subcutaneously immediately. It reduces anxiety, depresses the respiratory centre and reduces adrenergic vasoconstrictor stimuli thus allevating the symptoms.
4. Injection Frusemide (80 mg) intravenously. It shall relieve pulmonary oedema and by its vasodilator action reduce venous return.
5. If patient has not received digoxin during the last fortnight. Injection Digoxin or Lanatoside C be given slowly (0.5-1 mg) under electrocardiographic control.
6. Injection Aminophylline (0.24 g) given intravenously slowly in 10 minutes is effective in not only relieving bronchospasm but also acts as diuretic increases renal blood flow and improves cardiac contractility. Rapid injection of Aminophylline is known to produce hypotension and anaphylactic shock. Drug may be repeated 6 hourly.
7. In patients not responding to the above regime intravenous nitroprusside may be employed (20-30 ugm per minute in infusion).
8. Rotating tourniquets are sometimes applied to the extremities to reduce venous return.

Above are the emergency measures. Attempt be made once the patient has come out of the crisis, to treat the underlying cause and any precipitating factors which may be operative.

HYPERTENSION

It is difficult to define what is normal blood pressure for an individual since it is dependent on a number of factors. Conventionally hypertension may be defined as rise in blood pressure levels more than the normal for that age and sex.

But what is meant by blood pressure? Blood pressure is the product of the amount of blood pumped by the heart (cardiac output) and the resistance to the flow of this blood by the vascular bed (peripheral resistance). Systolic blood pressure is chiefly determined by the force of contraction of the left ventricle, heart rate, preload and afterload while diastolic pressure is controlled by the peripheral vascular resistance which is dependent on the lumen of vessel and its thickness and neurohumoral mechanisms.

There appears to be no general agreement as to what constitutes the upper limit of normal pressure levels. There is a wide variation in blood pressure figures and from infancy to sixth decade there is a gradual increase in levels. At birth the blood pressure is about 60-75/40, during childhood 90-100/50, at puberty 100-120/60, during adult life the average levels are 120-140/80 and at the age of 60 and beyond the levels can go upto 140-160 systolic and 80-90 mm diastolic.

Variations in the blood pressure figures may take place in the same person at different times during the day depending on the activity, rest, exertion, excitement or sleep phases. Generally speaking systolic blood pressure levels beyond 150-160 mmHg and diastolic levels beyond 90 mmHg in an adult are abnormal.

Blood pressure tends to fall with rest and so recordings of a pressure when a person gets out of bed in the early morning on awakening are usually on the lower side and this is termed as basal blood pressure while casual blood pressure recordings are the one taken at any time of the day under any condition irrespective of environmental factors.

Since basal blood pressure is recorded when the patient has had complete physical and mental rest it is a good index of the individuals normal levels. Sometimes it becomes difficult to draw a line between normal and abnormal blood pressure levels because blood pressure figures for one individual may not be normal for another at that age.

Normally there is a gradual rise of blood pressure as age advances. In elderly persons with a normal heart, there is disproportionately greater increase in systolic pressure compared to diastolic pressure since the blood vessels loose their elasticity due to aging process. Out of the two levels it is diastolic levels which are important and significant as the harmful effects of the pressure levels are concerned. Depending on blood pressure levels, hypertension

has been graded as follows:

Normotensive. Systolic below 140 mmHg and diastolic below 90 mmHg.

Border line. Systolic 140-160 mmHg and diastolic 90-95 mmHg.

Hypertension. Systolic above 160 mmHg and/or diastolic above 95 mmHg.

Further hypertension is classified as mild (diastolic 90 to 105 mmHg) moderate (diastolic 105-120 mmHg) and severe when diastolic levels are above 120 mmHg. There are a number of persons who are labelled as "pre-hypertensives" and whose blood pressure figures are normal at one time but on the higher side at another time. In majority of such people there are temporary factors like excitemenet, emotions and nervousness playing their part. Such people's blood pressure levels react violenlly to stress and strain and every passing day makes it more worse and a day comes when pressure in these hyper-reactors remains permanently raised.

Prevalence. Hypertension is widely prevalent all over the world and millions of people all over the world suffer from it and its consequences. Hypertension targets major organs in the body and predisposes to coronary heart disease, cerebrovascular disease and renal disease along with being a major factor of left ventricular dysfunction and congestive heart failure. The true prevalence of the disease in various parts of the world may be difficult to assess but on an average 10 to 15 per cent of the population suffers from it. Prospective epidemiological studies have emphasized the importance of hypertension as a precursor of cardiovascular morbidity and mortality and a factor promoting death and disability. The total mortality is about doubled and cardiovasculr mortality tripled among hypertensives as compared to normotensives in the general population.

Classification of hypertension.

Hypertension may be broadly classified as:

1. Primary or essential hypertension
2. Secondary hypertension.

Causes of hypertension

1. Acute or transient hypertension

a. Acute glomerulonephritis
b. Toxaemia of pregnancy
c. Acute intermittent, porphyria

2. Paroxysmal hypertension

a. Phaeochromocytoma

Causes of persistent hypertension

1. Renal diseases

a. Chronic nephritis
b. Chronic pyelonephritis
c. Congenital polycystic kidney
d. Diabetic Kimmelstiel-Wilson disease
e. Post-toxaemic hypertension
f. Renal tumours

2. Involvement of renal vessels

a. Renal artery stenosis
b. Collagen disorders, polyarteritis nodosa, DLE, scleroderma

3. Endocrine disorders

a. Cushing's syndrome
b. Adrenocortical tumors
c. Acromegaly
d. Phaeochromocytoma
e. Thyrotoxicosis
f. Conn's syndrome
g. Hyperparathyroidism

4. Miscellaneous

a. Coarctation of aorta
b. Adverse reaction to drugs e.g. oral contraceptives corticosteroids, ACTH, sympathomimetic amines.

Of all the impressively large number of diseases which produce hypertension these account for not more than 10-15 per cent of all cases of hypertension while the rest basically belong to primary or essential hypertension.

Etiology of essential hypertension. A number of risk factors like body built, heredity, race, sex, obesity, hormonal and emotional disturbances etc. are known to play their role in the causation of hypertension.

Heredity. Heredity has been incriminated in the causation of hypertension though no distinctive gene markers are available. One concept is that

hypertension is transmitted by a single dominant gene, an individual who inherits a dominant gene from one parent and a recessive gene from the other parent would develop hypertension while those who received dominant genes from both parents would certainly develop hypertension and that too in severe form. The other concept is that hypertension is inherited on a multifactorial basis i.e. there are a large number of different genes and one of their phenotype expressions is hyprtension.

Role of heredity is significant in more than 70 per cent of the patients suffering from essential hypertension. High blood pressure tends to run in families. Blood pressure levels tend to be higher at all ages in the first degree relatives of all persons with essential hypertension. Almost all patients with hypertension are the descendents of one or more grand parents or great grand parents who had this disease. There is very strong history of deaths due to cardiac diseases in such families. Figures of hypertension are three times as frequent among siblings of hypertensives as compared to those with normal blood pressure. Siblings of hypertensives inherit a defect in renal excretion of sodium in the transport of sodium across the cell membrane. Thus children of hypertensive parents have a fall in sodium excretion as compared to children of normotensive parents indirectly suggesting a relationship of the genetic influence on renal sodium excretion via sympathetic system.

Factors in the aetiology of hypertension
1. Heredity
2. Age
3. Sex
4. Race and environment
5. Obesity
6. Emotional factors
7. Constitution
8. Physical activity
9. Salt intake
10. Smoking
11. Alcohol
12. Neurogenic and humoral factors

Age. Blood pressure levels rise with age and 40 to 60 per cent of people beyond the age of 50 have got raised levels. Rise may be mainly in systolic levels and it is more so in people above the age of 60. Compared to people in urbanized societies there are certain communities living in New Guinea Bahámas, Panama and some pacific islands where blood pressure does not rise with age. This contradicts the theory of aging.

Sex. High blood pressure is slightly more common in females as compared to men for that age group yet women stand the pressure levels better than men and morbidity of the disease is much less. There is an observation that men of upper strata of society and women from lower socioeconomic group are more prone to the development of high blood pressure.

Women on oral contraceptives are likely to develop hypertension. In such women number of factors like sodium retention due to oestrogen activity with resultant fluid retention, increased blood volume and cardiac output are associated.

Race and environment. There is no doubt that people in more affluent and industralized societies suffer from a higher incidence of hypertension. The phenomenon of hypertension is global. People who migrate from less industralized societies to industralized one, develop hypertension sub-sequently. Certain communities like Africans, Negroes, Chinese, Red Indians and Puerto ricans have rather less incidence of high blood pressure amongst them but in the same people when they migrated to more urbanized societies, the incidence went up. Observations on British men blood pressure levels have shown that their levels were strongly influenced by where they lived for most of their lives then by where they were born and brought up.

Similarly urban populations have high blood pressure readings as compared to neighbouring rural population. Migration from rural areas to urban areas in the same country has been associated with rise in blood pressure levels. These factors are proobably due to accelerated environmental changes, urbanization and rapid cultural, social, emotional or ococupational stress.

Obesity. There is more than a casual relationship between obesity and high blood pressure. Obese are more prone to suffer from hypertension since not only they carry extra load of fat but also have insulin resistance, high levels of lipids and glucose which are all interconnected. Blood pressure levels tend to be highest in those with central or upper body obesity. Sustained hypertension develops in those who are over weight at a rate two and one half times compared to those not overweight. In fact in obese people hypertension may be a compensatory effect to meet the increased burden on the heart which may not keep pace in size and weight with the growth of the body.

Emotional factors. Emotional stress has a great role to play in the causation of hypertension and this action is mediated by autonomic nervous system stimulation with resultant release of norepinephrine. Long continued and sustained emotional stress especially due to anger, fear or resentment brings about a rise in blood pressure. Again it has been observed that people with subnormal assertiveness, suppressed hostility, aggressiveness and obsessive compulsive traits are more liable to suffer from hypertension.

Emotional disturbances like fear, anxiety and certain psychological traumas may sometimes serve as initiating factors in the development of hypertension.

Constitution. High blood pressure is by large more common in people who are short, stocky and have ruddy complexions. This does not mean that only such type of people are affected. In fact constitution of this type and obesity go side by side, hence this inferance. A number of hypertensives may be either of thin lean or normal built.

Salt intake. Role of salt intake in the causation of hypertension is significant. It has been well accepted that hypertension and its complications are greater in societies which habitually consume higher amount of sodium in their diet. Societies where intake of dietary salt is less with low incidence of age related increases in blood pressure are often more of primitive and isolated one. The average consumption of sodium upto 250 mg or less per day along with adequate quantities of potassium and calcium in the diet is ideal and safe from predisposing to hypertension. But most of the people take much more quantity of sodium in their diet. Though correlation between sodium intake and blood pressure levels is significant yet salt restriction role in lowering blood pressure levels is not universal among all individuals. Younger subjects appear to have less changes in blod pressure levels with the manipulation of salt balance than elderly subjects. At initial stages salt restriction may be helpful but once hypertension is established, alterations in salt intake has its own limitations.

Physical activity. Lack of physical activity and leading a sedentary life are important factors in the development of hypertension. Leading an active life combined with diet control and weight reduction shall go a long way in prevention of hypertension.

Exercise need not be strenous but, what shall matter is the regularity. Those who adopt more of a couch potato. Syndrome culture i.e watching T.V. slouched up in bed or chair most of the time and those who do not take active part in vigorous sports have greater risk of developing hypertension.

Smoking. Smoking in either form (cigarette, bidis, hooka, cigars) is injurious and predisposes to the development of hypertension probably through the nicotine induced release of norepinephrine from adrenergic nerve endings.

Alcohol. Excessive ingestion of alcohol and its related forms by its pressor effects, increases the cardiac output and heart rate possibly because of increased sympathetic activity and raises blood pressure levels. Even in small quantity alcohol raises blood pressure levels and in large quantity it may be responsible for hypertension in significant number of cases. A linear relationship irrespective of other factors has been observed between blood pressure and amount of alcohol consumed.

Neurogenic and humoral factors. Increased sympathetic activity is suspected to be of significance in causing rise in blood pressure. Beta sympathetic activity increases plasma renin levels and cardiac output while alpha sympathetic activity increases peripheral resistance. This is one aspect to explain hypertension while humoral mechanism is supported by a number of substances which are known to account for hypertension in experimental studies (renin-angiotensin system). Renin, an enzymatic substance formed in juxtaglomerular cells of the kidney which is stimulated by changes in blood pressure, is released into the blood stream, it acts on circulating alpha globulin called Angiotensingen to form angiotensin I which is further converted to angiotensin II by an enzyme located in the vascular beds of lungs, kidneys, testes and brain. Angiotensin II exerts a powerful vasoconstrictor act by its direct action on peripheral blood vessels. In addition it stimulates the secretion of aldosterone which effects the reabosrption of sodium by the renal tubules and thus fluid retention.

High plasma renin activity is an important factor in 5-10 per cent cases of essential hypertension especially young hypertensive.

Apart from role of kidney in renin-angiotensin pathway deficient production of renal vasodilator substances (bradykinin or prostaglandin) is another factor in the aetiology of hypertension.

Pathology. Main pathological changes in hypertension are born by the heart and peripheral blood vessels. In early stages cardiac output is normal and as the blood pressure levels rise, peripheral arterial resistance increases. This leads to thickening of wall of small arteries, arteriolar narrowing and development of atheroma in coronary, cerebral and renal vessels and other larger vessels. As hypertension advances, impairment of renal blood flow and renal functions develops. The work of the heart increases in proportion to peripheral vascular resistance and this increased load on the heart leads to cardiac dilatation and hypertrophy. Reduction in renal perfusion with decreased glomerular filtration and deficiency in renal excretion of sodium and water shall predispose to development of congestive heart failure. Most cases of hypertension if untreated progress to left ventricular failure, cerebral haemorrhage, myocardial infarction, malignant hypertension and renal failure.

Clinical picture. Mild cases of hypertension are asympatomatic and hypertension in majority of people is detected accidentally on routine medical check up or physical examination for an insurance policy. Symptoms when present may be manifold like headache (severe, throbbing) giddiness palpitation, tiredness and ringing noises in the ears. Many persons unaware of their disease may present with bleeding from the nose which may be early signal warning that they suffer from raised blood pressure. A few patients may present with involvement of target organs and present either with congestive heart failure. Stroke, cerebral haemorrhage, myocardial infarction and even kidney failure. High blood pressure produces definite harmful effects as regards the frequency and extent of atherosclerosis. The incidence of coronary heart disease is very high in hypertensives.

Physical examination in early stages shows heart size to be within normal limits. Later on as heart enlarges, left ventricular hypertrophy is suggested by a forceful, heaving apical impulse, second aortic sound is loud and acentuated. Murmurs are usually absent but a systolic murmur due to functional mitral insufficiency may be heard. Pulse is good and bounding. A gallop rhythm may be heard at lower end of sternum indicating left heart failure. Blood pressure is persistently elevated.

Secondary hypertension will have different clinical picture depending on the underlying disease. Coarctation of aorta will have hypertension in the upper limbs and feeble femoral pulses with radiofemoral delay.

Clinical profile of a hypertensive

1. Symptoms of headache (throbbing), palpitaiton, giddiness, tiredness and ringing noises in the ears.
2. Presentation with stroke, myocardial infarction, cerebral haemorrhage and kidney failure and symptoms referable to these systems.
3. In early stages heart within normal limits. Later on heart enlarges. Forceful heaving apical impulse, second aortic sound is loud and accentuated. Mitral systolic murmur due to functional mitral insufficiency. Gallop rhythm at lower end of sternum indicating early left heart failure.

Kidney disease may be in the form of acute nephritis (hypertension, oliguria and peripheral oedema) chronic glomerulonephritis (hypertension, renal failure). Chronic pyelonephritis (recurrent urinary tract infection). Polycystic disease of kidney (bilateral renal masses palpable). Diabetic nephropathy (diabetes, hypertension, oedema over legs and feet) collagen disorders (evidence of collagen disorders like pigmentation over face (DLE) changes in skin (scleroderma). Renal artery stenosis (presence of bruite over the abdomen lateral to the umbilicus or over the renal arteries). Of the endocrinal causes, cushings syndrome has a striking moon shaped face, hirsutism in females, obesity and purplish striae over the abdomen in addition to hypertension.

Adrenogenital syndrome has precocious puberty, acne, deepening of voice and accelerated musculo skeletal development, while cases of Conn's syndrome (primary hyperaldosteronism) have severe form of hypertension, parasthesia, headache, polyuria and polydypsia, muscular weakness and severe degree of hypokalemia.

In phaeochromocytoma, hypertension is either paroxysmal or episodic in nature and patient may present with headache, palpitation, sweating and flushing. In early stages hypertension is paroxysmal but later on it becomes established.

Physical examination in all cases due to secondary form of hypertension shall vary depending on the nature of underlying disease and some cases may be having features of cardiac decompensation or complications.

Progress of a case of hypertension. The precise level of blood pressure is not necessarily the most important criteria of severity of the disease. This is basically assessed by assessing cardiac, renal function and state of the changes in optic fundus.

A case of mild hypertension and those with blood pressure levels under contral with drugs carry good prognosis. Cases with malignant hypertension, hypertensive encephalopathy cardiac failure, cerebrovascular accidents, coronary heart disease and renal failure carry poor prognosis. 60 per cent of cases of hypertension die from cardiac failure and associated cardiac complications, 30-35 per cent from cerebrovascular accidents and 5-10 per cent from renal failure. Severity of hypertension and its prognosis has been graded as follows:

Grade I Fundus grade I, no cardiac renal or cerebral complications. Slight to no symptoms. B.P. range 150-200 mm systolic 100 mm diastolic.

Grade II Fundus grade II, III but no cardiac, renal or cerebral complications. Symptoms are little like headache, giddiness. Urine shows albuminuria, blood pressure from 180-220 systolic, 100-120 mm diastolic.

Grade III Fundus grade II, III. Frequent headaches, fatigue, dysponea, B.P. ranges systolic 150-280 mmHg. Diastolic 120-140 mmHg. Cerebral, cardiac or renal complications may be present.

Grade IV Symptoms like severe Headaches, confusion, vertigo. Breathlessness are common. Fundus grade IV, cardiac, cerebral or renal complications. B.P. ranges systolic 240-280 mmHg and diastolic levels above 140 mmHg.

Based on the above, cases of hypertension with grade III and grade IV carry poor prognosis and mortality in this group ranges from 75-90 per cent.

Complications. Hypertension involves target organs in the body and a number of serious complications develop.

Cardiac. Left ventricular failure and congestive heart failure are important complications. Coronary heart disease is more common in hypertensives since process of atherosclerosis is being accelerated. It

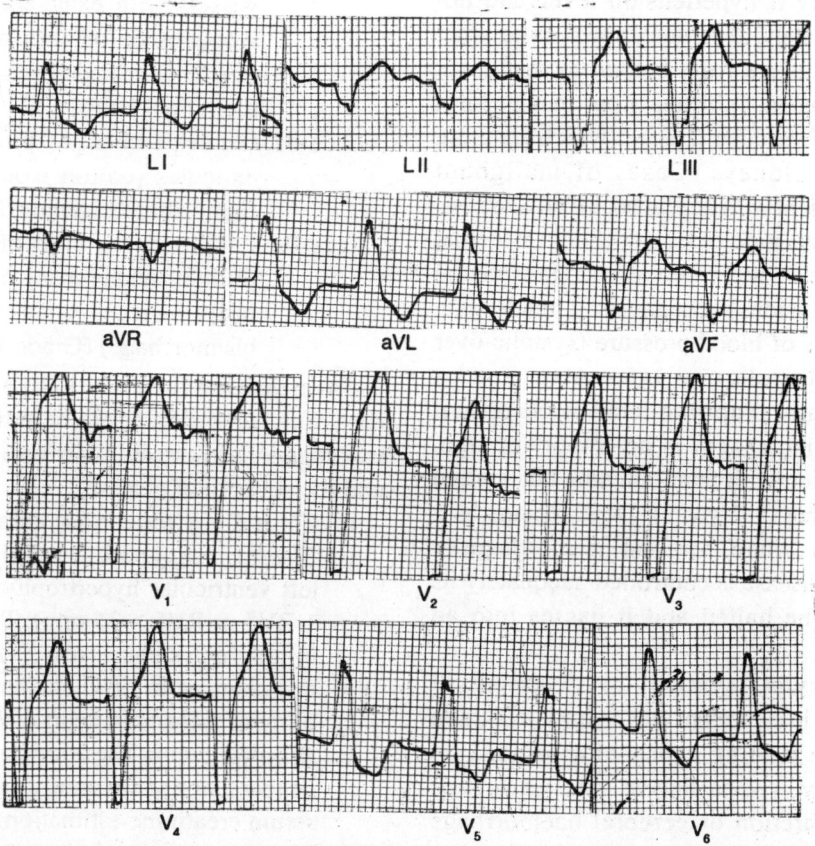

Fig. 4.29. Left Bundle Branch Block. A case of hypertension may show this pattern. A wide notched R wave with depressed ST segment and T wave inversion is seen in L I, aVL, V$_5$ - V$_6$. QRS duration is prolonged to 0.12 secs and VAT 0.1 secs.

may be in the form of angina pectoris, myocardial infarction and even sudden death.

Hypertensive encephalopathy is a serious complication and is due to rapid rise of blood pressure to very high and dangerous levels. Patient complains of severe throbbing headache, nausea, vomiting, giddiness, visual disturbances, convulsions, parasthesia, paresis and loss of consciousness. Hypertensive encelphalopathy develops more in cases of malignant hypertension and there is spasm of cerebral arteries with cerebral oedema and ischaemia. Most of the neurological disturbances are as a result of sudden rise in blood pressure levels. Lowering of blood pressure reverts the attack provided there is no irreversible damage.

Malignant hypertension is serious entity which develops in any patient with severe hypertensive disease especially if hypertension levels are not controlled adequately. It is not known as to what determines the change from benign to malignant form of hypertension. It differs from benign form in the intensity of vascular changes which are more marked in the kidneys. Cases of malignant hypertension present with headache, breathlessness, visual impairment, giddiness, dependent oedema, hematuria, epistaxis and cerebral changes (mental confusion, convulsions). Diagnosis is made with accelerated levels of blood pressure (systolic over 220 mmHg and diastolic over 140 mmHg). Fundus grade IV changes. Papilloedema with retinal exudates or haemorrhages is an important sign. Rapid deterioration with fatal outcome takes place within a short time (1-2 years). Death occurs as a result of cardiac failure, cerebral haemorrhage or renal failure. If disease is controlled adequately its onslaught may be halted and it passes into an inactive phase.

Central nervous system. Involvement of cerebral arteries in hypertensives is quite common and strokes are leading cause of morbidity in hypertensives. Involvement may be either as cerebral thrombosis. Infarction or cerebral haemorrhage which carries poor prognosis.

Renal. Arteriolar degeneration is more severe in renal vessels leading to renal ischaemia and subsequent impairment of renal functions. Earliest evidence of renal involvement is the presence of albuminuria and renal functions show diminished tubular concentrating power. Rise in blood urea may take long time to appear. With deterioration of renal functions, renal failure develops rapidly.

Retina. Vascular lesions secondary to hypertension may be responsible for haziness of vision, progressive deterioration of vision or sudden loss of vision. Examination of the fundi gives useful information about the severity of hypertension and a correct assessment is made. The changes in fundi are graded as follows (Keith-Wagener criteria).

Grade I Mild narrowing or sclerosis of the retinal arteries and increased reflectiveness (Silver wiring).

Grade II Moderate to marked narrowing of vessels with exaggerated light reflex. Appearance of arteriovenous nipping due to crossing of retinal arteries over the retinal veins.

Grade III Grade II changes plus soft to fluffy exudates (cotton wool exudates) and flame shaped haemorrhages.

Grade IV Papilloedema or choking of the disc (bulging and blurring of the edges of the optic disc) with exudates and haemorrhage) (Grade III).

Investigations of a case of hypertension. Every case of hypertension has to be submitted to certain investigations to assess involvement of target organs and the severity of disease.

a. *Chest X-ray* for cardiac enlargement.

b. *Electrocardiogram.* It is helpful in assessing left ventricular hypertrophy and strain (SV1 + RV5 or RV6 > 35 mm). T wave inversions in left ventricular leads. Evidence of ischaemic changes in ECG shall suggest the possibility of ischaemic heart disease.

c. *Renal functions.* These are assessed by urinalysis (presence of albumin, casts) blood urea and serum creatinine estimation.

d. Blood sugar to exclude associated diabetes.

Serum cholesterol and complete lipidogram to assess cardiovascular risk factors.

In addition to the above, in young hypertensives further investigations have to be done to exclude any operative cause responsible for the disease. Tests for renal pathology shall include urine analysis for evidence of bacteria. Urine culture and testing sensitivity of the organism to various antibiotics. Presence of hyaline and granular casts shall suggest chronic nephritis. In addition finding of low fixed specific gravity of urine will be further pointer. Plain X-ray abdomen (for renal stones) intravenous pyelogram (to assess kidney size, its architecture, and functions). Ultrasound of abdomen. Blood urea and creatinine levels when elevated mean advanced renal pathology. For renal artery stenosis, differential renal function tests and aortography is indicated.

In suspected coarctation of aorta, aortography or MRI will demonstrate the lesion. For cases where endocrinal causes are suspected like phaeo-chromocytoma, measurement of serum or urinary catecholamines metabolites (VMA), regitine test, MRI are required. Plasma cortisol levels and plasma aldosterone assay are needed to support the diagnosis of Cushing's syndrome and primary aldosteronism.

In fact every cases of hypertension especially secondary hypertension should have relevant investigations performed to diagnose the aetiological factor.

Management. Every case of hypertension should be treated since persistently raised levels of blood pressure are going to produce deleterious effects on the various organs of the body and reduce the rate of survival. Depending on the levels of blood pressure, treatment shall vary. Any body with diastolic blood pressure levels above 100 mmHg must receive treatment. In young hypertensives efforts be made to locate the cause and treat it since a treatable cause shall improve the morbidity of disease. Attempt be made to bring down blood pressure levels to near normal levels and maintain them. In fact treatment of hypertension should start early in life. People who are likely to fall more prone to get hypertension later on life include siblings and children of hypertensive patients, persons with a high normal blood pressure levels, and children of parents who suffer from coronary heart disease,

diabetes, stroke and hypertension with strong family history. In all such people, change in life style must be ensured from very young age so that they do not fall prey to the disease. Management of a case of hypertension shall be:

1. General measures
2. Drug therapy

General measures. All hypertensives who are suffering from borderline hypertension or mild early cases, genernal measures may be adopted and these may successfully bring down the blood pressure levels without drug therapy. Otherwise also general measures shall help in reducing blood pressure in established cases to some extent.

1. Weight reduction especially in obese must be enforced. For this weight control diet be advised.
2. Salt in the diet be restricted. Extra salt in the food must be completely banned.
3. Regular exercise is advised in all patients. Patient be advised to lead an active physical life. Strenous exercises are not to be advised (Isometric exercises) since these put a strain on the cardiovascular system. Mild exercises (isotonic) like walking, swimming are advised.
4. Patient must have adequate periods of rest and sleep. Tension and stress be avoided. This can be achieved by various behavioural modification therapies like yoga transcendental meditation and biofeed back and relaxation techniques.
5. Excessive use of alcohol and its related products must be restricted. Smoking has to be avoided.

Drug therapy. All patients of hypertension where blood pressure levels are persistently raised have to have drug therapy for its adequate control. A number of drugs are available and type of drug to be employed shall depend on number of factors. Treatment in every case is individualised.

For mild hypertensives: treatment is usually started with a diuretic or a beta blocker or a calcium channel blocker. For severe forms of hypertension a combination of two drugs is required. It is called a stepped care programme. Common drugs used for treatment of hypertension are:

Diuretics. These cause slight fall in blood pressure and are effective in mild and early cases. They not only inhibit reabsorption of sodium but also increase cardiac output and decrease peripheral vascular resistance. Since they have got week antihypertensive effect, combined treatment with other drugs potentiates their blood pressure lowering effects.

Commonly used diuretics are hydrochlorthiazide 100 mg per day, Chlorthalidone 50-100 mg per day. These reduce potasium levels in body resulting in hypokalemia. Potassium supplements have to be given in people on long term diuretic therapy.

Potassium sparing diuretics (Spironolactone 25 mg thrice a day: Amiloride 5 mg per day) are weak diuretics, mild antihypertensives and are mainly used in combination with other diuretics.

Beta-adrenergic blocking drugs. These are now the most forequently used drugs next to diuretics. They decrease heart rate, force of contraction and cardiac output lowering arterial pressure when there is increased cardiac sympathetic nerve activity. In addition their action is by blocking adrenergic nerve mediated release of renin. Beta-adrenergic receptors are of two types—Beta-1 (receptors located in heart and kidneys) and Beta-2 (receptors in bronchial tree and blood vessels). Based on this we have non-selective beta blocking agents acting on both beta-1 and beta-2 receptors (e.g. propranolol) and one which are cardioselective acting mainly on beta 1 receptors (metoprolol: atenolol: acebutolol). Non-selective beta blockers may possess both membrane stabilising and intrinsic sympathetic activity thus drug having only membrane stabilising action is Propranolol while that with intrinsic sympathetic activity shall be Pindolol.

Propranolol was used extensively as an effective antihypertensive drug (dose 40-160 mg) per day in divided doses. Side effects include bradycardia, tiredness, G.I. upset.

Cardioselective beta blockers are preferred when patient has diabetes, or bronchospasm. Metroprolol (100-200 mg) in divided doses.

Atenolol (50-100 mg) per day.
Acebutolol (400-800 mg) per day in divided doses.

All the beta-blockers produce some degree of bradycardia and are contraindicated in the presence of cardiogenic shock, heart block, congestive heart failure and are to be used with caution in cases of diabetes, bronchial asthma and reduced cardiac reserve.

Pindolol, a potent B-blocker with prominent intrinsic sympathomimetic activity has been used in patients who develop bradycardia due to propranolol. Dosage 10-30 mg per day in divided doses. Again it is not to be used in the presence of A-V heart block, bradycardia, bronchial asthma and cardiac failure. There is chance of rebound hypertension on withdrwal of the drug.

Calcium channel blocking drugs. These are effective anti-hypertensive in addition to being anti-anginal drugs. They reduce blood pressure by increasing myocardial oxygen supply, increase in coronary blood flow and exert a potent vasodilator effect on peripheral blood vessels to lower both systolic and diastolic blood pressure levels. Commonly used drugs in this group are:

1. *Nifedipine.* Dosage 10-20 mg twice a day. Side effects include headache, dizziness, flushing, peripheral oedema palpitation and nasal stuffiness. Drug is contraindicated in acute myocardial infarction, cardiogenic shock, pregnancy and be used with caution in diabetics and those with oedema. Some patients may develop increased attacks of angina at the time of starting the drug.

2. *Felodipine* suitable for mild to moderate hypertension. More effective when used in combination with B-blocker. Dose 5-10 mg per day.

3. *Nitrendipine.* Long-acting second generation calcium channel blocker useful in mild to moderate hypertension. Dose 10-20 mg per day once daily in morning. Side effects include headache, flushing, oedema, palpitation.

4. *Amlodipine.* It is a dihydropyridine calcium channel blocker whose therapeutic effect is

being mediated by peripheral and coronary vasodilatation, increasing cardiac output, decreasing peripheral vascular resistance and thus lowering mean arteral pressure. Dose 5-10 mg once a day. It is an effective and safe antihypertensive. Side effects include headache, flushing, oedema, lethargy, fatigue, palpitation and somnolence.

5. *Diltiazem.* It is a weak antihypertensive but is effective antianginal. Dose 30 mg two-three times a day. Not recommended in bradycardia, heart block.

6. *Verapamil.* It is more effective antiarrhythmic agent than antihypertensive though this effect stems from a decrease in peripheral vascular resistance. Dose 40-80 mg three times a day. Drug is contraindicated in cardiovascular shock, conduction disorders and in left heart failure.

Alpha-1-adrenergic blockers. These are balanced vasodilators producing reduction in peripheral vascular resistance and thus are effective in lowering blood pressure. Cardiovascular reflexes are not impaired by their use. Side effects include postural hypotension, drowsiness, headache, marked weakness.

Prazosin is the commonly used drug in this group. Dose 0.5 mg thrice daily increasing to 1 mg 2-3 times daily. Anti-hypertensive effect is enhanced if the patient is already on diuretic therapy. Because of resultant postural hypotension, use of this drug in hypertension is limited.

ACE inhibitors. Angiotensin converting enzyme inhibitors function by competetive inhibition of angiotensin II and making angiotoensin inactive and thus paralysing renin-angiotensin system. The drug has a vasodilator effect lowering the systemic vascular resistance and blocking the degradation of bradykinin down grading the adrenergic activity and resultant lowering of blood pressure. Ace inhibitors do not increase heart rate and thus are ideal in the presence of congestive heart failure accompanying hypertension. They are indicated in all grades of essential hypertension, renovascular hypertension but are contraindicated in aortic stenosis, outflow obstruction, and renal artery stenosis. Side effects include dry cough, headache, dizziness, fatigue, angioneurotic oedema, hypotoension and sometimes temporary exaggeration of renal failure. Common drugs in this group are:

1. Enalapril maleate. Dose 5 mg once a day. Maximum 40 mg once a day.
2. Lisinopril. Start with 5-10 mg once a day and gradually increase but not more than 20-40 mg per day.
3. Captopril. It is used generally in combination with a diuretic or a beta blocker. It is considered safe in asthmatics and diabetics. Effective in hypertension resistant to other drugs. Dose 25 mg three times a day gradually increasing to 100 mg three times a day.
4. Ramipril. It is a long acting ACE inhibitor reduces both supine and standing blood pressure without significant alterations in pulse rate. Dose 2.5 mg daily. Maximum 10 mg per day. Side effects include light headedness, fatigue, constipation and urticaria.

A. Angiotenen II Receptor Blockers

These include losartan, irbesartan, telmisartan and eposartan. These drugs are less potent than ace inhibitors in reducing blood pressure but improve cardiovascular outcome in patients of hypertension associated with heart failure and type 2 diabetes with nephropathy.

Losartan potasium. It is an angiotensin II receptor (type AT1) antagonist and blocks the vasoconstrictive and aldosterone secreting effects of angiotensin II by its selective blockade. It is effective in mild to moderate hypertension alone or in combination with other antihypertensives. It should not be used along with potassium sparing diuretics. Dose 25-100 mg once or twice a day. Maintenance dose 50 mg a day. Side effects include headache, dizziness, diarrhoea, myalgia, oedema.

Other drugs in this group include irbesartan (Dose 150 mg once or twice a day) Telmisartan (dose 40 mg once daily). Side effects include hyperkalemia, renal dysfunction, angioedema etc.

B. Other antihypertensive drugs:

1. Methyldopa. It is a moderately effective anti-

hypertensive which decreases total peripheral resistance with little effect on cardiac output. It acts centrally to reduce sympathetic outflow. Dose 250-500 mg given orally four times a day. Adverse side effects include dry mouth, fluid retention, nasal congestion, postural hypotension, hepatitis, lethargy and reduced mental activity.

2. Reserpine. One of the earliest used antihypertensive drug. It is an alkaloid derived from the roots of Rauwolfia serpentina (Sarpgandha). It is a mild antihypertensive which acts both by central and peripheral mechanisms, and acts slowly taking 2-3 weeks to produce full effect. Dosage 0.1 to 0.5 mg orally daily. Side effects include nasal stuffiness, depression, weight gain, postural hypotension, parkinsonism and suicidal tendencies.

3. Hydralazine. It is a direct acting arteriolar vaso dilator thus reducing total peripheral vascular resistance. It causes greater reduction of diastolic than systolic B.P., produces reflex tachycardia and increases renal and coronary blood flow. Mainly indicated in moderate to severe hypertension not controlled by first line of drugs. Dose 25-50 mg once to thrice a day. Side effects include facial flushing, headache, dizziness, muscle cramps, oedema, palpitation.

4. Sodium nitroprusside. It is a rapidly acting vasodilator with a brief duration of action. It rapidly lowers blood pressure and is mainly indicated for the treatment of hypertensive emergencies. Its mode of action is by reducing total peripheral resistance as well as cardiac output by reducing venous return. Dosage is 50 mg dry powder freshly dissolved and added to 500 5% glucose and infused intravenously at rate of 0.1 mg/minute and titrated upwards with the response. Once the desired result is achieved the drug is withdrawn. Side effects include severe hypotension, palpitation, nausea, vomiting, weakness and psychiatric disturbances.

Principles of anti-hypertensive therapy.

Every case of hypertension has to be individualized. A mild case of hypertension initially should be treated with a diuretic and if not controlled then drugs like Atenol or Nifedipine or Amlodipine be added. Mild to moderate hypertension will be controlled by any of the above drugs or ACE inhibitors especially when complicated by diabetes, congestive failure or renal impairment.

Severe hypertension may require use of these drugs including a peripheral vasodilator like hydralazine. The basic aim of therapy should be to achieve ideal or near normal control of blood pressure levels and these levels should be main-tained. Uncontrolled blood pressure is likely to involve target organs and increase morbidity as well as mortality.

Treatment of hypertensive encephalopathy.

Hospitalise the patient. Sedate with diazepam (10 mg I/M). Lower blood pressure with injection serpasil 1 mg I/M stat and to be repeated as required. Injection Lasix 80-120 mg I/V to relieve pulmonary oedema. O2 inhalations. Once acute emergency is controlled, patient is to be evaluated and appropriate oral anti hypertensive drugs prescribed.

Prognosis in a case of hypertension shall depend on:

1. Co-existing coronary heart disease.
2. Aetiological factors like renal disease, diabetes.
3. Control of blood pressure whether adequate or not.
4. Presence of complications like retinopathy, left heart failure and renal dysfunction.

Patients who maintain adequate control of blood pressure by drugs, change in life style, avoidance of smoking, control in weight, and lead an active physical life carry good prognosis and have reduced chances of developing complications like stroke, myocardial infarction and congestive failure.

CORONARY HEART DISEASE

Coronary heart disease is one of the most common causes of death and cardiac morbidity in middle and elderly age groups. It involves men more as compared to women before menopause and the incidence is almost same both in men and women after menopause. It strikes men at the prime of life when they are needed most. Though the disease is more common in affluent societies yet people in poor social working class are equally at risk. The exact cause of coronary heart disease is not very clear but a number of factors, preventable and non-preventable are known to play their role.

Risk factors of coronary heart disease

1. **Non-modifiable risk factors**
   a. Age and sex
   b. Genetic predisposition
   c. Personality
2. **Modifiable risk factors**
   a. Blood lipids
   b. Smoking
   c. Hypertension
   d. Diet
   e. Diabetes mellitus
   f. Obesity
   g. Physical activity
3. **Miscellaneous**
   a. Emotions
   b. Soft water
   c. Trace elements

Non-modifiable risk factors:

Age and sex. As age advances atherosclerosis progressively develops and in fact more than 90 per cent of cases of coronary artery disease are due to atherosclerosis which may even start at an early age.

Women before menopause are almost protected against coronary artery disease because of protective effect of female hormones and this protection goes away after menopause sets in.

Men are more prone to suffer from coronary artery disease as they have no natural protection.

Genetic predisposition to coronary artery disease is revealed by several members of the family suffering from it. Presence of a positive family history of sudden death, myocardial infarction, angina or cerebrovascular accidents points to the genetic predisposition.

Personality. Coronary artery disease is more prevalent in type A personality which is characterized by traits of aggressiveness, ambition and competetiveness. These people are over ambitious, workacholics and always striving to reach the top. Patients with type A personality are more prone to suffer from the disease as compared to people with type B personality (converse of type A, more relaxed and sedate).

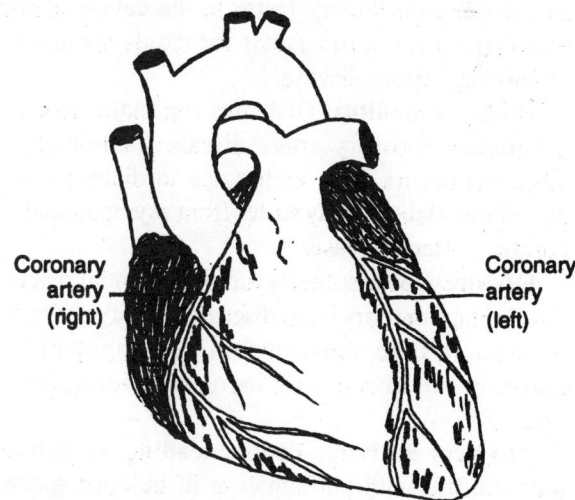

Coronary artery (right)

Coronary artery (left)

Fig. 4.30. Diagram of heart showing the coronary arteries.

Modifiable risk factors:

Blood lipids. There is a direct relationship between coronary artery disease and levels of circulating lipids, and amongst them high levels of cholesterol, low levels of high density lipoproteins (HDL) are definately associated with atherosclerosis as compared to high levels of triglycerides. Lipids circulate in the blood in the form of lipoproteins i.e. alpha lipoproteins (high density lipoprotein HDL) beta lipoprotein (low density lipoproteins LDL) and pre beta lipo proteins (very low density VLDL). HDL is good cholesterol and its rise favours protection while LDLis a bad cholesterol and favours atherosclerosis. Lowering of cholesterol by diet, change in life style and by drugs lowers the risk of coronary artery disease.

Smoking. Smoking in any form is associated with increased risk of developing coronary artery disease and this is because of nicotine and carbon monoxide present in smoke. More the number of cigarettes smoked more is the risk of developing disease.

Hypertension. Elevated blood pressure levels both systolic and diastolic increase the risk of coronary artery disease as well as progression of atheroma.

Diet. A diet rich in total calories, total and saturateed fats, refined sugar and cholesterol acts as a major contributory factor in the development of atheroma and a risk factor for the development of coronary artery disease.

Diabetes mellitus. Diabetics run major risk of developing coronary artery disease. Pathological atheroma occurs at an earlier age in diabetes and patients of diabetes may suffer from asympatomatic coronary artery disease.

Obesity. Obese subjects run the potential risk of developing coronary heart disease. Obesity not only impairs cardiac function but development of coronary atherosclerosis increases mortality in obese.

Physical activity. People leading an active physical life with participation in outdoor sports have less chance of developing coronary disease as compared to people who lead a sedentary life. Exercise and physical activity have a protective effect against developing the coronary disease.

Other risk factors. Industralization and urbanization have brought their own ills. Rapid transition from primitive to westernized mode of life makes the community more prone to heart disease. Emotional factors like prolonged stress, anxiety gout, oral contraceptives and use of soft water (low in calcium and magnesium salts) makes the incidence of coronary artery disease on the higher side as compared to those using hard water. Lack of trace elements like chromium as well as antioxidant vitaminis (Vit.C, E and A) is also known to have some role.

To sum up, of the various risk factors, a lot shall depend on the individual since, in some, hereditary and genetic factors may play main role while, in others, host of other factors shall play their part. Overall changes in lifestyle may prevent the onslaught of disease.

Hyperhomocysteinemia has also been proved to be an independent risk factor in the causation of coronary heart disease though its exact role is still not conclusively proved. Plasma homocysteine is a graded risk factor for the incidence of myocardial infarction and stroke and persons with hyperhomocysteinemia benefit from increased folate intake by dietary means or by use of vitamin supplements.

Pathology. Coronary heart disease is the result of generalized atheroma and involvement of coronary arteries leading to myocardial changes indicative of myocardial ischaemia. Myocardial ischaemia results when there is imbalance between myocardial oxygen demand and supply. Because of atherosclerosis there is plaque formation in the intimal and subintimal regions of the arteries, with haemorrhage into the atherosclerotic patch, ulceration and formation of thrombi leading to coronary stenosis. Occlusion of coronary artery may result due to sluggish blood flow, endothelial injury, platelet aggregation and occlusive thrombi from complicated atherosclerotic plaques as a result of fissuring, ulceration, haemorrhage or rupture.

Damage to the myocardium due to sudden coronary occlusion shall be differnt than the chronic ischaemic process, when anastomotic channels may form in the distribution of the coronary artery involved. Myocardial infarction is the result of sudden occlusion of a coronary artery resulting in acute ischaemia and myocardial necrosis.

Clinical presentations of coronary heart disease

1. Angina pectoris
2. Acute myocardial infarction
3. Sudden cardiac death
4. Chronic ischaemic heart disease
5. Coronary disease presenting with complications like acute left heart failure, cardiac arrhythmias, congestive failure.

Clinical presentation. Coronary heart disease may present in various forms and these are:

1. Angina pectoris
2. Acute myocardial infarction
3. Sudden cardiac death.
4. Chronic ischaemic heart disease

5. Coronary heart disease presenting with complications like Acute left heart failure, cardiac arrhythmias and congestive failure.

ANGINA PECTORIS. It is a symptom complex characterized by substernal discomfort, pain or oppression produced by reversible myocardial ischaemia. Classically patient has pain situated in retrosternal region, radiating to precordium inner side of left arm, shoulder and to back. Pain may be mild, severe but often choking or crushing type brought about by exertion, after a heavy meal and walking in cold weather, accompanied by sweating, uneasiness and fear. This pain is relieved by rest or by use of nitrates.

Forms of angina pectoris

1. Decubitus angina
2. Nocturnal angina
3. Prinzmetal's angina
4. Intractable angina
5. Unstable angina

Attacks of anginal pain are of short duration and location of pain is often variable. Many people have only discomfort located to the arms, others may have pain in the jaw or pain located to right arm. Commonest cause of angina is coronary atherosclerosis. Other causes include aortic stenosis, syphilitic aortitis and arterial hypoxemia.

Forms of angina. *In addition to classical form of angina pectoris other variants may be seen:*

1. Decubitus angina: Angina when patient lies down in recumbent position.
2. Nocturnal angina: It occurs at night and wakes up the patient from sleep.
3. Prinzmetal's (Variant) angina: A form of angina which occurs at rest. Electrocardiogram taken during pain produces ST segment elevation. It is produced by spasm of coronary artery.
4. Intractable angina: Repeated attacks of anginal pain occurring at frequent intervals and often make physical activity difficult.
5. Unstable angina: It includes angina which is progressively worsening and may be present at rest. Unstable angina often can be interre-

lated with intractable angina. It is more severe, brought by little physical activity, persists for longer times, and response to therapy is poor.

Physical examination. There are hardly any physical signs in a case of angina except sometimes during the attack tachycardia or bradycardia may be seen. A gallop sound may be heard during the attack.

Diagnosis. A case of angina pectoris is primarily suspected with a typical history of attacks of pain or discomfort in chest wall, radiating to the arms. Pain is squeezing choking or smothering in nature brought on by exertion and relieved by rest. Tests include electrocardiogram which is usually normal though during an attack, transient ST segment depression or elevation may be seen.

Exercise ECG. When resting ECG is normal, exercise ECG (Masters two step test and double masters test) after giving specified exercise on steps is recorded. In case, two step test is negative, then double exercise is given and records observed. S-T segment depression of 2 mm or more and T wave changesshall favour a positive test.

Treadmill test (TMT). In this procedure the extent of exercise is quantified by giving exercise on a treadmill or using bicycle ergometer. Idea is to achieve maximal or submaximal heart rate depending on the age of the patient. The stress electrocardigram shows ST segment response (amount of exercise at which these changes occur, how long they persist after exercise). Factors which interfere with the interpretation are such as bundle branch block, left ventricular hypertrophy, blood pressure response and appearance of chest discomfort.

A positive test is diagnosed when ST segment depression is 2 mm or more, Horizontal depression of ST segment of more than 0.08 seconds. J junctional depression, appearance of inverted μ wave, inversion of 'T' wave from the normal resting ECG and development of arrhythmias. TMT is not indicated in a case of unstable angina or those with a suspicion of myocardial infarction. A positive TMT shall indicate the degree of myocardial insufficiency and severity of coronary atherosclerosis.

Cardiac scintigraphy. Thallium-201 uptake test is useful when exercise test is equivocal.

Coronary angiography. It is indicated (i) when patients symptoms of angina are not very clear cut, (ii) angina is not responding to medical therapy, (iii) unstable angina, (iv) abnormal exercise ECG and (v) when surgical intervention is desired.

Cardiac enzymes. SGOT/SGPT, LDH, CPK are within normal limits.

Treatment of angina pectoris

1. General measures. Change in life style: Amount of saturated fats and cholesterol in diet to be reduced. Avoidance of over weight, active and passive smoking. Regular exercise be done. Mental tension be avoided.
2. Drug therpy
   a. Aspirin
   b. Nitrates
   c. Beta-blockers
   d. Calcium channel blockers
3. Surgical treatment
   a. Percutaneous transluminal angioplasty (PTCA)
   b. Coronary artery bypass grafting (CABG)

Management of angina pectoris:

General measures. Life style of the patient must be structured in a way that if there are coexisting diseases like diabetes and hypertension these must be adequately controlled. Amount of saturated fats in diet be redued. Weight reduction be ensured if over weight. Avoid both active and passive smoking. Regular exercise to improve the cardiac oxygen supply but strenous exercises which may provoke angina be avoided. Patient must change his life style from type A to type B personality: Situations which create tension and anxiety be avoided. Ensure adequate periods of rest and sleep.

Drug therapy:

Aspirin. Low doses of aspirin (75-150 mg) should be given in all patients. It shall reduce platelet adhesivness.

Nitrates. These are the main line of therapy. They bring relief from angina by dilating epicardial coronary vessels and increasing blood flow in coronary collateral vessels. The activity of these agents depends on their quick absorption through the mucous membrane and thus giving relief.

Commonly used drug is Isosorbide dinitrate available both as sublingual tablets (5 mg and 10 mg chewable tablets) and long acting (5,10,30 mg tablets). Whenever a patient experiences a discomfort or anginal attack on exertion, he should immediately stop activity and place a tablet of sorbitrate sublingually under the tongue. Discomfort generally disappears quickly. For patients with anginal attacks Tablet Sorbitrate one tablet (10 mg) 6 hourly orally is to be taken. Intravenous nitrates (0.6mg/hr) are used in the treatment of unstable/intractable angina.

Nitroglycerine available in ointment form is also used. Dose is 1/2 inch applied in the skin to start with and it can gradually be increased to 6 inches. Side effects of nitrates include headache, flushing tachycardia, dizziness and postural hypotension. Nitrates are also available in the form of metered dose aerosol spray (400 ug per spray) to be used as an emergency measure during the attack. If a patient of angina does not get relief immediately a second dose of nitrate may be given but if relief still does not occur in 10 minutes, evaluation for acute myocardial infarction or unstable angina be carried out.

Beta blockers. These are important drugs in the treatment of effort angina and especially useful when given along with nitrates. Beta blockers act by reducing heart rate, and force of cardiac contractility and thus reduce the myocarodial oxygen demand.

Commonly used beta blockers are propranolol (20 mg twice daily and increasing the dose gradually) Atenolol (50 to 100 mg perday) Metoprolol (50 to 100 mg twice a day). Dosage of beta blocking drugs is adjusted in a way that heart rate does not go down below 60/minute. Sudden withdrawl of the drug may precipitate either an attack of acute myocardial infarction or induce an arrhythmia.

Side effects include fatigue, depression, G.I. upset, cold extremities, heart block. These drugs can worsen bronchial asthma, intensify insulin and oral antidiabetic drugs induced hypoglycaemia and also induce left heart failure.

Calcium channel blockers. Calcium inflow into the myocardial cells is blocked by these drugs and hence its utilization with the result that coronary arteries dilate, do not go into spasm and myocardial oxygen demand is reduced.

Drugs in this group are Nifedipine (10-20 mg twice a day) verapamil (40-80 mg twice a day) Diltiazem (30 mg thrice a day). Side effects include headache, dizziness, flushing leg oedema. In some patient on Nifedipine because of tachycardia sometimes frequency of anginal attacks may increase.

Verapamil and Diltiazem may produce bradycardia and conduction disturbances as well as worsen left ventricular failure. Calcium channel blockers are more useful when combined with nitrates.

Plan of treatment. To start with patient is put on nitrates and if no relief is obtained then either beta blockers or calcium channel antagonists are combined. If adequate relief is not obtained and patient gets repeated attacks of angina then coronary angiography is performed. If patient has got single vessel disease, then percutaneous transluminal angioplasty (PTCA) is performed. If more othan one vessel i.e. triple vessel disease of coronary arteries is present then bypass surgery should be planned.

Unstable angina. It is a severe form of angina where picture is of acute myocardial infarction with absence of classical ECG changes except ST segment suggestive of subendocardial ischaemia. It is often labelled as Crescendo angina, acute coronary insufficiency and intermediate coronary syndrome.

Angina may be present at rest as well as with minimal exertion and is not relieved by nitrates. ECG changes of ST segment depression may disappear if the relief from pain occurs but their persistence indicates subendocardial infarction.

Treatment is by bed rest, nitrates, oxygen,

calcium channel antagonists, sedation aspirin and intravenous heparin. Fibrinolytic therapy is often considered if myocaridial infarction is suspected. In patient with failure of medical therapy urgent angiography is performed and depending on the outcome either angioplasty or bypass surgery planned.

Variant angina (Prinzmetal's angina). This angina occurs at rest and has characteristic ST segment elevation in ECG during the attack. Often the pain may be severe and is asociated with cardiac arrhythmias provoked by the attack. This angina is due to coronary spasm. Treatment is by nitrates and calcium channel antagonists. Beta blockers should not be used in a case of prinzmetal's angina since these produce vasoconstriction of coronary arteries, increase coronary tone and may worsen angina.

Surgical treatment is generally not required in such cases as medical therapy generally gives desired relief.

Asymptomatic coronary artery disease. This is not uncommon since 25 per cent of patients with acute myocardial infarction may not be detected and patients are unaware of it. Some of them may present with sudden death or with cardiac irregularities. It may be difficult to detect such people except by carrying out exercise induced electrocardiograms in persons with strong family history of hypertension. Diabetes, strokes, sudden deaths or those who suffer from one of these disease or by population surveys in people above the age of 50 years.

Ischaemic cardiomyopathy. It is as a result of severe coronary insufficiency resulting in diffuse fibrosis of the myocardium and severe degree of myocardial dysfunction. Most such patients present with cardiomegaly and congestive heart failure. There generally is no history suggestive of angina or myocardial infarction.

SILENT MYOCARDIAL ISCHEMIA

Although traditionally angina pectoris is the classical clinical manifestation of myocardial ischemia and coronary artery disease yet a great number of cases of coronary artery disease remain silent until the onset of severe morbid clinical event. Episodes of asymptomatic (silent) myocardial ischemia occur far more frequently than symptomatic episodes. As the treatment is almost always guided by symptomatic episodes, there is often under treatment of recurrent ischemia. Detection of silent myocardial ischemia in acute phase of infarction gives insight into the subsequent events after recovery from acute myocardial infarction.

Silent myocardial ischemia is an objective evidence of disease which is documented by direct or indirect measurements of left ventricular function. It is classified into three clinical types.

Type 1 includes persons with ischemia who are asymptomatic and had no signs or symptoms of any cardiovascular disease. Type II includes persons who are asymptomatic after myocardial infarction but still show evidence of ischemia. Type III consists of patients with both angina and silent ischemia. The precise mechanism responsible for the condition is not known but factors ranging from abnormal threshold to perception of painful stimuli, differences in the severity and duration of transient ischemic episodes as well as extent of collateral coronary circulation have been put forward.

Silent myocardial ischemia can lead to cardiac arrhythmias acute myocardial infarction or sudden death. Test for its detection include. Treadmill test, holter monitoring, radionuclide angiography and haemodynamic monitoring.

Since cases have hardly any symptoms it may be difficult to diagnose such cases. Majority of these patients exhibit S.T. segment depression during exercise testing and these episodes are precipitated during minimal physical activity and mental and emotional stress.

All patients of silent myocardial ischemia should be treated with anti-anginal drugs.

ACUTE MYOCARDIAL INFARCTION

Acute myocardial infarction is one of the common-est medical emergency carrying with it high degree of mortality. In a great number of cases myocardial infarction occurs at rest, during sleep in 10 per cent of cases or after heavy exertion, or severe emotional stress. Further risk factoors include unstable angina, variant angina and hypoglycemia which may culminate into an attack of acute myocardial infarction.

Clinical picture. A patient of myocardial infarction may present with features of chest pain, restlessness, sweating or a rapidly developing acute left heart failure or with features of cardiac arrhythmias like ventricular tachycardia, fibrillation or supraventricullar tachycardia.

Classicially pain of myocardial infarction is constricting squeezing or oppressive, its intensity varying from severe agonizing intolerable pain to a dull pain or discomfort.

Pain is often present over the chest and radiates to both arms but more to the left arm. It may radiate to the scapula, back neck or jaws. Sometimes there may be first pain in the arms which later on travels to the chest or precordium. Occasionally a case of myocardial infarction has agonising pain in the epigastric region which may sometimes be mistaken as a case of acute abdomen.

Duration of pain varies lasting from a few minutes to half an hour. A case of angina may find pain not responding to usual nitrates which he may be taking.

Accoompanying symptoms include sweating, a sensation of profound weakness, cold extremities, nausea and vomiting.

Physical examination. Patient is anxious and in distress. There is restlessness. Extremities are cold and sweating. Face has got pallor arnd an anguished look.

There may be fall of blood pressure (Hypotension) and sometimes the blood pressure may be normal or high if patient is hypertensive.

Most patients develop fever about 101-102°F 12-24 hous after an infarction because of tissue necrosis.

Heart shows tachycardia but there may be bradycardia if there is inferior wall infarction.

Syncopal attacks may occur.

There is muffling of heart sounds. A gallop rhthm may appear. If there are features of acute left heart failure, patient is acutely breathless unable to lie in bed. Chest shows bilateral crepitations. Venous pressure is raised.

Pericardial friction rub may be heard in some patients on the second or third day especially if it is a transmural infarct.

Clinical features of acute myocardial infarction

1. Symptoms. Chest pain (constricting, squeezing intensity varying from severe agonising pain to dull pain or discomfort). Pain present over precordium, substernal region, rediating to left or both arms, back and shoulder.
   Sweating, restlessness, apprehension of an impending doom. Marked weakness. Nausea, vomiting, diarrhoea.
2. Physical examination. Weak peripheral pulse: Cold and sweating extremities pallor on face. Anguished look. Fall of blood pressure (hypotension), tachycardia or bradycardia, heart sound muffled. A gallop rhythm may appear. Syncopal attack may occur. Fever 12-24 hours after an attack of infarction because of tissue necrosis. Pericardial rub on second or third day.

Pathology. Myocardial infarction is due to occlusion of coronary artery and is generally confined to left ventricle and may be in the form of a transmural infarct which traverses the endocardium into subepicardial myocardium or a subendocardial infarct which is generally confined to one half to one third of the left ventricle.

Most commonly affected vessel is anterior descending branch of the left coronary artery. The location of the infarct depends on the vessel effected.

1. Left anterior descending coronary artery. Its involvement leads to damage of anterior wall of left ventricle and two thirds of interventricular septum.
2. Left circumflex coronary artery. Result is damage to lateral and posterior wall of left ventricle.

3. Right coronary artery: Its occlusion produces damage to inferior posterior wall of left ventricle and posterior one third of interventricular septum.

The infarcted portion is pale which becomes evident in 18-24 hours and by second to fourth day the necrotic portion becomes more sharply defined. By tenth day colour changes are well developed, the infarct is soft, yellow and may contain blood. Over course of time pale grey scarring takes place and by the end of sixth week, infarcted tissue is completely replaced by scar tissue. On an average healing of infarct takes 6-8 weeks depending on the size of the infarct.

Investigations:

Non-specific tests. A rise in polymorph cells along with leucocytsis may occur within few hours after the onset of pain and persists for few days. Rise in erythrocyte sedimentation rate occurs. But generally after 24 hours.

Cardiac enzymes:

1. After infarction there is release of large amount of enzymes into the blood. There is rise of SGOT/SGPT (AST & ALT) levels within 8-12 hours, reaching peak levels in 24-48 hours and may fall to normal levels by 3-4 days (normal levels 5-40 IU/L). These enzymes are not specific since their rise may occur with damage to kidney, liver, lungs etc.
2. Serum lactic dehydrogenase (LDH). Levels of this enzyme start rising by 12-24 hours, reaching maximum at 3-4 days and remain so for two weeks (normal values 20-200 IU/L). This enzyme is not only raised in myocardial infarction but also in diseases of liver, skeletal muscle and red blood cells.

Creatinine phosphokinase (CPK). It is more specific. It rises after infarction in 6-8 hours, reaching its peak in 24 hours and declines to normal within 3-4 days. Normal values are 20-200 IU/L. Among the three isoenzymes of CPK, the rise in MB-CK is specific for myocardial infarction.

Elevation of enzymes correlates with the extent of infarction. Even when electrocardiogram is not specific, enzyme levels may help to diagnose.

Except for MB-CK all other enzymes are also elevated in other diseases like those of liver, renal diseases, Pulmonary embolism, muscular diseases, shock. Haemolysis and skeletal disorders.

Faise positive rise in enzyme levels is also seen.

Rise in enzyme levels after myocardial infarction

Enzyme	Rise after	Peak	Duration
1. CPK (MB)	4-6 hours	12 hours	48 hours
2. LDH	12 hours	2-3 days	7-10 days
3. SGOT/SGPT	12 hours	1-2 days	3-4 days

Electrocardiogram. It is a very valuable test and taken within a few hours of symnptoms suggestive of myocardial infarction shows diagnostic changes in majority of patients (80-95%).

Presence of infarction is shown by appearance of a deep broad, Q wave, elevation of ST segment and T wave inversion.

ST segment and T wave changes are as a result of myocardial injury and ischaemia. At the site of injury ST segment is elevated while ST depression is seen in an opposing lead. This is termed reciprocal ST depression.

Localization of infarct. Depending on changes in ECG it may be possible to localize the infarct.

Anterior myocardial infarction:

1. Q_1T_1 pattern in limb leads (L1 and L2) and extremity leads aVL.
2. Convex ST segment in leads V1-V3.
3. QS complexes or abnormal Q waves in precordial leads.

Anteroseptal infarction. ST segment elevation V1-V4.

Inferior and lateral wall infarction. Q_3T_3 pattern in lomb leads (LII, LIII) extremity leads (aVF). ST segment elevation: T wave inversion in V5-V6.

Transmural infarction. ST segment changes V1-V6.

Subendocardial infarction. ST segment

depression and T wave inversion in leads recorded from the overlying epicardial surface.

Complications. A number of complications may arise in a case of myocardial infarction. Some patients presenting feature may be in the form of acute left heart failure, shock or arrhythmia. First 24-48 hours following an infarction are the critical phase though no patient is declared out of danger till a week has passed. Complications may be immediate or delayed. In the acute phase various complications encountered are:

1. Arrhythmias especially ventricular (ventricular tachycardia, fibrillation) Atrial fibrillation ventricullar premature beats, sinus bradycardia, supraventricular tachycardias, severe grades of conduction disturbances like heart block, cardiac arrest.
2. Acute left heart failure: pulmonary oedema.
3. Cardiogenic shock.
4. Rupture of papillary muscle leading to acute mitral incompetence.
5. Rupture of interventricular septum leading to sudden acute left heart failure.
6. Cardiac rupture at the site of infarct leading to haemopericardium, cardiac temponade and death.

Complications of acute myocardial infarction

1. Immediate
   a. Acute left heart failure.
   b. Acute peripheral circulatory failure
   c. Cardiac arrhythmias (sinus bradycardia, atrial fibrillation, supraventricular tachycardia, multiple ventricular extrasystoles, ventricular tachycardia, ventricular fibrillation, various degrees of heart block).
   d. Cardiac rupture leading to haemopericardium and death.
   e. Cardiac stand still/sudden death.
   f. Rupture of papillary muscle leading to mitral incompetence.
   g. Rupture of interventricular septum.
2. Delayed
   a. Thrombophlebitis leading to pulmonary embloism.
   b. Pericarditis
   c. Ventricular aneurysm

7. Pericarditis occurs within first few days after an infarction especially of anterior wall. There is an acute chest pain with presence of pericardial rub.
8. Thrombophlebitis and resultant pulmonary embolism due to prolonged bed rest and immobilisation. Venous thrombosis is as a result of venous stasis.

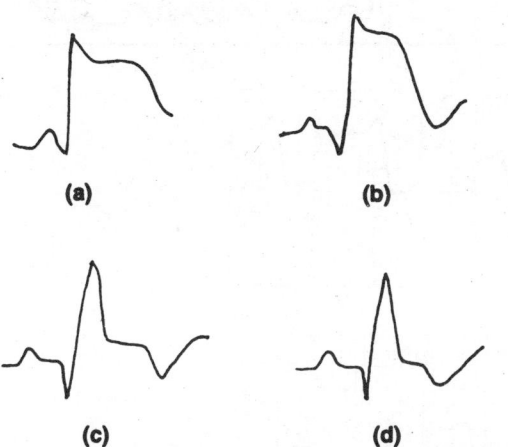

(a)   (b)

(c)   (d)

Fig. 4.31. Sequence of changes in infarction. (a) ST elevation occurs within first few hours. Sometimes it may be delayed. (b) ST elevation is followed by T wave inversion and development of abnormal Q waves (broad and deep (> 2mm). (c) ST elevation is marked but gradually assumes a typical shape over 24–72 hours. (d) T wave inversion may persist indefinately as well as Q waves.

Delayed complications include ventricular aneurysm and Dressler's syndrome. It is an auto immune mediated reaction occurs weeks to months after an acute attack of infarction. Dressler's syndrome is characterized by fever, arthralgia, pericarditis, pleurisy and in some cases with pericardial effusion.

Management. Management of a case of acute myocardial infarction depends on the stage at which the patient presents and state of the patient. Wherever facilities are available patient should be admitted in ICCU because it would be essential to monitor heart rate. Blood pressure, respiration and look for the development of arrhythmias like ventricular tachycardia ventricular fibrillation or multiple ventricular extrasystoles. since their early

detection has a great bearing on the prognosis of the case.

Some centres have mobile coronary care vans where staff is trained to manage cardiopulmonary resuscitation. Cardiac monitoring is done in every case and in uncomplicated cases it is usually done for 48-72 hours.

Relief of pain. First measure to be adopted in every case is relief of pain. For this Injection Pethidine 100 mg with Injection Phenergan 25 mg S/C is administered. If pain is not relieved within 15-30 minutes Injection morphine 15-20 mg is given either I/V slowly or S/C since it shall not only relieve pain but also anxiety. Another drug for relief of pain is Injection Pentazocine 30 mg/ml to be given intramuscularly. Only drawback with this drug is development of physical dependence on repeated use.

Oxygen therapy. Oxygen is administered preferably by a mask. Continuous oxygen gives relief from pain by improving myocardial oxygen supply.

Drugs. If there is no hypotension, Sorbitrate 10 mg every 6 hourly is given. This is supposed to limit the infarct size. Aspirin/Dispirin is a safe antiplatelet drug. Sedation in the form of diazepam 5 mg, twice a day to relieve anxiety. In patient with cardiogenic shock, persistent pain and extensive transmural infarcts, anticoagulation is employed especially if there is danger of thrombembolism due to immoblization. Injection Heparin 10,000 units I/V 6 hourly by continuous infusion. Constant monitoring is required.

Fibrinolytic therapy. These agents are of benefit in reducing infarct size as well as ventricular damage especially if administered during the first 6 hours after an acute attack. They are of benefit in restoring coronary artery blood flow, reducing mortality and salvaging the myocardium.

Three fibrinolytic agents commonly used are Streptokinase, Urokinase and Tissue, type plasminogen activator.

Streptokinase. It is the most commonly used fibrinolytic agent. Dose 750,000-1.5 million IU intravenously in infusion over 1 hour. Dosage of

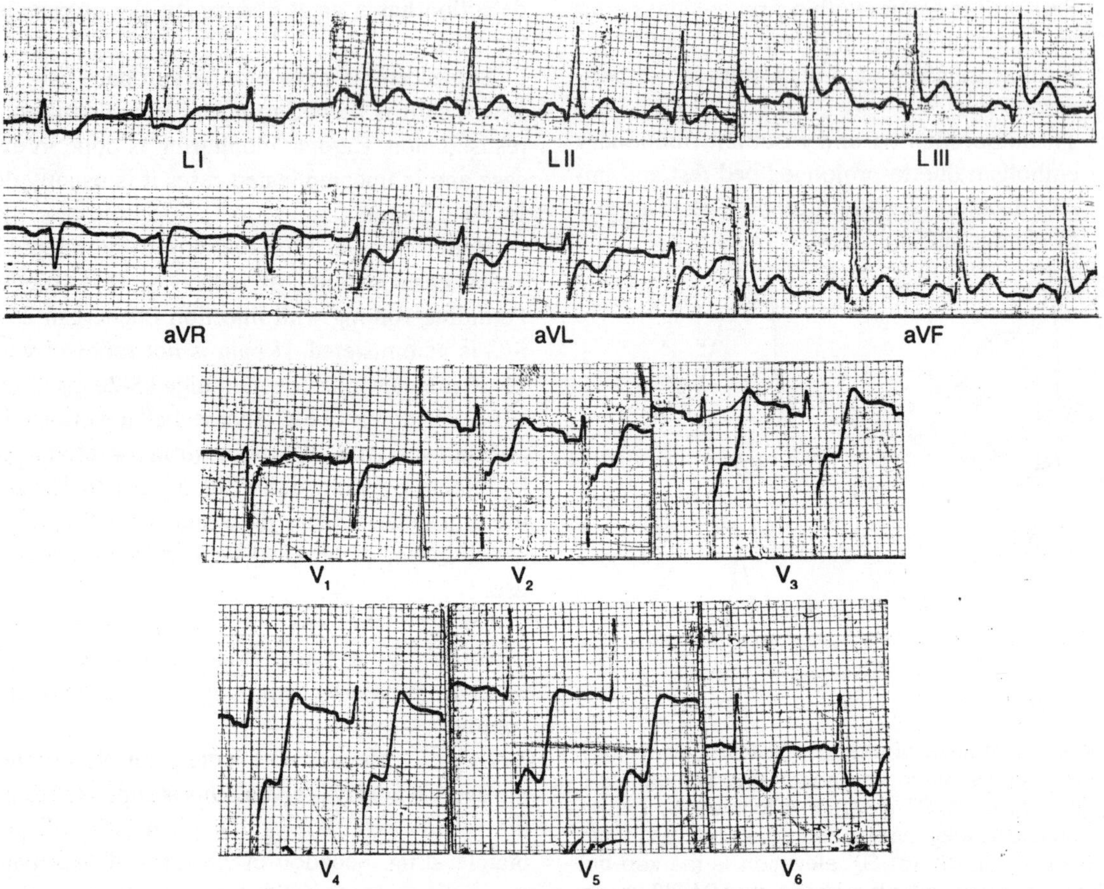

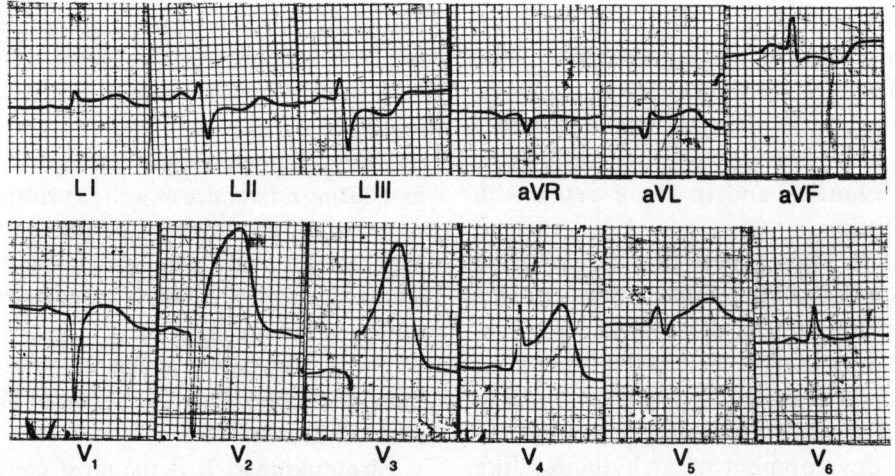

Fig. 4.32. Acute Subendocardial Infarction: There is marked diffuse ST segment depression with T wave inversion recorded in a patient with acute pain in chest. ST segment depression in most prominent in L I, V_2 - V_6.

Fig. 4.33. Acute Myocardial Infarction (Early Phase): There is ST segment elevation in anterior precordial leads (V_1 - V_4) and L I, aVL with depression of ST segment and T wave inversion L II, LIII, aVF.

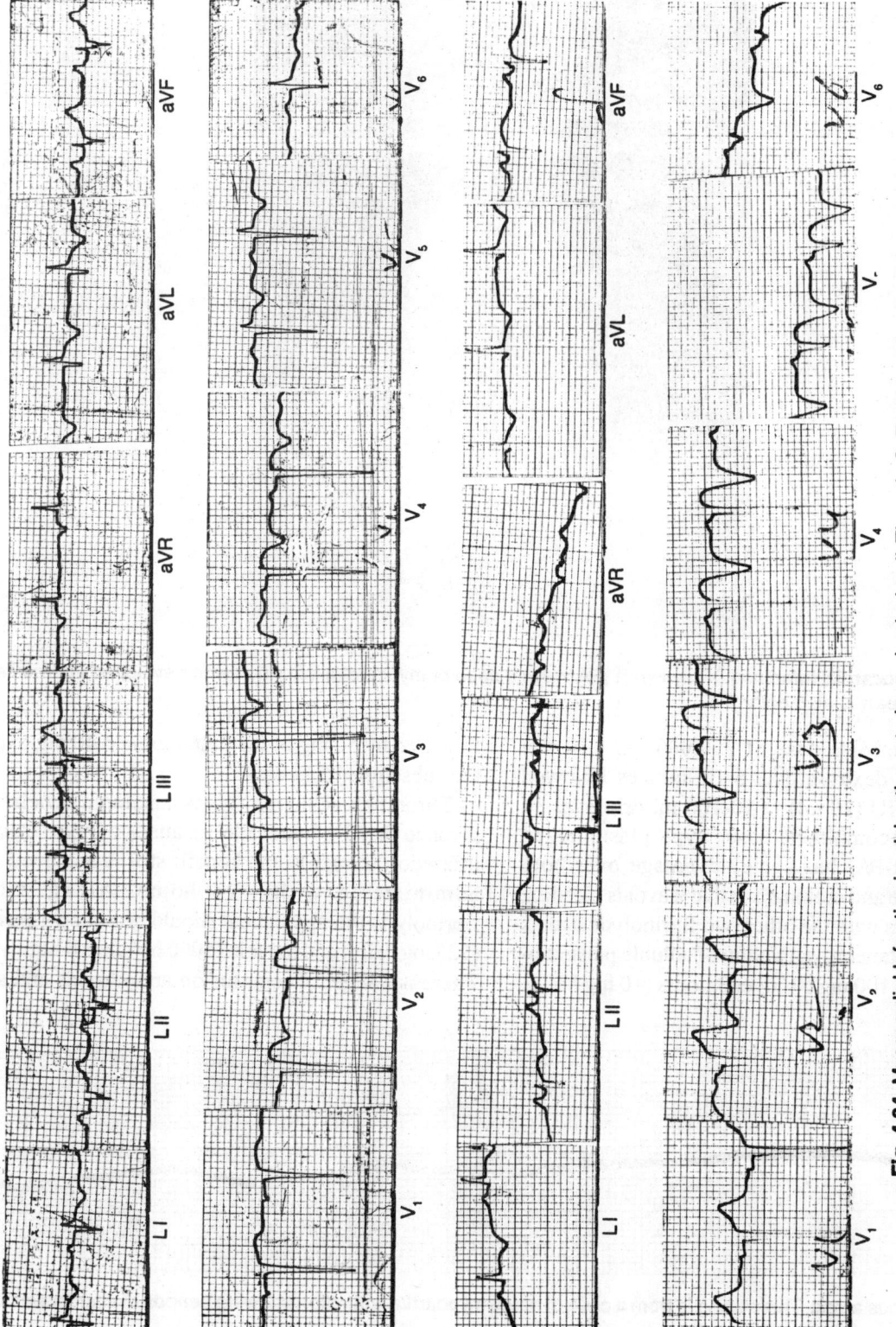

Fig. 4.34. Mycocardial Infarction involving the anterior and apical wall: There is Q_1 T_1 pattern involving L I, L II, aVL. Qs wave V_1 - V_4 and deep Q wave with qR complexes in V_5 - V_6. There is ST segment elevation in ant. Precordial leads. Abnormalities in inferior leads reflect involvement of apical and lateral wall of heart.

Fig. 4.35. Mycardial Infarction (Transmular): There is elevation of ST segment with T wave inversion V_2^* - V_6 leads.

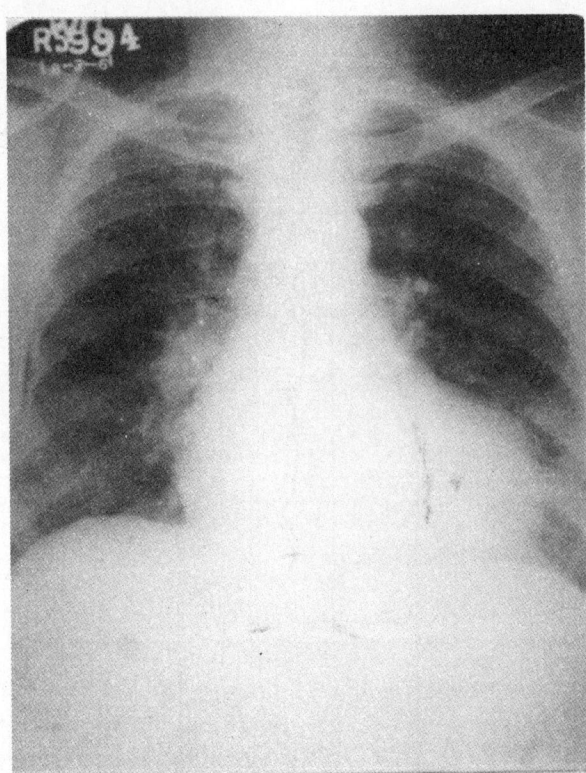

Fig. 4.36. Myocardial Infarction: X ray Heart (PA View) a case of myocardial infarction who developed ventricular aneurysm. Heart is also enlarged.

urokinase is bolus dose of 250,000 I.U. (10 ml) dissolved in dextrose over 5-10 minutes followed by 250,000 IU (10 ml) in 50-100 ml drip over 30 minutes. Recombinent tissue type plasminogen activator (rt-PA) has some advantage over both streptokinase and urokinase in that it avoids bleeding which occurs with the other two fibrinolytic agents due to simultaneous activation of soluble plasminogen. Dose is 100 mg I/V over 3 hours (10 mg bolus,

followed by 50 mg in the first hour and 40 mg over the subsequent 2 hours).

Thrombolytic therapy gives maximum benefit if given in first 3-6 hours after an attack of myocardial infarction though some benefit still is achieved if administered within 24 hours. Along with fibrinolytic therapy patient should be put on aspirin (325 mg daily) and heparin (5000 I/V units 6 hourly). There is danger of reperfusion arrhythmias and so

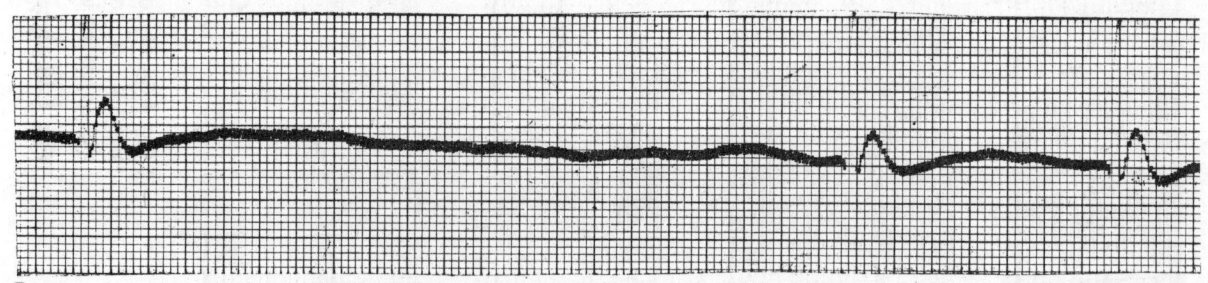

Fig. 4.37. Sinus arrest. This tracing is from a case of acute myocardial infarction showing periods of sinus asystole.

patient should be monitored during and after therapy for next 48 hours.

Contraindications to fibrinolytic therapy are active gastrointestinal bleed. Recent surgical procedure or trauma within preceding 10 days, severe hypertension, subacute bacterial endocarditis, history of cerebrovascular accident, bleeding disorders, purpura, pregnancy. Special care should be taken in diabetics and those with hepatic or renal impairment. Repeat administration of these agents is generally not recommended within 3 months.

Bed rest. Complete bed rest is enforced in the first 48 hours after an attack of infarction and by third day patient can sit up in bed for 1-2 hours. Ambulation shall depend on the state of heart and presence or absence of any complications. In a stable case, if there are no attacks of chest pain, patient be encouraged to go to the attached bath room on the 10th day or so. Movements in room are permitted and generally patient is discharged on the 12th day. Unnecessary immobilization is not good.

Diet. Diet should be low caloric liquid in the early part of illness and semisolid during the next few days. Easily digestible, soft diet in small quantities with less fats and salt is advised. Gradually as the general condition improves patient starts taking almost normal diet. Patient must have a tension free environment. A restful sleep must be ensured. Unnecessary visitors must not be allowed to disturb the patient. Since patient is on bed rest, liquid or semi solid diet, he/she is likely to suffer from constipation. Patient must not strain while passing stools. Problem should be explained to him and constipation be treated with a mild laxative.

Limiting size of the infarct. Size of the infarct depends on site of occlusion and collateral blood supply to the damaged tissue. Infarct size can be limited by proper rest, oxygenation control of arrhythmias, and adequate employment of various therapeutic agents. Though it is important not to employ measures which may alter the supply-demand balance of the infarct, yet drugs like beta blockers (Propranolol, metoprolol) calcium channel blockers (verapamil) if used for long periods because of their effect in reducing myocardial

requirement of oxygen can prevent not only reinfarction but also reduce mortality. Benefit occurs if these drugs are started early in a case of myocardial infarction. These are contraindicated in the presence of hypotension, shock, heart block.

Rehabilitation after myocardial infarction. Ambulation after an attack of myocardial infarction is gradual. Generally it takes 6-8 weeks for the infarct to heal and if the progress of the patient has been good, on an average the patient is able to resume normal activity in 10-12 weeks time. Persons who resume their normal routine as early as possible their chances of remaining healthy are excellent.

But any physical effort which puts a strain on the heart be avoided such as lifting heavy objects, climbing stairs, car driving. Light exercise in the form of walks is encouraged. Light walking programme which does not put undue stress on the heart is desirable.

Patient should be advised not to over eat. A well balanced diet containing proteins, fresh fruits and vegetables be taken. Food rich in cholesterol and saturated fats (ghee, butter) be avoided and fats of polyunsaturated and monosaoturated variety (safflower oil, corn oil, olive oil be substituted). Patient should rest after a meal and not take a walk after a heavy meal.

Smoking be avoided. Alcohol only in moderation is permitted. Patient be explained his illness and advised to avoid both physical and mental stress. He should be encouraged to keep all excitement and emotions under control.

Surgery for heart. If a patient after an attack of myocrdial infarction adopts various measures to change his life style as well as takes adequate amount of drugs, and still goes on having repeated anginal attacks or substernal discomfort or where quality of life suffers, these are the type of patients where interventional procedures are planned. Such a patient is submitted to stress testing (TMT) Thallium scan and coronary angiography. Depending on whether patient has single vessel or triple vessel disease, patient is submitted to surgical procedures. Various surgical prcedures employd are:

Percutaneous transluminal coronary angio-

plasty (PTCA). It is employed in patients with proximal stenosis of one or two coronary vessels. A catheter is passed into the narrowed coronary artery and across the stenosis to be dilated, a small balloon catheter is advanced over the guidewire and into the stenosis. By repeated inflations the stenosis is decreased and narrowed segment of the artery is widened. Sometimes a stent is placed after opening the obstructed part of coronary artery.

Angioplasty is comparatively safe and simple procedure. Major complictions are rupture of the artery, dissection or thombosis of the occluded vessel. Restenosis of the artery may occur in 20-40% of cases within six months of the procedure. Primary success may be obtained in 80-90% of cases. Patients who do not develop restenosis within first year after angioplasty results for next 4-5 years are good and most such patients do well. Sometimes during angioplasty procedure because of complications emergency bypass surgery may be required in small percentage of cases.

Overall angioplasty is comparatively a safe procedure, less expensive and patients stay in hospital after procedure is generally for two to three days and he can resume his active life in a short time.

Coronary stenting

Two main limitations of coronary angioplasty are acute coronary occlusion and restenosis occurring during the first 6 months after angioplasty. To decrease the rate of restenosis, several devices have been designed to achieve the largest acute luminal gain and minimum late luminal loss. A stent (wired coil placed in the blocked lumen after angioplasty) shows significant decrease in the restenosis rate.

An ideal stent should exert sufficient radial force to effectively support the vessel and maintain an appropriate lumen diameter and it should be flexible enough along its long axis to adopt to torturous coronary anatomy and should remain stable after being positioned. Moreover the stent should be long lasting, non-thrombogenic and be rapidly covered by neoendothelium. Most of the stents do not meet all the criteria. Of the various stents being used include self-expanding stents (Medinvent vall stent).

Balloon expandable stents (Palmaz-Schatz stent: Gianfurco-Rubin stent: Medtronic-Witkor coronary stent) and thermal expansion stents. Contraindications to stenting include funnel shaped lesions, vessel diameter less than 3 mm, lesions situated less than 10 mm from the left main coronary artery, tight bend in the target segment and insufficient blood flow anticipated through the stent.

Complications after stenting includes stent displacement, coronary perforation, bleeding, infection, spasm and stent thrombosis. But despite stenting restenosis does occur.

The use of anti-thrombotic agents after this procedure are advocated to prevent the formation of thrombi.

Coronary artery bypass surgery (CABG). It is employed in people who have more than one coronary vessel blocked (triple vessel disease) or where there is failure of angioplasy. The operation is relatively safe and mortality is almost one percent.

In this either a venous or arterial graft is used to bypass the blocked coronary arteries. CAVBG (coronary artery vein bypass grafting) involves taking a vein from one or both the legs usually saphenous vein and connecting to the ascending segment of aorta and the other end to coronary artery beyond the obstruction so that now pure blood reaches the myocardium having bypassed the diseased obstructed coronary artery.

When arterial graft is used it is either one or both of internal mammary arteries. Generally left mammary artery is used. The whole course of artery is separated and the other end is implanted in the coronary artery distal to the obstruction. Result is flow of uninterrupted blood supply to the heart with resultant improvement in cardiac function. Blocking of venous graft takes place in 10-20% of patients in the first year after surgery and this incidence falls as time passes with the result that in persons who maintain graft without any problem incidence of blockage of graft within the next five years is only 2 percent.

Long-term results with arterial graft are good and the graft remains patent for a longer time as compared to venous grafts.

Mortality in patients of coronary artery disease after surgery is reduced and this is especially so in those with triple vessel disease. Relief from anginal pain is good and the person can now lead a more active trouble free life.

After surgery the person must take adequate precautions about weight control, diet, physical exercise, smoking and avoidance of stress and strain. Daily intake of aspirin (50-100 mg) Dipyridamole (75-100 mg) is advised. Restenosis of the graft may take place after a few years and may require a repeat by pass operation.

Though there are no special contraindications to this procedure but results after surgery are definately good in persons less than 70 years of age, those without any cmplications and coexisting diseases like diabetes and hypertension and with good cardiac function.

Laser angioplasty. Use of laser or rotablators by use of diamond tipped devices is another method short of bypass surgery. Procedure is less traumatic and results are good.

Management of complications. A number of patients of acute myocardial infarction are likely to develop life threatening complications which require immediate management.

Cardiac arrhythmias. Common arrhythmias are ventricular tachycardia, ventricular fibrillation, multiple frequent ventricular premature beats (more than 6 per minute or R-on-T). Atrial fibrillation, sinus bradycardia varying degrees of heart block, and supraventricular tachycardias. All arrhythmias require correct and prompt management.

Cardiogenic shock. It is a serious emergency with a mortality of more than 90 per cent. There is hypotension peripheral circulatory failure and low left ventricular falling pressure. Treatment is by continuous oxygen, careful administration of fluids and use of vaso pressures (Dobutamine 2.5 to 10 ugm/kg per minute).

Left heart failure pulmonary oedema. When acute shall require oxyen, digoxin, diuretics and ACE inhiibitors.

Cardiac rupture. It is a sudden complication most likely to occur during the first week. There is development of cardiac temptonade and shall require emergency cardiac surgery. Mortality is very high.

Thromboembolism. Prolonged immobilisation in bed in all patients of myocardial infarction prpedisposes to thromboembolic complications. Preventive measures in all patients like passive leg exercises be encouraged. Prophylactic anticoagulants use shall reduce the incidence further.

Prognosis. Mortality in a case of acute myocardial infarction is variable. Almost 50 per cent of cases may die within first hours after the attack because of cardiac standstill, development of life threatening arrhythmias and lack of emergency medical support. Adverse prognostic factors are:

1. Cardiogenic shock
2. Acute left heart failure
3. Ventricular arrhythmias (V-tachycardia/fibrillation)
4. Age more than 70 years.
5. Poor myocardial function
6. Heart blocks
7. Poor family history.

Prognosis shall definately be good in those who do not have coexisting diseases like diabetes, hypertension or those without genetic predisposition, absence of family history of heart disease. Serum cholesterol and lipid levels low and those who adopt a changed healthy life style.

REFRACTORY HEART FAILURE

In practice one often comes across case of congestive cardiac failure which defies the conventional line of treatment and is a real problem to tackle. Presence of such a condition is termed as refractory or intractable heart failure which is a poorly defined term but in its usual usage it conveys a distinct clinical state when despite all the therapeutic measures adopted, the patient of congestive heart failure fails to respond or ceases to respond and the heart failure persists or progresses. Often a distinction is made between refractory heart failure and intractable heart failure, the latter term being reserved for cases of myocardial damage where because of prolonged and persistent heart failure the myocardium is unable to respond to therapy and fails to act as an effective pump. But such a distinction seems rather arbitrary since both the terms are synonymous.

Once one confronts a patient with intractable heart failure then one must critically reviw the case for there may be some error in diagnosis or there may be some posible reversible and irreversible factors which are operative and thus the failure of the condition to improve. Often some complications arise as a part of congestive heart failure or as a result of the treatment which might be responsible for causing the refractory failure.

Broadly the possible causes of refractory heart failure can be looked into under two broad groups. *Firstly* conditions which simulate heart failure may be in acute form like acute massive pulmonary embolism, cases of status asthmaticus with associated coronary heart disease, acute viral pneumonia, acute intoxications like kerosene oil poisoning petroleum fuel ingestion, aluminium phosphide poisoning. Severe anaemia developing acutely after massive gastrointestinal bleed and extensive metastasis in lungs.

Similarly chronic conditions which may produce a picture resembling refractory heart failure shall include severe degree of obesity producing cardio-respiratory embarrassment, advanced stage of chronic obstructive lung disease with resultant picture of chronic cor pulmonale, endocranial disorders with cardiac involvement such as myxoedema, thyrotoxicosis etc. These conditions have been alluded to since more often one may be presented with a picture simulating congestive heart failure which is refractory to treatment.

But the most important aspect is that when one is confronted with the problem of refractory failure. First of all one must look into the clinical picture of the case along with all the usual investigations. If necessary go over the full picture of the case and evaluate your diagnosis. It is quite likely that one may be treating the patient with wrong diagnosis and in fact it may not be a true case of congestive heart failure but one of the above conditions which is simulating heart failure.

After having satisfied one self with the correctness of diagnosis, there are factors which complicate cardiac disease and may be leading to refractoriness of heart failure.

Broadly these important factors shall include often over looked causes of heart disease, surgical correctable conditions of heart like tight mitral stenosis, aortic stenosis, infective endocarditis, severe degree of infection/sepsis, recurrent pulmonary embolisation, electrolyte imbalance, incipient renal failure etc. Let us look at some of these factors:

1. Multiple pulmonary emboli. Recurrent pulmonary emboli are an important factor since only in less than 10 per cent of patients of pulmonary embolism there are classical signs and symptoms. Unexplained deterioration in a patient of congestive failure who had previously been stable, presence of tachycardia and tachyponea may help to suspect this condition. This is especially in a case of severe congestive failure lying confined to bed for a long time or one with cardiac rhythm irregularities.

2. Chronic arrhythmia with tachycardia. One of the commonest irregularity to complicate cardiac failure is Atrial Fibrillation. Patients with cardiac failure have poor cardiac reserve and therefore any arrhythmia which results in compromise of cardiac function is poorly tolerated and leads to refractoryness of heart failure. At the same time one must not over look the fact that aggressive treatment of cardiac failure with diuretics and digoxin can be an important cause of cardiac arrhythmias especially digitalis induced atrial tachycardia with 2:1 A.V. block which if not recognised in time may prove fatal. A persistent fast atrial fibrillation is an important cause of unresponsiveness of the patient of congestive failure.

3. Bacterial endocarditis. This is one condition which is often over looked. Majority of cardiac patients may have only low grade fever, persistent anaemia and in the presence of intractable failure one should look into this cause. If only one keeps this condition in mind and looks for other signs like splinter haemorrhagès, osler nodes, splenomegaly, change in character of murmur and microscopic hematuria then the diagnosis can be clinched.

4. Infections. Any persistent infection in the body like chest infection, (bacterial/viral) urinary tract infection can be important causes of refractory heart failure. Tachycardia consequent to elevated temperatues is poorly tolerated by patients with cardiac failure.

5. Valvular Lesions. Adequate treatment of valvular lesions may achieve control of patients with refractory cardiac failure. Evidence of silent mitral stenosis, mild aortic regurgitation may have been over looked. Cardiac failure in patients with tight mitral valve disease, aortic stenosis and tricuspid stenosis may not respond till surgical intervention is done.

6. Constrictive pericarditis. This condition has to be distinguished from restrictive form of cardiomyopathy which is often difficult. Response to digitalis and diuretics is poor. Characteristically ascites is an early feature. Oedema of feet develops latter. Dysponea is minimal and orthoponea is unusual. A pericardial knock, normal cardiac size, prominent 'Y' descent in the jugular venous pulse and calcification of pericardium may provide useful clues. Clearly therapy of cardiac failure in such cases is unrewarding.

7. Pericardial effusion. It results in systemic venous congestion. There are signs of poor pulse pressure, pulsus, paradoxus, raised jugular venous pessure, decreased cardiac pulsation and cardiomegaly. Adequate treatment of effusion leads to control of venous congestion.

8. Rupture of chordea tendinae. Spontaneous rupture of chordea tendinae may occur in cases of coronary heart disease, resulting in myocardial failure. Such patients are often resistant to treatment because of poor cardiac reserve.

9. Cardiac tumours. Cardiac tumours are important causes of intractable heart failure. Commonest cardiac tumour is atrial myxoma which gives rise to paroxysmal episodes of heart failure due to blockage of mitral or tricuspid valves. Infiltrative tumours of the heart like metastasis from

leukaemias, lymphomas are important as being responsible for refractory cardiac failure.

10. Infiltrative disease of myocardium. Haemochromatosis, sarcoidosis, glycogen storage disease etc can all lead to refractory heart failure. Diagnosis can be established if the basic disease is diagnosed by appropriate investigations.

11. Disorders of thyroid function. Hyperthyroidism is an operative factor when the manifestations of hyperthyroidism are predominantly cardiac and hyperthyroidism is not apparently detected. In the pesence of pre-existing heart diease this may lead to refractory heart failure. Unexplained persistent or paroxysmal atrial fibrillation may be an important pointer towards over activity of thyroid.

12. Myxoedema. Patients with poor thyroid function manifest with hypertension, cardiac enlargement, poor myocardial contractility and even picture of congestive failure. Many a times such cases are not correctly diagnosed and they do not respond to therapy for congestive cardiac failure. Correct diagnosis and treatment shall result in dramatic improvement.

13. Avitaminosis. Severe degree of malnutrition, anaemia may lead to congestive heart failure and in cases of pre-existing cardiac disease may render the cardiac failure refractory. Beri beri heart disease is also an important cause especially in people who suffer from thiamine deficiency.

14. Digitalis toxicity. Digitalis over dosage is a common cause of refractory heart failure though it may appear contradictory to some since digitalis is an important drug in the management of congestive failure. Inadequate and over dosage of the drug are important factors responsible for refractory heart failure. The usual symptoms of digitalis toxicity like nausea, vomiting, loss of appetite are common to idientify. All type of arrhythmias may arise like bigeminy, atrioventricular block, paroxysmal atrial tachycrdia with 2:1 A-V block multiple ventricular extrasystoles etc. Out of all these digitalis induced tachycrdia with 2:1 A-V block is most dangerous. Non-responsiveness of a patient with congestive failure with either under or over dosage of the drug must be thought of in a patient on digoxin who suddenly shows signs of deterioration of failure, with development of tachycardia suspect digitalis toxicity.

15. Electrolyte disturbances. Electrolyte disturbances result in decreased response to diuretics and similarly changes in pH result in decreased activity of drugs. Hypokalemia as a result of aggressive diuretic therapy results in potentiation of digitalis toxicity. Other important electrolytes to be taken care of are calcium and magnesium. So monitor the electroytes regularly in a patient of congestive failure. Hyponatremia, a late manifestation of refractory heart failure, is due to aggressive diuresis with resultant reduced glomerular filtration rate.

16. Rheumatic activity. In a case of valvular heart disease presence of rheumatic activity shall be responsible for non-responsiveness of the heart failure, so look for signs of rheumatic activity in a case of valvular heart disease.

17. Renal failure. Incipient renal failure is another important factor. Patients of azotemia shall fail to respond to therapy until and unless azotemia is corrected.

In addition to the above factors, patients of cardiac failure may go into end stage myocardial failure which should always be considered an important factor in the causation of refractory heart failure.

Management. Management of a case of intractable refractory heart failure shall call on the acumen of the physician and his/her treating skills. Attempt be made to find out the probable factors which might be responsible and operative in the causation of intractable failure. A thorough clinical examination be done to review the diagnosis. Patiet be investigated for anaemia (haemoglobin, peripheral blood film) infections (X-ray chest, total and differential leucocyte count), renal profile (blood urea, serum creatinine, complete urine examination including urine for culture, plain X-ray abdomen), thyroid functions (T3, T4, TSH, radioactive iodineo uptake), X-ray heart (PA view), fluoroscopy, electrocardiogram) and echo-cardiography. In addition serum electrolytes, blood gas analysis, lung scan (for pulmonary embolism), blood culture for exclusion of subacute bacterial endocarditis, C-reactive proteins (rheumatic activity), serum assay for digoxin levels.

In sum total the patient should be investigated from all probable angles to arrive at operative factors. It is essential that all therapeutic measures be carried out with meticulous care in order to succeed. Broadly the management shall be:

1. Bed rest. Adequate bed rest if not already enforced must be adhered to. The patients activity must be linked with advice to exercise his limbs in bed to prevent development of venous thrombosis. Diet should be soft, nutritious and low in salt content preferably not more than 200 to 500 mg daily.

2. If there is infection in the lungs adequate antibiotics cover be given. Urinay tract infection be corrected. If obstructive uropathy then relief of obstruction will achieve control in these patients.

3. Where a smouldering bacterial endocarditis is detected appropriate antibiotics be given depending on blood culture. Important thing is to give the antibiotic cover for six weeks.

4. Where persistent heart failure is due to tight mitral valve and other surgically correctible congenital cardiovasocular conditions, it is desirable to undertake the corrective procedures after suitably controlling the congestive failure.

5. If thyroid functions are involved, thyroid replacement therapy will result in dramatic improvement. In cases of hyperthyroidism, antithyroid drugs or thyroid ablation by radio-isotopes/surgery will tend to control the cardiac failure.

6. Anaemia due to any cause should be corrected. Patients of beri-beri will show dramatic improvement with thiamine. Anaemia be corrected with proper haematanics. In very severe form of anaemia, blood transfusion (packed cells) shall help.

7. Cardiac tumours are hardly fit for surgery by the time the patient comes to the physician. Resection is possible in few cases. Radiation

and chemotherapy may provide some palliation. In infiltrative diseases of myocardium, therapy be directed towards the basic disease. Haemochromatosis is amenable to treatment with iron-chelating drugs like desferroxamine.

8. Intractable heart failure when complicated with digitalis overtoxicity requires withdrawal of digoxin, stoppage of diuretics, use of potassium and antiarrhythmic drugs like phenytoin (dilantin).

9. Electrolyte disturbances including changes in pH should be corrected. This line of action shall depend on whether there is evidence of severe hyponatremia/acidosis/alkalosis. Diuretic therapy may have to be temporarily stopped.

10. Where there is persistent heart failure due to recurrent pulmonary emboli, relief of heart failure may be obtained by use of anticooagulants (Heparin).

11. In addition to specific measures for all patients of intractable heart failure, use of potent symphthomimetic amines (Dopamine or Dobutamine) will result in increase in cardiac output with fall in pulmonary wedge pressure. Vasodilator therapy and ACE inhibitors are useful adjuvants in improving cardiac function along with Inotropic agent like Amrinone given orally or intravenously. ACE inhibitors produce an improvement in many of haemodynamic parameters resulting in increase in cardiac output and cardiac index as do the indices of stroke work and volume while nitrates shall reduce preload and afterload. The end result shall be improvement in heart failure.

Above are some of the broad guidelines in the management of a case of refractory heart failure but sooner or later a stage shall come when heart failure becomes non-responsive because of the end stage myocardial failure.

DISORDERS OF HEART BEAT (CARDIAC ARRHYTHMIAS)

Heart rate and rhythm is controlled by a number of factors ranging from body metabolism, exercise, environmental temperature, emotional state and balance of cardioinhibitory (vagal) and cardioaccelator forces (sympathetic).

Any irregularity associated with heart beat whether in rate or rhythm constitutes disorder of the heart referred to as arrhythmia. Cadiac arrhythmias assume significance since they can range from a very benign manifestation (occasional premature beats) to life threatening emergencies (ventricular tachycardias/fibrillation). Many a times cardiac arrhythmias may be the first manifestation of an underlying cardiac ailment but arrhythmias may occur in the presence or absence of organic heart disease.

Aetiology of cardiac arrhythmias

1. *Anxiety*
2. *Excessive* intake of tea, coffee, alcohol, tobacco
3. *Metabolic factors.* diabetic acidosis, hypoglycaemia, hypercalcaemia
4. *Endocrinal disorders.* Hyperthyroidism, hypothyroidism, phaeochromocytoma, hyperaldosternosim.
5. *Electrolyte disturbances.* Hypokalemia, hyperkalemia hyponatremia, alterations in magnesium levels.
6. *Infections.* Septicaemia.
7. *Drug toxicity.* Digitalis, diuretics, tricylic antidepressants, phenothiazine, antiarrhythmic drugs.
8. *Organic heart ailments.* Ischaemic heart disease, hypertension, valvular heart disease, congenital heart disease, myocarditis, chronic cor pulmonale.

Aetiology. Aetiologically arrhythmias may be produced by a number of factors ranging from anxiety, varying degrees of sympathetic stimulation (excessive intake of tea, coffee, alcohol, tobacco) metabolic factors (hyperthyroidism, hypothyroidism, hypercalcaemia, hyper-aldosteronism, phaeochromocytoma, diabetic acidosis hypoglycaemia) Electrolyte disturbances (hypokalaemia, hyperkalemia, hyponatremia, alterations in magnesium levels). Infections and toxic states, drugs like digoxin, diuretics, tricyclic anti-depressants, phenothiazines antiarrhythmic drugs like procain amide, quinidine etc. and organic heart ailments like ischaemic heart disease, hypertension, rheumatic heart disease, chronic cor pulmonale, myocarditis, and degenerative or congenital heart disease.

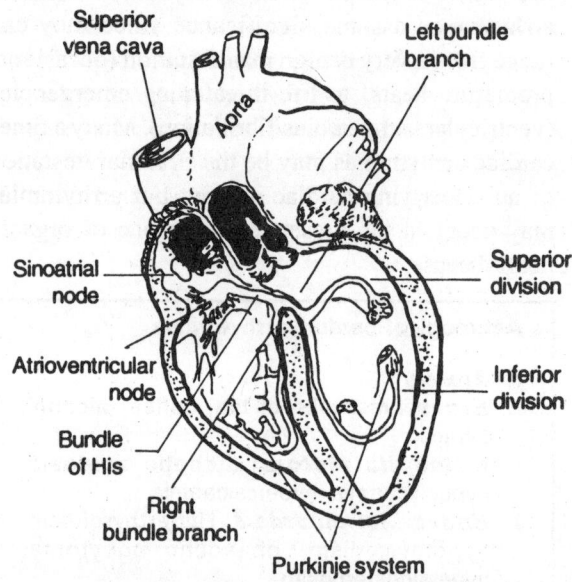

Fig. 4.38. Conducting system of heart.

Classification. Disturbances of rhythm have been classified in various ways. Disturbances of rhythm may involve the SA node (sinus bradycardia/tachycardia, SA heart block), Atria (premature beats atrial tachycardia, atrial flutter/fibrillation). A-V node (A-V heart block, A-V dissociation) and ventricles (ventricular premature beats, ventricular tachycardia/fibrillation). An arrhythmia may be benign or pose a life threatening situation which only means that accurate recognition of a cardiac arrhythmia should be considered as a challenge since prompt recognition and institution of therapy at the appropriate time shall go a long way in reducing the morbidity and mortality in the individual.

General management. The basic approach to the management of cardiac arrhythmia is to make an accurate diagnosis of the underlying cardiac condition and of the arrhythmia.

A detailed history for any previous attack suggestive of cardiac ailment, drug intake like digitalis or other drugs which could induce arrhythmia must be taken. Factors which could induce an arrhythmia like electrolyte disturbances, infections toxic states, metabolic and endocrinal factors should be considered.

Physical examination for signs of congestive failure, hypertension, presence of cardiac murmurs, clicks, gallops, peripheral pulses and neck veins for irregular venous 'a' waves should be carefully done. A 12 lead electrocardiogram is generally an adequate tool to make the diagnosis. In any ECG recording not only the rhythm should be identified but also various other parameters like Axis, heart rate, character of P waves. P-R interval QRS complexes and T waves, measurement of QT and R-R interval should be evaluated. Constant cardiac monitoring of an arrhythmia is very often required not only from prognostic but also from therapeutic point to evaluate the action of therapy. Special techniques like intracardiac potential recording from the atria, bundle of his and ventricles associated with the use of programmed stimulation techniques are not usually required and the diagnosis of an arrhythmia depends primarily on surface electrocardiography.

Management of arrhythmias. It should be looked in the light of total state of the patient. Any factors which may be acting or aggravating the state must either be removed or corrected. Electrolyte disorders must be gone into and adequate measures instituted to correct them. Toxic and noxious influences should be removed.

To decide whether the said arrhythmia warrants treatment in the context of the particular clinical situation prevailing shall depend on the clinical judgement and assessment of the gravity of the arrhythmia. One must understand the course of treatment and the use of specific antiarrhythmic drugs. Other approaches to management than the use of drugs like cardioversion, D.C. shock, programmed stimulation with pacemarkers must be considered. One of the view has been that treatment and/or suppression of any particular arrhythmia is only justified if the consequent improvement in symptoms, morbidity and mortality outweight the risks and inconvenience of treatment. This may not be accepted in totality since every arrhythmia which (a) Produces symptoms, (b) Is life threatening, requires treatment. Once the arrhythmia in a patient is recognised adequate treatment be instituted at the earliest. It shall be governed by the nature of the arrhythmia, the haemodynamic effects it produces and the state of the heart.

Clasification of cardiac arrhythmias

1. **Disturbance of impulse formation.**
   a. *Disturbance of sinus mechanism*
      1. Sinus arrhythmia
      2. Sinus bradycardia
      3. Sinus tachycardia
   b. *Disturbances of atrial contraction*
      1. Atrial premature beats
      2. Paroxysmal atrial tachycardia
      3. Atrial flutter
      4. Atrial fibrillation
   c. *Disturbances of ventricular contraction*
      1. Ventricular premature beats
      2. Paroxysmal ventricular tachycardia
      3. Ventricular fibrillation
2. **Distrubance of impulse conduction.**
   a. Sinoatrial heart block
   b. Atrioventricular heart block
      Incomplete
      1. First degree
      2. Second degree
      3. Wenkebach's phenomenon
   c. Complete or third degree heart block
   d. Bundle branch block

Premature beats (Extra systoles or ectopic beats). Premature beats are one of the commonest arhythmia and are so common that probably there shall be hardly any person who has not had extra systoles at one time or the other in his/her life time. In a large number ofcases these are benign and there may be no evidence of any organic heart disease. Exercise may cause premature beats to disappear both in normal and diseased hearts but if these beats persist they are indicative of an organic heeart disase like rheumatic heart disease, ischaemic heart disease, infections, hypertesion, anoxic pulmonary heart disease etc. Conditions of anoxia, physical stress, excessive tobacco, coffee, alcohol, tea intake and use of drugs like digitalis, quinidine etc may be other factors responsible for the production of ectopic beats. Extra systoles may be either supraventricular (Atrial, nodal) or ventricular in origin and the treatment shall depend on a numberof factors.

Supraventricular ectopic beats. In majority of the patients atrial premature beats are quite innocous and require no treatment. There may be no symptoms but when symptoms appear like discomfort in the chest, precordial pain or the patient feels a catch in his heart beat it may require treatment.

Since atrial premature beats are most often associated with beign conditions the underlying causative factor should be corrected.

Remove any source of infection. Electrolyte imbalance if present should be corrected. Some of the patients are addicted to excessive intake of either tea, coffee, alcohol or smoking. This should be looked into. If the patient is on any of the drugs which are known to produce ectopic beats these drugs should be withdrawn. Reassure the patient. A small dose of phenobarbitol 30 mg twice a day or diazepam 5 mg twice shall go a long way in sedating the patient and removing anxieity.

If all the above measures fail and the extra systoles are persisiting and multiple then specific drug therapy should be instituted. Institution of treatment shall be important if a patient with acute myocardial infection or after cardiac surgery develops frequent atrial premature bears since this shall be a warning to the subsequent development of either atrial flutter or fibrillation. Digoxin 0.25 mg given orally twice a day is the first choice. It may not be the ideal anti-arrhythmic for the correctrion of supraventricular ectopics but it improves myocardial contractility and improved myocardial function may result in lesser number of ectopics. Alternatively quinidine (quinidine sulfate 200-400 mg) orally every 6 hours be employed. Longer-acting quinidine preparations (quinidine gluconate 324 mg tablet) may be administerd every 8 to 12 hours. Side effects of quinidine like gastrointestinal disturbances, cinchonism and E.C.G. changes (prolonged Q-T interval) be watched.

Procainamide (Pronestyl 500 mg) can also be employed in a total dose of 2-3 gms per day given every 6 hours. It is equally effective and has cardiac depressant effect leading to prolongation of Q-T interval.

Propranolol (Inderal) is also an effective antiarrhythmic agent especially when the extra systoles are related to increased sympathetic activity like exercise, emotions or myocardial ischaemia. Dose shall range from 10-40 mg three or four times a day. Dosage of propranolol required to control the ectopic beats is variable and after a test dosage it has to be gradually increased to the level of tolerance but in no case the total dosage should exceed more than 200 mg per day. Beta blockers have their side effects and may trigger off potential bronchial asthma, diabetes and congestive heart failure.

Disopyramide (Norpace) 150 mg four times a day is also an effective drug. Its effect is variable. It induces myocardial depression (prolongation of Q-T interval) and may aggravate congestive heart failure. Diphyenyl hydantion (Dilantin 100 mg tablet) is a weak anti-arrhythmic drug. A loading dose of 1 gm on first day 500 mg on second to fourth day and then afterwards 300-400 mg per day in divided doses is recommended. The drug has to be withdrawn slowly. Its main indication is when the extrasystoles are digitalis induced.

Prognosis in a case of supraventricular extra systoles is good depending on the underlying condition and the presence of these is no bar to leading an active normal life.

Causes of ventricular premature beats

1. Excessive smoking, intake of alcohol, tea and coffee.
2. Coronary artery disease
3. Acute myocardial infarction
4. During anaesthesia
5. Rheumatic heart disease
6. Digitalis toxicity
7. Congestive heart failure

Ventricular premature beats. Premature ventricular beats are of more concern even when asymptomatic since they are associated with sudden cardiac death. This type of irregularity is more common than atrial beats and can also occur in healthy persons increasing in frequency with advancing age. Excessive smoking and intake of tea, coffee, alochol has been blamed in some people and stoppage of their use seems to help the patient.

But ventricular premature beats are commonly seen in a patient of coronary artery disease especially during the acute attack of myocardial infarction, congestive heart failure, cardiomyopathy, during anaesthesia and following digitals toxicity. Simple, single focus ventricular premature beats carry little risk but it is the presence of multiple multifocal ventricular ectopic beats which are dangerous and may induce ventricular tachycardia/fibrillation and sudden death. VPBS have to be treated urgently if:

1. VPBs are frequent and more than 6 in a minute
2. Multifocal in nature or coming in pairs
3. Runs of VPBs
4. R-on-T pattern of VPBs.

Treatment. If the above type of condition exists, the patient should be treated. If patient on digoxin stop the drug and give potassium supplements. Those with disturbing symptoms the following drug treatment is suggested.

Lignocaine (Lidocaine, Xylocard). This drug remains the drug of choice and in urgent situation a bolus dose of 50-100 mg (1 mg/kg body weight) by slow I/V route over a period of 5-10 minutes is given. Bolus is followed with 1 G in 500 ml of infusion solution by I.V. drip at the rate of 10-40 drops/minute (1-4 mg/minute). Special care should be taken in case of cardiac decompensation, liver damage, hypotension shock and in very old people. In patients with known hypersensitivity to amide group of local anaesthetics, serious conduction disturbances. A-V blocks and bradycadia the drug should not be administered. ECG control must be maintaind by constant monitoring.

Mexiletine hydrochloride (Mexitil) is the next line of therapy. It is useful for the treatment of ventricular ectopic beats such as those found after myocardial infarction, after digitalis and idiopathic states.

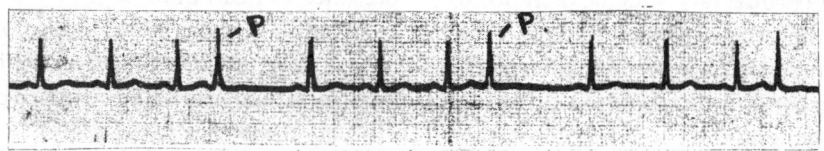

Fig. 4.39. Atrial Premature Complexes. These result due to an impulse arising in a ectopic focus somewhere in the atria. Contour of P wave shall depend on the focus of origin of Impulse. QRS complex generally in normal Atrial premature complexes (Marked P) are seen.

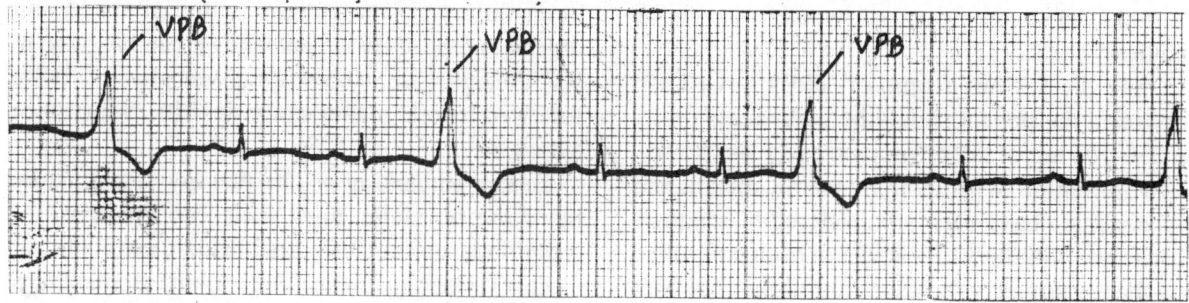

Fig. 4.40. Premature ventricular Complexes. These are arising from a single focus. QRS complex is broad, prolonged and followed by a compensatory pause.

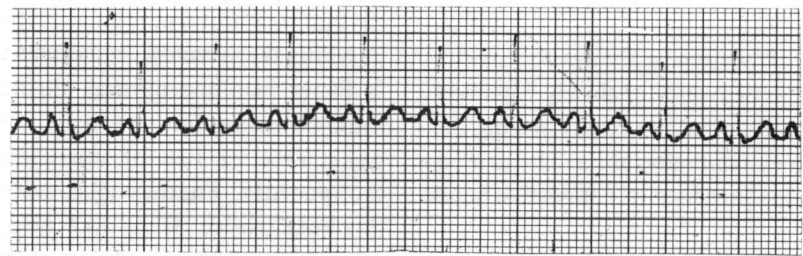

Fig. 4.41. Atrial Tachycardia. Heart rate varies from 140–220 beats/minute. In this recording heart rate regular 150/minute.

In cases where it is desirable to reach sufficient blood levels of the drug, initial loading dse is recommended especially with I/V administration. Initial dose of 100-250 mg (equivalent to 2-5 mg/kg body weight) given at a suggested rate of 0.5 ml per minute. Follow this with 500 mg in 500 ml 5% dextrose saline I/V infusion over 3-4 hours (2.0 mg/kg body weight).

Maintenance therapy with 250 mg in 500 ml 5% dextrose saline at rate of 1 ml per minute. This has to be continued depending on patients response.

As the arrhythmia gets controlled then switch on to oral capsules (150 mg capsule three times a day).

Side effects include drowsiness, confusion, nausea, hypotension, sinus bradycardia, hiccups etc.

Quinidine sulphate given orally in a dose of 200-400 mg every six hours. It being a cardiac depresant, it depresses cardiac excitability, slows down A-V nodal and intraventricular conduction. It is contraindicated in the presence of complete heart block, in acute infections and extensive myocardial damage. Quinidine not withstanding its side effects, is an effective oral agent for the control of premature ventricular beats. Intravenous administration leads to fall of blood pressure and severe degree of hypotension.

Procainamide (Pronestyl) is the next choice of antiarrhythmic drug for the urgent control of VPBs if there is known sensitivity to lidocaine or the patient fails to respond to the adequate dosage of the drugs. It is given initially I/V in a bolus dosage of 50-100 mg followed by intravenous slow administration of the drug (500-1000 mg) ECG control should be monitored and the maximum dose should not be exceeded. The drug carries the risk of producing severe degree of hypotension, shock and heart blocks.

Once the serious forms of VPBs have been controlled the patient should be maintained orally on 250-500 mg of the drug given every 4-6 hours.

Propranolol. When both lidocaine, mexitil and procainamide have been administered in adequate dosage and still the VPBs have not been controlled and there is urgency for their control the trial with propranolol should be considered. The usual dose is 0.5-1 mg given I/V every 5 minutes slowly but total dosage should not exceed 5 mg. When found effective, the patient is usually controlled within a dose of 3 to 5 mg.

Intravenous use of the drug be always done under cardiac monitoring and given very slowly. Injection Atropine 0.4 mg be given before administering the drug to prevent excessive bradycardia. The drug is contraindicated in the presence of congestive heart failure.

If all the above measures fail then the patient may require pacing.

But for the patient who has got distressing ventricular premature beats which require treatment though not urgently then the following line of treatment can be adopted. First use Mexitil or Quinidine. Other drugs are:

Disopyramide (Norpace). Given orally in a dose of 100-150 mg every six hourly is an effective drug. Since it induces myocardial depression it is contraindicated in the presence of congestive heart failure.

Diphenyl hydantoin. It is the drug of choice when ventricular premature beats are digitalis-induced or when there is contraindication to the use of Lidocaine, Mexitil, Pronestyl, Propranolol like the presence of congestive heart failure or there is presence of heart blocks.

Dilantin is given I/V in a dose of 50 mg/minute upto a total of 1000 mg in 24 hours. Once the urgency is over, patient be switched over to oral drug (100 mg three-four times a day).

Digoxin. Though it may look a strange situation but digoxin which is a very important aetiological factor in the causation of VPBs, shall be the drug of choice when VPBs, are associated with congestive heart failure. If the patient is undigitalised and urgency of the situation demands it can be given in I/V dosage (0.25-0.5 mg) given slowly. It be followed by oral maintenance dose (0.25 mg twice a day).

Before embarking on the therapy of premature beats the physician must look into the cause of arrhythmia, correct the probable toxic metabolic, or electrolyte derangements. The anti-arrhythmic drugs must be selected with due care keeping in view their probable toxic effects and contraindications. Once the actue stage is over the patient shall have to be controlled on maintenance therapy and the cardiac rhythm monitored at regular intervals.

Sinus tachycardia. It denotes that the heart rate is faster than the normal intrinsic rate with the impulse arising from SA node. Usually in an adult heart rate of 110 or more constitutes sinus tachycardia. Factors like exercise, emotions, anaemia use of drugs like atropine, sympathomimetic agents (epinephrine, salbutamol). Thyroid hormones and acute toxic states like fever, severe degree of infections, respnse to haemostatic mechanisms like hypotension haemorrhage or shock and organic heart disease, thyrotoxicosis, congestive heart failure shall be responsible for the induction of tachycardia. In majority of the patients where the heart rate is not very high (120-140/mt) there are no symptoms but in some there are complaints of palpitation, restlessness and even in some complaint of chest pain. Patient is generally apprehensive.

It is important to recognise the condition. ECG confirms the diagnosis. Rhythm is regular P-R interval is usually shortened and there are regular R-R complexes. Carotid sinus massage may slow down the rate temporarily.

Causes of sinus tachycardia

1. Exercise
2. Emotions
3. Fever
4. Anaemia
5. Blood loss/shock
6. Drugs (atropine, epinephrine, salbutamol, thyroid extract, nifedipine).
7. Thyrotoxicosis
8. Organic heart disease
9. Congestive heart failure

Treatment of the condition is directed towards the treatment of under lying condition. A small dose of diazepam (2-5 mg) shall go a long way in alleviating the apprehension. If tachycardia is associated with congestive heart failure digitalis and diuretics are indicated.

In cases where there is no apparent cause to explain the tachycardia, propranolol 20 mg twice or thrice a day shall benefit the patient provided there are no contraindications to the use of drug like congestive failure, diabetes, bronchial asthma etc.

Paroxysmal-supraventricular tachycardia. It is a common condition often seen in young healthy individuals without any apparent heart disease. There is a rapid succession of cardiac impulses which arise from an irritable ectopic focus in the atrium. Patient gets attacks of tachycardia which come suddenly, last for brief periods and often are terminated spontaneously. Diagnosis is made from the history of paroxysms of attacks of palpitation. Heart rate varies between 180 to 250 beats per minute and is regular. ECG shows T wave slightly modified with fusion with P wave which is often buried in QRS complex or ST segment. P waves in

Causes of paroxysmal supraventricular tachycardia

1. Idiopathic
2. Acute myocardial infarction
3. Rheumatic heart disease
4. Cardiac catheterization
5. Digitalis toxicity
6. Electrolyte abnormalities.

atrial tachycardia may be identified by the use of oesophageal leads or recording precordial leads from the right side in the third interspace.

Most of the times, PAT being a benign condition terminates spontaneously but if it causes distressing symptoms and haemodynamic embarrassment, emergency medication must be instituted. This is equally important if PAT is present in a patient with underlying heart disease like myocardial infarction, rheumatic heart disease or in patients with. Wolff Parkinson-White syndrome (WPW syndrome) or during cardiac catheterization and cardiac surgery. Digitalis is an important cause of paroxysmal atrial tachycardia with atrioventricular block and if not recognised early, the arrhythmia may prove fatal.

Before instituting therapy one must correct any underlying toxic, metabolic or electrolyte abnormality since these are known to induce attack of atrial tachycardia.

Treatment

During the attack. In majority of the patients of PAT where there is no organic basis sedation and assurance followed by physical manouvers like asking the patient to lean forward with his head bent down, to expire forcibly with glottis closed after a deep inspiration (Valsalva manouver). Quite often drinking sips of water, coughing or inducing vomiting terminates the attack. Applying pressure on eye balls with the eye lid closed may be helpful but it shall be done with caution in cases with suspected glaucoma or those using contact lenses.

Carotid sinus massage is a very useful procedure but before doing it one must be doubly sure that both the carotids are pulsatile. The patient in a recumbent position with his head extended and turned slightly to the side, the carotid sinus on the right side is first massaged for upto 10 seconds and if not successful then massage is repeated on the left side. Massage should be done lightly with two or three fingers and direct pressure on the artery avoided. While doing carotid sinus massage do constant cardiac auscultation by means of a stethoscope since there is often a risk of inducing cardiac stand still or syncope if the carotid massage is unnecessarily prolonged. If the physical measures fail then drugs should be administered.

Verapamil. It is the first line of therapy. Dose is 5-10 mg slowly I/V at a rate of 1 mg per minute. It can be repeated after 30 minutes if required.

Digoxin. Digoxin has been the drug of choice for the termination of an acute attack. It is administered intravenously slowly in a dose of 0.5 mg. It is important that the patient receiving digitalis should not have been previously digitalised. Cedilanid (Lanatoside C) another short acting preparation of Digoxin is preferred since it acts rapidly, is quickly eliminated and is less hazardous. Dose is 0.8 to 1.2 mg given I/V slowly as a bolus dosage. Again it can be repeated in 30 to 60 minutes if required.

Propranolol. It is an effective therapy after trial with verapamil and digoxin has failed to restore normal sinus rhythm. Dose is 0.5 to 1 mg/minute I/V in five minutes period upto a maximum of 10 mg. Propranolol should be used with caution since it may exacerberate congestive failure and can also produce bradycardia or A-V block.

Phenytoin sodium (Dilantin). It is especially indicated when PAT is associated with Digitalis-induced 2:1 A-V block. Dose is 50 mg/minute I/V to a total dose of 1000 mg.

Adenosine. It is an effective drug. Initial dose is 3.5 mg given as rapid intravenous bolus. If first dose does not eliminate PSVT within 1-2 minutes, 6 mg should be given as rapid I/V bolus. If it still does not eliminate PSVT, then 12 mg. be given, additional doses are not recommended.

Lidocaine. If all the previous drugs have been unsuccessful, Lidocaine may be employed initially in a bolus dose of 50-100 mg (1 mg/kg) given over 1-2 minutes followed by an infusion at the rate of 1-4 mg/minute, the total dose not to exceed 500 mg in 24 hours.

Cardioversion. If drug therapy fails and there is haemodynamic embarrassment causing syncope, myocardial ischaemic or congestive heart failure, D.C. cardioversion should be employed and is the treatmet of choice.

While doing cardioversion in a case of supraventricular tachycardia start at the lowest potentially effective energy. A DC shock of 20-100 joules is generally sufficient in correcting the rhythm.

Before giving DC shock, patient should be sedated with Diazepam given slowly I/V (5-10 mg). Blood pressure be maintained and airways patency be ensured.

In a patient developing PAT who has already been digitalized, DC shock may be risky so rapid atrial pacing may be employed.

Prevention of recurrent attacks. Once an acute attack of PAT has been terminated attempt should be made to prevent its recurrence. Many a times this may not be easy since in a large number of patients the underlying cause may not be found. As a general principle patient must avoid, all those factors which could precipitate an attack. Excess use of tea, coffee, alcohol and smoking should be curbed. Such patients must avoid excessive fatigue, exertion and emotional tension.

For prevention of further episodes any of the following drugs be employed orally (i) tablet verapamil 40 mg thrice a day or (ii) tablet propranolol 10-40 mg thrice a day or (iii) tablet digoxin 0.25 mg twice a day.

If the above drugs fail then disopyramide or quinidine or amiodarone be given a trial. In majority of the cases the patient is relieved of further attacks. Maintenance therapy by oral drugs has to be continued for a minimum period of 3-6 months and in some cases even continued upto a period of one year.

If drug therapy fails, temporary or permanent pacing may be required. The pacemaker is activated when tachycardia occurs and interrupts the re-enterant pathway. In very selected cases who resist treatment, surgical interruption of the abnormal conducting pathway may be attempted.

Paroxysmal atrial tachycardia with block. This is an arrhythmia which if not recognized can often prove fatal and invariably occurs in a patient who while receiving digitalis develops an increase in the ventricular rate. Atrial rate is usually between 120-250 beats per minute and there is isoelectric interval

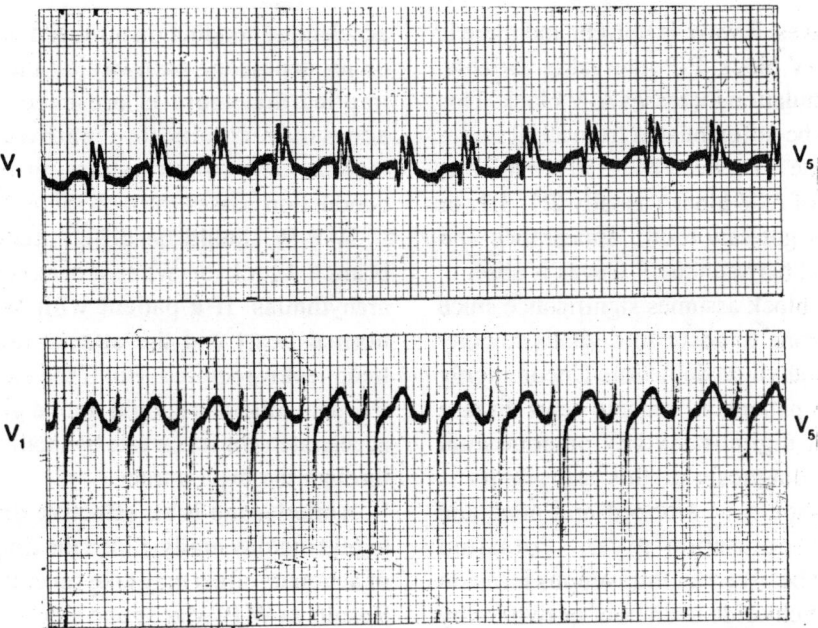

Fig. 4.42. Paroxysmal Supraventricular. Tachycardia. A regular narrow complex atrial tachycardia, Heart rate 188/ minute there is fusion of T and P waves.

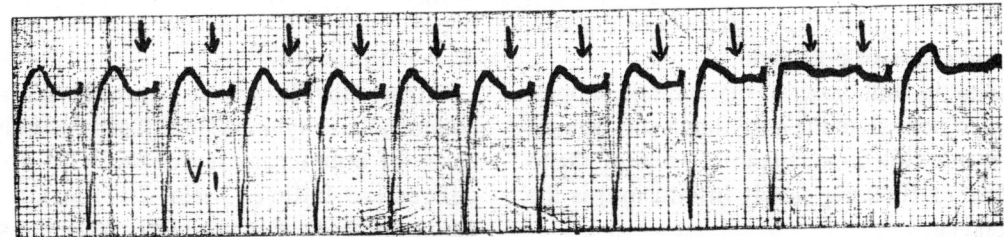

Fig. 4.43. Atrial Tachycardia with 2:1 A-V Block.

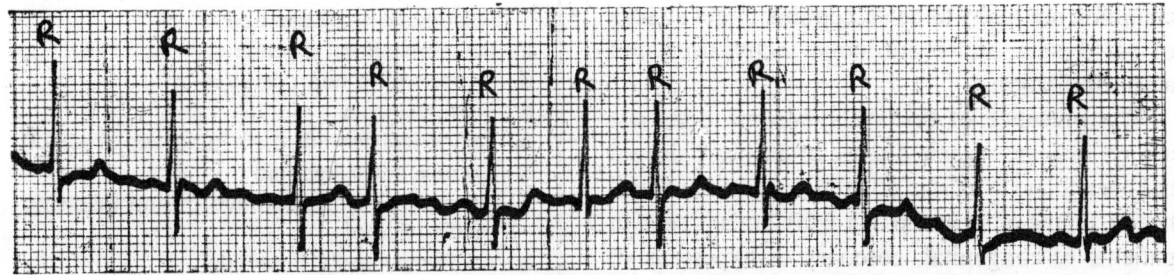

Fig. 4.44. Atrial Fibrillation. R-R Interval is irregular. Atrial waves are replaced by fibrillary waves.

between the P waves. P wave is upright and there is commonly 2:1 A-V block. P-P interval is variable. Carotid sinus stimulation increases A-V block. This arrhythmia has to be differentiated from atrial flutter where the atrial rate is between 250-350 per minute, variable degrees of A-V block (usually 2:1, 3:1, or 4:1). P wave has got saw tooth, appearance and isoelectric interval between the P waves is absent.

PAT with A-V block assumes significance since it is especially prone to occur in digitalis toxicity associated with potassium depletion. Uncommonly it may be seen in patients of organic heart disease without apparent digitalis toxicity or potassium depletion. Once diagnosis of this arrhythmia is made, digitalis should be stopped and adequate supplements of potassium given. Potasium supplements may be given by intravenous infusion (3 G of potassium chloride in an hour or two) or by oral route (2 to 8 G of potassium chloride in 24 hours). In a large number of patients of congestive failure on digitalis the development of this arrhythmia can be prevented by giving adequate supplements of potassium salts with diuretics. Early recognition of the arrhythmia is equally important since it responds quickly to withdrawl of digitalis and administration of potasium.

If despite the withdrawl of digoxin and supplementation of potassium the arrhythmia still persists then phenytoin (Injection Dilantin 50 mg/minute to a total dose of 1000 mg slowly in infusion) is the drug of choice.

Wolff-Parkinson-White syndrome. A condition characterised electrocardiographically by a short P-R interval and prolonged QRS complex. This arrhythmia is significant since patients with this condition are likely to be susceptible to get attacks of paroxysmal supraventricular tachycardia and atrial fibrillation.

The presence of W-P-W syndrome does not always indicate organic disease of the heart since it has been found to exist in 60 to 70 per cent of normal hearts. Of the other group this arrhythmia is seen in patients of congenital, coronary or hypertensive heart disease.

The underlying mechanism may be an accelerated conduction through the normal pathway or an accessory pathway or the concept which implies that there is presence of one or more accessory conduction pathways (paraseptal mechanism) which bypassing the normal A-V conduction passes through the A-V node.

W-P-W should be differentiated from bundle branch block or when co-existing with other arrhythmias. If a patient with W-P-W has got a normal heart and the attacks are infrequent no treatment is required. But if the attacks become too frequent, digitalis should not be given since it may accelerate ventricular rate by facilitating conduction through the bypass tract.

Amiodarone is an effective drug. Dose is 300 to 600 mg/day orally. Since the drug has long range of action its effect may take several days to develop. Results in W-P-W are good since it suppresses both normal and aberrant pathway. Side effects include induction of bradycardia and A-V block. Prognosis in cases of W-P-W syndrome is good but frequent attacks of long duration both in normal and diseased hearts shall not indicate favourable prognosis. Surgical intervention in the form of ablation of bypass tracts allows success in refractory cases of W-P-W syndrome.

Atrial fibrillation. It is probably one of the commonest arrhythmia since it is frequently seen in cases of organic heart disease with or without congestive failure. Atrial fibrillation may be paroxysmal or established (attacks occur suddenly and last a few seconds, minutes or days). Often atrial fibrillation has continued for months or years.

Causes of atrial fibrillation

1. Rheumatic heart disease
2. Ischaemic heart disease
3. Hypertensive heart disease
4. Thyrotoxicosis
5. Congenital heart disease (atrial septal defect)
6. Chronic cor pulmonale
7. During and postoperative period following cardiac surgery
8. Acute myocardial infarction

Uncommonly atrial fibrillation has been seen in

the absence of organic heart disease (Lone atrial fibrillation). Of the various cardiac ailments the arrhythmia is most commonly seen in cases of rheumatic heart disease (especially mitral valve disease) ischaemic and hypertensive heart disease, thyrotoxicosis, congenital heart disease and chronic cor pulmonale. Atrial fibrillation is often seen in the first week following acute myocardial infarction and it may be seen only in brief paroxysms which may subside of their own. It is also not infrequently seen during surgery and in the immediate post operative period especially in elderly patients and those undergoing cardiac surgery. Diagnosis of atrial fibrillation depends on an irregularly irregular pulse with an irregular heart (Atrial rate greater than 350 beats/mt and ventricular rate varying from 100 to 160 beats per minute). Heart may not show a murmur. There is absence of presystolic character of the diastolic murmur in mitral stenosis. ECG shows an irregular rhythm with rapid oscillations (400 to 700 per minute), P wave being replaced by 'f' (fibrillary) waves.

Before treating a case of atrial fibrillation one must evaluate:

1. Underlying cardiac ailment
2. Presence or absence of congestive heart failure
3. Whether fibrillation is paroxysmal or established and if so its duration
4. Left atrial size
5. Ventricular rate
6. Effect of atrial fibirillation on haemodynamics.

Treatment to a large extent shall be guided not only by the above factors but attempt made to treat the underlying cause. Thus if thyrotoxicosis is the underlying condition, anti-thyroid drugs must be given.

Treatment is to be aimed at slowing the ventricular rate and in restoring the sinus rhythm.

Drugs. Digitalis is the first choice since it not only slows the rate but may also convert it to sinus rhythm. In a patient with congestive failure and not already on digoxin, rapid digitalization is performed (injection digoxin 0.25 mg I/V slowly, to be repeated

after six hours until the ventricular rate falls to 60-80/minute). Total dose of digoxin in 24 hours by injections route should not exceed 1.25 mg.

Once digitalization has been achieved patient should be put on oral digoxin (tablet digoxin 0.25 mg twice a day or 8 hourly). Dosage of digitalis has to be altered depending on the age of the patient (less in elderly people) and degree of heart failure. Presence of failure also requires use of diuretics. If there is associated anaemia, hypopotassaemia or infection it should also be simultaneously treated. It is not possible to achieve normal sinus rhythm with digitalis alone in majority of the patients. Then quinidine is the drug of choice for the conversion of atrial fibrillation to a normal rhythm. This is required to achieve improvement in cardiovascular dynamics and to prevent embolic phenomenon. Combined therapy with digitalis and quinidine is employed and when both drugs are used in combination, the deleterious effects of the other are prevented. Digitalis will be effective for the control of failure and ventricular rate. Once this is achieved, quinidine should be added to convert the rhythm to normal. Dosage of quinidine is 200-300 mg orally four hourly. This dose may further be reduced to six hourly and continued for two to four weeks or longer depending on the tendency of the heart to revert to atrial fibrillation.

Cardioversion. There may be some cases where atrial fibrillation is producing serious cardiac embarrassment in the form of hypotension or is poorly tolerated and requires urgent control. Cardioversion (DC shock) is the treatment of choice. In such emergency, situation, patient should be put on anticoagulants and 100 mg of lignocaine I/V over two minutes prior to cardioversion must be administered.

If patient is already on digoxin, it should be withdrawn for 24-48 hours prior to cardioversion because of the danger of ventricular arrhythmias likely to develop following DC shock.

In cases of chronic established atrial fibrillation elective cardioversion has been attempted. Patient should be anticoagulated for two to three weeks prior to this procedure. But in all such cases especially if the left atrium is very large and if fibrillation is of more than six months duration, chances of recurrence of atrial fibrillation after cardioversion are there.

But if the factors are favourable and once sinus rhythm has been restored after DC shock this has to be maintained by drug therapy.

Tablet Digoxin 0.25 mg twice a day be administered. But if ventricular rate is not well controlled (60-80/mt) propranolol (60-80 mg/day in divided dose) or verapamil 40-80 mg twice or thrice a day be administered. Presence of severe degree of congestive failure shall be a contraindication to the use of these drugs. When atrial fibrillation is of long standing and not contributing significantly to poor haemodynamic status of the patient it may be left alone and only drug therapy be employed. Cardioversion is not of much help. If atrial fibrillation follows acute myocardial infarction, and there is danger of acute cardiac embarrassment, cardioversion may be attempted followed by I/V use of digitalis or verapamil. After wards normal sinus rhythm is maintained by the oral use of one of these drugs.

Atrial flutter. It is an uncommon arrhythmia as compared to atrial fibrillatin. Aetiologically it is seen in cases or rheumatic heart disease, acute rheumatic fever, coronary heart disease, acute infectious states, thyrotoxicosis and occasionally in cases with congenital heart disease. On clinical examination the pulse in atrial flutter is regular in contrast to atrial fibrillation where the rhythm is irregularly irregular. Atrial rate varies from 240 to 300 beats per minute. There is either 2:1, 3:1 or 4:1 block and the ventricular rate varies from 60 to 150 depending on the degree of A-V block. Carotid sinus massage does not interrupt the arrhythmia but increases the block and slows the ventricular rate. But this returns to original rate when the pressure is removed. Diagnosis of atrial flutter is made by electrocardiogram which shows characteristic flutter waves (saw-toothed P waves) without any isoelectric line between the P waves. Atrial rate ranging from 240 to 300 and ventricular rate of 120 to 150 with 2:1 A-V block. Atrial flutter generally requires to be differentiated from sinus tachycardia, paroxysmal atrial tachycardia, atrial fibrillation and ventricular tachycardia.

```
Causes of atrial flutter

1.  Rheumatic heart disease
2.  Coronary heart disease
3.  Thyrotoxicosis
4.  Congenital heart disease
5.  Acute infectious states
6.  Acute rheumatic fever
```

Treatment:

Digitalis is the drug of choice. If patient not already on digitalis, administer digoxin 0.5 mg I/V slowly. The important action of digitalis shall be slowing of ventricular rate by increasing the A-V block. It may convert atrial flutter into atrial fibrillation which may revert to normal sinus rhythm.

After I/V medication with digitalis patient should be put on oral digitalis (0.25 mg twice a day or 8 hourly). Inadequate digitalization may be cause of failure. Very occasionally digitalis may convert flutter to sinus rhythm without the intervention of fibrillatioon. If digoxin fails to convert the flutter to sinus rhythm then quinidine is the second drug of choice. Quinidine sulfate 200-300 mg orally four hourly is often successful. Quinidine slows the rate of flutter by its direct effect on the atrium but can increase ventricular rate if not given in combination with digoxin.

Propranolol. In cases where quick action is required and there is no congestive failure, propranolol may be given I/V at a rate of 1 mg every five minutes (5-10 mg) followed by maintenance by oral route (20-40 mg three times a day).

Verapamil. Its indications for use are the same as for propranolol. Dose is 5 mg I/V slowly followed by oral maintenance dose of 40-80 mg thrice a day.

Both propranolol and verapamil have an effect of converting atrial flutter to sinus rhythm by increasing A-V block and slowing ventricular rate. Sometimes flutter may be converted to fibrillation before reverting to normal sinus rhythm.

Cardioversion. In case a patient of atrial flutter

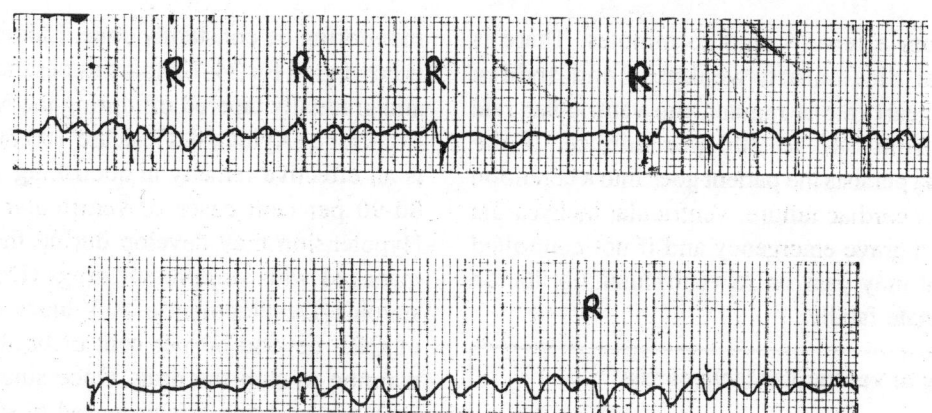

Fig. 4.45. Flutter Fibrillation R-R. Interval is irregular but atrial waves are more coarse giving a saw tooth appearance.

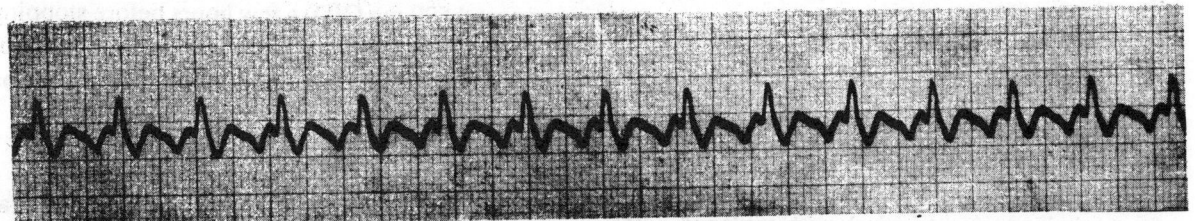

Fig. 4.46. Atrial Flutter. Atrial rate is regular at 250/mt. There is characteristic saw tooth appearance.

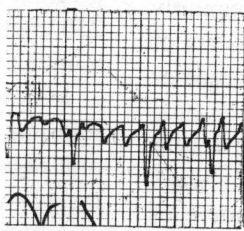

Fig. 4.47. Atrial Flutter with 4:1 A-V conduction.

shows evidence of haemodynamic embarrassment, DC shock is the treatment of choice (dose varying from 25 watts sec to 400 watts sec). In majority of the cases either sinus rhythm is restored or patient's flutter gets converted into fibrillation which is managed by the use of anti-arrhythmic drugs.

In a patient where flutter occurs because of digitalis, rapid atrial pacing is employed. Prognosis of a case with atrial flutter shall depend on the condition of the myocardium, response to treatment and the persistence of flutter. Recurrent attack of flutter makes the prognosis unfavourable.

Paroxysmal ventricular tachycardia. It is a serious type of arrhythmia and almost always occurs in the presence of serious myocardial disease. The important conditions are acute myocardial infarction, hypertension, cardiomyopathy, severe infection (diphtheria, rheumatic fever) during procedures like cardiac catheterization, angiography, surgery, anaesthesia and severe degree of digitalis toxicity. Rarely paroxysmal ventricular tachycardia has been seen in patients with apparently normal heart. Generally a patient getting attacks of ventricular tachycrdia may have brief episodes lasting from a few seconds to minutes. There is substernal discomfort, weakness and sudden collapse, heart rate is regular, the ventricular rate ranging from 140 to 200 per minute. If the tachycardia persists the patient goes into a condition of shock or cardiac failure. Ventricular tachycardia is always a grave emergency and if not controlled the patient may pass on to ventricular fibrillation and terminate fatally.

Causes of ventricular tachycardia

1. Acute myocardial infarction
2. Hypertensive heart disease
3. Cardiomyopathy
4. Severe infections
5. Myocarditis
6. During cardiac catheterization, angiography, anesthesia
7. Digitalis toxicity

Diagnosis of ventricular tachycardia is invariably made by electrocardiogram which shows paroxysms of ectopic beats (ventricular) with widened. QRS complexes (0.12 secs and more). The ventricles are beating reglarly at rates ranging from 140 to 200 per minute while Atria are also beating regularly but more slowly and nearly always independent of ventricles. In doubtful cases oesophageal leads or his bundel electrocardiography helps in establishing the diagnosis. Once diagnosis of ventricular tachycardia has been made, treatment is always instituted as an emergency measure. Choice of treatment shall depend on the underlying cause (myocarodial infarction). Haemodynamic status of the patient (hypotension, shock, congestive failure, precordial discomfort etc). Apart from the specific drug therapy, patient may require coincidental administration of vasopressor drugs. In desprate condition, electric cardioversion is indicated.

Drugs. Lidocaine. It is the drug of choice. Dose is 50-100 mg (1 mg/kg body weight) I/V given as a bolus dose. It may be repeated once or twice at an interval of 5 to 10 minutes. If required, but not more than 300 mg during one hour period. Afterwards, lidocaine infusion should be started at the rate of 1-4 mg/minute to prevent recurrence. Cardiac

monitoring be constantly done. Lidocaine infusion is continued for 24-72 hours as per the requirement and gradually tapered off during the next 24 hours. Lidocaine (Xylocard, Gesicard 100 mg/5 ml amp.) is an effective remedy in abolishing arrhythmia in 80-90 per cent cases of ventricular tachycardia. Hypotension may develop during therapy and be managed with vasopressor drugs (Dopamine) and steroids. Development of A-V block and widening of QRS beyond 50 per cent of basic control is a warning to stop the drug. Once sinus rhythm has been restored and it is proposed to stop the use of lidocaine patient should be put on oral antiarrhythmic drugs (Disopyramide 100-150 mgm six hourly or quinidine 300 mg six hourly or pronestyl 500 mg QID) a few hours before stopping I/V infusion of Lidocaine to prevent recurrence of arrhythmia. Maintenance therapy may have to be continued for periods ranging from 3-6 months.

Other drugs:

Mexiletine. If lidocaine fails to control ventricular tachycardia then Mexiletine, a drug chemically and pharmacologically similar to lignocaine should be given. It is given by intravenous route. Dose is 200-250 mg/minute followed by I.V. infusion of 1 mg/minute over 1 hour.

Maintenance is 0.5 mg/minute by intavenous infusion. Once arrhythmia controlled, switch on to oral capsules (150 mg thrice a day). Side effects include hypotension, bradycardia and accentuation of A-V block. Drug has got exceollent response in ventricular tachycardia following post myocardial infarction or during cardiac surgery.

Procainamide. It is an effective therapy specially after the failure of lidocaine. Slow intravenous infusion of 25 mg/minute to a total of one gm procaine amide (1 gm dissolved in 100 ml of 5% glucose in distilled water and administered at the rate of 2 or 3 ml per minute). Once the tachycardia is controlled then I/V infusion is continued at the rate of 4-6 mg/minute. Procaine amide may cause hypotension and A-V block. If marked prolongation of QRS complexes (more than 50% or P-R interval is prolonged the drug has to be discontinued).

Quinidine. It has the same range of action as procainamide. Quinidine gluconate (0.5 to 1.0 gm) diluted in 50 to 100 cc of 5% glucose in distilled water is given by I/V route slowly in over 30 minutes to an hour under electrocardiographic control. Hypotension and accentuation of A-V block are serious side effects of the therapy.

Phenytoin. If ventricular tachycardia is digitalis induced then Diphenyl hydantoin is the drug of choice. Dose is 100-200 mg I/V slowly in three to five minutes and may be repeated after 15 minutes if required. Total dose is one gram.

Propranolol. It is the second line of therapy. Dose is one mg I/V to be given slowly and repeated at five minute interval upto a maximum of three mg. It may exaceberate congestive heart failure and cause A-V block, bradycardia or bronchospasm.

Cardioversion. If the arrhythmia fails to respond to drug therapy or the condition of the patient is desperate (circulatory collapse, hypotension or shock). DC shock (100 to 200 joules) be applied immediately. Cardioversion is successful in majority of the patients. While applying DC shock one must synchronize the shock to QRS to prevent ventricular fibillation.

Other measures. In addition to antiarrhythmic drugs, DC shock, patient must be sedated by the use of 5-10 mg diazepam given I/V slowly and at the same time monitoring blood pressure and respiration. This shall not only sedate the patient but also allay anxiety. Blood pressure must be maintained at adequate levels by the use of vasopressors (mephetamine/noradrenaline/dopamine) and steroids. O_2 be administered continuously at the rate of six to eight litres/minute. Metabolic acidosis be prevented by I/V administration of 100 ml of 0.5% sodium bicarbonate solution. Electrolyte abnormalities if present must be corrected. Management of ventricular tachycardia must be done as a grave emergency and adequate therapy in proper dosage must be administered. Patient must be treated as a whole and not only the arrhythmia. Once the crisis is over, patient be put on long term oral drug therapy (mexiletine/procainamide/quinidine/phenytoin) of one or more of these drugs to prevent recurrence of the arrhythmia.

Polymorphous ventricular tachycardia (Torsades de pointes). It is a rare type of ventricular tachycardia characterised by variable shape of QRS complexes and is often confused with ventricular fibrillation. This arrhythmia may stop suddenly and then a long Q-T interval is noticed while in sinus rhythm. During the episode of arrhythmia the rate ranges upto 300 beats per minute. Aetiologically a number of antiarrhythmic drugs have been known to be responsible for it.

Treatment is by I/V infusion of isoproterenol (1 to 4 ugm per minute). It shall increase the sinus rate and decrease Q-T interval. Over drive pacing of right atrium or ventricle may abolish the arrhythmia if drug thereapy fails.

Ventricular fibrillation. It is one of the most serious cardic arrhythmia and is closely allied with cardiac arrest and is often the terminal cardiac event before death.

Causes of ventricular fibrillation

1. Acute myocardial infarction
2. During surgical procedures
3. Electrocution
4. Digitalis toxicity
5. Under anaesthesia

Aetiologically ventricular fibrillation follows an attack of acute myocardial infarction, during surgical procedures, under anaesthesia, electrocution, toxic doses of drugs (digitalis, quinidine) or as terminal event in a variety of diseases. Ventricular fibrillation is characterized by irregular, uncoordinated rapid fibrillary twitchings of the ventricles leading to almost ineffectual functioning of the ventricles and zero cardiac output. Patient may exhibit attacks of Adams stokes syndrome with syncope and periods of asystole. There is sudden disappearance of pulse, blood pressure and heart sounds with signs of collapse and a shock like state associated with convulsive seizures. Diagnosis is confirmed by electrocardiogram which shows rapid regular or irregular oscillations representing bizarre QRS complexes, the rate ranging from 150 to 300 per minute.

Treatment. Ventricular fibillation is a dire emergency and requires very urgent detection and management. Defibrillation must be done immediately. One or two blows with the closed fist should be given in the middle of the sternum till defibrillation is done. In some cases it may restore sinus rhythm. Defibrillation is done with high energy levels (200 to 400 joules). At the same time patients electrolyte or metabolic abnormalities, acidosis or hypoxia be corrected as well as diazepam given to allay anxiety. If necessary a second counter shock at the same energy level be delivered. If ventricular fibrillation is refractory to electrical defibrillation Bretylium 5 mg/kg I/V by slow infusin may increase success of defibrillation.

If successful defibrillation, patient be put on maintenance drug therapy (Lidocaine, Mexiletine, Bretylium or Procainamide).

Sinus bradycardia. When heart rate falls below 60/mt it is called bradycardia but bradycardia does not cause any symptoms till the heart rate falls below 50/mt. The impulse here arises from the S.A. node normally and it can be seen in healthy adults, athletes and during pregnancy. Pathologic conditions like coronary heart disease, myxoedema, raised intracranial pressure, obstructive jaundice and drugs like digoxin, beta blockers, procainamide, quinidine etc. shall be the other important causes. Usually there are no symptom but in very slow rates there may be attacks of dizziness or syncope.

Diagnosis is made by ECG which shows a very slow heart rate with long T-P interval.

Causes of sinus bradycardia

1. Normally present in athletes and healthy adults
2. Pregnancy
3. Coronary heart disease
4. Myxoedema
5. Raised intracranial pressure
6. Obstructive jaundice
7. Drug-induced (digitalis, beta-blockers, procainamide, quinidine)
8. Sick sinus syndrome

Treatment. Symptomatic since sinus bradycardia does not require any treatment. If there is any underlying pathological cause, it should be treated.

If symptomatic, injection atropine 0.4 mg I/V or S/C be administered followed by oral administration of atropine like drugs (probanthine).

Sick sinus syndrome. Often called sinoatrial dysfunction it manifests by multiple arrhythmias like intermittent sinus arrest, sinus bradycardia, junctional rhythm, escape rhythm with attacks of paroxysmal atrial tachycardia or atrial flutter/fibrillation. Patients with this arrhythmia suffer from episodes of alternative bradycardia and tachycardia, hence called tachycardia-bradycardia syndrome. Since there are periods of both slow and fast heart rates, patient suffers from syncopal attacks and chest pain.

This syndrome generally results from myocardial infarction, ischaemic and hypertensive heart disease, rheumatic, congenital heart disease, cardio-myo-pathy, infiltrative diseases like collagen, sarcoidosis, amyloidosis etc. Most of the patients are either middle aged or elderly persons. Rarely there may be no evidence of any organic heart disease.

Diagnosis of this arrhythmia may be quite tricky. Suspicion should arise if one observes varying arrhythmias in any elderly person like sinus bradycardia or unexplained slow fibrillation with occasional period of sinus arrest or atrial tachy-cardia. Long term electrocardiographic monitoring may establish the diagnosis.

Treatment of choice is permanent ventricular pacing which will take care of bradycardia as well as permit suppression of tachyarrhythmias with use of drugs like amiodarone, digoxin, propranolol or verpamil. For severe bradycardia, atropine or isoproterenol may be employed temporarily. Atrial pacing is not preferred since A-V conduction disturbances are likely to exist in patients of sick sinus syndrome.

Heart blocks. Any condition which gives rise to either a temporary or permanent interruption in conduction of cardiac stimuli in the region of the A-V node, SA node, the node itself or the bundle of His adjacent to the node constitutes the condition

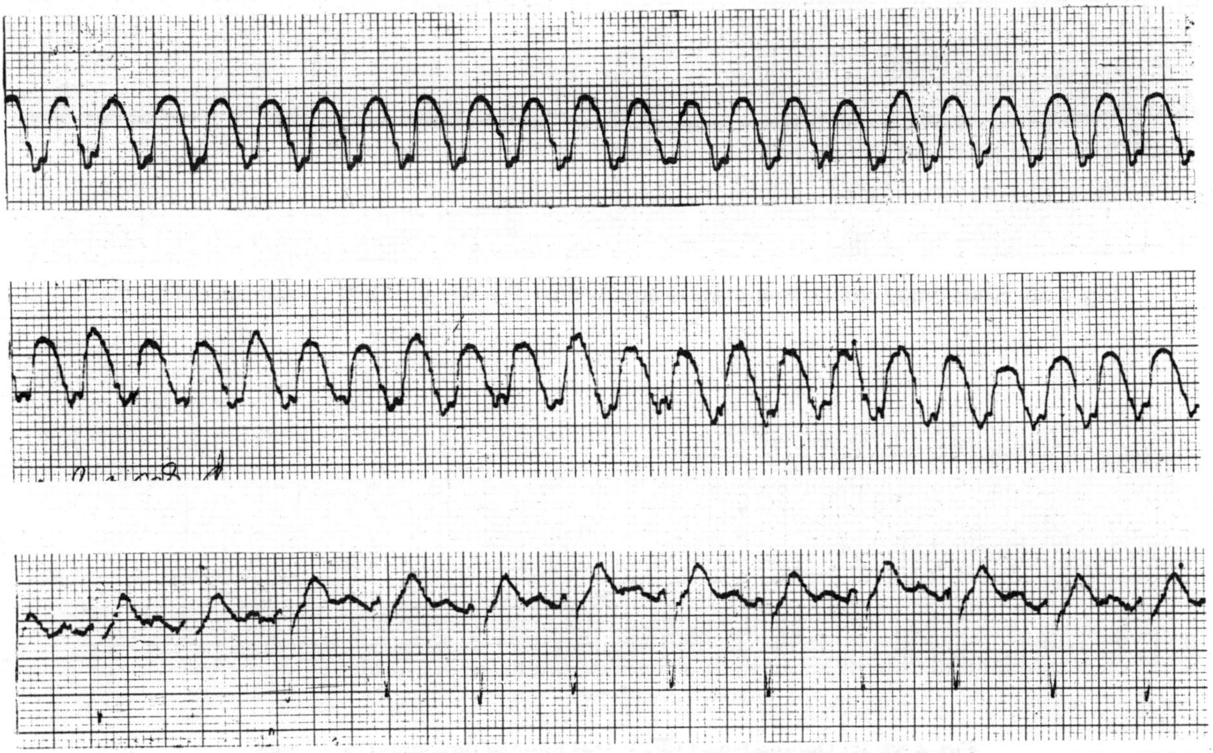

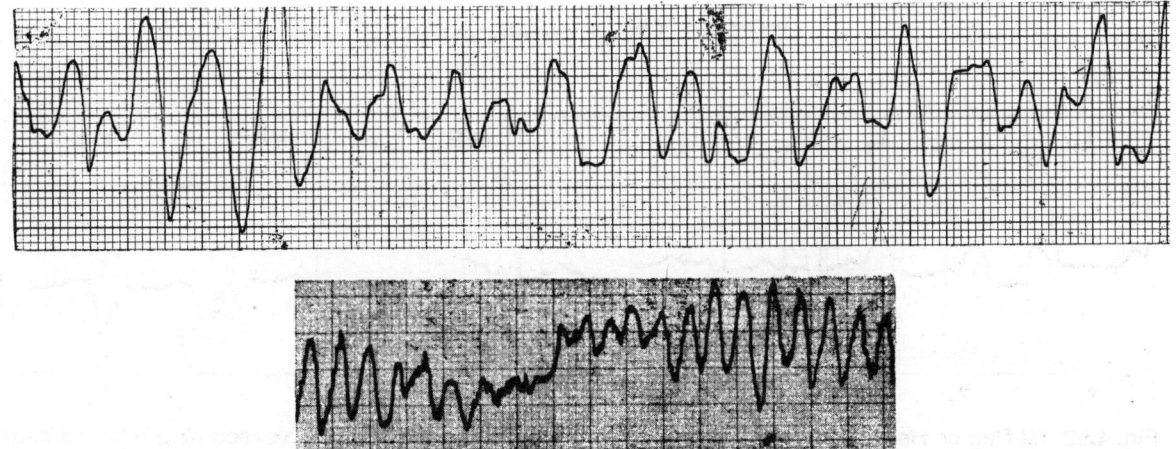

Fig. 4.48. Ventricular Tachycardia. First strip shows ventricular tachycardia in a case of acute myocardial infarction. Ventricular rate is approximately 166/mt. The QRS complexes are wide bizarre shaped. Second strip recorded after patient was administered lignocaine. Rhythm did not revert to normal. DC shock of 200 Joules was then administered. Ventricualr tachycardia reverted to sinus rhythm (3rd strip).

Fig. 4.49. Polymorph Ventricular Tachycardia degenerating to ventricular fibrillation.

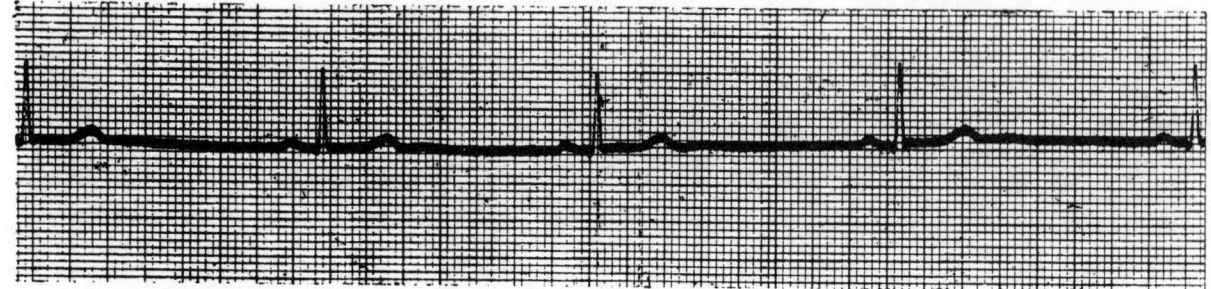

Fig. 4.50. Sinus brady cardia. Heart rate is about 40/mt. P wave and QRS complexes are normal.

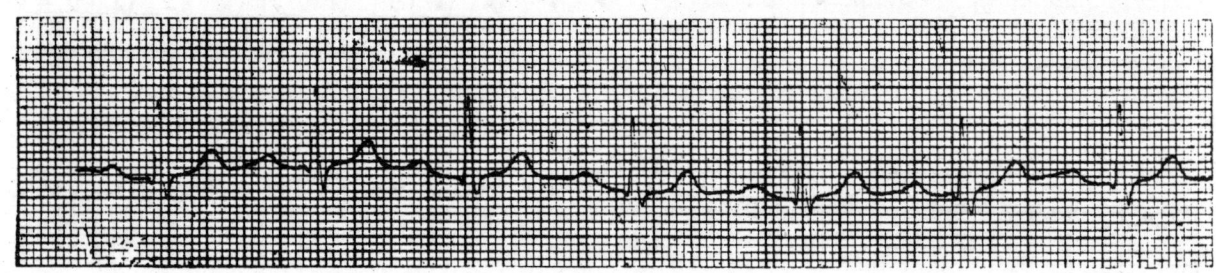

Fig. 4.51. Ist Degree Heart Block. P-R Interval prolonged (> 28 secs.).

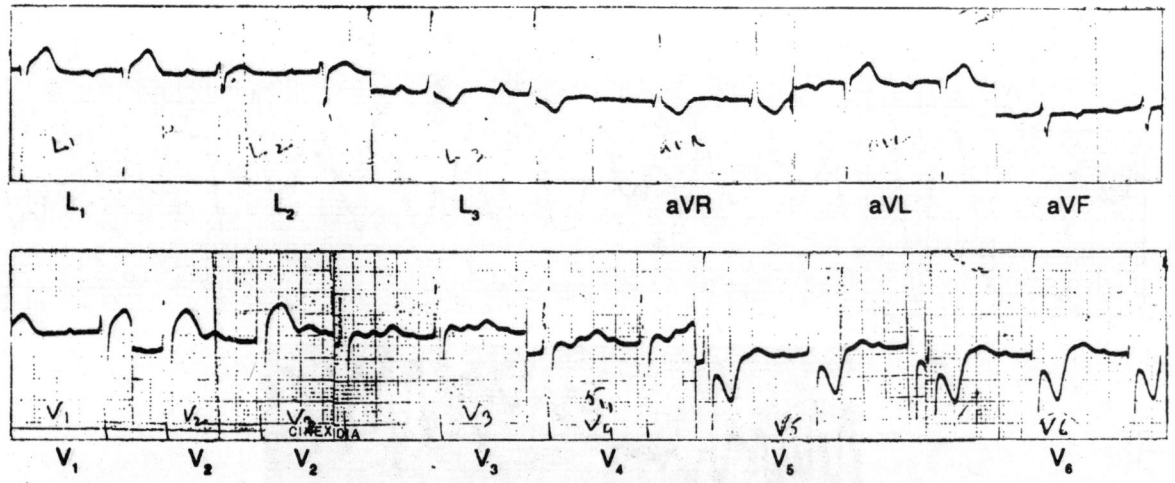

L₁ L₂ L₃ aVR aVL aVF

V₁ V₂ V₂ V₃ V₄ V₅ V₆

Fig. 4.52. 1st Degree Heart Block with Left Ventricular Hypertrophy and Strain. This recording is from a case of ischaemic heart disease. P-R interval is prolonged (0.28 secs.) Deep S wave V_1 + tall R waves V_5 - V_6 (SV_1 + RV_5 or V_6 > 35 mm). There is inversion of T waves L III, V_5 - V_6 indicating left ventricular strain.

called heart block. Sometimes the block may exist only in the distal portions of the conduction system i.e. right or left bundle branches of bundle of His or anterior or posterior fascicles. Proximal blocks are generalrly consideed benign while the distal ones (fasicular blocks) are more serious in nature. Heart blocks may come on acutely or be of chronic in nature. Aetiologically the common causes are acute myocardial infarction, hypertension, rheumatic and coronary artery disease, acute infections likie diphtheria, rheumatic fever, typhoid, viral infections and over dosage of drugs like digitalis, quinidine, beta blockers and calcium channel blockers etc. Congenital heart blocks are seen in degenerative conditions as well as in persons with congenital anomalies.

Diagnosis of heart blocks is made by conventional electrocardiography and sometimes with the aid of bundle of his electrocardiography. *Approach to the patient with heart block shall depend on:*

1. Whether the block is acute and has developed rapidly.
2. Whether there are any symptoms like syncopal attacks or Adams-Stokes seizures.
3. What are the underlying causes and if the precipitating factor can be reversed.
4. Effect of block on the haemodynamics of heart. If cardiac embarassment or danger of developing life threatening complications, then the treatment must be instituted at the earliest.

Atrioventricular block. It indicates impaired conduction of impulses from atrial to the ventricles.

It may be partial or complete. Partial heart block is either first degree or second degree (Mobitz type I and type II).

First degree A-V block. It is characterised by prolongation of the P-R interval to 0.21 secs or more. There is impaired conduction in the A-V junction proximal to the bundle of His. It is asymptomatic and diagnsis is made only by electrocrdiogram. First degree block is seen in patients of acute rheumatic fever, myocarditis, myocrdial infarction (inferior) degenerative or vascular diseases. Occasionally it

may be seen in normal hearts due to increased vagal tone and then requires no treatment. Drugs like digitalis, quinidine are important culprits. For first degree block underlying cause should be treated. If patient is on digoxin, withdraw the drug and give potassium supplements. In case the vetnricular rate is slow, Injection Atropine 0.4 mg S/C be administered besides treatment of the underlying disease.

Second degree A-V block: it is of two types:

a. Mobitz type I (Wenkebach's phenomenon). There is progressive prolongtion of the P-R interval until a point is reached at which no ventricular complex follows the P wave (dropped beat). The P-R interval shortens considerably after the dropped beat and then lengthens progressively from cycle to cycle until the dropped beat occurs again. Generalaly the ratio is 2:1 but may be 3:2 or 4:3.

Wenkebach's phenomenon is usually transient in nature and is often seen in cases with digitalis toxicity or in patient of myocardial infarction. It requires no treatment except of the cause unless there are haemodynamic disturbances or the block increases.

b. Mobitz type II. It is a more serious type of block. The P-R interval is normal or increased but constant and the beats are dropped at regular intervals. QRS is often prolonged and there is right bundle branch block and associated hemiblock.

The block is either 2:1, 3:1 or 4:1 but sometimes there may be irregular ratio. This type of partial heart block assumes significance since it may suddenly pass on to complete heart block. Patients with Mobitz type II block may suffer from syncopal attacks which may come rather suddenly. Common causes are myocardial infarction, calcific aortic stenosis, congenital heart disease (ventricular septal defect) and diffuse disorders of the myocardium. Treatment of the block is by atropine by I/V or S/C route if the ventricular rate is slow. In patients with bifascicular block, mobitz type II or threatened appearance of complete heart block permanent pacing should be done.

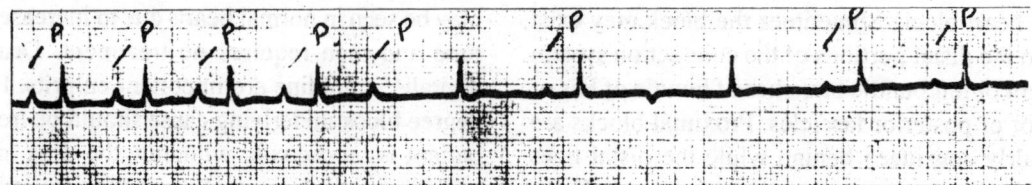

Fig. 4.53. Second Degree A - V Block (Wenkebach's Phenomenon). Here sinus impulses are conducted to the ventricle with progressive increase in P-R intervals until an impulse fails to be conducted.

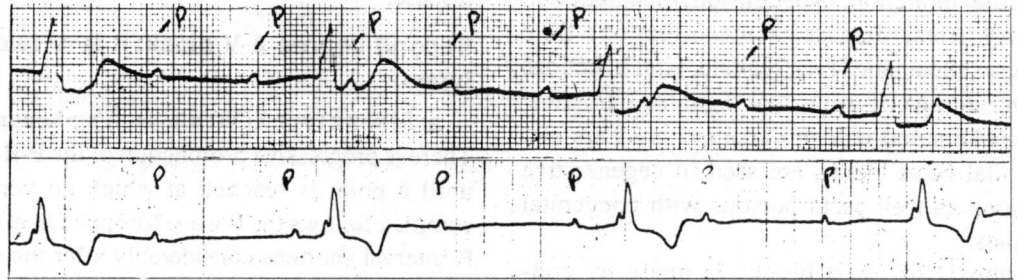

Fig. 4.54. Complete Heart Block. Here atria and ventricles are beating independently of each other. Ventricular rate is 30/mt. QRS complexes are wide and notched.

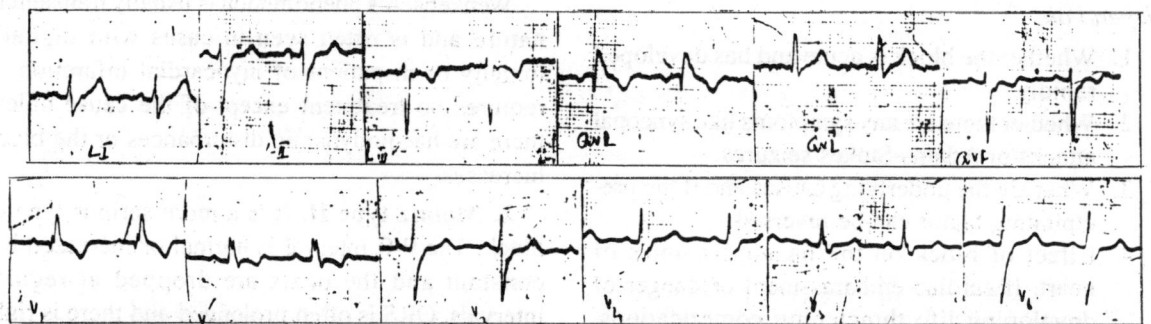

Fig. 4.55. Right Bundle Block. The wide S waves in L I, V_4 - V_6 and R wave in leads V_1 - V_2 are typical of right intraventricular conduction delay r' RS pattern in V_1 - V_2 is typical.

Third degree (complete) A-V block. It may be transient or established though the latter is the one commonly seen. There is complete A-V dissociation with the result that the atria and ventricles are beating independently of each other. Both the atrial and ventricular rhythms are essentially regular, the atria being faster than the ventricles. In the electrocardiogram. QRS complexes bear no relationship to the P waves. When the pace maker is in the A-V node or bundle of his, the QRS complex is normal while if it is below the bifurcation of the bundle of his, the QRS complex is prolonged,

notched or slurred. Diagnosis of complete heart/ block is made when heart rate is 20 to 40 per minute. There is increase in systolic and decrease in diastolic pressure. Intensity of first heart sound is changing (Cannon sounds) and atrial 'a' waves are seen in the neck. Electrocardiogram confirms the diagnosis. Management of a case of complete heart block shall depend on whether the block has developed acutely or is chronic in nature.

Acutely developing heart block. If heart block develops with a serious underlying heart disease its significance should be recognised. Thus heart block following acute myocardial infarction and myocarditis in cases of severe infections (Diphtheria, Viral, typhoid and rheumatic fever) is a serious emergency and requires immediate treatment. Treatment may be directed on the following lines if there are attacks of syncope, dizziness or Adams stokes seizures.

Causes of complete heart block

1. Congenital
2. Acute myocardial infarction
3. Myocarditis
4. Drug toxicity (digitalis, quinidine, beta-blockers)
5. Degenerative disorders involving conducting tissue.

Corticosteroids. Prednisolone 15-20 mg three or four times a day preceded by Injection Dexamethasone 2-4 mg I/M six hourly for first 24-48 hours. Steroids are useful since they reduce edema around the conducting system.

Isoproterenol (Isuprel). It is the drug of choice for managing the case of complete block. It increases the heart rate, the stroke volume, coronary blood flow and the amplitude of myocardial contractions. Isuprel acts predominantly on the sinus and atrioventricular node but has the least tendency to induce ventricular fibrillation. Drug is given at a slow I.V. infusion (2-4 mg in 500 ml of 5% Glucose) at the rate of flow adjusted 10 to 20 drops per minute (ventricular rate should be aimed at 50 beats per minute and this can be achieved by adjusting the rate of flow and concentrate of the drug in infusion). The infusion is maintained for 24-48 hours and then tapered off. It is then replaced by four to six hourly I/M injections of 0.2 mg Isoproterenol and finally by sublingual tablets (5-10 mg) every one to six hours depending on clinical response and the cardiac status.

Other drugs employed are ephedrine (15-30 mg) and Atropine 1 mg I/V six hourly). If the drug therapy is unsucessful and the patient is showing repeated syncopal attacks (Adam's Stokes) emergency transvenous pacing be instituted. The question of inserting a permanent cardiac pace maker has to be evaluated subsequently.

Chronic complete heart block. The common causes of complete heart block which is an established one include coronary heart disease following an attack of myocardial infarction, degenerative processes, involving the conducting fibres of the heart or occasionally it may be congenital in nature. Most of the cases of complete heart block are asymptomatic and require no treatment. But when patient of a complete heart block gets attacks of dizziness vertigo or syncope or has high grade block, definative therapy must be instituted. Drugs are employed to increase the heart rate as well as to prevent recurrence of Adams Stokes fits.

Ephedrine (30 mg three to four times a day) is the usual form of therapy. Isuprel (5-10 mg tablet) sublingually every one hour till the ventricular rate rises is a better drug. It not only increases the cardiac rate, the stroke volume, the amplitude of myocardial contraction but has the least tendency to produce ventricular fibrillation. Sustained action isoproterenol tablets (30-60 mg) three times a day may be used. If required Isuprel may be administered subcutaneously 0.2 mg every one to six hours or as a continuous intravenous infusion (one mg of the drug in 200 ml of 5% glucose) at rate of about 10-15 drops per minute.

Steroids. Role in chronic heart block is controversial but are employed in patients getting recurrent attacks of Adams Stokes fits especially in patients with heart block following myocardial infarction. Dose 60-120 mg prednisolone in divided doses in 24 hours.

Cardiac pacing. If the drug therapy fails or the Adams Stokes fits are not controlled, permanent cardiac pacing should be instituted. Demand pacemaker may be a better choice.

Bundle branch block. These are better termed intraventricular conduction defects and may be either right or left, complete or incomplete or trifascicular or bifascicular blocks. Right bundle branch (RBBB) block may be seen normally in elderly or in cases of chronic cor pulmonale. Left bundle branch block (LBBB) is always seen in organic heart disease like hypertension, coronary heart disease. Cases of bundle branch block are asymptomatic and require no treatment except that of the underlying condition. Bilateral bundle branch block trifascicular or bifascicular block associated with varying degrees of A-V heart block are known to have poor prognosis. Such patients will require temporary pacing followed by permanent pacing.

To conclude. Cardiac arrhythmias present a variable clinical picture. Some are symptomatic while the others are asymptomatic and therapy as well as management of the cardiac dysfunction shall depend on the underlying cardiac condition, the safety of the arrhythmic therapy and individual assessment of each patient vis-à-vis various measures to be adopted.

CHAPTER 5

Diseases of the Respiratory System

1. Tests of respiratory function
2. Acute bronchitis
3. Chronic obstructive pulmonary disease
4. Emphysema
5. Bronchiectasis
6. Chronic cor pulmonale
7. Pneumonia
8. Bronchopneumonia
9. Lung abscess
10. Eosinophilia
11. Pulmonary embolism
12. Pulmonary tuberculosis
13. Respiratory failure
14. Bronchial asthma
15. Disease of pleura
16. Pleural effusion
17. Empyema
18. Pneumothorax

Respiratory system is an important system of the body and its diseases constitute a major chunk of the various body's ailments and are responsible for increased degree of morbidity and mortality. With increasing environmental pollution there is a substantial rise in respiratory diseases like chronic bronchitis, emphysema and bronchial asthma.

A detailed history and physical examaination are important in making a diagnosis of respiratory disorders. But a number of systemic disorders like collagenosis, malignancy, endocrine, haematological and renal disorders may manifest with respiratory symptoms and similarly carcinoma of lung may show extra pulmonary manifestations like osteoarthropathy, neuropathy and myopathy. Exposure of persons to certain noxious dusts like silica, coal, asbestoss, cotton dust is responsible for causing occupational lung disease. These persons suffer because of their occupation and constant exposure to the hazardous dusts and have complaints of breathlessness and asthma like picture. So in every case a detailed personal history, occupational, family history, history of smoking and contact with patients of tuberculosis must be enquired into.

Some of the common symptoms include cough with or without expectoration and breathlessness, haemoptysis, weight loss, loss of appetite and pain in chest.

Cough is an important feature in a respiratory case and may be dry or accompanied with expectoration. Cough in fact is a defence mechanism by which respiratory passages are kept clear, by bringing out any secretions lying in respiratory passage and also preventing entry of any foreign material.

Sudden onset of cough in the form of paroxysm may occur when a foreign body is inadvertently inhaled. Similarly spasmodic attacks of cough occur in whooping cough (in children) bronchial asthma, bronchogenic carcinoma when a growth is pressing on the bronchus. A distressing painful cough may be as a result of diseases of lung (pneumonia) or pleurisy. The timing of cough, character and quantity of sputum expectorated also helps in diagnosing the condition. A patient suffering from chronic sinusitis and bronchitis has symptoms most marked in the early hours of morning. A cough in which large amount of material is expecotrated with change of posture suggests bronchiectasis or lung abscess. Large amount of purulent sputum is present in bronchiectasis, lung abscess and necrotizing pneumonia. A foul smelling, mucopurulent sputum is present in fulminating infections of the lungs by Fusiform, K. pneumoniae and H. influenzae organisms. A currant jelly appearance of sputum occurs in bronchogenic carcinoma while a streak or blood stained frothy sputum may be seen in pulmonary oedema.

Common causes of cough shall include infections of the respiratory tract (acute/chronic bronchitis, bronchiectasis, pulmonary tuberculosis, broncho-genic carcinoma. smoker's cough, occupational lung diseases) extrapulmonary causes (left heart failure, enlarged mediastinal glands, mediastinal tumours, substernal thyroid, diaphragmatic pleurisy sub-phrenic pathology). Sometimes cough may be psychogenic in origin and occasionally wax in the ear may cause irritating cough due to vagal nerve irritation.

Dysponea or breathlessness is a common symptom of respiratory and cardiac diseases. To start with it is present at exertion and as the disease progresses it may be present even at rest. Patient of bronchial asthma, chronic bronchitis with emphysema, diffuse interstitial fibrosis of the lungs. Lobar or bronchopneumonia, pneumothorax and pleural effusion are likely to have dysponea as a predominant symptom.

Dysponea may start suddenly in cases in massive or rapidly developing pleural effusion, spontaneous pneumothorax, pulmonary embolism, massive collapse of lung while chronic form of breathlessness is seen in pulmonary tuberculosis, chronic bronchitis with emphysema, bronchial asthma. Inspiratory type of breathlessness may be seen in obstruction below the larynx, narrowing of bronchioles as in cases of bronchial asthma. Inspiration in bronchial asthma is in the form of short gasps while expiration is prolonged.

Presence of fever, toxaemia in the presence of breathlessness shall suggest superimposition of infection while presence of oedema over legs and feet, cyanosis, raised jugular venous pressure shall suggest right heart failure secondary to diseases of lungs. In elderly patients often dysponea may be due to coexisting cardiac disorders like hyper-tension, ischaemic heart disease.

TESTS OF RESPIRATORY FUNCTION

In making a definitive diagnosis of patients with respiratory disorders a wide choice of diagnostic procedures is available. These vary considerably and some may produce discomfort to the patient but wherever tests are required they should produce minimal risk to the patient.

X-ray chest. Both posteroanterior (PA) and lateral views are important. Every case with respira-tory problem must have X-ray chest as a routine. In an X-ray chest one looks for shape of the chest wall (emphysema) bony cage, level of diaphragm (elevated in subdiaphragmatic patho-logy). Hilar shadows, vascular shadows, presence of any lesion in the lungs (infiltration, consolidation, cavitation, fibrosis) costophrenic angle (blunting in minimal pleural effusion) and presence of pleural effusion.

Many times asymptomatic cases are diagnosed on routine X-ray chest. Importance of X-ray chest can not be minimized in any case. It is especially important in pneumonic consolidation, lung abscess, bronchogenic carcinoma, pulmonary tuberculosis, hilar lymphadenopathy, pleural effusion, mediastinal growths and metastatic tumours.

Flouroscopy. It shows visualization of the chest contents in a dynamic rather than static manner. Movements of diaphragm are observed (restricted in subdiaphragmatic pathology, paradoxical movements in phrenic nerve lesion) whether the lesion is pulsatile (aneurysm) and precise location of a lesion is observed.

Tomography is a technique in which serial radiographs representing a slice of the lung at different depths is obtained. Tomograms help in identifying the lesion in its entire thickness which was not appreciated on routine X-ray chest. Tomography is useful in cases with cavity. Calcification, hilar adenopathy and abnoormalities

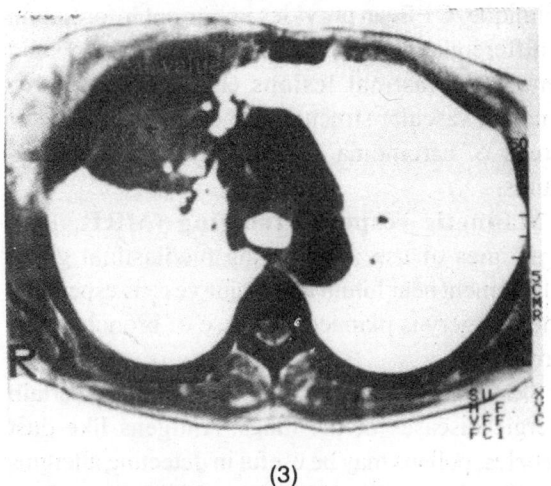

(3)

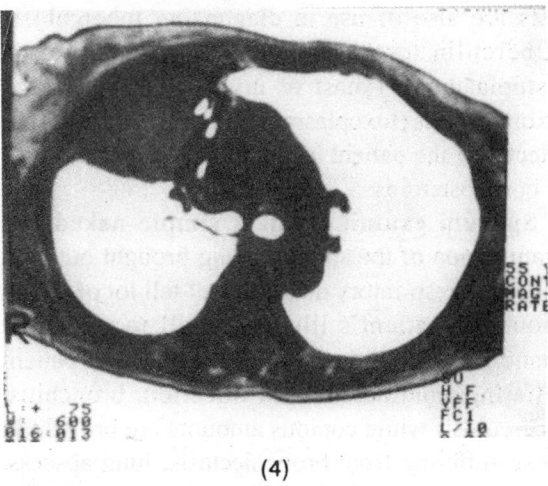

(4)

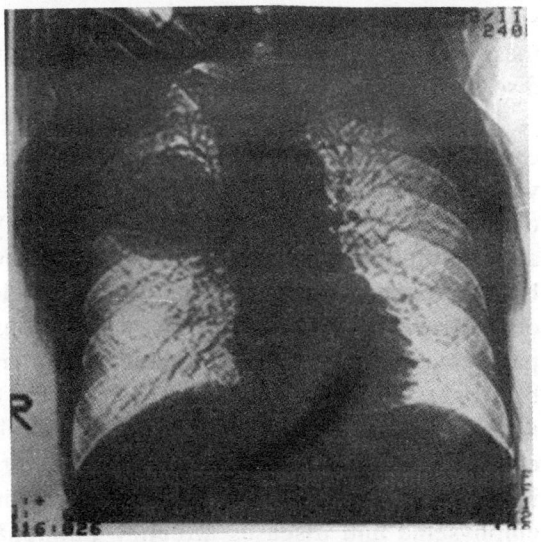

(1)

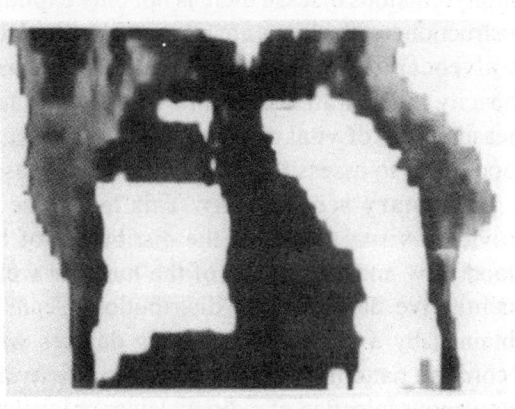

(2)

Fig. 5.1-4. CT Scan Thorax: There is a large mass with areas of necrosis present in anterior segment of right upper lobe. The mass is extending upto the chest wall anteriorly and medially reaching upto the hilum. Suggestion of destruction of Adjacent Ribs. Small specks of calcium present in the mass. Right upper lobe bronchus is compressed and pushed medially. Retro caval, Paratracheal lymph nodes are enlarged on right side and appear necrotic. Left lung is clear. This is a case of Bronchogenic Carcinoma Right Upper Lobe with spread to regional and paratracheal lymph nodes. CT Scan is required to assess the spread of carcinoma.

in shape of major bronchi as well as in identifying primary lesion.

Thoracic computed tomography (CT Scan). It is of great value and an important non-invasive technique. CT Scan provides important information in differentiating encysted pleural fluid from solid tumor, mediastinal lesions (lymphadenopathy, tumours, vascular structures) and for assessment of spread of carcinoma in the lungs, bronchus and glands.

Magnetic response imaging (MRI). It is sometimes of use in detecting mediastinal gland enlargement near hilum and major vessels especially when surgery is planned in a case of bronchogenic carcinoma.

Skin tests. These are of use in detecting certain allergic diseases of the lungs. Antigens like dust particles, pollens may be useful in detecting allergins and allergic conditions like bronchial asthma. Skin tests are also of use in diagnosing tuberculosis (tuberculin test), sarcoidosis (Kveim's test), histoplasmosis (yeast or mycelial antigen) and toxoplasmosis (toxoplasmin skin test). Skin tests are effected if the patient is already on antihistaminics or corticosteroids.

Sputum examination. A simple naked eye examination of the sputum being brought out by a patient of respiratory disease shall tell lot of things about the patient's illness. Small to moderate quantities of sputum are brought out by a patient suffering from acute chest infection, bronchitis, tuberculosis while copious amounts are brought in those suffering from bronchiectasis, lung abscess, pulmonary tuberculosis.

Colour of the sputum, odour and the presence of blood shall provide valuable clues. Purulent sputum indicates infection and its large quantities are expectorated in bronchiectasis, lung abscess, pulmonary tuberculosis. Sputum is rusty in pneumonia, blood-stained in pulmonary oedema, prune coloured in malignancy, blackish in coal miner's lung disease and anchovy sauce like in amoebic liver abscess rupturing into the lung.

A foul-smelling offensive sputum indicates infection with anaerobes, Staphylococcus, fusiform bacilli, Klebsiella pneumoniae and Pseudomonas pyocyaneous infections. Carefully stained smears of the sputum should be examined for identifying the causative organisms in bacterial pneumoniae,

tuberculosis and fungal infections. Direct smear of the sputum should be made for gram-negative organisms and acid-fast bacilli.

Culture of sputum is indicated for isolation of organisms and their sensitivity to various antimicrobial agents. Exfoliative cytology of the sputum is useful in the diagnosis of carcinoma of the lung.

Sometimes fungal infections shall require special culture. Occasionally fibrinous casts (fibrinous bronchitis) fragments of ruptured hydatid cyst (daughter cysts) may be seen in sputum.

Pulmonary function tests. These tests serve as diagnostic guides about the capacity of lungs as well as their function. Normal values vary with the age, sex and height of the patient. Repeated values of these tests are required to assess the progress of the disease.

Tests of ventilatory function include peak expiratory flow rate (PEFR) forced expiratory volume (FEV1) and forced vital capacity (FVC). In obstructive airways disease both FEV1 and FVC are reduced. Total lung capacity (TLC) as measured by a spirometer is either normal or increased in obstructive lung disease and decreased in pulmonary parenchymal disease. Measurements of arterial blood gases tells about diffusing capacity of the lungs as well as about diseases affecting alveolar-capillary bed or pulmonary vasculature. This is important in diffuse interstitial fibrosis of the lung, emphysema and diseases affecting pulmonary vasculature. In patients suffering from chronic emphysematous disease there is not only expiratory obstruction but the lungs are hyperinflated and there is alveocapillary block with reduced diffusing capacity. Out of all the respiratory function tests, measurement of vital capacity is a simple test and good guide to assess the progress of the disease.

Pulmonary scintigraphy. This technique can provide a visual image of the disribution of both blood flow and ventilation of the lungs as well as quantitative data on such distribution. Scans are obtained by a variety of scanning devices which record the pattern of pulmonary radioactivity after intravenous injection of radionucleides or inhalation of gamma emitting radionuclds. This procedure is useful in parenchymal lung disease, Pulmonary embolism and for detection of neoplasia, inflammatory diseases in the lungs or mediastinal lymph nodes.

Invasive procedures:

Bronchoscopy. It involves introduction of a flexible fibreoptic bronchoscope and directly visualising tracheobronchial tree, and studying various abnormalities like malignancy, granulmatous lesions and other pathological lesions. A biopsy forceps, cathether or brush is passed through the endoscope and thus brushing aspiration of secretions for culture and cytological examaination and a transbronchial lung biopsy from any suspicious lesion can be obtained. In addition to diagnostic use of bronchoscope it is also useful for removal of foreign body, aspiration of secretions in patients with airways obstruction or atelectasis. Broncho alveolar lavage is another procedure performed through a bronchoscope and is useful in diagnosing P. carini pneumonia and other infections.

Bronchography is useful for the diagnosis of bronchiectasis and identification of congenital and acquired forms of tracheobronchial abnormalities.

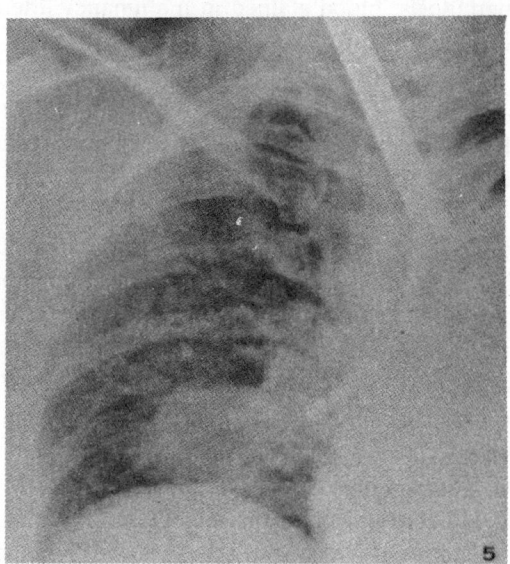

Fig. 5.6. Bronchoscope reaching a growth in the lower lobe of right lung.

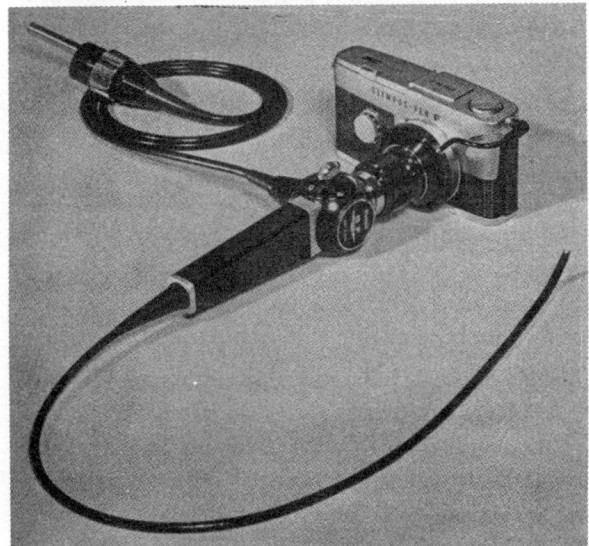

Fig. 5.5. Photograph of a Bronchofiberscope.

Bronchography. Radio-opaque material is injected into the tracheobronchial tree through bronchoscope or via a catheter. Catheter and position of the patient is adjusted in such a manner that all portions of the tracheobronchial tree are coated.

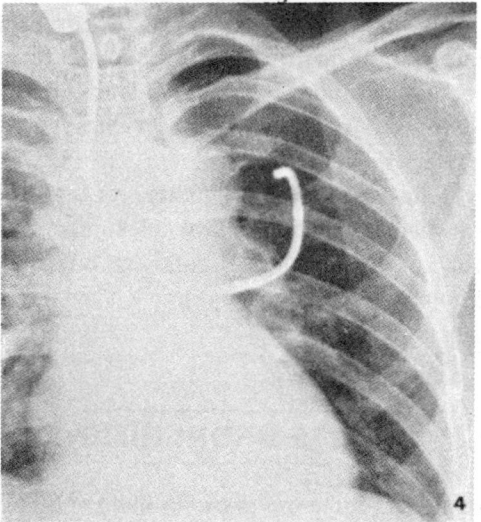

Fig. 5.7. Bronchoscope in the orifice of upper division bronchus of left lung.

Pleural aspiration. Aspiration of pleural fluid through intercostal spaces in mid axillary line in area of maximum dullness is done both for diagnostic as well as therapeutic purposes in patients with pleural effusion. Pleural fluid is examined for its protein content cell count, bacteriological examination and cytology. Pleural fluid is straw coloured in tuberculosis, blood stained in malignancy. Pleural biopsy is an important method of confirming the aetiological diagnosis. Abraham's punch biopsy needle is the one commonly employed. Bleeding, infection, pleural shock and bronchopleural fistula are the likely complications with this procedure.

Lung biopsy. Sometimes in a suspected lung malignancy or an undifferentiated lesion in the lung where other diagnostic measures fail, a thoracotomy is performed and an open lung biopsy done. Closed lung biopsy has also been carried by means of transbronchial aspiration and cutting needles through a fibreoptic bronchoscope. There is high incidence of complications through this procedure and often the biopsy specimen is inadequate.

Mediastinoscopy. This method involves study of mediastinal glands since they receive lymphatic drainage from the lungs. This is important in such diseases as carcinoma, sarcoidosis and granulomatous infections. This is accomplished by use of a mediastinoscope introduced from an incision made at the base of neck anteriorly. Inspection and biopsy of the glands is carried out. It is a low risk procedure and useful in patients of pulmonary malignancy.

Scalene node biopsy is another procedure where scalene nodes are biopsied from left supraclavicular region. Scalene node glands are enlarged in carcinoma lung. Malignancy stomach and testicular tumours.

ACUTE BRONCHITIS

It is an acute infection of the bronchi and may be caused by infection with organisms such as Streptococcus, pneumococci, haemophilus influenzae, friedlander's bacillus or primarily viral in origin.

Causes:

1. More prevalent in damp and foggy climates.
2. Descending infection from nasal sinuses.

3. Inhalation of irritant gases or fumes.
4. Common in debilitated individuals, extremes of age and those with poor immune responses.
5. Specific bacterial infections often following or superimposed over a viral infection.

Symptoms:

1. *Toxaemia.* Malaise, fever, ill health, tachycardia.
2. *Respiratory.* Feeling of rawness over the chest. Cough on first day is irritating and later on it becomes mucoid to mucopurulent. Breathing in early stages may be increased. Sometimes in severe cases paroxysms of cough may occur.

Physical signs. Signs of toxaemia (fever, tachycardia, malaise, respiratory rate slightly increased), flushing of face. On auscultation vesicular breath sounds with prolonged expiration. Sometimes sonorous or sibilant rhonchi may be heard. Crepitations are heard at the base when secretions collect in the lungs.

Complications. Most cases of acute bronchitis get cured if adequately managed. Complications in some cases may include bronchopneumonia, aspiration pneumonia and atelectasis of lung lobule. Some persons especially those who are cigarette/hooka smokers may get repeated infections and develop chronic bronchitis.

Investigations. No specific investigations are required until or unless basic underlying disease is suspected. Polymorphonuclear leucocytosis may be seen in purulent infection. X-ray chest be done to exclude bronchopneumonia, lung abscess or pneumonia.

Treatment:

In dry stage

1. Rest in bed.
2. Nourishing diet, soft and nutritive food.
3. Tincture benzoin Co. inhalations.
4. Application of Vicks Vaporub over the chest.
5. Cap. Amoxycillin 250 mg 8 hourly for 4-5 days.
6. Tablet Aspirin or Paracetamol twice a day. Cough sedative mixture like Linctus codeine

to suppress dry cough (1 teaspoon BD). Protect the patient from draught.

In moist stage. When patient is bringing out large amount of expectoration antibiotics like Amoxycillin and Cloxacillin (500 mg 8 hourly) for 4-5 days. For person where expectoration is more purulent sputum culture be done and appropriate drug given.

Expectorant mixture with sodium or potassium iodide to bring out the secretions.

General measures like bed rest, good nourishing diet.

Convalescent stage. Gradually activity resumed. Diet increased.

Prognosis. It is good. Complications mainly occur in debilitated patients or those with poor nutrition and immunity. Course of the disease generally is short unless acute bronchitis is superimposed over pulmonary tuberculosis or complicating any major ailment.

CHRONIC OBSTRUCTIVE PULMONARY DISEASE

It may be defined as a condition in which there is chronic obstruction to air flow within the lungs as assessed clinically or by physiological measure.

It is a common denominator of many lung diseases. There is obstruction to air flow due to chronic bronchitis and/or emphysema accounting for vast majority of patients.

It refers to large number of patients with cough, expectoration, dysponea and progressive respiratory impairment. The main disorders under it are:

1. Chronic bronchitis
2. Emphyema

Risk factors of chronic obstructive airways disease:

1. Heavy smoking
2. Community air pollution, dust, chullas smoke, industrial fumes, ill-ventilated houses, and bronchial irritants.
3. Occupational hazards, exposure of workers to inorganic/dust particles.

4. Childhood respiratory illnesses
5. Recurrent upper and lower respiratory tract infections.
6. Deficiency of glycoprotein alpha-1-antitrypsin associated with advanced emphysema, clearly established in case of homozygots deficiency (genotype zz). Patients with zz pi type have emphysematous form of COPD.

Pathogenesis of chronic obstructive airways disease. Three important factors:

1. Bronchial obstruction
2. Hyperinflation of the lungs and gradual loss of pulmonary elasticity.
3. Overdistension and inevitable rupture of alveoli leading to reduction in capillary bed.

CHRONIC BRONCHITIS

Chronic bronchitis is of world wise distribution and is associated with great degree of morbidity and mortality. Though the disease may start at any age yet it is more common in middle age and men are affected more as compared to females. Disease is more common in cigarette smokers, lower socio-economic group and people who live in dusty, cold and damp climates.

Though chronic bronchitis and emphysema are two distinct entities but often both conditions merge into each other and are referred to chronic obstructive lung disease where there is obstruction to the flow of air in the pulmonary airways. Chronic bronchitis may be defined as a condition where there is persistent productive cough for at least three consecutive months in at least two consecutive years.

Factors contributing to chronic bronchitis

1. Cigarette smoking
2. Air pollution and climatic factors
3. Infections
4. Occupation
5. Familial and genetic factors
6. Alpha-1-antitrypsin deficiency

Chronic bronchitis may be subclassified into

chronic catarrhal bronchitis where patient passes small amount of mucoid sputum while in chronic suppurative bronchitis large quantities of muco-purulent sputum is passed. Both these forms intermingle with each other and are different stages in the evolution of disease.

Aetiology. A number of factors act as contributing to chronic bronchitis and since emphysema is the main cause of irreversible airways obstruction, the same factors operate in both groups.

Cigarette smoking. Smoking in any form (bidi, cigarette, hooka) is an important cause. Damage produced in the lungs is directly related to the number of cigarettes etc. smoked per day and its duration. Prolonged smoking impairs ciliary movements, produce an acute increase in airways resistance leading to considerable obstruction in small airways and as a result of infiltration by neutrophil granulocytes in airways there is release of enzymes elastases and proteases which have been incriminated in the production of emphysema. Smoking amongst sufferers of chronic bronchitis is probably the most important factor and may interact with other factors.

Air pollution and climatic factors. Climatic factors such as temperature, humidity, cold and foggy climate are important factors. Cold air has a deleterious effect on the pulmonary functions even in normal persons. Inhalation of dust, fumes from motor vehicles, industrial pollution have important aetiological significance. Chronic irritation of the respiratory passages by the smoke particularly from the cow dung cakes in poorly ventilated houses is an important contributory factor in our country.

Infections. Repeated respiratory infections with bacteria, viruses and mycoplasma lead to inflammation of the bronchioles with disruption of smaller airways, air trapping, aggravation of damage to bronchopulmonary segments and chronic respiratory obstruction. Whether infection per se produces chronic bronchitis is difficult to say but it is accepted that repeated and frequent attacks of respiratory illness increases morbidity in patients of chronic bronchitis. Release of enzymes and disruption of respiratory bronchioles predispose to perpetuation of the condition leading to the production of emphysema.

Occupation. Chronic bronchitis is more common in those engaged in hazardous industries, workers in mines like coal, silica and those who are exposed to both organic, inorganic dusts as well as irritant gases. In such people the respiratory passages are under constant irritation.

Familial and genetic factors. Chronic bronchitis may run in families. Genetic and immunological factors are also important. Children and other members of the family may suffer to some extent because of environmental pollution at home and surroundings.

Alpha-1-antitrypsin deficiency. Deficiency of alpha-1-antitrypsin enzyme has been associated with emphysema which is of relatively early onset and predominantly localized to base. It is genetically transmitted deficiency with autosomal dominant fashion. Persons who are homozygous and have this deficiency suffer from severe emphysema during third and fourth decades of life but heterozygous subjects also have a higher incidence of emphysema particularly when they have been smoking over a long period of time. Enzymes present in purulent sputum are inhibited by alpha-1-antitrypsin and in those with deficiency of this enzyme, it leads to break down of lung tissue. This may be another way to explain development of emphysema in young persons.

Pathology. The most characteristic pathology in chronic bronchitis is hypertrophy and hyperplasia of mucus-producing glands. This results in over production of mucus which contributes to airflow obstruction in the larger airways. Smaller airways show even more airways obstruction because of coexistant emphysema. There is loss of tissue support, increased mucosal secretions, oedema, mucosal and submucosal inflammation, congestion, bronchospasm, peribronchial fibrosis with resultant distortion of the airways and narrowing of smaller airways. This is further aggravated by repeated infections and chronic irritation by cigarette smoke, dust etc. In fact it is a vicious circle, the problem being worsened by air flow obstruction.

Clinical features. A case of chronic bronchitis presents with recurrent bouts of cough which may be dry to start with but subsequently patient starts bringing out sputum mucoid to mucopurulent. Cough may occur in paroxysms or is constant more in the early hours of morning. Patient's symptoms are worsened in cold months or due to sudden change of temperature. Often patient complains of sense of tightness in chest. With advancing disease patient complains of breathlessness and asthma-like picture may develop. Fever and toxaemia appear when infection supervenes. Sputum becomes mucopurulent and may be copious in amount. Sometimes a streak of blood may appear in sputum due to severe bout of infection.

Physical signs. These will depend on the stage at which the patient presents. In early stages, except for occasional rhonchi, harsh breathing and few crepts there are no other signs.

As the disease progresses, emphysema may supervene when chest expansion is poor, it tends to assume a barrel shape, an inspiratory position and respiratory excursions are considerably diminished. Accessory muscles of respiration start working and there is tachypnoea.

Investigations:

1. X-ray chest (PA view) in early stages may be normal but later on it shows widening of intercostal spaces, ribs placed more horizontally, diaphragm displaced downwards and some patients may show patches of pneumonia.

2. Sputum examination (smear and culture).

3. Pulmonary function tests. There is evidence of pulmonary airways obstruction. Forced expiratory volume (FEV1) expressed as a ratio of forced vital capacity (FEV1/VC) shows a low value. Maximal voluntary ventilation (MVV) and maximum expiratory flow rate (MEFR) are also diminished. Increased airways resistance tends to increase the functional residual capacity (FRC) and residual volume of the lung (RV). Because of poor ventilation and ventilation perfusion defects there are blood gas changes.

4. Electrocardiogram. If cor pulmonale develops then P. pulmonale and evidence of right ventricular hypertrophy.

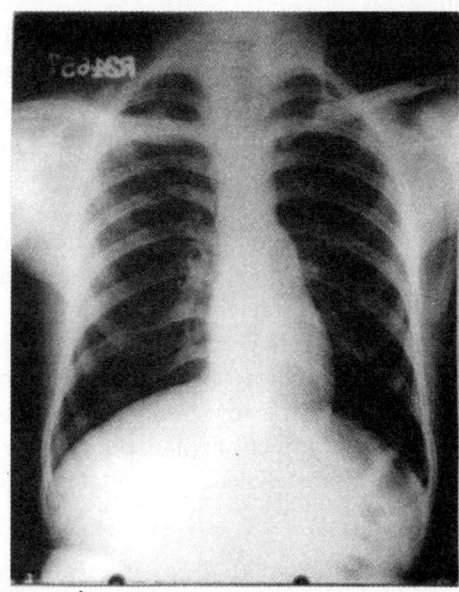

Fig. 5.8. X-ray Chest (PA View) Case of chronic bronchitis.

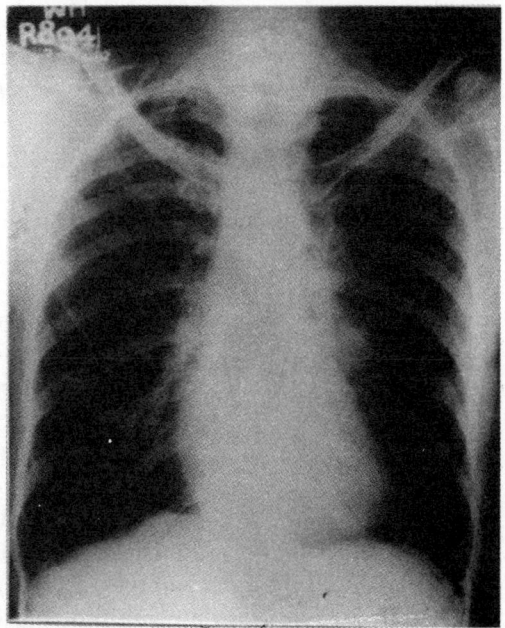

Fig. 5.9. X-ray Chest (PA View) Case of chronic bronchitis and emphysema. Translucency of lung field increased. Bronchovascular markings prominent.

Diagnosis. It is based on long hisitory of cough, recurrent respiratiory infections and physical findings. Further confirmation is done by investigations.

Chronic bronchitis has to be differentiated from bronchiectasis, bronchial asthma and sometimes from pulmonary tuberculosis. Very often features of bronchospasm are present and the whole picture may be combination of chronic bronchitis, emphysema and asthma-like features.

Course and prognosis. If the source causing chronic bronchitis is not controlled in early stage, the disease follows a relentless course.

Over a number of years, emphysema develops which subsequently leads to involvement of right side of heart leading to chronic cor pulmonale. Repeated chest infections and poor respiratory reserve may ultimately lead to respiratory failure.

Management:

1. Remove the cause if possible of source of chronic cough like unhealthy tonsils, chronic sinusitis and oral sepsis.
2. Smoking in any form must be stopped. Patient should avoid damp and foggy places, cold wintry months by moving to warm places. Dust, pollution and environmental allergens be avoided.
3. Body's resistance be increased. Anaemia if present be treated.
4. Deep breathing exercises to improve lung function and increased exercise tolerance.
5. Weight reduction if obesity or overweight.
6. Infections be totally avoided. Respiratory infections must be treated promptly. A broad-spectrum antibiotic should always be started. Cap. Amoxycillin 500 mg 8 hourly for 7 days is the usual course, since common pathogenic organism are *H. influenzae* and *Streptococcus pneumoniae* which respond well to the drug. But sputum culture can be got done especially if the patient is getting recurrent episodes of infection and appropriate antibiotic prescribed.
   Drugs like theophyllines are very useful. If some degree of bronchospasm then theo-phylline/aminophylline/salbutamol are used. Where person is expectorating large amounts of sputum an expecotrant mixture should be prescribed. If cough is dry and troublesome, a cough sedative like Linctus codeine especially at bed time.
7. Steam inhalation to open up the bronchi and improve lung function.
8. O_2 inhalations intermittently if patient is showing progressive breathlessness. It shall improve pulmonary ventilation and exercise tolerance.

Prognosis in chronic obstructive pulmonary disease (COPD)

1. Closely related to intial levels of functional impairment of lungs.
2. If initial levels of ventilatory capacity are held constant, other features of illness such as resting pulse rate, clinical or ECG evidence of chronic cor pulmonale, blood gas abnormalities, pulmonary diffusing capacity and levels of nutrition are related to subsequent survival.
3. Survivors live approximately for 10 years when FEVI is 1.4 liters. 4 years when FEVI falls to 1 liter and little more than 2 years when FEVI nears 500 ml.
4. When another adverse feature in addition to low FEVI, median survival decrease by 25-35%.
5. High pulmonary vascular resistance associated with poor prognosis.

EMPHYSEMA

Emphysema has been defined as pathological enlargement in the size of air spaces of the lung distal to the terminal bronchioles with destruction of their walls. In contrast to this, enlargement of air spaces, not accompanied by destruction is called over inflation or hyperinflation.

Emphysema is classified according to the pattern of involvement of acinus, the lung unit distal to the terminal bronchiole. The two most important forms of emphysema are:

a. Centrilobular emphysema where there is involvement of proximal acinus sparing distal air spaces. But with progression of the disease process, dilatation and destruction of walls of distal alveoli may occur. This form of emphysema is common in cigarette smokers and more severe in the upper as compared to lower zones of lobes.

b. Pan acinar emphysema where the entire acinus is involved with progressive enlargement of alveoli and alveolar ducts and almost loss of distinction between the two.

Quite often this distinction between two forms of emphysema is not present and a combination of two forms of emphysema is present in those dying from chronic obstructive airways disease and sometimes one type may predominate over the other.

In addition to the above two forms of emphysema which is more of a pathological classification, two other forms of emphysema are described.

1. Compensatory emphysema. It is not true form of emphysema and actually is dilatation of al-veoli following loss of lung substance as that following lobectomy. It is not emphysema in true sense since there is no destruction of sep-tal walls.
2. Senile emphysema seen in elderly people. Because of changes in chest skeleton due to old age, the lungs expand to fill the pleural cavity. Since there is no destruction of septal walls it is also not emphysema but senile hy-perinflation.

Aetiology. All those factors which cause chronic bronchitis shall also operate in case of emphysema. Certain occupations like furnace blowers, gold smiths, use of wind instruments predispose such people to develop emphysema. All those conditions where forced expiratory effort is required, make the person easy target for the condition.

Pathology. The lung in emphysema is inflated, there is abnormal enlargement of air spaces while there is thinning and destruction of the septal walls Lungs lose their elasticity with lack of elastic recoil leading to collapse or narrowing of the intrapulmonary airways. As the alveoli distend, septa rupture and alveoli may join to form air cysts. Most

often emphysema is panacinar involving both the central and peripheral parts of the acinus. There is diffusion block with subsequent fall in arterial oxygen saturation. The loss of lung elasticity results in an increase in total lung volume as well as decreased exchange of gases. The pulmonary vascular bed is progressively decreased and hypoxia acts as a potent stimulus for pulmonary vasoconstriction and pulmonary hypertension.

Clinical features. Clinical picture in a case of emphysema is continuation of chronic bronchitis like picture with the addition of progressive dysponea which becomes steadily more as the disease progresses.

There are two types of patients suffering from emphysema. Type A refers to pink puffers who have minimal cough and expectoration while dysponea is the predominant respiratory symptom. Congestive heart failure or chronic cor pulmonale is infrequent. Despite significant impairment of pulmonary diffusing capacity, these patients have near normal blood gas tensions.

Clinical presentation of cases of emphysema

Symptom	Type A (Pink puffers)	Type B (Blue bloaters)
Cough	Minimal	Predominant
Expectroation	Minimal	Copious
Dysponea	Predominant feature	Mild
Cyanosis	Absent	Present
Cor pulmonale	Infrequent	Common
Odema	Not common	Oedema on dependant parts
Jugular venous pressure	Not raised	Raised
Hypoxaemia	Mild	Moderate to severe
Diffusing capacity of lungs	Decreased	Relatively within normal limits

Second type (Type B) have chronic bronchitis as the predominant disease and start with early picture of cor pulmonale. These patients are called "Blue bloaters" and have marked blood gas abnormalities though the pulmonary diffusing capacity is relatively within normal limits. There is marked pulmonary arterial hypertension, carbon dioxide retention and a picture of cor pulmonale. The degree of emphysema in such patients is mild to moderate.

Clinically patient is breathless and its degree varies with the extent of involvement. Accessory muscles of respiration are working. There is tachyponea. Pulse is good and bounding.

Type A patient is not cyanosed. Congestive failure is generally not seen.

Type B patient is cyanosed, blue, bloated, with peripheral oedema, enlarged liver, and jugular venous pressure is raised.

Chest commonly is barrel shaped. Precussion note is hyper resonant. Liver and cardiac dullness often is obliterated. Auscultation shows prolonged vesicular breathing with rhonci and crepitations. Pulmonary second sound is loud if pulmonary hypertension is present.

Investigations:

1. Blood shows raised levels of haemoglobin. PCV is elevated. There is polycythaemia.
2. X-ray chest shows widened intercostal spaces, ribs placed more horizontally. Diaphragm is displaced downwards. Increased translucency of lung fields. Emphysematous bullae may be seen.
3. Pulmonary function tests show reduction of forced expiratory volume (FEV1) to forced vital capacity (FVC). Peak expiratory flow rate (PEFR) is also reduced. Blood gas analysis shows dimiunation of arterial oxygen (PaO_2) and increase in carbon dioxide levels ($PaCO_2$). Respiratory acidosis with fall in plasma bicarbonate levels develops. Presence of hypokalemia and other metabolic factors further complicate the picture.
4. Electrocardiogram in cases of emphysema for detection of chronic cor pulmonale. Early changes are P. pulmonale (tall spiky P wave) clockwise rotation of the heart and subsequently right ventricular hypertrophy or right bundle branch block pattern (rSR').

Complications. A case of emphysema is likely to develop a number of complications. These include:

1. Respiratory failure supervenes as the disease progresses and is often associated with increased cardiac output. There are features of drowsiness, confusion, respiratory depression and patient has evidence of involvement of vital organs like heart, kidney and cerebral dysfunction.
2. Chronic cor pulmonale where there is involvement of right side of heart secondary to emphysema leading to features of right heart failure.
3. Development of emphysematous bullae which sometimes enlarge and rupture leading to pneumothorax.

Complications in emphysema

1. Respiratory failure
2. Chronic cor pulmonale
3. Emphysematous bullae rupture leading to pneumothroax

Course and prognosis. Once emphysema develops patient follows a downhill course. Progress of the disease can be halted to some extent by removing the patient from atmospheric pollution, stopping smoking and treating any infection especially respiratory at the earliest. Mild cases of emphysema with due care and precautions can lead a long span of life.

Management. *Basic principles are:*

1. Treat the underlying cause and if possible any chronic source of infection in the upper respiratory airways be removed.
2. Patient should be taken away from cold climate and all possible factors of environmental pollution be removed.
3. Smoking in any form must be stopped. A patient with emphysema must also avoid passive smoking.
4. Breathing exercises be advised. An abdominal binder is sometimes useful in giving support and increasing levels of diaphragm.
5. Respiratory infections be prevented and prompt antibiotic treatment be instituted at the earliest sign of infection. Ampicillin/Amoxycillin are the preferred antibiotics.

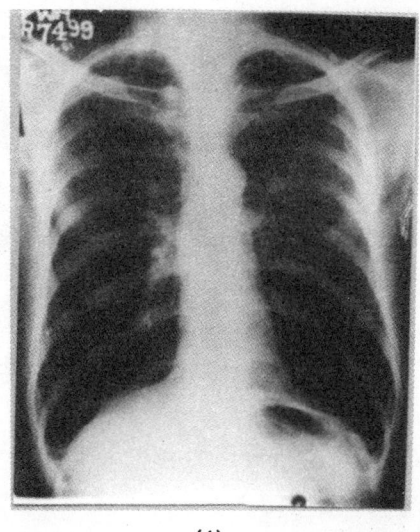

(1)

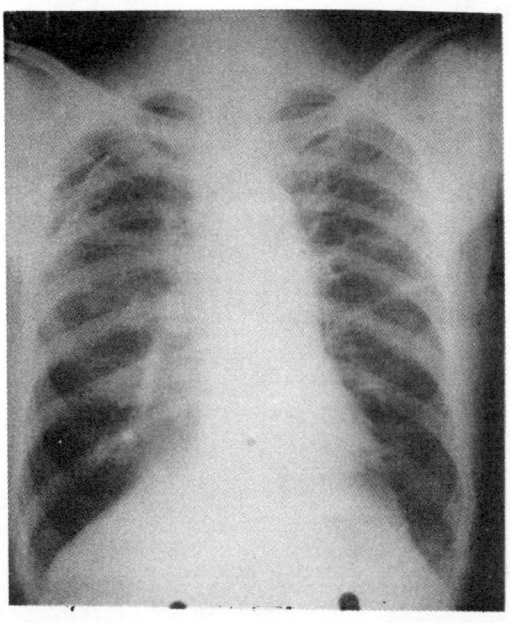

(2)

Fig. 5.10.1-2. *Chronic bronchitis with emphysema.* 1. X-ray chest (PA view). Case of chronic bronchitis with emphysema. There is increased translucency of lung fields. Ribs are placed more horizontally. Widening of intercostal spaces. Diaphragm displaced downwards. Heart is tubular. 2. X-ray chest (PA view). Case of chronic bronchitis with emphysema. There are increased reticular markings. Presence of small pneumothrorax in upper part of right lung is due to rupture of an emphysematous bullae.

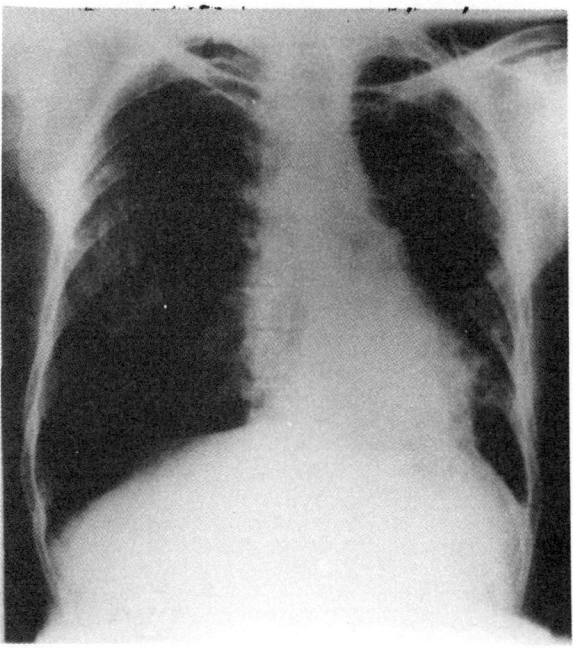

Fig. 5.11. X-ray chest (PA view): There are multiple small cavities in the left lung. Base of right lung has honeycombed appearance.

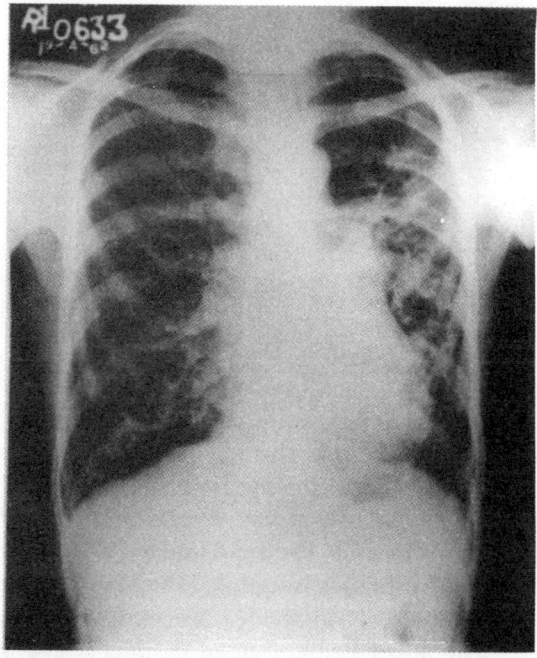

Fig. 5.12. X-ray chest (PA view). Honeycombed appearances in right base and left mid zone suggestive of bronchiectasis.

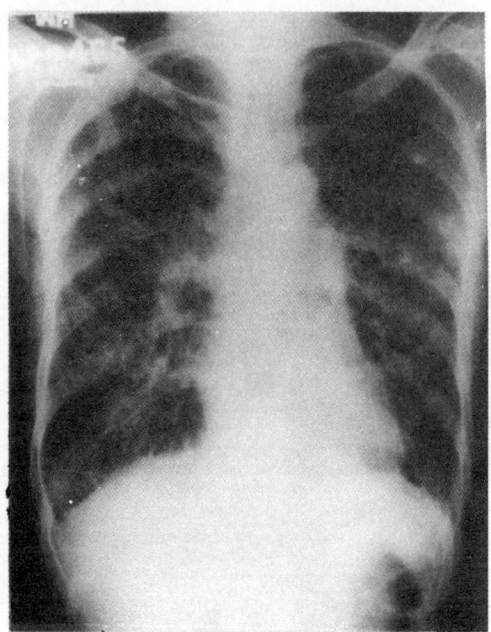

Fig. 5.13. X-ray Chest (PA view). Left lower part of lung shows bronchiectasis. Some of it is being overshadowed by cardiac shadow.

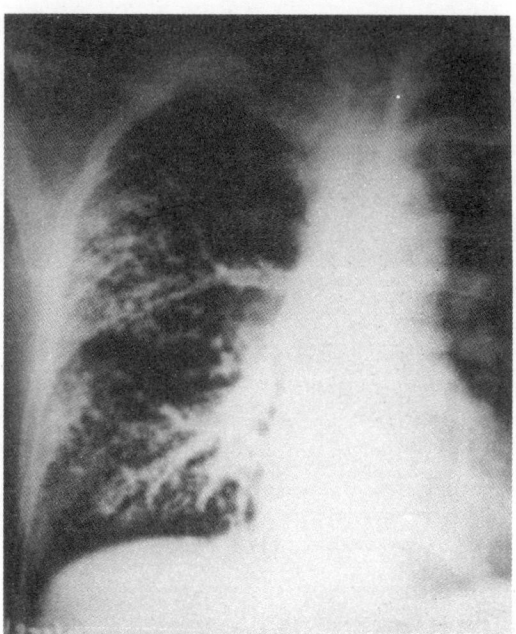

Fig. 5.14. X-ray Chest (Bronchogram) A radio opaque dye has been injected through bronchoscope. Bronchiectasis of right lower lobe is well demarcated.

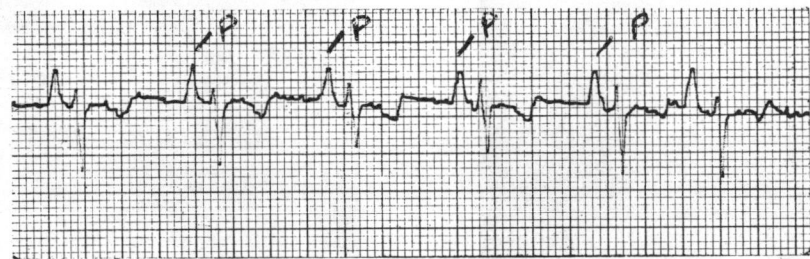

Fig. 5.15. P wave in case of chronic cor-pulmonale. It is Tall, Spiked P Pulmonale.

6. Bronchodilators are of use when bronchospasm is present. Theophylline and salbutamol are the drugs employed.

7. In patients with severe respiratory insufficiency and bronchospasm a trial of corticosteroids is useful (Tablet Prednisolone 30 mg daily in divided doses). Cortisteroids can also be administered by inhaler and are useful since by inhalation systemic effects of steroids are minimized.

8. O_2 inhalations intermittentely are useful in cases of emphysema. Where respiratory insufficiency is marked, continuous oxygen therapy is employed.

BRONCHIECTASIS

It may be defined as irreversible dilatation of one or more bronchi, where patient suffers from repeated bouts of cough with excessive expectoration of purulent or mucopurulent sputum. The bronchial walls are inflamed, thickened and irreversibly damaged with impairement of mucociliary mechanism.

Actiology: Bronchiectasis is generally secondary to disease of the bronchi, where obstruction and infection play an important role. Obstruction may be intrinsic (Plugs of mucus retained in the lumen of the bronchi contributing to mucosal injury or inhaled foreign body) or extrinsic (Pressure from enlarged glands probably tubercular at the hilum of the lung, or a tumour or aneurysm pressing on the bronchus). This leads to localized pulmonary collapse which results in increased traction on the bronchial wall which coupled with inspisated secretions in the lumen of bronchi, weakness of the bronchial wall (result of stagnant, secretions, inflammation and cumulative effects of proteolytic enzymes contributing to tissue necrosis) and raised intrabronchial pressure lead to irreversible dilatation of bronchi.

Children who suffer from measles or whooping cough and get repeated bouts of cough they are liable to get bronchiectasis especially if they suffer from pneumonia. Cases of influenza who have pulmonary complications also subsequently get bronchiectasis.

Conditions of lung parenchyma which may cause bronchiectasis include unresolved pneumonia, broncho pheumonia and lobular collapse. Bronchiectasis may be localized or diffuse. Localised form is caused either by broncho pulmonary infections or by obstruction of bronchi. Pulmonary infections are important cause of bronchiectasis in children and these include Measles, whoping cough, pulmonary tuberculosis and infection with adenovirus or respiratory syncital virus. Localised endobronchial obstruction and recurrent aspiration of secretions are other important causes of localized bronchiectasis. Diffuse bronchiectasis involving multiple lobes is as a result of inherited or acquired defects in the defense mechanism of the respiratory system. These include congenital or acquired hypogammaglobulinemia, cystic fibrosis and dyskinetic ciliary syndrome.

Absence of IgA and /or IgG neutralizing antibodies against viruses in tracheobronchial secretions predispose to recurrent infections.

Patients of Kartageners syndrome, a rare condition characterized by a combination of situs inversus, agenesis of frontal sinuses, suffer from recurrent chest infections and bronchiectasis.

Sometimes pleural conditions such as pleural adhesions associated with pulmonary fibrosis and empyema lead to prolonged collapse of the lung followed by bronchiectasis.

Though there is no specific age when bronchiectasis may occur but in large majority of patients disease starts in childhood and it is repeated respiratory infections which worsen the condition.

Pathology. Bronchiectasis commonly affects lower lobe bronchi. It is mainly confined to left side followed by the right side. Next in order of frequency is the lingula and right middle lobe. Upper lobe bronchiectasis is not common and generally follows apical tuberculosis.

There are four stages in the pathogenesis of disease and these range from localized collapse of lung leading to secondary bronchial dilatation (2) weakening of bronchial wall as a result of cumulative effect of proteolytic enzymes and products of inflammation. When stagnation of secretions in bronchi occurs. Septic organisms produce tissue necrosis (3) Increased pressure on the walls of bronchi due to accumulated secretions behind an obstruction and lastly the traction exerted on the wall of bronchi by contracting tissue in the fibrosed being.

Morphologically bronchiectasis has been divided into saccular or cystic form and cylindrical or fusiform forms. Saccular form generally affects the major or proximal bronchi. It is generally localized and may be found in any part of the lung but is common in lower lobes and near the base. Cylindrical form is characterized by uniform dilatation of several bronchi and subsegmental bronchi. Bronchial dilatation in fusiform variety is irregular and may show a beaded appearance.

Clinical features. The disease generally has an insidous course and the patient has history of chronic cough with bringing out of mucoid to mucoprulent sputum. There is often history of exanthematous illness in children. Cough in well developed cases is raspy. The quantity of sputum passed varies daily, its quantity and consistency changing depending on the presence of infection. Postural relationship of cough is very important. It is more when the patient bends forward or lies down. This occurs especially when the patient awakes in the morning as due to overflow of secretions, large quantities accumulate during the night.

Patient may suffer from attacks of broncho spasm. Sputum is often foul swelling and may be blood tinged. Sometims haemoptysis may occur. Patients breath is malodorous. Constitutional symptoms like fever. lassitude, fatigue and poor health are present when patient has acute exaceberation. There is evidence of chronic malnutrition and the growth of the child may be affected if the disease manifests in childhood.

Physical examination shall depend on the degree and extent of disease. In early stages except for persistent crepts at bases of lungs there may be no physical signs. As the disease progresses well marked clubbing of fingers (drumstick character) develops. There may be localized flattening or retraction of chest over the affected area. If there is a large bronchiectatic cavity, bronchial breath sound are heard with coarse crepitations.

With advanced disease patient may develop chronic cor pulmonale or pulmonary hypertension. Chief complications include septic broncho-pneumonia, cerebral abscess, secondary. Amyloid disease of kidneys, liver, empyema and purulent pericarditis.

Diagnosis. In a well developed case, history and physical findings are characteristic. Further confirmation is made by:

(i) Radiology of chest: It will show cystic lesions varying in size from 1-2 cm with or without fluid levels, generally present at lung bases.

(ii) CT scan of chest is a sensitive method to de tect bronchiectasis especially the sacculai form.

(iii) Bronchography is not advocated until it is re- quired to define the distribution of disease.

(iv) Fiberoptic bronchoscopy may be required to evaluate segmental disease and atelectasis of collapsed areas of lung.

(v) Pulmonary function tests. These are impaired and show a mixed pattern of obstructive and restrictive functions.

Treatment. It is mainly directed at controlling infection and providing adequate drainage of secretions. Postural drainage is an important method of treating all such patients and should be done at least twice a day. There is no fixed time limit to the procedure and is to be done as long as the patient tolerates.

Sputum should be examined for the type of organism and sensiturity tests carried out. Type of antibiotic employed shall vary on sputum culture. Antibiotics must be given in adequate dosage and for proper time. Generally ampicillin / Amoxycillin / cephalosporins / trimethoprim - sulphamethoxazole are employed. If there is bronchospasm broncho-dilators are administered. For thick sputum use of expectorants containing potassium iodide is employed. Smoking in any form is prohibited. Breathing exercises are advised to strengthen respiratory muscles.

Most patients of bronchiectasis are managed on medical lines but in a case with localized bronchiectasis who suffers from recurrent chest infections or haemoptysis, resection of the affected segment (lobectomy) is carried out. Before carrying out surgery assessment of respiratory functions must be made.

CHRONIC COR PULMONALE

It is defined as involvement of the right side of heart with or without right sided heart failure secondary to disease of chest, lung, Bony cage and pulmonary vasculature. Two fundamental factors are involved in the pathogenesis of the diseases ie hypoxia and obliterative changes in the pulmonary vascular bed (obliterative pulmonary hypertension). The two fac-tors are interrelated and one may be primary in one disease and secondary in another. Hypoxia may be produced by any disease which interferes with the oxygenation of blood in the lungs and a number of factors ranging from emphysema, fibrosis of lungs and alveocapillary block operate while pulmonary hypertension may arise as a primary disease and secondary to disease of pulmonary arterioles.

Two main types of causes operate in chronic cor pulmonale ie due to chronic emphysema. Secondary to chronic bronchitis (with or without emphysema). Bronchial asthma, bronchiectasis, tuberculosis. Bony cage abnormalities etc and the other is diseases involving pulmonary vasculature (pulmonary hypertension).

Incidence. Chronic cor pulmonale is widely prevalent and its incidence runs parallel with that of chronic bronchitis. Repeated chest infections, smoking, dust, cold climate, smoke from cow dung, and pollution in environment play important role in the causation of disease. It involves both sexes equally though it is more common in males because of their increased exposure to environmental pollution as well as their smoking habits. Workers in mines (coal, mica, stone crushers) in course of their work over the years fall easy prey to occupational lung disease leading to cor pulmonale.

Pathology: There are two broad factors involved in the pathogenesis of chronic cor pulmonale i.e. chronic obstructive emphysema and pulmonary hypertension. In the former there is retention of carbon dioxide while in the later there is obliteration of pulmonary vascular bed, which though may not be extensive enough to raise the pulmonary pressure during rest but during effort or accentuated hypoxic states there occurs a sharp increase in cardiac output and pulmonary hypertension.

Chronic obstructive emphysema produces increase in residual air which exceeds 35 percent of the total lung capacity, at the same time increasing work of breathing and reducing maximum breathing capacity. This results in reduction in arterial oxygen saturation and increase in carbon dioxide content. The kidney tends to retain becarbonate leading to a state of chronic hypercapnoea and respiratory acidosis. Hypoxaemia further produces increased blood volume and polycythaemia. Peripheral and

cerebral vasodilatation occurs due to increased arterial carbon dioxide tension.

As a result of obliterative changes in the pulmonary vascular bed pulmonary vaso constriction and hyper kinetic circulation, right ventricular failure occurs. Result of all the patho physiological changes is enlargement of the right side of heart (Right atrium and right ventricle) and dilatation of the main pulmonary artery. When the disease further progresses and right ventricle dilates, tricuspid incompetence results.

CAUSES OF CHRONIC COR PULMONALE

1. Chronic emplysema with or without bronchitis
2. Emphysema secondary to diseases of lungs
   (a) Bronchial asthma
   (b) Bronchiectasis
   (c) Pneumoconiosis
   (d) Pulmonary tuberculosis
3. Disease of bony cage
   (a) Kyphoscoliosis
   (b) Bony deformity of chest.
4. Disease causing pulmonary fibrosis
   (a) Diffuse interstitial pulmonary fibrosis or Hamman Rich syndrome
   (b) Radiation fibrosis
   (c) Scleroderma
   (d) Pneumoconiosis Silicosis, Asbestosis
   (e) Diffuse carcinomatosis / reticulosis
   (f) Sarcoidosis
5. Diseases leading to pulmonary hypertension
   (a) Primary pulmonary hypertension
   (b) Secondray pulmonary hypertension
      (i) Diseases of pulmonary arterioles (Polyarteritis nodosa, sarcoidosis, scleroderma, schistomiasis
      (ii) Lesions of pulmonary artery

Clinical features. In the clinical presentation of a case of chronic cor pulmonale there are three stages (i) uncomplicated emphysema without cardiac involvement (ii) compensated cor pulmonale and (iii) decompensated disease with evidence of right heart failure.

There is history of chronic cough with or without productive cough and breathlessness on exertion. Orthoponea is uncommon. Physical findings show a barrel shaped chest with diminished respiratory excursions. Percussion note is hyperresonant with liver or cardiac dullness either diminished or obliterated. Ascultation reveals diminished breath sounds with prolonged expiration and wheezing sounds and crepitations. There may be polycythaemia and central cyanosis, clubbing of fingers may be present. The duration of uncomplicated stage of emphysema lasts for about 5 years.

As the disease progresses, exertional dysponea becomes more marked and may be present even at rest. The extremities are warm and capillary pulsations may be present at the pulp of the fingers. Signs of right ventricular hypertrophy are generally masked by emphysema. There is parasternal lift of an hypertrophied right ventricle. The heart sounds are muffled. Pulmonary second sound is accentuated and split indicating pulmonary hypertension. A right ventricular heave may be palpable in the epigastrium suggesting right ventricular hypertrophy.

As the patient progresses into decompensated stage of chronic cor pulmonale, cyanosis becomes marked. Neck veins become distended and palpable with a visible giant 'a' wave. Liver is enlarged and tender. A positive hepatojugular reflex is an important sign of right heart failure. Systemic venous congestion and dependant oedema herald the development of congestive heart failure. Retinal venous engorement and papilloedema may be present. Ascultation of the heart reveals split and accentuated pulmonary second sound, a proto-diastolic gallop rhythm and pansystolic murmur at lower end of sternum.

Patient now is more breathless, disorientated and may have psychosis because of cerebral anoxia.

The duration of decompensated stage will vary and patient may go back into compensated stage depending on how well he is treated. Most patients of chronic cor pulmonale succumb to inter-current infections and progressive respiratory insufficiency.

Investigations:

1. **Chest X-ray:** It is an important non-invasive test. Chest radiographs shows increased translucency of the lung fields with widening of intercostal spaces, ribs placed more horizontally and diaphragm pushed down. There is dilatation of pulmonary artery and its branches. Right ventricle is enlarged.

2. **Electrocardiogram:** There is right axis shift with right axis deviation. Evidence of right ventricular hypertrophy (depression of RS-T segment with inversion of T waves in V1-V2 and appearance of tall R waves in these leads). Tall spiky P waves (P pulmonale) in leads II, III and aVF. Incomplete right bundle branch (rSR) pattern may be present. Cardiac arrhythmias are uncommon.

3. **Pulmonary function tests:** Forced vital capacity is reduced (FVC) as well as forced expiratory volume (FEV_1). There is fall in oxyen saturation, with reduction of PaO_2 and increase in PCO_2.

4. **Echocardiography.** It shows enlargement of right ventricular cavity in relation to that of left ventricle, thickness of right ventricular wall is increased. Peak regurgitant tricuspid flow and pulmonary regurgitation flow is measured by doppler echocardiography.

5. Haemoglobin and packed cell volume for assessment of polycythaemia, they are usually raised. Total and differential leurocyte count, and sputum examination (culture and sensitivity) for type of organisms.

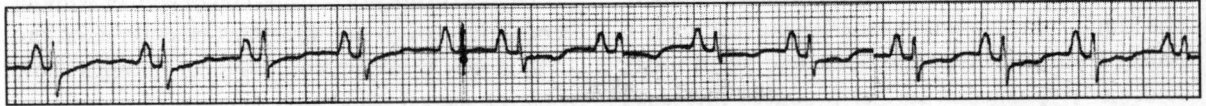

Fig. 5.16. E.C.G. in a case of chronic cor-pulmonable, showing P Pulmonale (Tall Peaked P waves)

Treatment

The main principles are:

(i) Chronic cough and episodes of chest infection be treated by the use of appropriate antibiotics. This shall prevent the progression of disease. Where there is bronchospasm, bronchodilators be used. Aminophylline/deriphyllin are useful drugs both as bronchodilators and respiratory stimulants.

(ii) Oxygen therapy is beneficial but should be used cautiously, since high concentration may lead to carbon dioxide retention thus inhibiting respiration. Oxygen is administered intermittently through a venture mask designed to deliver 24% oxygen. An intermittent positive pressure breathing apparatus with full humidification is used during periods of greatest pulmonary insufficiency. In patients with long standing disease, long term oxygen therapy is advocated.

(iii) Congestive Heart failure shall require both digoxin and diuretics Digitalis is used to increase the cardiac output and contractility which though is high but relative to patient needs is low. Small doses of digoxin should be administered and monitored carefully, since heart is very sensitive to digoxin and there is danger of starting cardiac arrhythmias. Of the various diuretics frusemide is useful. Its dose (40-80 mg) should be regulated depending on the degree of congestive failure. Potassium supplements are given to prevent potassium loss. Earlier on carbonic anhydrase inhibitor (Acetazolamide) was preferred because of its effect on bicarbonate excretion. Since it may transiently intensify acidosis, loop diuretic like frusemide is preferred.

(iv) Because chronic cor pulmonale is a consequence of chronic pulmonary disease, the main therapy should be aimed at improving pulmonary functions. Patient should avoid smoking and dusty atmosphere. Respiratory infections should be promptly treated. Patient should avoid contact with persons known to be suffering from colds and respiratory illnesses. Some patients benefit from breathing exercises. Patients nutrition must be maintained by giving good nourishing diet.

PNEUMONIA

Pneumonia may be defined as inflammation of the lung parenchyma caused by different organism ranging from bacteria to viruses. Pneumonia generally refers to an acute infection caused by specific organisms, the patient presenting with acute illness, high fever, toxaemia and cough.

Pneumonias are generally of two forms, lobar pneumonia where entire lobe or a large portion of lung is involved resulting in total lobar consolidation while in bronchopneumonia there is either patchy or lobular involvement of the lung along with bronchi and bronchioles.

Aetiology. A number of agents are responsible for causing pneumonia but the commonest form of pneumonia is caused by pneumococci.

Acute specific pneumonias. *Various causes are:*

1. Bacterial. *Steptococcus pneumoniae, Mycoplasma pneumoniae, Klebsiella pneumoniae, Staphylococcus aureus, H. influenzae, Mycobacterium tuberculosis, Legionella pneu-mophila.*

2. Viral and associated with influenza, measles, primary atypical pneumonia.

3. Rickettsial infection

4. Fungus

5. Chemical (irritant gases)

6. Radiation.

Aspiration pneumonia. It may be diffuse (bronchopneumonia) or localized (pneumonitis) and follows aspiration of infected material from the upper respiratory passages or material regurgitated from the stomach or aspirated from outside like in drowning.

Pneumococcal pneumonia. It is disease of middle-aged adults, males predominating as compared to females. The disease is equally common in young children as well as elderly age group. Persons suffering from debilitating illnesses, starvation, immunosuppressed (AIDS or treatment with anti-cancer drugs), alcoholic excess, exposure to chill are some of the conditions which predispose to it. Any previous attack of pneumonia does not confer any immunity but may be responsible for repeat attack.

The organism responsible commonly is pneumococcus (type I, II, III or VII) which together accounts for more than 50 per cent of all cases. Often other organisms such as streptococci, staphylococci, H. influenzae or other gram-negative organisms are also present and produce picture of lobar pneumonia.

Pathology. There is invasion of the lung by the bacteria with their rapid proliferation resulting in vascular engorgement and inflammatory exudates in the effected alveoli. The effected lobe is heavy, red and congested. This is followed by a stage of red hepatization when inflammatory exudate containing a large number of neutrophils, red blood cells and fibrin fills up the alveoli. In the stage of grey hepatization (consolidation), the capillaries are less congested, the lung tissue although still solid is softer in consistency and less friable. There is disintegration of leukocytes and red blood cells as well as accumulation of fibrin within the alveoli. The final stage of resolution takes place if there are no complications. The exudate within the alveolar spaces is either absorbed through lymphatics or expecotrated out by coughing. The lung parenchyma returns to its normal spongy state. The whole process may take variable time depending on the virulence of the organism and immunity of the patient. Pleural reaction also resolves in similar manner. In those with virulent form of disease complications like abscess formation in lung, Empyema or bacterial dissemination leading to meningitis, arthritis, pericarditis, endocarditis etc. may develop.

Clinical features. It is acute onset with fever and chills along with toxaemia and malaise. To start with cough is dry, irritating often accompanied with pain in the chest. By second or third day sputum which was viscid, thick and difficult to expectorate now may become more abundant and is rusty or pinkish in colour.

Organisms responsible for pneumonias

1. Bacterial. *Streptococcus pneumoniae, Staphylococcus aureus, Klebsiella pneumoniae, H. influenzae, Mycoplasma pneumoniae, Mycobacterium tuberculosis, Legionella pneumophila.*
2. Viruses
3. Rickettsial
4. Fungus

In ill patients, headache, sleeplessness and delirium appear. Patient has got tachycardia and tachypnoea. Respiratory accessory muscles are working and alae nasi appear to move more rapidly. There is dysponea and often cyanosis. Fever is high and continuous, persisting in untreated cases for period ranging from 7-10 days. Crisis which generally occurs by the seventh day results in fall of temperature to normal or even subnormal levels. There is relief from toxaemia and overall improvement in general symptoms. Sometimes crisis may be preceded by pseudo crisis where though there is fall of temperature yet little improvement in general condition. Defervescence by lysis may also occur when temperature falls but takes two to four days to reach normal levels.

As compared to acute onset in a case of lobar pneumonia often there may be insidious onset of disease preceded by upper respiratory catarrh, the course and mode changed as a result of antibiotic therapy.

Physical signs. These will vary with the stage of disease at which the patient presents. There is rise in pulse and heart rate. Alae nasi are in action. Presence of herpes on the lips is quite common. In early stages, movements of chest are restricted. Precussiosn note over the affected area is diminished. Breath sounds are harsh with prolonged expiration and few crepts are present.

By second or third day when consolidation is present signs include limitation of movement on the affected side, increased vocal fremitus and impaired precussion note over consolidation. Breath sounds are bronchial (tubular) and occasionally a few crepts may be audible. Vocal resonance is increased.

Bronchophoney and whispering pectoriloquy are marked over the consolidation. A pleural rub may be heard due to pleural involvement.

During the period of resolution, the bronchial breathing disappears and normal breath sounds appear. But there are coarse crepitations during both phases of respiration.

Above physical signs are if the patient has not been treated with antibiotics but with the advent of antibiotics the clinical picture including physical signs may not follow the classical pattern.

Laboratory investigations. There is leucocytosis with polymorphs ranging from 85-90%. Sputum on gram staining shows pneumococci. Blood culture is positive in 30-40% of patients in early stages before antibiotics administration. X-ray chest (PA view) shows a homogenous opacity in the lung depending on which lobe involved.

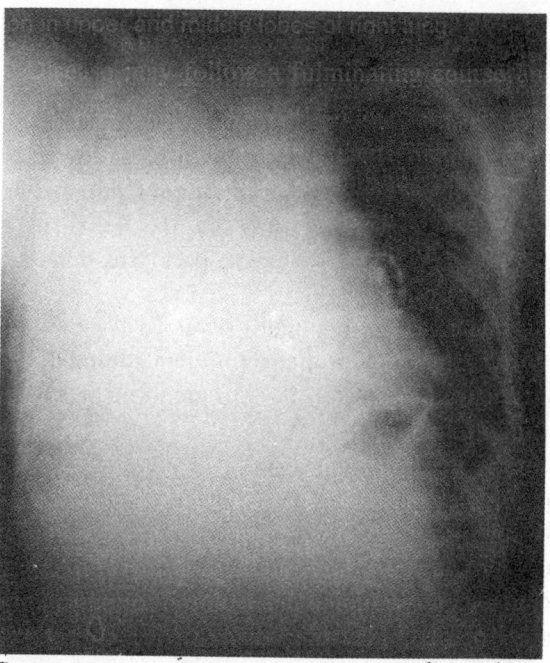

Fig. 5.18. X-ray Chest (PA View) showing opacification in right lung due to pneumonia.

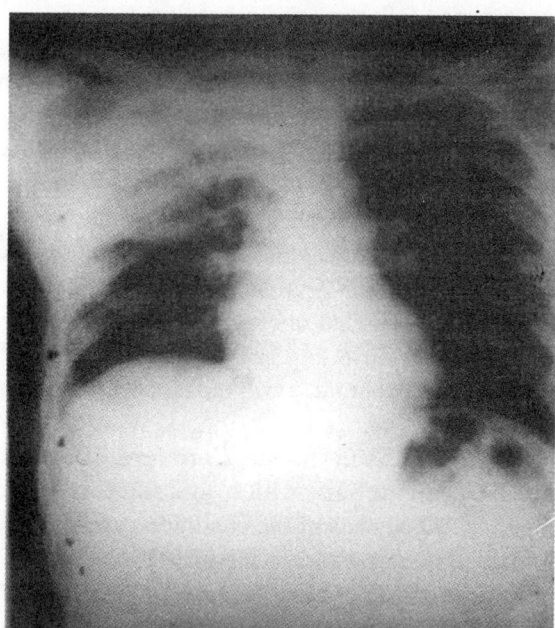

Fig. 5.17. X-ray Chest (PA view) Pneumonia of right upper lobe. There is opacification of upper lobe.

Complications. Pneumococcal pneumonia may be a serious ailment especially in elderly and immunocompromised individuals. In some people resolution may be delayed and signs of consolidation persist for weeks.

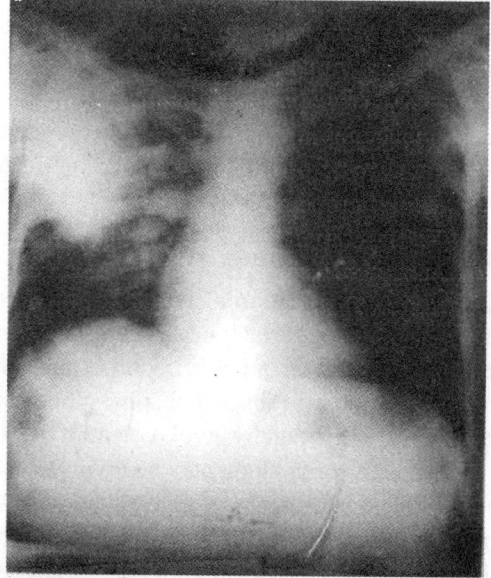

Fig. 5.19. X-ray Chest (PA View) showing consolidation in upper and middle lobes of right lung.

Disease may follow a fulminating course and

involve adjacent structures as well as major organs in the body. In lungs, there may be abscess formation while pleura shows pleural effusion and empyema. Cardiac involvement means grave prognosis. There may be pericarditis, myocarditis, endocarditis and cardiac failure. Gastrointestinal complications are uncommon and may be in the form of acute dilatation of stomach, paralytic ileus and peritonitis.

Pneumococcal meningitis develops in some cases and carries poor prognosis. Other complications include arthritis, parotitis, otitis media, nephritis and venous thrombosis.

Differential diagnosis. In a classical case of pneumonia diagnosis may not be difficult. But it has to be differentiated from number of acute conditions. A case of influenza may start in similar manner but examination of sputum with history suggestive of sore throat shall differentiate it.

Acute fevers such as typhoid and typhus may simulate pneumonia at the onset but clinical profile as well as investigations shall differentiates them. Pleural effusion is another condition to be considered. Pulmonary infarction may have same physical signs but the presence of cardiac disease absence of fever and blood stained sputum with breathlessness shall suggest the condition. Where meningeal irritation is present, it may have to be differentiated from tubercular or pyogenic meningitis. Further CSF examination including culture shall differentiate the condition.

Other forms of pneumonia:

Staphylococcal pneumonia. It generally follows secondary to previous viral illness. It may also sometimes arise as a complication of septicaemia from a carbuncle, perinephric abscess or some other lesion in the body. There is patchy involvement of the lung and several areas of the lung may be involved at the same time. There are areas of consolidation in one or more lobules. These break down to form thin walled cavities or abscesses. This type of pneumonia is often seen in intravenous drug users. Rupture of thin walled cavities may lead to pneumothorax, empyema and pleural effusion. Staphylococcal ab-

scesses may result in various parts of the body due to pyaemia.

Streptococcal pneumonia. It follows streptococcal infection of the throat but may also complicate influenza or parainfluenza infection of the respiratory passages. The course of the disease is severe and there is more toxaemia malaise, and ill health.

Klebsiella pneumonia (Friedlander's pneumonia). It usually occurs in elderly patients causing high degree of morbidity and mortality. Patients who are suffering from debilitating illnesses like diabetes malignancy, malnutrition are more prone to suffer from it. There is sudden onset of illness with fever, rigor and chills. Cough is productive and the sputum is gelatinous, purulent and blood stained. Disease follows a severe fulminating course and sometimes it may prove fatal. Prostration and cyanosis are often present. Lung abscess may follow acute pneumonia.

Tubercular pneumonia. It is of insidious onset and patient is not very ill. Diagnosis is arrived at on failure of a case of pneumonia to respond to antibiotic therapy. Sputum examination shall confirm the diagnosis when acid fast bacilli are demonstrated. If diagnosed early it carries good prognosis.

Viral pneumonia. Not very common. May be caused by influenza A virus or adenovirus or Rota virus. It is of gradual onset with headache, fever, chills and dry irritating cough. There is often a prominent sore throat and lymphadenopathy may be seen.

Physical signs in the lungs are few. These are signs of pneumonia which are scattered and migratory. Diagnosis of the condition can be made by detection or culture of the virus from sputum. Serum antibody rises can be seen by complement fixation, ELISA or radioimmune assays.

X-ray chest shows fleeting shadows either in miliary or lobular lesions.

Haemophilus influenzae pneumonia. It is often a secondary invader in a person suffering from chronic bronchitis and presents with fever, pain in throat, marked prostration and generalized aches and pains.

Pneumonia is either wide spread, diffuse or in the form of patchy lobular consolidation. Diagnosis is based on finding a yellow green sputum where organisms of H. influenzae can be demonostrated.

Aspiration pneumonia. It is as a result of aspirating respiratory secretions or gastric which have regurgitated into the respiratory pasages. Aspiration pneumonia commonly occurs in patients of coma, following general anaesthesia, drowning, violent contraction of abdominal muscles forcing gastric contents into respiratory passages, Cardiac achlasia, pyloric obstruction, oesophageal stricture and bulbar palsy. Often the patient presents with low grade pyrexia but when large volumes of secretions or fluid has been aspirated, a more serious profile may be seen. A picture of consolidation which may be massive is seen. Most often right lower lobe is involved. If appropriate treatment in the form of treating underlying cause is not undertaken a case of aspiration pneumonia may go into lung abscess formation. In massive consolidation following aspiration of large amount of secretions, patient may choke to death.

In addition to use of broad spectrum antibiotics given parenterally, aspiration of secretions has to be done either by a sucker or bronchoscope. Patient is encouraged to cough out the secretions. Underlying condition has to be treated energetically. In a comatosed patient, frequent change of sides shall help in the prevention of pneumonia.

Primary atypical pneumonia (Mycoplasma pneumonia). This is the type of pneumonia caused by mycoplasma, which differ from bacteria in that it is devoid of a rigid cell wall. This infection is generally common in close knit communities like hostels, institutions, boarding, schools. Since spread of infection is by droplet infection clinical presentation is in the form of pyrexia, acute or subacute tracheobronchitis. There is headache, fever, malaise, sore throat and dry cough. Disease is self limiting, the course generally running to two weeks. In mild cases, temperature falls by lysis in three to four days while in more severe form fever may last for a week or more.

Very severe infection may present with marked

toxaemia, meningoencephalitis, myocarditis, rashes, haemolytic anaemia and arthralgia. Physical signs include fever, signs of consolidation in one or the other lower lobe, presence of coarse crepitations and wheezing sounds. Diagnosis is based on demonstration of organism in sputum. Total and differential leucocyte count is normal though ESR is raised. Complement fixation test and rise in cold agglutinins in the serum especially during the first or second week of illness are further confirmatory tests. Mycoplasma antibodies (1gM and 1gG) are present in acute and convalescent stage.

X-ray chest shall show bronchial thickening with increased reticulation extending from hilum and maximum at periphery. Small homogenous opacities not corresponding to any lobe or segment may be seen.

BRONCHOPNEUMONIA (LOBULAR PNEUMONIA)

It is in the form of patchy consolidation of the lung and often follows bronchitis. It is more common at extremes of life - in infants and young children following or as a complication of measles, whooping cough and other exanthemata as well as viral infections. Elderly persons or those suffering from debilitating illnesses like carcinoma, AIDS, malnutrition, chronic bronchitis, chronic alcoholics and those on immunosuppressive drugs are more prone to suffer from it.

Though many organisms can cause bronchopneumonia yet the common ones are H. influenzae, staphylococci, streptococci and pneumo-cococi. Rare organisms include Pseudomonas, Proteus, rickettsiae, viruses and fungi.

Pathology. There are patchy areas of inflammation and consolidation in one or both lungs and most of the lesions are generally confined to lower lobes. The bronchioles are involved and there are secretions or exudate which block these and produce small areas of lobular collapse and consolidation. The areas of consolidation may conllude and result is larger areas of consolidation. Bronchioles and consolidated alveoli are filled with inflammatory exudate and epithelial cells. Occasionally area around the consolidated alveoli may become distended and show compensatory emphysema. With treatment the consolidation resolves but sometimes leaves behind residual areas of fibrosis.

Clinical features. Initially picture is that of acute bronchitis with malaise, fever and cough with or without expectoration. Overall the presentation is insidious but clinical picture is determined by the underlying condition and virulence of the organism. In children the picture is more severe, characterized by rapid rise of temperature, breathing difficulty, cyanosis and restlessness. In elderly people picture is equally grave with marked tachycardia, tachypnoea, restlessness and delirium.

Physical signs in a case of bronchopneumonia are those of bronchitis with prolonged expiration, wide spread rhonchi and medium to coarse crepitations present all over, but more at the bases. Occasionally patches of tubular breathing may be present at site of consolidation.

Cases of bronchopneumonia recover but in some cases where disease is more fulminating, bronchiectasis, fibrosis, lung abscess or empyema may be resultant sequlae.

Diagnosis of bronchopneumonia is based on clinical picture. X-ray chest shows patchy areas of consolidation present in one or both the lungs. Course of the disease is variable. Secondary bronchopneumonia has a more prolonged course.

Prognosis generally is good and recovery complete. But very old debilitated people, and young infants where the disease is fulminating prognisis is poor and mortality is high. Rising pulse, cyanosis, delirium and breathlessness carry poor prognosis.

Prognosis in a case of pneumonia. Most cases of pneumonia with adequate treatment carry good prognosis and recovery is complete. But number of factors govern the prognosis.

1. Age. Extremes of age i.e. infants and old people carry poor prognosis.
2. Presence of chronic debilitating diseases like malignancy, diabetes, malnutrition, cardiovascular respiratory and kidney diseases carry unfavourable prognosis. Immuno-compromised patients, chronic alcoholics and those on cytotoxic drugs have high mortality.
3. Type of organism producing the disease and extent of underlying lung condition are equally important. There is high mortality with pneumonia type III, klebisellae or frieclander's infection.
4. Rising temperature, fall in blood pressure with rising pulse and respiratory rate, marked restlessness, delirium, dehydration and cyanosis are poor signs.
5. Development of complications like pericarditis, myocarditis, meningoencephalitis carry poor prognosis.
6. Poor immunity and lack of response of body to infection in the form of leucopenia, subnormal temperature in the presence of toxaemia are grave signs.

Management of pneumonia. Management of a case of pneumonia requires both general and specific measures. All cases of pneumonia should be nursed carefully looking to hydration, nutrition and general care. Patient should be encouraged to cough and bring out expectoration. For unproductive cough, cough suppressants like Linctus codeine is to be given. Analgesics for any pleuritic pain. Attention should be paid to oral hygiene especially in elderly patients and those suffering from debilitating illnesses. For respiratory distress O_2 therapy should be given preferably through a face mask.

Specific therapy. In every case of pneumonia sputum should be examined by grams stain and culture done. In view of the acuteness of the condition antimicrobial agents must be started immediately without waiting for culture report.

Commonly employed drugs are Injection Penicillin (one lac units I/V six hourly), Injection Ampicillin (500 mg - 1 gm I/M or I/V six hourly), Injection Amoxycillin (500 mg - 1 gm I/M or I/V eight hourly), Injection Ciprofloxacin (500 mg I/V twice a day). For more severe infection Injection Cefotaxime (1 gm I/V twice daily) is employed since it is a broad spectrum cephalosporin effective against Klebsiella. H. influenza, Salmonella organisms.

Where anerobic infection is suspected to be present, Injection Metrogyl 500 mg I/V eight hourly be administered. Change in antimicrobial therapy may be made depending on response of the patient's drug sensitivity and sputum culture report.

Once the acute stage subsides, patient can be switched on to oral antibiotics (Ampicillin/Amoxycillin/Ciprofloxacin/Cotrimoxazole/Erythromycin). Treatment must be continued till there are no signs in chest and X-ray chest is clear. Inadequate treatment and premature stoppage of treatment shall leave behind a lung abscess.

LUNG ABSCESS

It is localized pyogenic infection of the lung characterized by suppuration, destruction of lung parenchyma with cavitation and formation of abscess.

Patient suffering from chronic debilitating diseases are more prone to suffer from this condition. The common organisms which reach the lungs either by inhalations or by spread from suppurative processes nearby or via blood stream include streptococci, staphylococci, pneumococcus, Friedlander's bacillus, and fusiform bacilli.

Causes:

1. Aspiration of infected material which occurs in patients after oral surgery, anaesthesia, coma and alcoholic intoxication. Secretions from infected tonsils sinuses and carious teeth and aspiration of gastric contents shall be other important cause.

2. As a complication of pneumonia when the organism is virulent, patients immunity is low and treatment has been inadequate. Mycotic infections of the lung may also lead to abscess formation.

3. Septic embolism from infective endocarditis or secondary infection of pulmonary infarction.

4. Bronchial obstruction especially in a case of bronchogenic carcinoma where a bronchus is obstructed and distal part of lung gets atelectasised and collection of secretions with impaired drainage leads to abscess formation.

5. Necrosis and abscess formation of a growth in lung.

6. Rupture of amoebic liver abscess in the lung.

7. Bacterial involvement of the lung secondary to systemic pyaemia.

Commonest site for abscess formation is right lower lobe, while right upper lobe is the next in frequency followed by those on the left side. Lung abscess is generally single while multiple lung abscesses may be seen with staphylococci infection. Similarly embolic abscesses are often small and multiple and can be present in any part of the lung. Abscess due to extension from adjacent diseased area is large and single.

Pathology. The lung abscess shows necrosis and suppuration of lung tissue, the involved area is often enclosed by a wall with variable amounts of fibrous thickening. Generally an abscess is single and has large amounts of inflammatory cells (lymphocytes, plasma cells and macrophages) varying with the chronicity of the lesion. An abscess may rupture into the bronchus expectorating large amounts of pus and it may itself be filled with air. Sometimes a lung abscess may rupture into the pleural cavity producing empyema or pneumothorax.

Clinical features. Symptoms are those of cough, when patient is bringing out large amount of mucopurulent sputum. There is fever, malaise and signs of toxaemia. Chest pain occurs when pleura is involved. In majority of cases lung abscess follows an inadequately treated pneumonia and symptoms may merge with the earlier disease though now there is production of large quantities of purulent sputum which is foul smelling due to anaerobic organisms. Haemoptysis is common. Clubbing of the fingers is present. As the process becomes chronic patient starts loosing weight and appetite. Physical examination shows an ill patient, with clubbing of the fingers and toes, with swinging type of fever. There are signs of consolidation in the lungs. Often cavity signs may be present when abscess is communicating with a bronchus. Pleural rub may be present when pleura has been involved.

Investigations:

Total and differential leucocyte count shows leucocytosis with rise in polymorphs. Culture of the sputum is helpful.

Bronchoscopy shall point to the cause of lung abscess and bronchoscopic aspirations for gram's stain, cytology and cultures be carried out.

X-ray chest shall show a localised shadow with a homogenous density. Air fluid levels may be seen in cases where abscess is communicating with airway. Both posteroanterior and lateral X-rays of chest are carried out to locate the site of abscess.

> **Causes of lung abscess**
>
> 1. Aspiration of infected material from oral cavity, throat.
> 2. Complication of lobar pneumonia.
> 3. Bronchial obstruction as in bronchogenic carcinoma.
> 4. Embolic infection with cavity formation.
> 5. Necrosis and abscess formation of growth in lung.
> 6. Metastatic lung abscesses.
> 7. Rupture of amoebic liver abscess into lung.

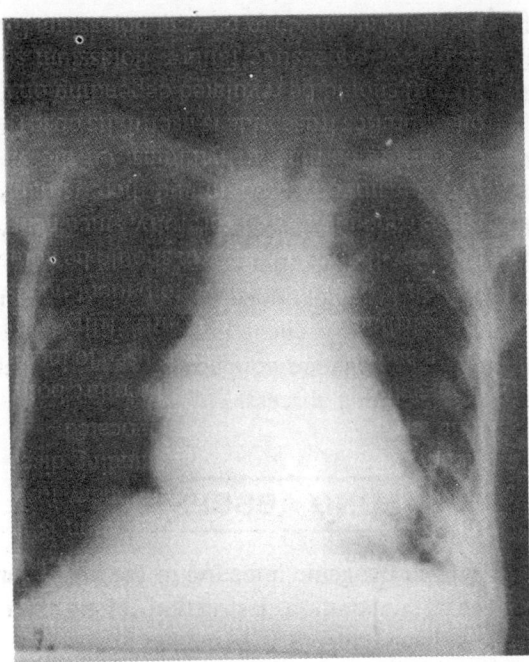

Fig. 5.21. X-ray chest (PA View) Case of lung abscess left lower base.

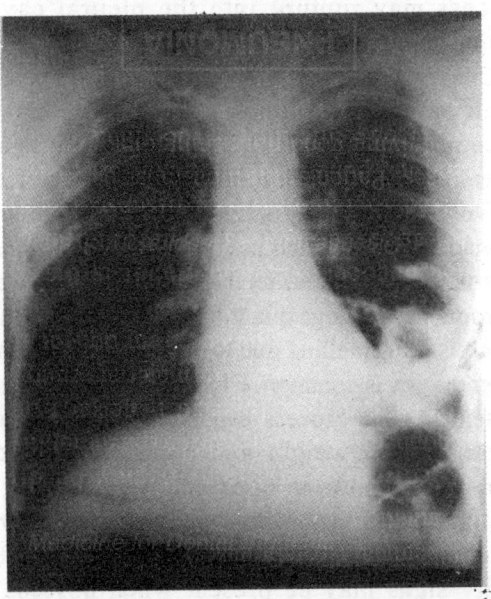

Fig. 5.20. X-ray Chest (PA View) A case of pneumonic consolidation with abscess formation in left lower lobe.

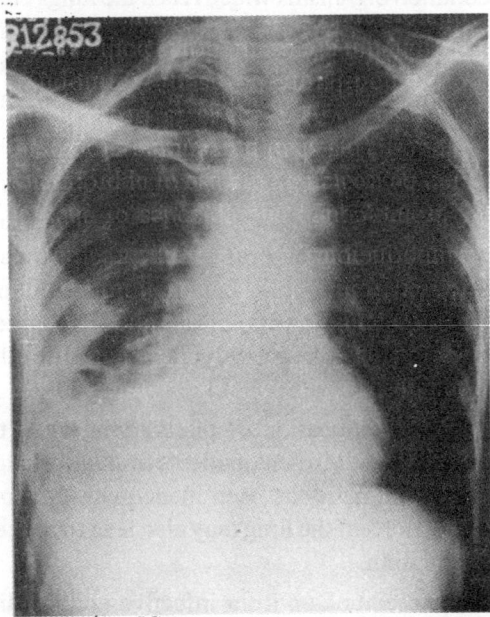

Fig. 5.22. X-ray Chest (PA View). Suppurative pneumonia with abscess formation in right lower lung. There is presence of both fluid and air in the abscess. Trachea is shifted to right side because of consolidation and fibrosis.

Complications. A number of complications may follow a lung abscess. An abscess may extend to surrounding stractures producing mediastinitis and pericarditis. Involvement of pleura shall produce pleurisy, empyema and pyopneumothorax if it ruptures into pleura. Severe haemoptysis may occur.

Extrapulmonary complications include brain abscess, cachexia and amyloidosis. A chronic form of lung abscess may leave behind bronchiectasis and chronic cavity with fibrosis.

Diagnosis of lung abscess shall depend on a careful history of illness and of predisposing causes. Radiology of the chest shall demonstrate a localised homogenous shadow. Sudden expectoration of large amount of purulent sputum in a patient with high fever, cough shall be suggestive of the condition.

A lung abscess has to be differentiated from pulmonary tuberculosis, bronchogenic carcinoma, bronchiectasis and cysts of the lung.

A positive sputum for AF-Bacilli with exudative or infiltrative lesion of the lung shall suggest pulmonary tuberculosis while bronchiectasis is more chronic, usually bilateral and X-ray shows honey combed appearances. In bronchogenic carcinoma there is history of weight loss, currant jelly sputum and hilar lymphadenopathy. Cysts of the lung are generally chronic in nature without acute manifestations except when a cyst has ruptured.

Treatment. Patient should be given good nutritious diet. Postural drainage be employed so as to evacuate and drain the abscess. Bronchoscopic drainage is also done in some cases. Intensive antibiotic therapy be employed depending on the sputum culture and drug sensitivity of the organism. Parenteral antimicrobial drugs like Ampicillin/Amoxycillin/Cephalosporins and Erythromycin are the commonly employed drugs but exact choice is made only after culture report is received. On an average a case of lung abscess requires four to six weeks of treatment.

In cases where there is failure of medical treatment and abscess defies treatment leaving behind a chronic abscess with fibrosis which is acting as a source of chronic infection in the lung. Surgical resection of the effected (segmental resection/lobectomy) lobe is done.

Prognosis in a case of lung abscess is on an average not bad because of availability of antimicrobial agents. Further course is governed by the underlying condition, virulence of the organism and its sensitivity and complications associated with the disease.

EOSINOPHILIA

Rise in eosinophils in blood to abnormal levels as a result of allergic reactions, parasitic, protozoal infections and hypersensitivity response etc. constitutes eosinophilia. A number of conditions produce eosinophilia and these are:

Parasitic infection. Hookworm, ascariasis, filaria, strongyloidosis, fascioliasis, trichuris.

Allergic disorder. Asthma, allergic rhinitis, hay fever, drug reactions (Aspirin, Penicillin, Nitrofurantoin, Iodides, Sulfanomides).

Skin disorder. Urticaria, eczema, pemphigus, psoriasis.

Pulmonary disorders. Tropical pulmonary eosinophilia, loeffler's syndrome, bronchopulmonary aspergillosis.

Malignant disorders. Eosinophilic leukaemia, Hodgkin's disease, lymphoma.

Miscellaneous. Eosinophilic gastoenteritis, sarcoidosis, hypereosinophilic syndrome, rheumatoid arthritis, SLE, polyarteritis nodosa.

Clinical feature. Cases of bronchopulmonary eosinophilia generally have mild symptoms in the form of dry cough, breathlessness and often mild fever. Where the cause is evident in the form of parasitic infection, allergic reaction to a drug, the disease is self limiting. In west, aspergillosis is a common cause of bronchopulmonary eosinophilia. The spores of Aspergilla Fumigatus which are present in the atmosphere throughout the year but more so in autumn months, when inhaled produce a form of allergic reaction in the form of bronchopulmonary features. Patient has features of breathlessness, wheezing, low grade fever and cough with expectoration. Blood count shows raised eosinophil count and IgE levels. Skin test is positive. There is presence of eosinophils and mycelia in the sputum. X-ray chest shows miliary mottling often simulating tuberculosis.

Treatment is by long-term steroids (oral prednisolone 60 mg per day in divided doses).

Hypereosinophilic syndrome. It is a multisystem involvement by eosinophilic infiltration. Typically patient has features of ill health, weight loss, dry cough and breathlessness. There is infiltration of various tissue by mature eosinophils. Pulmonary involvement is in the form of either interstitial lung disease or pleural effusion.

Cardiac involvement may lead to congestive cardiac failure. Treatment is by corticosteroids.

Loeffler's syndrome. It is as a result of migration of larvae of ascarias and other parasites through the lungs. There are features of cough, wheezing, fever and occasionally haemoptysis. Benign form of eosinophilic pneumonia may occur. Treatment is of the causative condition.

Tropical eosinophilia. A disease of tropical countries (India, Pakistan, Bangladesh, Sri Lanka, Malaysia, etc) is characterised by chronic cough, attacks of breathlessness, lassitude and weight loss with rise in eosinophil count in the blood.

Etiology. The most accepted cause of tropical eosinophilia is allergic reaction to filarial worms and both non-human and human filaria have been considered as aetiological factors. Of these human filaria probably Wucheria bancrofti is responsible. At one time mites and Helminthic infestations were suspected but now these have been excluded.

Pathology. Disease is common in hot, humid climate. There are no seasonal variations and commonly people in age group of 20-40 years fall victim to it. Besides hypereosinophilia there are circulating filarial antibodies and patients lack 1gG blocking antibodies against circulating microfilaria. Destruction of parasites intiate Type-I hypersensitivity reaction.

The changes in the lungs resemble that of viral pneumonia. There is infiltration by inflammatory cells, lymphocytes, histiocytes and eosinophils. Pathological lesion may be in the form of broncho-

pneumonia and interstitial fibrosis depending on the duration of the disease. Sputum examination may reveal epithelial cells and eosinophils.

Clinical picture. Clinical presentation is variable, Chronic cough of several weeks or months duration is the prominent complaint. Cough is more marked at night accompanied by wheezing and asthma like attacks. There is constricting sensation in the chest. Cough may be dry or may be accompanied by mucoid to mucopurulent sputum. Paroxysms of cough may end in a whoop. Main differentiation in acute attack is to be from bronchial asthma where generally the history of illness in family and allergy is present. In cases of tropical eosinophilia bronchial spasm is not always present.

Patient suffers from general debility, weight loss, low grade fever and malaise. Paroxysms of coughing often lead to sleeplessness and general fatigue. Patient is never seriously ill and chronic cases go about with vague ill health and asthma-like picture.

Examination of Chest may be negative. In some cases signs of bronchospasm (prolonged expiration and rhonchi) and crepitations may be heard over the bases of both lungs. Symptoms in cases of tropical eosinophilia are disproportionate to physical signs. Sometimes generalized lymphadenopathy and mild splenomegaly may be observed.

Investigations. Total leucocyte count ranges between 10,000 to 30,000 per cmm with eosinophils count ranging between 70-80 per cent. Other cells are present in normal number. Intercurrent infections may raise the polymorph count and decrease number of eosinophils. Eosinophils are mature and normal in appearance. Absolute eosinophil count range from 2000 to 10,000 cmm. ESR is raised. X-ray chest shows miliary mottling. Hilar shadows are irregularly enlarged and blurred. Lung fields may be transversely crossed with fine irregular branching striations. Changes on X-ray in the lungs are usually bilateral and are more prominent in basal region and mid zone. These shadows are more prominent in acute stage and tend to disappear with treatment.

Another test is filarial complement fixation test which is positive in majority of cases.

Diagnosis. It is based on clinical presentation,

blood picture showing high eosinophil count and characteristic radiological signs. It may have to be differentiated from simple and prolonged pulmonary eosinophilia which is due to transient allergic reaction to worms such as ascaris, ankylostoma, trichuris trichuria and drugs like aspirin, penicillin, sulphanomids PAS etc.

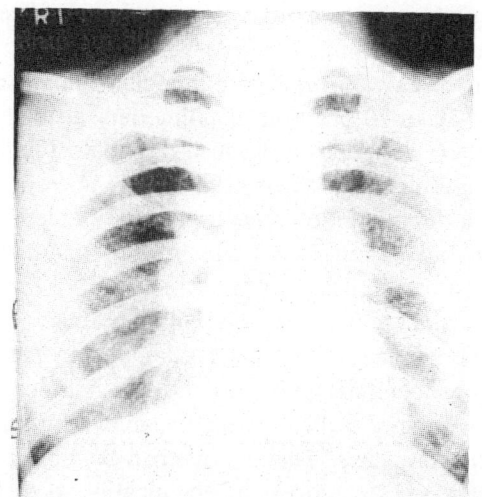

Fig. 5.23. Military Mottling in Tropical Eosinophilia

Allergic bronchopulmonary aspergillosis produces wheeze, cough fever and malaise as a result of allergy to Aspergillus fumigatus with rise in peripheral eosinophil count and a positive skin test. Other conditions associated with raised eosinophil count are Loeffler's syndrome (high eosinophil but low white cell count), Bronchial asthma and hypereosinophilic syndrome (fever weight loss, recurrent abdominal pain, persistent cough and congestive heart failure).

Very often eosinophilia may require to be differentiated from miliary tuberculosis because of radiological appearances. A case of pulmonary tuberculosis may have long drawn out history of ill health, wasting, evening rise of temperature and cough. Sputum may be positive for AFB. X-ray signs is tuberculosis are generally diffusely present. Mottling is more clearly defined and harder.

Course and prognosis. Prognosis in a case of tropical Eosinophilia is good. The course of the disease is benign and there are periods of remissions and relapses. Signs and symptoms take number of months to develop. Spontaneous recovery is common. The condition is not fatal.

Treatment. The drug of choice is diethyl carbamazine given in a dose of 5 mg per kg. body weight. In adults dosage is 3 tabs (50 mg tab) four times a day for 5 days. Side effects are minimal except for headache, nausea, vomiting.

In addition patient will require bronchodilators to relieve the bronchospasm. Sometimes coroticosteroids are employed.

Recovery after theraphy is good. Repeat course of the drug may have to be given after six weeks. A careful watch on clinical profile and Eosinophil count must be maintained by regular follow up.

PULMONARY EMBOLISM

Occlusion of the pulmonary vessel or its branches by a thrombus geting dislodged either from the peripheral veins or from the right side of the heart resulting in cardiac and circulatory effects depending on the size of the embolus constitutes pulmonary embolism. Pulmonary embolism is a common condition but is usually not diagnosed and often a great percentage of patients are only diagnosed after death. A number of conditions predispose to pulmonary embolism and these range from formation of clot in the systemic veins to formation of clot in the right side of heart.

Conditions predisposing to formation of pulmonary embolism:

1. Prolonged bed rest and immobilisation in bed due to medical or surgical problem, pelvic and lower limb fractures. Pelvic or abdominal surgery where pulmonary embolism is more common in second or third postoperative week.
2. Pregnancy, after child birth and women on oral contraceptive pills.
3. Congestive heart failure.
4. Carcinoma especially of the stomach or pancreas or any wide spread malignant process.

5. Haematological disorders such as polycythae-mia, leukaemias.
6. Atrial fibrillation where thrombus forms in the right atrium gets dislodged and goes into right ventricle. Embolisation is also common in cases with subacute bacterial endocarditis and right ventricular infarction.
7. Miscellaneous conditions include obesity, and straining at stools which may initiate the process of displacing the clot into circulation.
8. Diseases of lower extremity veins like thrombophlebitis.

Conditions predisposing to pulmonary embolism

1. Prolonged bed rest
2. Pelvic or abdominal surgery
3. Pelvic and lower limb fractures
4. Postpartum period
5. Oral contraceptives
6. Hypercoagulability states, polycythaemia
7. Atrial fibrillation
8. Congestive heart failure
9. Malignancy stomach or pancreas
10. Infective endocarditis
11. Obesity

Pathology. Generally there is pathology in the deep veins of the calf or pelvic veins or right side of the heart when a clot which has formed there gets dislodged detaches itself from its site of formation and produces obstruction of the pulmonary artery. Common site being bifurcation of the pulmonary artery with complete occlusion of one branch and partial of the other. Sudden death may take place when there is complete or almost complete occlusion of the pulmonary artery.

Haemodynamic disturbances shall depend on the size of the embolus. The bigger the embolus, more circulatory disturbances. The cardiac and circulatory effects of pulmonary embolism are because of mechanical circulatory obstruction as well as myocardial ischaemia. Embolic obstruction produces a zone of the lung tissue which is ventilated but not perfused. There is impaired gas exchange.

Loss of alveolar surfactant does not occur immediately and may take a few hours. Atelectasis and hypoxaemia may take 24-48 hours after embolisation to develop. Reduction in cross-sectional area of the pulmonary arterial bed leads to pulmonary hypertension and development of acute right heart failure. Extent of pulmonary obstruction is an important factor governing the circulatory disturbances. Humoral and or reflex influences also operate in certain patients.

In cases with massive pulmonary embolism at least 50 to 70 per cent of pulmonary arterial tree must be occluded to produce ciriculatory effects. As a result of this there is fall in output from right heart, diminution of venous return to the left heart with fall in left ventricular output resulting in myocardial ischaemia.

Small pulmonary emboli seldom produce serious cardiocirculatory disturbances though they produce pulmonary infarction in great majority. Vast majority of pulmonary emboli especially small may resolve within few days. This is governed by fibrinolytic system and the process of organization of emboli. Another factor is the development of bronchial arterial collateral circulation which develops in patients who have pulmonary infarction of some duration where not only blood supply to the infarcted area improves but also alveolar stability and resolution of atelectasis.

Clinical features. These will depend on the extent of pulmonary obstruction and acuteness of the process. A sudden massive pulmonary embolism may produce sudden death.

In a patient with a small embolus, symptoms may be mild in the form of low grade pyrexia, pain in the leg veins, breathlessness and pain in the chest. In those with submassive pulmonary embolism there is not only sudden onset of cough, dysponea but also chest pain and haemoptysis. It may take few days for the whole picture to crystalise. Physical examination shall reveal signs of atelectasis, a few wheezing sounds and rales. Pleural rub shall be present. Signs of pleural effusion may appear after few days.

A case with massive pulmonary embolism

presents with acute chest pain, breathlessness, faintness, dizziness shock and marked sweating with circulatory collapse. There may be haemoptysis, cyanosis, convulsions, mental confusion and even syncope. Physical examination reveals a rapid, thready pulse with cold extremities, pallor and low blood pressure. Signs of acute right heart failure (engorged neck veins, prominent a wave in the jugular venous pulse, hepatomegaly)may appear. Cardiac auscultation reveals a loud pulmonary second sound with wide spliting of second heart sound, systolic or continuous murmur generated by turbulence of blood flow in obstructed vessel.

General physical examination shall reveal thrombophlebitis in deep veins in about 50% of patients, which may be detected by Homan's sign, Pleural rub and fever when infarction has developed may be present.

Laboratory investigations:

1. Investigations like total and differential leucocyte count, ESR are not of much help. There may be leucocytosis as well as rise in ESR levels. Once infarction has developed, LDH levels are also raised.

2. X-ray chest is not helpful in all cases. A normal X-ray chest does not exclude diagnosis of pulmomary embolism. Positive signs include elevation of hemidiaphragm, abrupt or 'cut off' of a pulmonary vessel when traced distally, a wedge shaped opacity with base of the triangle towards the pleura, linear opacities suggestive of atelectasis. Differences in diameters of two pulmonary vessels also raises doubts about pulmonary embolism. Pleural effusion though small may be seen in late stages after 12 to 36 hours after embolization.

3. Electrocardiogram. It is helpful in some cases where massive pulmonary embolism has produced acute haemodynamic disturbances. Classical pattern shall be:

   (a) Prominent S wave in lead I and II. Q wave and T wave inversion in LIII. T wave inversion in V1-V4. Right axis shift right ventricular hypertrophy and right bundle branch block.

   (b) Tall and peaked P waves. Electrocardiographic changes are transient and last only for a few hours to days.

   (c) Pulmonary perfusion and ventrilation scintigram. Perfusion scintigraphs and use of radionucleides labelled with technetium 99 m are helpful in the diagnosis of pulmonary embolism when a nonperfused area but ventilated one shall suggest the condition. The test is simple and multiple scan views should be taken because lesions not seen in one view can be detected in others.

4. Lower extremity ultrasound (leus). Lower extremity venous ultrasound has an excellent sensitivity for diagnosing deep vein thrombosis. However a negative LEUS does not exclude pulmonary embolism because the thrombus can originate in pelvic, calf or upper extremity veins or the entire clot may have already embolized.

5. D-Dimer testing. Second generation D-dimer tests can be divided into qualitative (whole blood or immuno filtration) and quantitative (ELISA or tubidimetree) tests. A quantitative test result of 500mg/ ml or higher is considered positive. A result below 500 mg/ml is negative and rules out the disease. Likelihood of pulmonary embolism increases with very high D-dimer level. But a positive D dimmer test requires a confirmatory radiological study to establish the diagnosis of pulmonary embolism.

6. Ventilation/perfusion testing. V/Q scans in pulmonary embolism are very important especially in patients with normal chest X-rays. A normal scan virtually excludes pulmonary embolism.

7. CT scan. A multidetector CT scan can image the entire thorax. Computed CT angiography is faster than a V/Q scan or a pulmonary angiogram. This is an important diagnostic tool.

8. Pulmonary angiography. This is a specific method for providing anatomic information about the obstruction. Radiopaque material is injected through a cardiac catheter into the

pulmonary artery. Important finding shall be abrupt 'cut off' of a vessel at the place of obstruction and intraluminal filling defects.

9. Blood gas analysis. There is hypoxaemia, respiratory alkalosis and wide differences between alveolar and arteral PCO_2.

Signs and symptoms of pulmonary embolism

1. Chest pain
2. Tachycardia
3. Tachypnea
4. Low grade fever
5. Hypotension
6. Cyanosis
7. Unexplained shock
8. Haemoptysis
9. Jugular vein distension
10. Dizziness
11. Shock
12. Signs of acute right heart failure
13. Loud pulmonary second sound

Diagnosis of pulmonary embolism is made on a number of factors. Presence of thrombophlebitis in deep leg veins, prolonged bed rest and immobilization, cardiac irreglarity in the form of atrial fibrillation should be considered while keeping in mind clinical picture of precordial pain, breathlessness, and tachycardia in any patient who has undergone a recent major surgery or is confined to bed.

The condition especially in massive pulmonary embolism should be differentiated from acute myocardial infarction. Dissecting aneurysm of aorta, pneumoia, pleurisy. Electrocardiogram in such cases along with X-ray chest shall help in making the diagnosis.

Management. It shall be in the form of preventive as well as therapeutic.

Preventive. All patients who are confined to bed for long periods must have regular exercises of the lower limbs so as to prevent venous thrombosis. This may be in the form of physiotherapy and gentle massage of the limbs.

Therapeutic management:

1. O_2 to be administered continuously. If patient is in shock, initiate measures like use of intra-

venous fluid, vasopressor drugs (Dobutamine).

2. Anticoagulant therapy: It is the main stay of treatment both for prevention as well as extension of the thrombus and immediate inhibition as well as resolution of the embolus.

Drug of choice is Heparin 10,000-15,000 units I/V given initially with maintenance dose of 5000-10,000 units every 6 hourly. The drug can be given both by intravenous or deep intramuscular route but intravenous route is preferred. Dosage is adjusted by keeping clotting time (normal 5-7 minutes) two to two and half times the normal levels. Drug should be continued in acute stage (48-72 hours) and since long term anticoagulation is desired oral anticoagulants like Dindevan are switched on after tapering heparin.

Anticoagulant therapy is contraindicated in pregnancy. Peptic ulcer, bleeding disorders, hypertension, recent cerebrovascular accident and infective endocarditis. If bleeding due to heparin occurs it is controlled by stopping the drug, fresh blood transfusion and intravenous administration of protamine sulfate (dose 50 mg intravenously).

Thrombolytic therapy. Exact role of fibrinolytic therapy in pulmonary embolism is controversial. Thrombolytic agents are definately indicated since they hasten the resolution of venous and pulmonary emboli. Commonly Injection Streptokinase is employed. Dosage is 1,25,000 units by intravenous infusion in 200 ml of glucose in first 30 minutes followed by 75,000 units to 1,00,00 units intravenously hourly for next 24-48 hours.

Surgical management. Ligation of inferior vena cava or insertion of a greenfield filter device to protect against small emboli from travelling are method commonly employed. Emergency pulmonary embolectomy is carried out when there is failure of medical treatment and patient is in critical state. This is a specialised method and requires special care as well as approach.

Prognosis. Prognosis in a case of pulmonary embolism is governed by a number of factors like presence of underlying disease, predisposing cause and size of infarct. Massive pulmonary embolism carries poor prognosis. Early institution of therapy and resucitative measures makes the prognosis good in majority of cases.

PULMONARY TUBERCULOSIS

Pulmonary tuberculosis, also known as pthisis or consumption, is of worldwide distribution and at any time probably about 15-20 million people suffer from it. But it is a disease more of poor and developing countries where because of economics, poor social conditions, bad sanitation and hygiene, malnutrition more people fall victim to it than in people living in Western countries. Tuberculosis in the West is seen in immigrant people and those suffering from AIDS and conditions where body's defence mechanisms are low such as immunocompromised persons and those on immunosuppressive drugs.

Pathology. Causative organism is mycobacterium tuberculosis whose main forms are human, bovine, avian and reptilian. Tuberculosis in humans is caused by human type of organism which accounts for more than 98 per cent of all cases of tuberculosis.

The mode of entry of the organism in the body can be either by inhalation, alimentary ingestion and inoculation. Most common method of acquiring infection is by direct person to person transmission of air-borne droplets of organisms from an infected person to susceptible host. These organisms may be dormant in such people for a period of time and only when their body's defences are lowered that infection already present may activate itself and produce an active disease process. Tuberculosis flourishes where there is poverty, malnutrition and poor body's defence mechanisms.

Primary pulmonary tuberculosis is the first lesion which develops in a previously unexposed non-sensitized individual irrespective of the age. Reinfection of a sensilized person or reactivation of a primary dormant lesion is called secondary or post-primary tuberculosis.

The initial lesion after ingestion of tubercle bacilli which mainly occurs in the lungs constitutes primary tuberculosis. It commonly involves children and is in the form of subpleural lesion either in the lower part of upper lobe or upper part of lower lobe. The initial entry of the bacilli iniates non-specific inflammatory response which hardly produces any symptoms. Bacilli are transported to regional lymph nodes and parenchymal lesion in the lungs (Ghon focus) along with enlarged lymph nodes which may calcify over a period of time and this constitutes primary complex (Ghon's complex). In majority of children primary complex does not produce any symptoms except to induce sensitivity reaction which can be detected by tuberculin reaction. A positive tuberculin test may remain so for life.

A case of primary tuberculosis draws attention when a child may present with a non-specific pneumonia or bronchial obstruction because of enlarged hilar gland or low grade fever with pleural effusion. Primary complex heals leaving a calcified lesion. Bacilli may remain for years and may become reactivated when body's immunity falls as in malnutrition, debilitating disease and following severe forms of measles, whooping cough.

Cases of primary tuberculosis once progressive are always symptomatic. There are features of low grade pyrexia, loss of weight, ill health, failure to thrive and persistent cough. Transient pleural effusion (small), erythema nodosum (painful, reddish lesions over tibia). Pneumonia or segmental collapse of the lobe may be other features. Uncommonly the primary lesion may become active, caseation and cavitation occurs and widespread dissemination of the disease may take place producing miliary tuberculosis and in some cases meningitis. Postprimary tuberculosis develops when bacilli lying dormant in the body become active because of fall in body's defence system or because of infection by a large number of virulent bacilli or as a result of progression of primary lesion or spread of infection from lymph nodes through blood stream.

Secondary tuberculosis is mainly located in one or both apices of the lungs. The sites of active involvement are characterised by a granulomatous inflammatory reaction with both caseating and non-caseating tubercles. Initial lesion may be in the form of exudative pneumonia or a small patch of consolidation. This may enlarge with expansion of area of caseation and coalesce to form a big cavity. When erosion occurs into a bronchus, caseous material is expectorated leaving behind a cavity lined by fibrous tissue. Haemoptysis occurs when there is erosion of a blood vessel.

Spread of disease takes place through lymphatics and blood stream. Miliary tuberculosis indicates widespread dissemination. Endotracheal, endobroncheal and laryngeal tuberculosis develop when infected sputum is being coughed up while intestinal tuberculosis is due to swallowing of infected sputum. Systemic involvement of body organs occurs when infective foci in the lungs involve venous system to the heart and then via arterial system it spreads to the various organs in the body like heart, kidneys, liver, adrenals, meninges, and genital organs.

Clinical picture. Primary tuberculosis generally has no symptoms and often remains undetected. Children with primary tuberculosis may present with vague ill health, failure to grow. Cough and wheeze when a bronchus is being compressed especially in the middle lobe, a picture of collapse consolidation may develop. This may leave behind bronchiectasis (middle lobe syndrome). Spread of caseous material results in widespread dissemination of disease and resultant miliary tuberculosis.

Postprimary tuberculosis develops slowly over a period of time. It generally is in the form of malaise, loss of weight, persistent cough, loss of appetite and evening rise of temperature. Fever in early cases is transitory for a hour or so, comes in the evening accompanied with marked sweating. In some cases a persistent cough not responding to treatment draws attention towards the disease. Sputum may be mucoid or mucopurulent. Haemoptysis may occur in the form of either mild streak or profuse haemorrhage.

Hoarseness of voice with pain in throat indicates involvement of larynx. A pleural effusion or dry pleurisy or spontaneous pneumothorax or a pneumonic consolidation may be other modes of presentation. In females, amenorrhoea or oligo-menorrhoea are often early symptoms of tubercular infection.

Physical examination of the patient shall reveal a wasted, cachexic individual with rapid pulse rate and tachycardia. Examination of chest may reveal a long narrow chest, with hollowing in the infraclavicular region. There may be physical signs of collapse, consolidation, cavitation and fibrosis depending on the stage at which the patient presents. Some patients may have clinical picture of either a pleural effusion or pneumothorax.

Recovery in a patient of tuberculosis shall depend on the body's resistance, virulence of the organism, nutrition of the patient and adequacy of treatment. If not treated properly death may result either due to disease itself or an intercurent infection.

Clinical types of tuberculosis:

Acute tuberculosis. It is a severe fulminating form of tuberculosis where there is widespread dissemination of bacilli through the bloodstream. It may be in the form of a pneumonic lesion with dysponea and cyanosis or in the form of meningitis with severe headache and signs of meningeal irritation. Fever is irregular with wide variations in morning and evening temperatures. Prostration may be present. There is anorexia, tachycardia and features of toxaemia. Spleen usually is enlarged.

Diagnosis may be difficult in view of the wide variation of clinical presentation. Mantoux test is positive though in people with fulminating disease it may be negative. Sputum may contain organisms. X-ray chest will show diffuse scattered opacities throughout the lung fields (miliary mottling: snow storm appearances). In some cases transbronchial, liver and bone marrow biopsy may be done to confirm the diagnosis.

Chronic pulmonary tuberculosis. It is a more common presentation. Disease has an insidious onset, symptoms to start with are mild but gradually over a period of weeks or even months, patient starts showing features of evening rise of temperature, malaise, generalised weakness, night sweats and weight loss. Persistent cough with mucoid to mucopurulent sputum and sometimes blood stained is common.

Pulmonary tuberculosis commonly involves the apices of the upper lobes and superior segments of lower lobes. The extent of disease shall vary ranging from apical infiltration to cavity formation. Development of lesions shall depend on the progress of the disease. Parts of lung may be involved with spread of exudative lesion transbronchially leading to tuberculous pneumonia.

Chronic fibrocaseous form of tuberculosis is the common form where normal pulmonary architecture is lost with volume loss, fibrosis and there are areas of caseation, cavitation, nodular or miliary tubercles with upward contraction of lung. This form commonly involves the upper lobes while fibroid form involves upper third and sometimes whole lung. There is associated bronchiectasis which produces severe degree of mucopurulent sputum and haemoptysis.

Physical examination shall show generally a wasted individual with features of toxaemia. Clubbing of the fingers is generally present depending on the duration of disease. Signs in chest shall depend on the stage at which the patient is seen. In apical involvement a few crepts and a wheezing sound may be heard while with cavitation and fibrosis, a bronchial breathing (amphoric) with crepitations (medium to coarse) shall be present.

Physical signs of pleural effusion, pleurisy, pneumonia or pneumothorax may be present depending on at which stage the patient is seen.

Miliary tuberculosis. It is a disease of young children and adults and is as a result of widespread dissemination of tubercular infection via the blood stream. Entry of the organism into the bloodstream takes place either through lymphatics or erosion of a blood vessel by a caseating lesion either in the lung or a gland. Since it is a widespread dissemination, most of the major organs in the body including heart, brain, meninges, lungs, liver, spleen, eyes get studded with small tubercles varying in size from 1-2 mm in diameter. Later on they enlarge and may become confluent.

Clinically a case of miliary tuberculosis may start insidiously or acutely and presents with fever, anorexia, malaise, ill-health and toxaemia. Except for signs of toxaemia in the form of tachycardia, loss of weight, high fever there may be no physical signs in lungs in early stages. As the disease progresses there is enlargement of liver, spleen and generalized lymphadenopathy. Sometimes patient may develop tubercular meningitis with signs of meningeal irritation and headache and may be presenting feature in some cases.

Fever is irregular with wide variations in morning and evening temperatures. Prostration may be present. Diagnosis of miliary tuberculosis is made by a number of tests.

X-ray chest in early stages may be normal since very small tubercles are not seen in X-ray. But as the tubercles enlarge, lungs show typical snow storm appearances or miliary mottling (diffuse scattered opacities throughout the lung fields). Mantoux test may be positive in some cases. It is negative in cases with advanced form of disease.

Sputum examination for AFB is generally negative. Choroid tubercles when present in the eyes on ophthalmoscopic examination are diagnostic.

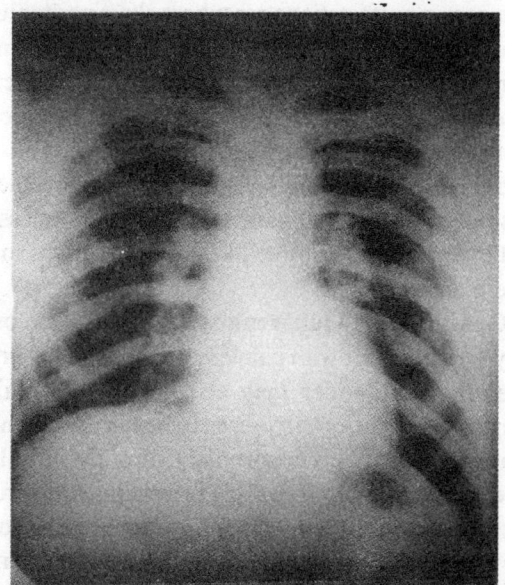

Fig. 5.24. Miliary Tuberculosis. X-ray Chest (PA View) showing miliary mottling (Snow storm appearances).

In cases where diagnosis is not established liver

or bone marrow biopsy is done when caseous lesions may be seen.

Differential diagnosis of miliary tuberculosis is from conditions like sarcoidosis, tropical eosinophila, pneumoconiosis and disseminated carcinomatosis. Miliary tuberculosis is a grave form of tuberculosis and without treatment it may prove fatal. Response to antitubercular therapy is good.

Extrapulmonary tuberculosis. Tuberculosis is one disease which involves almost all the major organs in the body ranging from heart to GI tract.

Tuberculous pericarditis. Pericarditis due to tuberculosis is one of the commonest involvement. It may be in the form of pericarditis, pericardial effusion and later on leads to constrictive pericarditis. Earliest sign is a pericardial rub and fever. As disease progresses effusion forms there and when it is massive cardiac tamponade may occur.

Gastrointestinal tract. Tuberculosis involves either as primary lesion due to swallowing of mycobacterium tubercle bacilli which get lodged in ileocaecal region and produce primary hypertrophic, ileoceacal tuberculosis. Secondary tuberculosis due to swallowing of infected sputum is more common. Common manifestations are tuberculous peritonitis, tabes mesenterica, tuberculous enteritis, chronic diarrhoea and fistula-in-ano as well as ischiorectal abscesses. Tuberculous involvement of liver does occur though not commonly.

Skeletal tuberculosis. Tuberculous involvement of spine (Pott's spine) paravertebral cold abscesses and involvement of joints like knees, and hips may take place.

Genitourinary tuberculosis. Renal tuberculosis may present either with painless hematuria or pyuria. Ureters and bladder may also be involved and sometimes ureteric strictures may be formed. In men tubercular epididymoorchitis and in females tubercular salpingitis resulting in sterility. Menstrual irregularities in women in the form of amenorrhoea are common. Genital tuberculosis of seminal vesicles, prostate in men and ovaries, uterus (endometrosis) in females also occur though the onset is insidious.

Meningeal tuberculosis. Tuberculoma in the brain and tubercular meningitis are very common complications and may leave behind a number of sequlae.

Adrenal tuberculosis is equally common producing a picture of Addison's disease. But it is seen either in long-standing cases of pulmonary tuberculosis or abdominal tuberculosis.

Miscellaneous. Tubercular lymphadenopathy, cutaneous lesions and involvement of the eyes (chorioretinitis and uveitis) are other sites of involvement. Tuberculosis also occurs with increased frequency in patients with silicosis and pneumoconiosis. Tuberculosis is more in patients who become infected with HIV and thus it is seen more frequently in patient suffering from AIDS.

Diagnosis. With the clinical profile of the disease and patients presenting with odd features like chronic ill health, low grade fever, persistent cough not responding to treatment, weight loss, anorexia, diagnosis of tuberculosis should be considered. Confirmation shall be dependent on further investigations:

1. Sputum examination for acid-fast bacilli: By direct smear examination (Ziehl-Neelsen stain). At least three smears must be examined before finally reaching a conclusion. When direct smear is negative sputum examination be done by concentration method using 24 hours collection of sputum. Further confirmation is done by sputum culture by animal inoculation which takes 4-8 weeks. If adequate amount of sputum is not available, bronchoscopic aspiration of secretions be made and submitted for smear and culture examination. Further examinations include laryngeal swabs and gastric lavage for AFB.

2. **Serology.** Though not commonly employed but in doubtful cases ELISA (Enzyme-linked immunosorbent assay) is carried out. Elisa is not very specific and has its own limitations.

3. X-ray chest is the simplest and most helpful.

4. Lymph node, pleural or peritoneal biopsy may be done to confirm the diagnosis in cases of tuberculous lymphadenopathy, pleural effusion and tuberculous peritonitis.

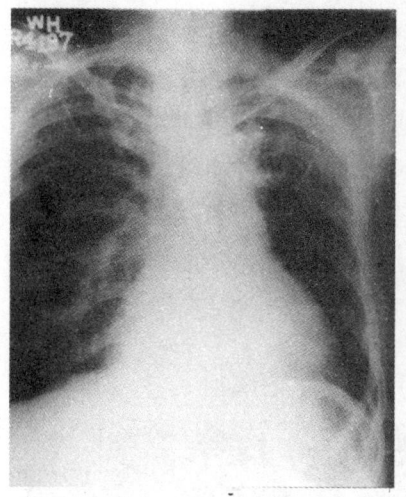

Fig. 5.25. X-ray Chest (PA View) A case of tuberculosis showing apical infiltration.

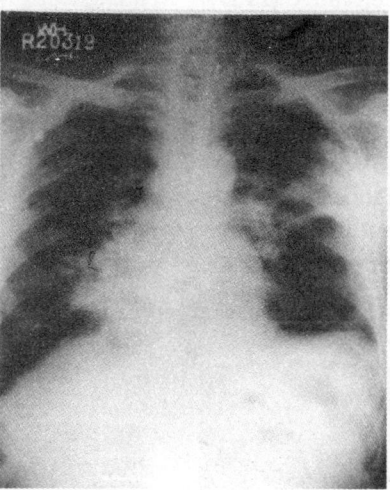

Fig. 5.26. X-ray Chest (PA View) A tubercular cavity in left mid zone. Pleural reaction is also present.

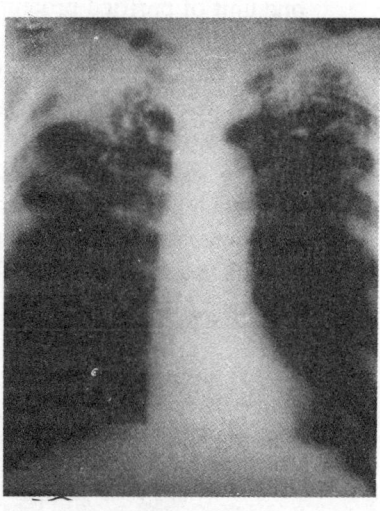

Fig. 5.27. X-ray Chest (PA View) Tubercular infiltration with breaking down in both apices. Calcified nodes are also seen.

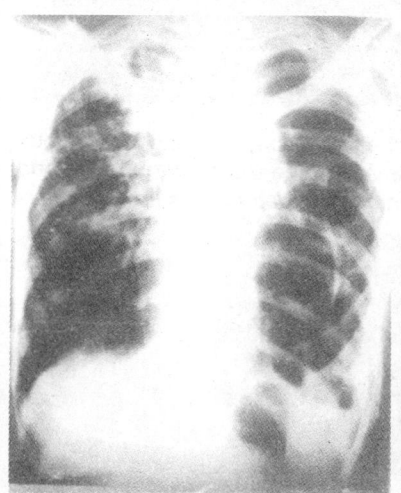

Fig. 5.28. X-ray Chest (PA View). There is tubercular infiltration on right apex. Left lung shows pleural effusion. There is obliteration of costophrenic angle due to effusion.

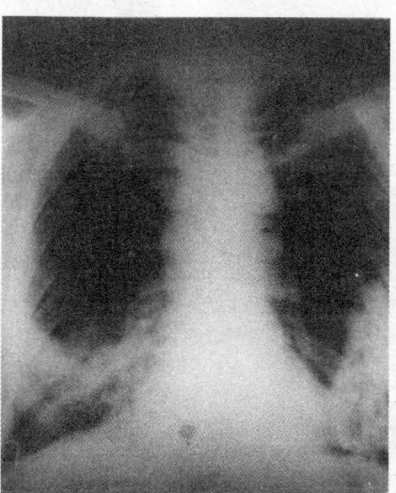

Fig. 5.29. X-ray Chest (PA View). Case of bilateral pleural effusion. Long standing tubercular effusions leave behind calcification seen here on left side.

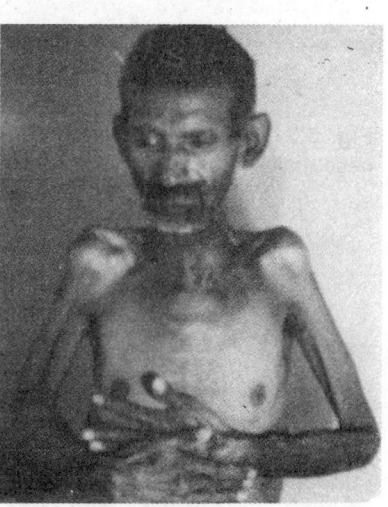

Fig. 5.30. Photograph of case of Koch's showing marked wasting and cachexia.

5. Tuberculin test. It is a test to recognise prior tubercular infection, and is done by injecting one unit of purified protein derivative (PPD) on the forearm and readings taken after 48 hours. Induration of more than 12 mm indicates a positive test. A negative test does not always exclude tubercular infection since it may be negative in patients of blood malignancies, malnourishment and those on immunosuppressive therapy. Tuberculin test is nonspecific and only indicates prior infection. Its sensitivity wanes with age.

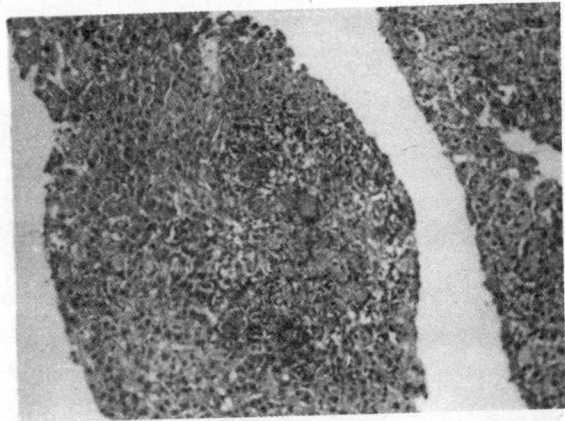

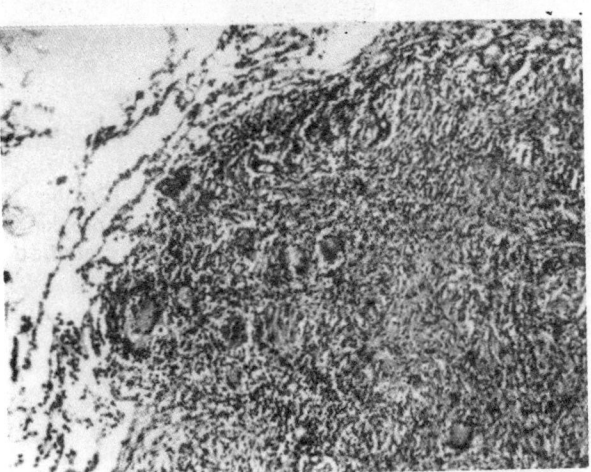

Fig. 5.31. Mesenteric lymph node biopsy showing caseation.

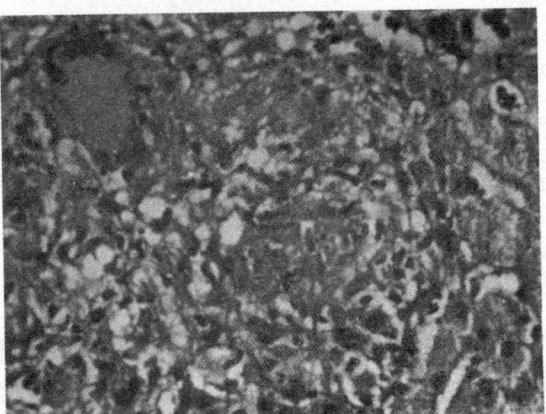

Fig. 5.33 and 5.34. Liver biopsy showing tuberculous caseating granuloma. In some areas fatty globules and tiny areas of chronic inflammatory cells are seen.

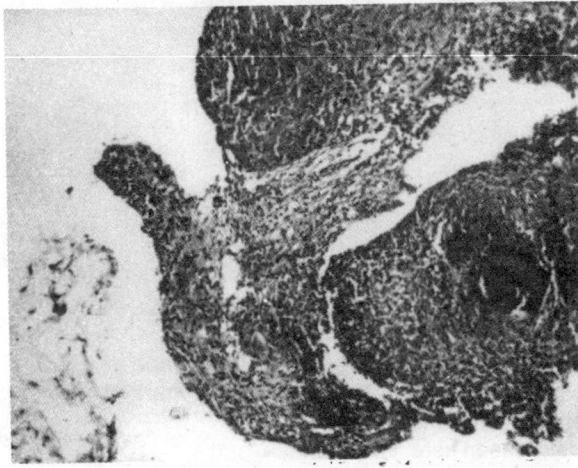

Fig. 5.32. Punch peritoneal biopsy showing caseous granuloma.

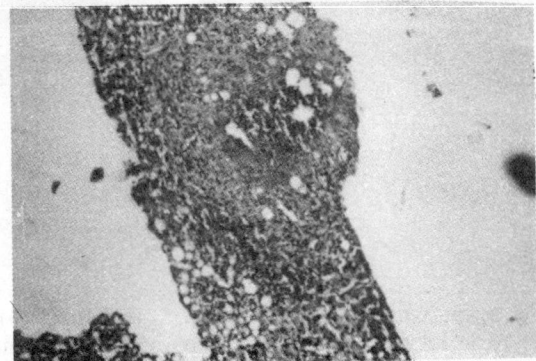

Fig. 5.35. Liver biopsy showing tuberculous caseating granuloma consisting of caseous material in the centre surrounded by chronic inflammatory cells, fibroblastic tissue and occasional giant cell.

6. Blood examination is not of much help. ESR is a good index of the activity of the disease process.

Treatment:

1. General. Adequate bed rest in an ill patient is advised. Degree of bed rest shall vary depending on the disease. Diet must be well balanced nourishing with high content of proteins, milk and vitamins. Since risk of spread to contacts especially in sputum positive cases is substantial, isolation at home, use of separate utensils and disinfection of items used by the patient be advised. Hospitalisation of patient is advised in an acute case, in the presence of complications like pneumothorax, severe haemoptysis, meningitis, Addisonian crisis, extreme cachexia and presence of debilitating diseases. It is preferable for the patient to avoid alcohol, smoking and any other drug abuse.

```
┌─────────────────────────────────────────┐
│  Chemotherapy of tuberculosis           │
│                                         │
│  Bactericidal drugs                     │
│                                         │
│   1.  Isonex (INH)                      │
│   2.  Rifampicin (R)                    │
│   3.  Streptomycin (S)                  │
│   4.  Pyrazinamide (Z)                  │
│   5.  Capreomycin (A)                   │
│   6.  Kanamycin (K)                     │
│                                         │
│  Bacteriostatic Drugs                   │
│                                         │
│   1.  Ethambutol (E)                    │
│   2.  Thiacetazone (T)                  │
│   3.  Ethionamide (ET)                  │
│   4.  Cycloserine (C)                   │
│   5.  Paraminosalicylic acid (PAS)      │
└─────────────────────────────────────────┘
```

Regimens of antitubercullar drugs:

Short-term course (6 months regimen)

For first two months. Isonex + Rifampicin + Pyrazinamide + Ethambutol or streptomycin

For next four months. Isonex + Rifampicin + Ethambutol or Streptomycin

Longer regimens (9 months - 12 months). Isonex + Rifampicin + Ethambutol or Pyrazinamide (for first two months)

For next 7-10 months. Rifampicin + Isoniazid

2. Drug treatment. Once a diagnosis of tuberculosis is arrived at treatment must be instituted immediately and its compliance ensured. Outcome of therapy shall depend on how strictly the drugs have been taken by the patient.

Conventional drug therapy. Initially it is triple drug therapy which consists of INH 300 mg once a day, Rifampicin 600 mg once orally supplemented by Ethambutol 800 mg once a day orally or Injection Streptomycin 1 g I/M once a day for first two months. These drugs are to be taken 30 minutes before breakfast since absorption of Rifampicin is interfered by food.

Continuous double drug therapy. It includeds INH 300 mg, Rifampicin 600 mg orally once a day Ethambutol 800 mg once a day or Injection Streptomycin 1 G I/M twice a week. The duration of this treatment is 18 months.

Short course treatment. It consists of two phases. An initial intensive treatment of first two months consisting of Isonex (300 mg), Rifampicin (600 mg), Pyrazinamide (1.5 g daily) and either Ethambutol (800 mg) or Injection Streptomycin (1 g I/M daily). A consolidated phase of Isonex Rifampicin and either Ethambutol (800 mg) daily or Injection Streptomycin (1 g d/m) twice a week be given for at least 4 months but preferably for 6 months.

Longer regimens. This comprises INH (300 mg) plus Rifampicin (600 mg) with Ethambutol (800 mg) or Pyrazinamide (1.5 gm) daily is given for first two months. For next 7-10 months two drugs rifampicin + isoniazid are given.

Most of the patients recover well with the drug regimens though relapse after completion of course is less than 1 per cent. Progress in the patient should be monitored by clinical assessment, conversion of sputum positive to sputum negative, and improvement in radiological signs.

A few cases may not respond to the treatment, because of the development of drug resistance. Therapy for drug resistant tuberculosis patient should be instituted with two drugs which the patient has not taken earlier and one of these two new drugs should be either Isonex or Rifampicin. Alternative drugs which can be used in resistant cases include Capreomycin sulphate (1 g I/M daily) useful when given along with INH or Ethambutol, Cycloserine (0.5-1 g/daily) and Ethionamide (250 mg orally twice a day with meals). Most of the drugs used as second line of treatment have number of adverse effects and require close monitoring.

Side effects of antitubercular drugs

Drug	Dose	Side effects
Streptomycin	1.0 g I/M (20-30 mg/kg),	Nephrotoxicity, ototoxicity ataxia, agranulocytosis
Isonex	300 mg daily (3-5 mg/kg)	Peripheral neuropathy hepatic injury, convulsions, dryness of mouth, epigastric distress
Ethambutol	800-1000 mg (25 mg/kg) daily	Blurring of vision, optic neuritis, nausea, vomiting, rash, periphenal neuropathy, liver impairment
Rifampicin	450-600 mg (10 mg/kg) daily	Nausea, vomiting, rash, peripheral neuropathy, liver impairment
Pyrazinamide	1500 mg (15-30 mg/kg) daily	Arthralgia, nausea, vomiting, malaise, toxic hepatitis
Capreomycin	1 g I/M daily	Tinnitus, vertigo, urticaria, skin rush, fever
Cycloserine	500 mg twice a day (15-20 mg/kg/day)	Dizziness, headache, tremors, visual disturbances, psychosis
Ethionamide	250 mg twice a day	Skin rash, purpura, anaphy- a day lactic shock, anorexia, nausea, vomiting, headache, postural hypotension

---

Adverse effects of drug treatment. As a general principle most of the antitubercular drugs used as first line of treatment are comparatively safe. Isoniazid may produce peripheral neuropathy which effect can be obviated to some extent by giving Pyridoxine 10 mg daily alongwith INH. Hepatitis may occur in small percentage of cases. Rifampicin produces liver damage which is judged by rise in enzyme levels. Sometimes an influenza like syndrome or thrombocytopenia may be produced. Side effects with Ethambutol are few. Most important is decrease in visual acuity and may produce optic neuritis which reverses once the drug is withdrawn.

Main toxic effect of Streptomycin is ototoxicity and may produce deafness as well as loss of vestibular functions. It is also nephrotoxic. Pyrazinamide is hepatotoxic and inhibits excertion of uric acid thus producing hyperuricaemia. Other side effects include nausea, vomiting and fever.

Cycloserine also produces nausea, vomiting, peripheral neuropathy, depression and psychosis. Capreomycin produces hearing loss, deafness, rashes, nitrogen retention and leucopenia.

Multidrug resistant tuberculosis. It is defined as resistance to more than one antitubercular drug. Multidrug resistant tuberculosis is on the increase. Inadequate therapy is the most common mode by which resistant organisms are acquired. Besides this patients with cavity lesions have a high frequency of resistance since they harbour greater number of organisms. The prevalence of MDR form of tuberculosis is an important cause of morbidily and mortlity form the disease.

A number of factors are known to play their role in causation of multidrug resistance and these range from spontaneous mutation, reduced catalase peroxidase activity to genetic basis.

Before one considers a patient to be suffering from MDR form of tuberculosis, a detailed history of previous treatment and names of drugs must be obtained. A general rule would be to suspect drug resistance in a patient who continues to remain sputum smear positive after four months of regular treatment with an established short course chemotherapy regimen. If necessary drug susceptibility studies should be done.

Further on these patients should be re-treated with atleast four drugs that patient has not received before and to which bacilli are likely to be susceptible. The number of drugs used shall vary depending on the extent of disease and the potency of available drug regimen.

Secondly a single drug should never be added to a failing regimen since it may lead to the sequential development of resistance to the drug that is being introduced. Two or more new drugs should always be added.

The retreatment should be initiated with small doses of each drug and then increased to the maximum as tolerated by the patient. This can be done in a period of 7 to 10 days. Though the optimal duration of retreatment is not clearly defined yet the treatment has to continue for atleast 12 months till the time when sputum culture becomes negative. Patients who are infected with organisms that are resistant to all or most of the first line antitubercular drugs (Isoniazid & rifampacin) are treated with drugs for 24 months after the sputum culture becomes negative.

The value of older drugs in the treatment of MDR tuberculosis has also to be emphasised. Patients who have not earlier received PAS or Thiacetazone can be successfully given these drugs with good results.

Patient with MDR tuberculosis may require 6-7 drugs including 2 to 4 second line drugs (Quinolones, ethionamide, cycloserine, amikacin, kanamycin etc).

The outcome for patients with MDR TB though is not very favourable. Treatment of MDR tuberculosis in immuo deficient patients is even more discouraging. The guidelines for treatment are similar to those recommended for HIV negative patients. Most of the strains in these patients (HIV infection or AIDS) are resistant not only to isoniazid and rifampacin but also to streptomycin and ethambutol. Despite aggressive treatment, prognosis in such cases is poor.

Multidrug Resistence: It is resistance to more than one antitubercular drug and is also defined as mycobacterium tuberculosis resistant to isoniazid and rifampacin with or without resistance to other drugs.

Prognosis. It shall be guided by the patient's underlying disease, body defence mechanism, nutrition of the patient, response to drug therapy and improvement in general condition as well as on radiological examaination. Poor response to treatment and emergence of drug resistant strains of mycobacterium tuberculosis portend poor prognosis.

Special precautions. Patients of tuberculosis with pregnancy require special care. Isoniazid is safe during pregnancy. So is ethambutol. Streptomycin should not be used because of risk of inducing ototoxicity in the foetus. Patients with renal failure as well as liver damage shall also present special problem. In these case dosage of Isoniazid be reduced and those with liver disease, Rifampicin and pyrazinamide have to be avoided. PAS (paraminosalicytic acid) in a dose of 8-10 gm in divided doses per day after meals may be given but again this drug is not to be given in patients with renal failure.

RESPIRATORY FAILURE

Failure of lungs to perform the normal function of gas exchange at rest or on exertion resulting in reduction in plasma arterial oxygen (PaO_2) and rise in plasma carbon dioxide concentration ($PaCO_2$) constitute respiratory failure. Broadly respiratory failure may be of two forms.

Type I or **acute hypoxaemic** respiratory failure which occurs in patients with extensive lung damage such as pneumonia, adult respiratory distress syndrome or fibrosing alveolitis. PaO_2 is decreased with normal or decreased $PaCO_2$.

Type II or **ventilatory failure** where there is failure of adequate ventilation with subsequent retention of carbon dioxide. Commonest cause is chronic bronchitis with emphysema where there is underventilation of the alveoli with resultant anoxaemia and hypercapnia. Here PaO_2 is reduced with $PaCO_2$ levels are high.

Normal respiration is governed by a number of factors ranging from functioning of respiratory center to process of ventilation and diffusion of gases in the lungs. Any process which interferes with any of these mechanisms shall produce respiratory failure.

Causes of respiratory failure. A number of causes are responsible for producing respiratory failure in acute or chronic form depending on the underlying disease.

Classification of respiratory failure

Type-I (Acute hypoxaemic failure) causes

1. Pneumonia
2. Adult respiratory distress syndrome
3. Pulmonary fibrosing alveolitis
4. Acute pulmonary oedema
5. Pulmonary embolism

   Arterial gases. PaO_2 is decreased but $PaCO_2$ is either normal or low.

Type-II (Ventilatory failure) causes

1. Chronic bronchitis: Emphysema
2. Chest wall deformities (kyphoscoliosis)
3. Respiratory muscle paralysis (Guillain-Barre syndrome)
4. Narcotic drug overdose
5. Failure of respiratory centre (bulbar polio, meningoencephalitis)

   Arterial gases. PaO_2 is reduced with high $PaCO_2$ levels.

---

1. Interference with the normal mechanism of the chest wall as in obesity, severe kyphoscoliosis, paralysis of the diaphragm or respiratory muscles.
2. Diseases of the lung such as chronic bronchitis with emphysema, restrictive lung disease (pulmonary fibrosis). Adult respiratory distress syndrome (ARDS), pneumonia, cardiogenic pulmonary oedema, Pulmonary embolism.
3. Diseases of respiratory centre: Overdosage of narcotics or sedative drugs. Neuromuscular disorders (Guillain-Barre syndrome), bulbar polio, injury to brain stem, encephalitis, meningitis.

Precipitating factors. Patients with chonic lung disease are likely to suffer from acute respiratory failure because of fulminating infection. This is more so when a patient is already on poor ventilating drive and infection leads to worsening of hypoxia with increased CO2 retention. Further patients of chronic respiratory disease may go to respiratory failure because of sedative or narcotics which may depress respiratory center. Sometimes conditions like

pneumonia, pneumothroax and massive pulmonary embolism may preciptiate acute respiratory failure.

Factors precapitating respiratory failure

1. Infection
2. Use of sedatives or narcotics
3. Pneumothorax
4. Massive pulmonary embolism

Clinical features. Acute respiratory failure manifests with features of hypoxia like headache, irritability, lack of sleep, confusion and progressive drowsiness. Subsequently patient goes into stupor and coma. Patient should be monitored for respiratory, cardiac functions along with signs of carbon dioxide retention (cyanosis, irritability, drowsiness). There is peripheral vasodilatation, warm extremitis, flushing and bounding pulse. In severe cass there is papilloedema, confusion, drowsiness, flapping tremors and even coma.

Monitoring of the patient. It is important to monitor the patient and for this blood gas analysis should be done to guide oxygen therapy and to monitor improvement of the case. A number of metabolic disturbances can result. Cases of chronic bronchitis and emphysema and those with venitlatory failure (type II) shall have high levels of PaCO2 and low PaO2 and because of retention of CO2 there is respiratory acidosis, though this to some extent is compensated by kidneys retaining bicarbonates. The process of oxygenation is mainly governed by the plasma arterial oxygen content.

Management of respiratory failures:

1. Respiratory failure is commonly precipitated by infection so broad spectrum antibiotics are indicated (Injection Amoxycillin 500 mg I/M or I/V 8 hourly or Injection Cefazolin 500 mg - 1 gm I/M or I/V 6-8 hourly or Injection Cefotaxime 500 mg - 1 gm I/M or I/V 8 hourly) and should be started at the earliest. In the meantime sputum be examined by Gram's stain and culture along with antibiotic sensitivity be done and suitable antibiotics be switched.
2. Patient should be encouraged to bring out

secretions by coughing. If secretions continue to accumulate then bronchoscopic aspirations be done. Many people prefer to do a tracheostomy which facilitates the removal of secretions. This also improves alveolar ventilation by reducing the dead space in the lungs.

3. Maintain hydration of the patient by intravenous fluids. Nutrition should also be taken care of.

4. In majority of patients there may be bronchospasm as well as poor ventilation. Injection Deriphylline (Theophylline + Etophylline) 1 amp I/V 6 hourly along with parenteral corticosteroids shall be beneficial. Another approach can be to give Injection Ampinopylline (0.24 g in 10 cc glucose) in intravenous infusion and given slowly over a period of 6 hours and monitored. Fall of blood pressure is an important side effect with use of Aminophylline which not only acts as a bronchodilator but also stimulates the respiratory center.

5. If patient is unconscious or drowsy as a result of severe hypercapnia. Injection Nikethamide 1 amp. intravenously slowly in drip can be given every 4 hourly till level of consciousness improves. This is only a temporary measure. Over dosage of the drug may produce convulsions.

6. Oxygen therapy: It is the main stay in the treatment of respiratory failure. It can be given by a nasal catheter or through a face mask. Oxygen should be administered continuously at a rate of 2-3 litres per minute. While giving oxygen it is important to monitar PaO_2 and as the respiratory center regains its activity, oxygen concentration be increased by giving oxygen at 4-8 litres/minute. Gradually as the patient improves, oxygen be given intermittently. While giving oxygen care be taken that PaO_2 levels go above 50 mmHg. If the above measures do not succed and carbon dioxide narcosis increases producing drowsiness and coma, mechanical ventilatory support will have to be instituted.

This is achieved by employing artificial positive pressure ventilation via the tracheostomy tube either mechanically by a ventilatory bag or mask. Further improvement is by use of volume cycled ventilators which give controlled ventilatory support. Intermittent positive pressure ventilation (IPPV) is ideally suited for patients of acute respiratory failure with signs of severe respiratory distress andthose with ventilatory failure as in narcotic drugs over dosage, and Guillain-Barre syndrome. This method also requires endotracheal intubation via tracheostomy. Side effects include pneumothorax, erosion of tracheal cartilage, infection, pneumomediastinum, rupture of lung, subcutaneous emphysema.

The net result of this method is often unpredictable. A serial monitoring of oxygen saturation and carbon dioxide tension of blood are of great use in monitoring the progress of the case.

Maintaining oxygen levels and ventilation in a case of respiratory failure buys time and in majority of patients they are able to tide over the crisis. For cases of chronic respiratory insufficiency since the lungs are irreversibly damaged and therefore because of inadequate ventilation there is going to be decreased $PaO2$ in blood, intermittent oxygen along with bronchodilators and frequent use of antibiotics shall be beneficial.

Prognosis in a case of respiratory failure shall be governed by the ventilatory capacity of the lungs, response of the patient to treatment and PaO_2 and $PaCO_2$ concentration in blood. Patients who are totally disabled from their disease, may not benefit by treatment.

BRONCHIAL ASTHMA

It is one of the commonest illness of the respiratory system and is widely prevalent all over the world. Bronchial asthma is defined as a clinical syndrome characterized by airways obstruction which is partially or completely reversible either spontaneously or with treatment. There is airways inflammation and increased responsiveness to a variety of factors both immunological and non-immunological.

Broadly bronchial asthma has been classified into:

1. Extrinisc or atopic where an external factor is identifiable. It includes people showing positive skin reaction to inhaled allergens with raised IgE levels. Family history of allergy is present. Usually starts in childhood or at an early age.

2. Intrinsic or cryptogenic: Here asthma starts in middle or later age and causative agent generally is not identifiable. No family history of allergy. Skin tests are negative and plasma IgE levels are not raised.

This classification is arbitrary since allergic factors play important part in both conditions.

Clinical profile of atopic (extrinsic) asthma

1. Early onset
2. Episodic
3. External factor (allergen) identifiable
4. Family hisotry of asthma, allergy
5. Seasonal incidence
6. Attacks occur at any time
7. Positive skin tests
8. Raised levels of IgE

Clinical profile of intrinsic (non-atopic) asthma.

1. Late onset
2. Non-episodic
3. Causative agent not identifiable
4. No family history of asthma or allergy
5. Non-seasonal
6. Attacks mostly at night
7. Skin tests are negative
8. Plasma IgE levels are not raised

Aetiology. Aetiology of bronchial asthma is multifactorial and a number of factors play their role in its causation.

1. *Allergy.* It plays an important role in the causation of extrinsic asthma. Often these patient have history of allergy, hay fever, allergic rhinitis, urticaria etc in their families. In some asthma is frequently seasonal when there are allergens in atmosphere like pollens, dust particles and this is the type common in young children and adults. At the same time non-seasonal particles like animal feacal particles, feather and fungal spores present in the environment can also provoke asthma. The exact mechanism by which these inhaled particles can cause asthma is not known but depends on antigen-antibody reaction on the surface of pulmonary mast cells.

2. *Occupation.* There are certain occupations like soldering, industrial, varnishing, industrial coating, metal refining (Platinum chrome nickel), millers and grain handlers where development of asthma follows, exposure to certain chemicals and reagents which are being produced there. The degree and predisposition to developing of asthma shall depend on the level and duration of exposure of the person and to the development of specific IgE antibodies.

3. *Drugs.* Certain drugs like aspirin, beta-adrenergic antagonists and NSAIDs compounds. Indomethacin, Mefenamic acid and coloring agents are associated with the induction of asthma in a susceptible individual.

4. *Infections.* Respiratory infections especially viral (rhinovirus, influenza virus, syncytial virus) are often responsible for producing acute exacerberation of asthma. Exactly how infections cause asthma is not known but probably inflammatory changes in the airways and weakening of host defense mechanism make the respiratory passage more susceptible to exogenous stimuli.

5. *Environment.* Environmental pollution from vehicle fumes, industrial gases and other waste products are important causes of promoting asthma. This is especially so in densely populated urban and industrial areas. The air pollutants ozone, nitrogen and sulfur dioxide especially the last one produce most deleterious effects.

6. *Exercise.* Mot asthmatics get worse by strenuous physical activity. Exercise in a large number of asthmatics acts as a trigger mechanism. Interestingly attack occurs at end of exercise period. Similarly exposure to cold air during winter, sking ice skating also act as

provocative agents. This is because of thermal changes brought into the bronchial mucosa by cool dry air which results in hyperemia and engorgement of the bronchial circulation. Cooling and dryness of the epithelial lining of the bronchi, brings an attack of asthma. Of all exercises swimming in indoor heated pools is safest since patient now does not inhale dry and cold air.

7. *Emotions.* Emotions do have some role to play in the aetiology of asthma. Psychological stress does interact and influences asthmatic process. Excessive laughing is known to trigger an attack of asthma through vagal activity.

Pathology. Pathological features in cases of asthma include chronic inflammation and infiltration of the bronchial mucosa with hypertrophy and hyperplasia of smooth musculature. These changes are present in both symptomatic and asymptomatic cases of asthma. Release of various mediators such as histamine, leukotrine C4 and prostaglandin D2 (PGD2) from a number of inflammatory cells like mast cells, macrophages epithelial cells and eosinophils cause disruption of epithelial barrier producing airway hyper responsiveness with resultant bronchoconstricton producing an asthmatic attack.

Exposure to allergens which is a predominant aetiological factor produces a number of reactions which involve various cells (mast cells, macrophages, eosinophils) nerves (C-fibre afferent nerves) midiators (Histamine, prostglandins and leukotrines) and vascular mechanisms.

Majority of asthmatics are atopic and commonest reaction to an allergen is an immediate or early reaction which begins within minutes of contact with the allergen reaching maximum in 15-30 minutes after challenge and subsides by 1-2 hours. The mechanism involved here is degranulation of mast cells with mediator release.

Many asthmatics develop a more prolonged and sustained attack of broncho constriction beginning 4-6 hours after challenge and this lasts upto 24 hours. This late phase reaction responds poorly to bronchodilators and is associated with increase in bronchial hyperresponsiveness along with influx of neutrophils, macrophages and eosinophils into the airways. Such persons may show recurrent episodes of asthma subsequently.

Clinical picture. Cases of asthma have paroxysms of wheezing attacks coming suddenly in middle of night. Cough is a common symptom and often predominates the clinical picture. Many patients before an attack of asthma have sneezing, restlessness and irritability. Once attack occurs which consists of a triad of cough, breathlessness and wheezing, there is sense of oppression in the chest. Respiratory distress occurs. Respiration becomes audibily harsh and wheezing sounds are heard in both phases of respiration. Patient many times sits up in bed fighting for breath. There is marked anxiety, tachycardia, cyanosis, cold extremities, perspiration and systolic hypertension. Accessory muscles of respiration become visibly active.

As attack terminates, spasm gets less. Breathing improves and patient may cough out a little viscid sputum which often takes the form of casts (Curschmann's spirals). These when examined under microscope show epithelial cells, eosinophils and Charcot-Leyden crystals. Duration of an attack is variable. It may last from few minutes to a number of hours. When the attack fails to respond to treatment and patient is in a continuous state of paroxysms it is called status asthmaticus.

Physical signs. During an acute attack of asthma there is an anxious patient sitting up in bed, extremely breathless, gasping for breath and leans forwards holding sides of bed. Chest is fixed in position of inspiration. Accessory muscles of respiration are active. There is tachycardia, cyanosis and blood pressure levels are raised. Wheezing sounds are heard from a distance. Wheeze or rhonchi can be felt sometimes. Percussion note over lung is hyperresonant. Auscultation shows a short high pitched sound on inspiration and prolonged on expiration. There are sibilant and sonorous rhonchi present all over the chest. Crepitations may be heard in the presence of infection.

Clinical variants of asthma:

Exercise induced asthma. It is a form of asthma which is commonly induced in asthmatics after exercise, outdoor activities in cold weather and occurs after prolonged and continuous exercise. This provocation to an asthmatic attack afterexercise is probably present in all asthmatics. Many such patients subsequently develop recurrent episodes of airways obstruction independent of exercise. Heat loss from airways appears to be probably the cause. Such patients should be advised to take beta-2-agonist or cromolyn inhalations prior to exercising or outdoor sport.

Occupational asthma. It is one of the commonest form of asthma related to occupation of the person where he/she is exposed to specific allergens or sensitising agents. Asthmatic attack is brought on by air flow limitation and bronchial hyper responsiveness due to the environmental conditions at work place. In such patients change of environment is required as once sensitization sets in asthmatic attack may be triggered by minimal subsequent exposure.

Cough-variant asthma. Here cough is the main complaint and this cough is relieved by either a bronchodilator or avoidance of allergens. In such cases bronchospasm is not present during the attack. Treatment is the same as in other cases of asthma.

Nocturnal asthma. It is a problem in poorly controlled asthmatic patients. Nocturnal asthma is a distressing condition and occurs during later time of night often disturbing the patients sleep. The cause is attributed to physiological decrease in airways tone during sleep due to variations in catecholamines and cortisol secretions at night. In addition to other treatments in such patients focus should be directed towards use of drugs which have sustained action and can take care of asthma during the night and early hours of morning. Long acting theophylline and beta-2-agonist (Salmetrol) is helpful.

Aspirin sensitivity asthma. More than 50 per cent of adults with asthma experience severe attack of asthma after taking aspirin and other non-steroidal antiinflammatory drugs. Many of these patients have nasal polyps though exact relationship is not explainable. Presumed mechanism is inhibition of cycloxoygenase pathway by these drugs, with shunting of arachidonic acid causing over production of leukotrines, a powerful bronchoconstrictor.

Such patients must avoid these drugs and instead take drugs like acetaminophen.

Episodic asthma. Clinical picture is of mild asthma and patient gets infrequent asthmatic attacks. Episodic asthmatic attacks are brought on by acute respiratory infection, allergy or psychological stress.

Chronic bronchitic emphysema asthma syndrome. This is a persistent form of asthama with dysponea where acute attacks occur from time to time. Mucosa of bronchioles in such patients is inflamed and thickened. There are excessive mucosal secretions and elastic recoil of lung tissue is decreased. Destructive changes in the alveolar wall takes place. Hyper reactivity of the bronchi leads to attacks of asthma which are either moderate or of severe grades.

Investigations. These are non-specific and no single test is specific.

Blood examination shows rise in eosinophil count. Measurements of serum IgE levels when raised favour extrinsic type of asthma.

X-ray chest shows widened intercostal spaces, ribs placed more horizontally, diaphragm displaced downwards, increased translucenly of lung fields and heart placed more vertically.

Skin tests with various antigens may be done to locate the allergen.

Pulmonary function tests are done to assess the lung functions. Reduction of FEV1 or PEFR indicates that respiratory functions are involved. Measurements of PEFR (Peak expiratory flow rate) at variable times of the day shall help in the assessment of the extent of patient's disease.

Diagnosis. Diagnosis of bronchial asthma is based on typical history and physical signs (wheezing sounds and rhonchi on auscultation). Often there is long history of respiratory allergy starting at a young age, and attacks of asthma coming more in winter months. Main differentiation has to be done from conditions where there is associated paroxysmal attacks of dysponea. Tropical eosinophilia may mimic the condition. Here the history is short. Cough is more predominant symptom and physical signs of rhonchi comparatively are very much less. History is of short duration. There may be loss of weight. Blood count shows marked eosinophilia. X-ray chest shows miliary mottling. Cases of chronic bronchitis with emphysema and pulmonary tuberculosis may be associated wiht asthma like features but then the underlying condition shall differentiate them.

An important differentiation arises from cases of acute left heart failure (cardiac asthma) where there is paroxysmal dysponea and lungs show both rhonchi and crepitations. It is essential to differentiate the two conditions more so in an elderly person presenting with acute attack simulating bronchial asthma. In cardiac asthma presence of underlying heart disease (hypertension, ischaemic heart disease, aortic valve disease, mitral incompetence) shall be a pointer towards the diagnosis.

Complications. A case of bronchial asthma may develop a number of complications and these are:

1. Spontaneous pneumothorax due to rupture of bullae.
2. Emphysema leading to chronic cor pulmonale.
3. Bronchiectasis
4. Spontaneous rib fractures
5. Mediastinal emphysema
6. Anoxaemia.

Treatment. In a case of asthma treatment is mainly directed towards (i) treatment of an acute attack and (ii) maintenance therapy i.e. treatment between the acute attacks.

In addition attempt should be made to locate an allergen in the atmosphere, food, clothes, environment etc and treatment instituted. Any infection in the upper rerspiratory passages must be promptly treated. A graded exercise programme in the form of respiratory exercises be started to improve sense of well being. In people where psychological stress is playing a role, a sympathetic consideration be given and attempt made to solve the problems.

Differences between bronchial and cardiac asthma

Age	*Bronchial asthma*	*Cardiac asthma*
Age	Usually younger age Group	Middle-aged or elderly
Duration of illness	Long history	Generally short history
History of allergy	Present	Not present
Time of attack	Early hours of morning	First half of night
Pulse	Tachycardia	Pulsus alternans
Associated disease	Chronic bronchitis, tuberculosis	Hypertension, ischaemic heart disease, valvular heart disease
CVS	Heart size within normal limits	Heart size enlarged, gallop rhythm
Chest	Wheezing sounds and rhonchi all over the chest	Bilateral crepts more at bases. Occasional rhonchi

Drug treatment. A number of drugs are employed in the treatment of asthma but no single drug is effective against all the pathological processes responsible for the disease so multiple drug regimens are advocated.

Drug therapy during an acute attack. Sympathomimetic drugs. Adrenaline hydrochloride is one of the oldest drug employed to abort an attack. It is a potent bronchodilator and gives immediate relief. Dose 0.5 to 1 ml of 1 in 1000 aqueous solution to be given subcutaneously slowly. The effect of drug takes place within few minutes and lasts upto 4 hours. An oily prepration for prolonged action is also available. During an attack adrenaline is given by Hurst's method where a drop is administered every minute till attack subsides. By this method dose of adrenaline is minimized.

Adrenaline has to be used with caution in middle aged persons and can be dangerous in patients with hypertension. Ischaemic heart disease, hyperthyroidism and elderly patients. Side effects include palpitation, tremors and sometimes cardiac arrhythmias. Its use is now limited and given only in young asthmatics. Ephedrine is another sympathomimetic drug employed for the relief of paroxysms. Dose 15-30 mg 6 hourly in combination with Xanthine derivatives and phenobarbitone.

Beta-2-adrenergic agonists. There are selective beta-agonists and have less of cardio vascular side effects. Common in use are Salbutamol and Salmeterol. Salbutamol is commonly used in the dose of 2-4 mg 8 hourly or 12 hourly. It can be administered by a nebuliser (2-5 mg) or metered dose inhaler (100 micrograms per puff) 2 puffs 4 times a day. Patient must be instructed about the proper use of inhalers and taught to synchronise the puffs with inspiration in order to maximise the delivery of drug to lung. They reduce the velocity of aerosol and allow more drug to reach the lungs. Spacers are also available. Action is rapid and effective bronchodilation when used in metered dose inhalations. They are the drug of choice for all types of acute bronchospasm. When taken prophylactically they protect from broncho constrictive challenge but do not prevent the late asthmatic response.

Salmeterol is a long-acting B2 adrenergic agonist and is weaker than salbutamol. Its onset of action is slow (2½ hours to peak action) and duration is about 12 hours. Because of its slow mode of action it is not of much use in acute attack of asthma. Salmeterol is effective in nocturnal asthma, exercise induced asthma and preventing attacks of asthma. Drug is administered by metered pressurized inhalers in the dose of 1-2 puffs (1 puff 25 mcg) 12 hourly. It is useful in infants and children and is safe during pregnancy.

Terbutaline. It is similar to salbutamol in properties and use. Dose 5 mg orally twice a day or 0.25 mg subcutaneously and by inhaler (250 mcg). Peak action occurs in 10 minutes and lasts upto 6 hours.

Beta-2 agonists are the drug of choice for exercise induced asthma and acute emergency management. Side effects include palpitation and tremors. Their main drawbacks is that they may worsen asthma control because of diminished responsiveness if used regularly and their excessive use may increase the risk of death due to asthma.

Methyl xanthines. Theophylline and its related drugs have been used extensively but have weak action when used orally. Aminophylline is a stable mixture of theophylline and ethylene diamine and acts as a bronchodilator by its direct action on the bronchial smooth muscle. It inhibits late response to allergens in body but does not inhibit the release of mediators.

It is effective in relieving an acute attack of asthma and can be safely given in all groups including elderly and those with cardiac ailments. Dose is 240 mg diluted in 10 ml of 10% glucose to be given intravenously slowly over a period of 5-10 minutes. Side effects include nausea vomiting, headache, seizures and insomnia. Rapid intravenous injection has been known to produce circulatory collapse and cardiac arrhythmias even leading to death.

Corticosteroids. There are indicated for prompt relief in severe fom of asthma especially when not controlled by other bronchodilators. They act by reducing bronchial hyperirritability, mucosal oedema and by suppressing inflammatory responses.

For acute attack Injection Dexamethasone (4-8 mg) or Betamethasone (4-8 mg) are given intravenously as a bolus dose and repeated 4-6 hourly. As acute symptoms subside switch on to oral steroids (40-60 mg per day in divided doses). Aerosols or inhaled steroids are the ones now preferred for prophylactic use on regular basis since these have high topical and low systemic activity due to poor absorption. Inhaled steroids are required when effect of B. agonists starts diminishing and disease is progressive. They not only reduce dose of B. agonists but also increase peak expiratory flow rate. Inhaled steroids are available in metered dose (50 ug. 100 ug or 200 ug per metered dose) or as Rotacaps (with rotahler)100-200 ug powder per cap.

Mast cell stabilizer. Sodium cromoglycate: It is not a bronchodilator but acts by inhibiting degranulation of mast cells thus preventing release of chemical mediators like histamine, interleukin, etc. It is not of use during an acute attack but is used as a long-term prophylactic in patients not adequately controlled. Therapy with it is best included between attacks or during periods of relative remission. It is more likely to benefit atopic and exercise induced asthma. Therapeutic benefits occur slowly over a period of 2-4 weeks. Sodium cromoglycate is used as a inhaler (1 mg metered dose aerosol. 2 puff 4 times daily) or as nasal spray (2% aqueous solution 2 sequeezes in each nostril 4 times a day). Side effects include throat irritation and cough. Uncommon effects include nasal congestion, headache, dizziness.

Ketotifen. It is primarily an antihistaminic with some cromoglycate like action. It is not a bronchodilator and has anti-allergic effect and reduces respiratory symptoms in 50 per cent patients of bronchial asthma. Dose 1-2 mg/twice a day. Side effects include sedation dizziness, nausea, dry mouth and weight gain.

Leukotriene system inhibitors. Leukotrienes liberated during inflammation are potent bronchoconstrictors. Drugs that either inhibit leukotrine formation or block leukotrines receptors have been shown to reduce asthma symptoms. Zafirlukast, a leukotriene receptor antagonist has been found to be effective in prophylaxis and treatment of chronic asthma in children and young adults. Dose is 20 mg twice daily 1 hour before or 2 hours after meals.

AIMS OF ASTHMA THERAPY

1. Maintain normal levels of activity
2. Free from acute attacks of asthma
3. Maintain normal respiratory function
4. Prevent acute exaceberations

Inhalers and their use in asthma

Antiasthma drugs are also effectively used for inhalation than by the oral route since a much smaller dose of the drug is required. It is estimated that about 10 to 20 times of an oral dose of a bronchodilator is required to produce an equivalent response as by the inhaled route. The inhalation route delivers the drug directly to the target organ (lungs and alveoli) and thus produces a rapid therapeutic response.

In non-inhaled routes of administration the drug is absorbed into the blood stream and distributed to the lungs and other parts of the body as well but only a small portion of the drug administered reaches the lungs, the rest being distributed to the extra pulmonary sites. The inhaled drugs act on the target organ (lungs) and avoid the side effects of systemic administration.

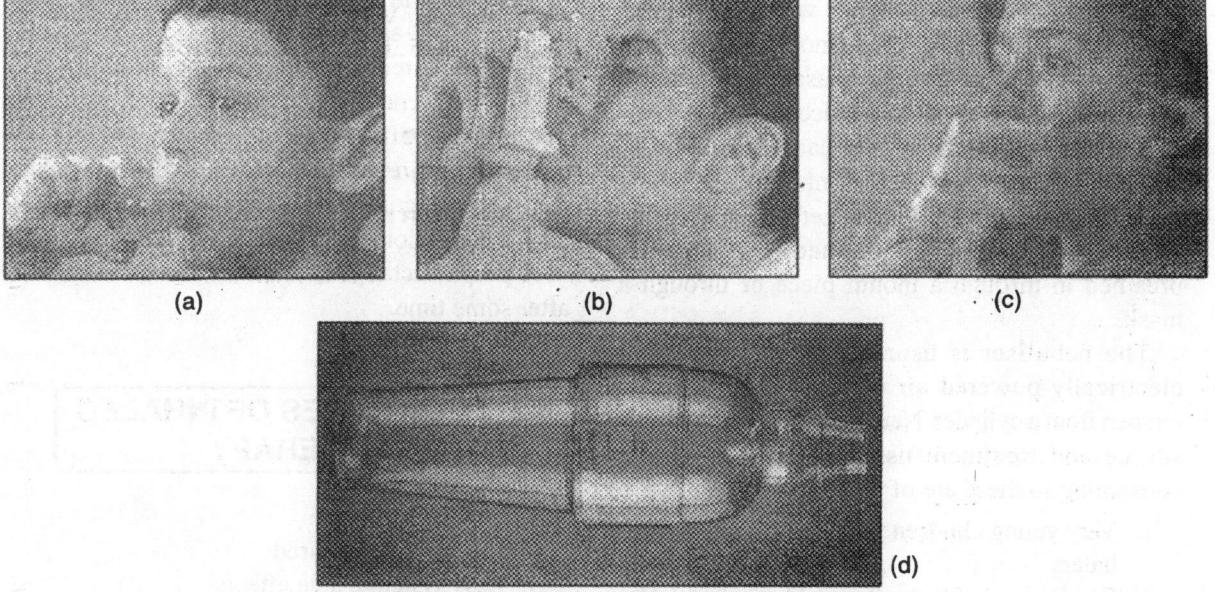

(a) (b) (c) (d)

Inhalation in bronchial asthma (Various devices)

Fig. 5.36. (a) Rotahaler (b) MDI's (c) Nebuliser (d) Space haler

Various devices are available for inhaling medicines for asthma relief and its prophylaxis.

The Metered dose inhaler (MDI) or pressurized aerosal

Here the medicine is suspended or dissolved in micronised form in a liquid propellant mixture and packed in a sealed container. When the canister is pressed, a metered dose of medicine is released through the mouth piece, hence the name Metered dose inhaler. This conventional metered dose inhaler is small compact and can be successfully used by adults and older children. Dose 1-2 inhalations 3-4 times a day.

Dry powder inhaler or Rota haler.

This method employs a dry powder system where micronised drug is mixed with a carrier substances and the mixture filled into a gelatine capsule (Rotacap) which is loaded into the inhaler device (called rotahaler) and is broken so that the powder is released and inhaled. The rota cap is pushed through a small opening in the base of the rotahaler. The rotahaler base is then twisted to split open the capsule before inhalation. The aerosol is generated by means of the energy contained in the inspired air, sucking through the mouth piece draws in a cloud of the powdered medicine which is breathed in. Rotacaps inhaler of salbutamol generally is of 200 mcg while that of beclamethasone dipropionate contains 200 mcg to be used twice a day.

Nebulisers. Nebulisation means generation of small droplets suitable for inhalation from a nebulising solution. The nebulizer produces a fine mist of the solution of the medicine which is breathed in through a mouth piece or through a mask.

The nebuliser is usually driven by a small electrically powered air compressor unit or by oxygen from a cylinder. Neubuliser requires a power source and treatment using nebulisers is time consuming so these are of value in:

1. Very young children who can not manage inhalers
2. For delivery of large doses of bronchodilators such as in acute severe asthma.

The basis of inhalation therapy is that the patient must learn the technique properly so that the inhaled drug reaches the intra pulmonary air ways. Various drugs for use through inhalation therapy include. Terbutaline, salbutamol, Budenoside, beclomethasone and a combination of these.

Spacehaler. It is useful for children and patients with poor coordination. The drug is inhaled by tidal breathing and is effective even at low air flows as in acute attacks and in children. The inhaler is fixed into the space haler device and shaken thoroughly so that the contents of the canister are properly mixed. Canister is pressed to release the required dose into chamber. Patient breathes out slowly and completely through mouth. Breaths out through the mouth piece, breathes in again slowly and deeply to ensure that all drug in the chamber has been inhaled. The advantage of space haler is that it does not require power supply as nebuliser and is easier to use. In conclusion one can say that relief after use of inhalation therapy is rapid. Inhalers are easy to handle and an asthmatic can help himself by their use within minutes. The beneficial effect of each dose lasts for 3 to four hours or even longer. Morover the drug acts effectively on the lungs and their side effects are minimal.

Summary of treatment of asthma. For acute attack. Beta-2-agonist inhaler. If no improvement then corticosteroids either intravenously or by inhaler. Intravenous injection of Aminophylline shall be further helpful. When attacks are frequent and not easily relieved by bronchodilators, inhaled steroids on regular basis are employed. In patients during remission ephedrine or salbutamol may be used prophylactally. Tolerance is known to develop after some time.

ADVANTAGES OF INHALED THERAPY

1. Quick onset.
2. Lesser dose required
3. Less systemic side effects
4. Targeted drug delivery

5. Ensures complete dosing

6. Preferred therapy in acute attack of asthma

Factors contributing to Nocturnal asthma

1. Position during sleep (Supine)

2. Exposure to dust, allergens in the bed

3. Collection of mucus in the air ways at night. Poor cough reflex.

4. Fall in body temperature especially in late hours of night.

5. Increased bronchoconstriction due to enhanced vagal tone.

6. Peak levels of histamine at night

7. Decrease in diameter of bronchi at night.

Treatment of Nocturnal asthma

1. Improve overall control of the disease

2. Inhaled steroids are effective in reducing attacks of nocturnal asthma because of their anti inflammatory effect.

3. Long-acting inhaled B2-agonists (Salmetrol)

4. Oral long-acting tablets of salbutamol or theophylline be given in the evening.

5. Avoid heavy meals in the evening.

Monitoring of Asthma Patient

Asthma monitoring is important in assessing the lung function as well as to assess the severity of the disease. Lung functions are determined by various tests but out of all these portable peak flow meters are of advantage in assessing lung functions in patients of asthma.

A peak flow meter for a patient with asthma is like a thermometer for a patient with fever. Peak flow or peak expiratory flow (PEFR) is a measurement of how fast and forcefully a person can blow out, thus assessing working of patients lung and severity of disease. PEFR is normal when a patient is well and ranges between600 to 750 liters / min while patients with asthma have peak flows between 200 and 400 l / min. A drop in peak flow is a warning of an impending attack. The patient uses a min-Wrights peak flowmeter which is a tubular device with a scale and indicator which shows peak flow readings. The patient breathes in deeply with mouthwide open and blows out as hard and fast as possible through the mouth piece of the meter and records the results. Patient is asked to repeat the test 2 to 3 times and records the highest of the three readings.

Asthma Classification in Adults and Children
(Classification based on symptoms and lung functions before treatment)

Asthma classification	Day time symptoms frequency	Night time symptoms frequency	Lung functions
1. Mild intermittent	2 days per week or less	2 nights per month or less	PEF or FEV1: 80 percent more of or predicted function
2. Mild persistent	More than 2 days per week but less than one time per day	More than 2 nights per month	PEF or FEV1: 80 percent or more of predicted function
3. Moderate persistent	Daily	More than 1 night per week	PEF or FEV_1: 60 to 80 percent of predicted function
4. Severe persistent	Continual	Frequent	PEF or FEV_1: 60 percent or less of predicted function

PEF - Peak expiratory flow

FEV_1 - Forced expiratory volume in one second.

Adopted from National Asthma eduction and Prevention Program. Guidelines for the diagnosis and management of Asthma. Expert Panel Report 2. USA Deptt. of Health and Human Services - 1997.

Peak flow readings before and after treatment help in measuring the effectiveness of the medicine.

DISEASES OF THE PLEURA

Pleura consists of visceral and parietal pleura. Visceral pleura covers the outer surface of the lung, lines the interlobar fissures and at the hilum continues with the parietal pleura which lines the inside of the thorax. The pleura are in apposition, the parietal pleura being richly supplied by capillaries and nerve endings. There is small amount of lubricating fluid between the two layers and when the amount of this fluid exceeds, 300 ml or more it is detected radiologically. When diseases of pleura occur the nerve ending located in the parietal pleura, get irritated and produce pain. Various diseases of pleura include pleurisy (Dry) pleural effusion, empyema and pneumothorax.

Pleurisy. It is inflammation of the pleura. When the pleural surfaces are inflamed at this stage it is called dry or fibrinous pleurisy. In some cases pleurisy recovers while in others it passes onto pleural effusion where fluid accumulates between the pleural surfaces.

Aetiology. Commonest cause of pleurisy is either idiopathic or due to pulmonary tuberculosis. Secondary causes include diseases of the underlying lung and these include pneumonia, bronchogenic carcinoma, Pulmonary infarction, collagen disorders (disseminated lupus erythematosus, rheumatoid disease) Hepatopulmonary amoebiasis, uraemia, injuries to chest wall and viral infections.

Clinical picture. There is acute pain on the chest where pathology is. Patient feels a sharp stabbing pain which becomes worse on breathing or coughing. Breathing is shallow and an unproductive dry cough is present. Signs of toxaemia and low to high grade fever is present. When pleurisy is complicating an underlying lung pathology features of that disease are present. Physical signs include diminished movements of the chest on affected side. A pleural rub is felt and on auscultation a grating sensation is heard which increases by pressure of chest piece of stethoscope. Pleural rub is not affected by coughing and is present in the acute stage. As disease process progresses, Pleural effusion appears and rub tends to disappear. Sometimes rub is heard over the upper level of effusion.

Investigations include X-ray chest which in early stages is normal. Later on slight haziness may appear. ESR levels are raised.

Treatment in primary cases is generally symptomatic in the form of rest in bed, and relief from pain by analgesics. In majority of cases, dry cough is very irritating. Syrup codeine phos. 1-2 tea spoonfuls twice a day shall give relief. Basic approach should be to treat the underlying pathology. Cases due to viral infections like coxsackie B virus generally clear up within a week.

PLEURAL EFFUSION

It is abnormal accumulation of fluid in pleural spaces. Normally pleura contains a very small amount of fluid which is not detected either clinically or by radiology. When amount of pleural fluid is more than 300 ml it is seen on X-ray while to be detected clinically amount should be minimum of 500 ml.

Causes of pleural effusion

Exudative pleural effusion

1. Pulmonary tuberculosis
2. Lobar pneumonia
3. Pulmonary infarction
4. Bronchogenic carcinoma involving pleura
5. Collagen disorders
6. Mesothelioma of pleura
7. Leukaemia, lymphoma
8. Amoebic liver abscess rupturing into pleura

Transudate pleural effusion

1. Congestive heart failure
2. Nephrotic syndrome
3. Anaemia, hypoproteinaemia
4. Cirrhosis of liver
5. Constricitive pericarditis
6. Meig's syndrome

Aetiology. Commonest cause of pleural effusion in India is tuberculosis but the other conditions which give rise to effusion are lobar pneumonia, pulmonary infarction, growths in lungs, leukaemias, septicaemia, chronic nephritis, collagen disorders, hypoproteinaemia congestive failure etc.

Classification of pleural effusion. Depending on the character of pleural fluid, pleural effusion may be classified as follows:

Transudate. Colour of fluid is pale-yellow or colourless, specific gravity 1.008-1.012. Fluid does not clot. Protein content is less than 3 gm%. There are occasional endothelial cells or none. Lactic dehydrogenase content is less than 200 I.U. Transudate is generally bilateral. Causes include congestive heart failure, cirrhosis of liver, Meig's syndrome, hypoproteinemia, severe anaemia.

Exudate. Colour of fluid is deep yellow, clots on standing, specific gravity more than 1.018, protein content generally is more than 4 gm%, cell content numerous lymphocytes, occasional RBC or polymorph. Lactic dehydrogenase content is more than 200 IU.

Exudate is a result of inflammatory process. Common causes include tuberculosis where the condition is primary. Secondary involvement of pleura occurs as a result of extension of inflammation from lungs like pneumonia, malignancy, pulmonary infarction, connective tissue disease, septicaemia, chronic nephritis, injuries to chest wall.

Haemorrhagic. This is exudative fluid mixed with blood. Other characters of the fluid are the same as in exudate except that it is well mixed with blood. Protein content of fluid is high and microscopic examination shows numerous RBCs. Causes include malignancy, tuberculosis, pulmonary infarction, trauma to chest wall, bleeding diathesis (purpura, haemophilia), rupture of aneurysm.

Chylous. Pleural fluid is opalescent and milky to look at. It is called chylous. Fluid contains large fat globules. The fluid clears up when shaken with ether. Chylous effusions are of three forms.

1. *Chylothorax.* Effusion is pure chyle and is a milky emulsion. Causes are injury to the tho-racic duct or its involvement by mediastinal glands or malignancy or filaria. Chylous fluid has fat globules seen on staining and is dissolved by fat solvent.

2. *Chyliform fluid.* In this the chylous fluid is not derived from thoracic duct but from either tubercullar involvement or malignancy of lung or pleura. Fluid is milky, contains small fat globules. Microscopically there are fat globules and leucocytes which are undergoing degeneration.

3. *Pseudochylous effusion.* In this the milky appearance is not due to fat but other particles (lecithin, globulin, calcium phosphate) which cause milky appearances. Causes are chronic effusions due to heart disease, chronic nephritis, tuberculosis and malignancy. Pseudochylous effusions are characterised by milky appearance but microscopic examination does not show fat globules and the fluid does not clear on adding ether or fat solvents.

Clinical features. Cases of pleural effusion may present generally in two forms: Acute or chronic.

Acute form comes in the form of acute pleurisy with constitutional symptoms like fever, toxaemia loss of appetite and ill health. Pain is present during the acute attack of pleurisy but as effusion develops the pain disappears. An acutely developing massive effusion will produce breathlessness and dry cough.

Chronic forms of pleurisy present with a picture of chronic ill health, low grade fever and loss of appetite. Physical signs on inspection include patient lying propped up in bed if effusion is massive. Movements of chest are restricted or diminished on the affected side. Inter cortal spaces are full and there may be slight bulge. Apex heat is displaced to the opposite side. Mediastinum is displaced and sternomastoid muscle on the side of mediastinal displacement is prominent (sternomastoid sign). On palpation movements of the chest on affected side are restricted. Trachea shifted to opposite side. Vocal fremitus is diminished or absent. Percussion note is stony dull. Dullness in its uppear border forms a curved convex line, it rising from spine, going maximum in axilla and again falling towards the front of chest, thus forming a S-shaped curve or Elli's line. If patient is examined while sitting upright, there is often a triangular area of dullness against the vertebral column on the sound lung, opposite the effusion (Grocc'o triangle). This paravertebral dull area is produced by the bulge of the fluid forming the effusion.

Physical signs of pleural effusion

1. Chest is prominent on the side of effusion. Intercostal spaces are full. Apex beat is displaced to the opposite side.
   Movements of the chest on effected side are restricted. Sternomaloid muscles on the side of mediastinal displacement are prominent (sterno mastoid sign).
2. On palpation movements of chest on effected side restricted. Vocal fremitus diminished. Trachea shifted to opposite side.
3. On percussion, stony dullness on the side of effusion. Rising dullness in axilla (S-shaped curve).
4. On auscultation, breath sounds are distant and weak or absent. If pulmonary collapse and patent bronchus, bronchial breathing is audible. Vocal resonance decreased. Aegophony and whispering pectoriloquy, above upper level of effusion.

On auscultation breath sounds are distant and weak or absent. Where there is pulmonary collapse and patent bronchi, bronchial breathing is heard. If the collapse is partial and bronchi are obstructed breath sounds are almost inaudible. No adventitious sounds are heard. Aegophony and whispering pectoriloquy is heard just above the upper level of fluid.

Investigations:

X-ray chest is the most essential investigation. It shall show obliteration of costophrenic angle. A dense shadow with curved upper border is present on the side where effusion is present. Heart is shifted to opposite side. Sometimes fluid is present in the inter lobar fissures and may give appearances of an intrapulmonary mass.

Diagnostic aspiration of pleural fluid is important. Pleural fluid generally is straw coloured. Protein content shall determine whether it is exudative or transudate. In exudate, fluid clots on standing, the protein content is more than 3 gm%. Cytology of fluid is equally important A marked preponderance of lymphocytes is suggestive of tuberculosis while presence of large number of polymorphonuclear cells indicates infection by pyogenic organism. Pleural fluid is stained by Gram's method and also culture done. Guinea pig inoculation is done for tubercular organisms. Blood for ESR shall show raised sedimentation rate.

Ultrasonography for detecting and locating effusion.

Pleural biopsy is done to confirm the diagnosis and establish aetiology.

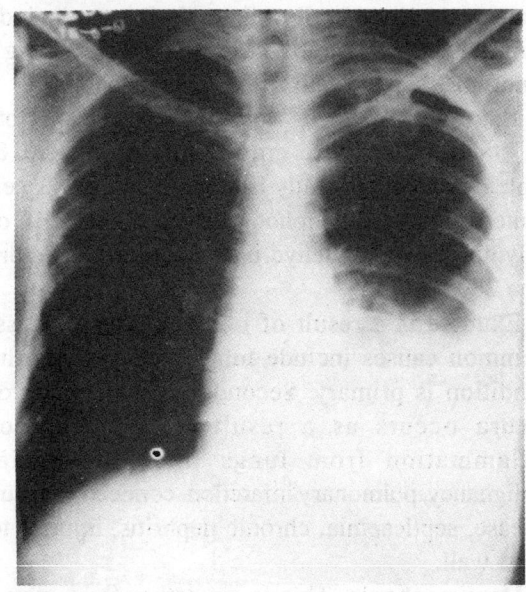

Fig. 5.37. X-ray Chest (PA View) Pleural effusion left side costophrenic angle obliterated.

Diagnosis. It is based on clinical presentation and physical signs as well as investigations like X-ray chest, pleural fluid examination (protein content cell count culture) and pleural biopsy. A case of pleural effusion may have to be differentiated from:

1. Thickened pleural where there is long-standing history of illness. Interspaces are narrowed and are not bulging. Percussion note is dull. No rising dullness, breath sounds are diminished. X-ray chest shows haziness. Upper level is not defined. Heart is not displaced.

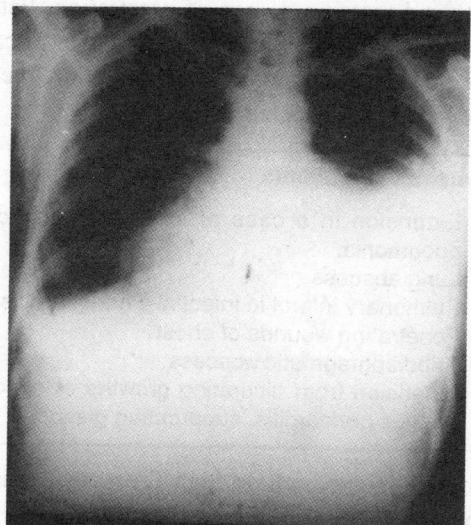

Fig. 5.38. X-ray Chest (PA View) Pleural effusion left side. There is shifting of trachea and mediastinum to right side.

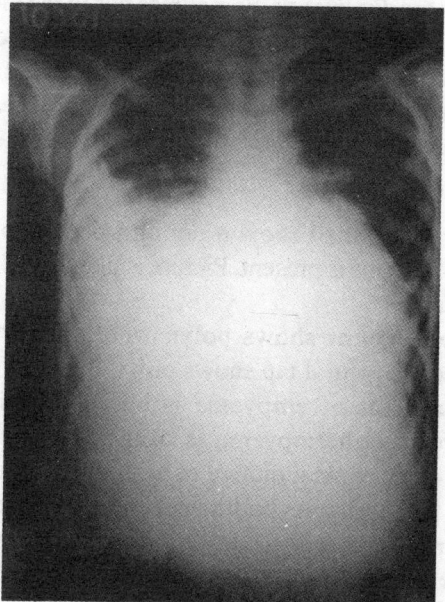

Fig. 5.39. X-ray Chest (PA View) A case of polyserositis tubercular in aetiology. There is pleural effusion, pericardial effusion and ascites.

2. Pneumonia. Acute onset with severe degree of toxaemia. Rusty sputum. Movements of chest limited. Percussion note impaired. Vocal fremitus may be increased. Bronchial breath sounds with medium to coarse crepts are present. Total and differential leucocyte count shows polymorph leucocytosis. X-ray chest shows consolidation.

3. Hydropneumothorax:. There is presence of both fluid and air in the pleura. It often complicates pleural effusion. Intercostal spaces are bulging. Radiology of chest clinches the diagnosis.

4. Bronchogenic carcinoma. when associated with pleural effusion. History of haemoptysis, weight loss, toxaemia, dry hacking cough and weight loss, marked cachexia with lymphadenopathy in supraclavicular region. X-ray shows shadow of growth.

Treatment. In majority of cases (90%) the underlying cause is tuberculosis while in a small percentage other causes operate. Treatment in such cases is along the line of that illness. In tuberculous effusion, all four drugs (Isonex, Rifampicin, Pyrazinamide and Ethambutol) have to be given for the first three months and then on three drugs (Isonex, Rifampicin, Ethambutol)for six months.

Aspiration of pleural fluid. *Indication for aspiration:*

1. If pleural fluid is large and producing marked dysponea.
2. Cardiac and respiratory embarrassment.
3. Failure of effusion to get absorbed after 2 weeks despite therapy.
4. Secondary infection with severe degree of toxaemia.
5. Bilateral pleural effusion producing breathlessness.

Pleural aspiration is done generally from the seventh space in the posterior axillary line. Too much of fluid should not be removed at one sitting. Removal of one to 2 pints of pleural fluids is safe. If while aspirating there is discomfort or cough, aspiration must be stopped. Too rapid aspiration may produce pulmonary oedema.

Risks of paracentesis are pleural shock, air embolism and introduction of air while aspirating producing hydropneumothorax. In cases of malignant pleural effusion, fluid accumulates rapidly. Symptomatic relief is obtained by instilling a sclerosing agent such as tetracycline into the pleural space after aspiration.

Complications. Permanent collapse of the lung may persist in cases of pleural effusion of long standing. Pleural effusion may resolve leaving behind a thickened pleura. Miliary tuberculosis with dissemination to other organs may occur. There may be Thrombosis of pulmonary vessels and pulmonary embolisation leading to sudden death.

Prognosis. In a case of pleural effusion where cause is treatable, prognosis is good. In cases of tubercular effusion though recovery is complete yet after some years some of these cases may develop pulmonary tuberculosis. Uncommonly cases of massive effusion may die suddenly due to cardiac failure, pulmonary oedema or embolism.

EMPYEMA

Empyema means presence of pus in the pleural cavity. The fluid is turbid and full of pus. Empyema generally complicates a case of pneumocal pneumonia where infection is extension from the lung in a case of lobar or bronchopneumonia. Other pulmonary causes include tuberculosis, lung abscess, gangrene or septic infarct in infective endocarditis. Further penetrating wounds of chest wall, fractured ribs, and spread from adjacent structures like subdiaphragmatic abscess, suppurating glands, ulcerating growths of oesophagus, pericarditis, septicemia are other responsible factors. Primary empyema is uncommon and is mainly due to pneumococcal infection. Empyema may develop in the course of acute fevers such as measles, scarlet fever, etc. Causative organisms most commonly responsible are pneumococcus and streptococcus. Less common organisms are staphylococci, H. influenzae, B. coli and Friedlander's bacillus.

Clinical picture. In majority of cases the clinical picture is that of primary cause and the picture of empyema is masked. Attention is drawn to it when a patient recovering from primary disease suddenly develops high fever, toxaemia, malaise, rigors,

sweats and extreme degree of prostration. Patient gets intermittent fever going up to 104°F. In cases where the cause is pneumococcal infection, picture is like that of lobar pneumonia.

Causes of empyema

1. Extension in a case of lobar or bronchopneumonia.
2. Lung abscess
3. Pulmonary infarct in infectinve endocarditis
4. Penetrating wounds of chest
5. Subdiaphragmatic abscess
6. Extension from ulcerating growths of oesophagus pericarditis, suppurating glands.

Physical signs include high fever, tachycardia, pallor, cachexia and severe degree of toxaemia. Chest shows signs of pleural effusion with bulging intercostal spaces, and restricted movements. Percussion note is dull. Trachea is shifted and heart displaced to opposite side. On auscultation breath sounds are diminished. Sometimes pus in the pleural cavity may track through an intercostal space and produce a fluctuating swelling on the chest wall simulating a superficial abscess. This is called Empyema necessitatis.

Investigations:

X-ray chest shall show a uniform density on the side where pus is present. Picture is like that of pleural effusion.

Blood count shows polymorph leucocytosis. Diagnostic pleural tap shows pus.

Diagnosis of empyema is based on clinical picture though empyema is overlooked since in many cases clinical picture of primary disease may mask it. Suspicion should arise when a case with primary disease with pleural effusion fails to respond to treat-ment and starts deteriorating. Three examinations are essential to establish the diagnosis, X-ray examination, blood count and a diagnostic aspiration of chest. Pleural tapping shall show presence of thick pus-like fluid which should be sent for Gram's stain and culture.

Treatment. The principles of treatment are:

1. Treat the primary cause.

2. Pus from pleural space should be removed since delay in its removal will prevent reexpansion of the lung and prolong toxaemia. Pus should be examined and organisms identified as well as cultured for sensitivity to various antibiotics. Depending on the sensitivity of the organisms antibiotics (Penicillin/Ampicillin/Amoxycillin/Ciprofloxacin) in heavy doses should be administered round the clock. Antibiotics may be instilled into pleural space at the end of aspiration. In case pus is thick and is difficult to aspirate it can be liquidifed by instillation of proteolytic enzymes like Streptokinase and Streptodornase. Surgical drainage of pus through introduction of a intercostal catheter and its constant drainage is required when pus accumulates rapidly. In cases of chronic empyema, where pus is thick and adhesions have formed and sinus is failing to close, rib resection with decortication is advocated.

Complications and sequelae. An untreated empyema portends very grave prognosis. But at the same time an inadequately treated empyema leads to chronic empyema. Chronic empyema results due to inadequate drainage of pus. Persistence of the infection results in chronic ill-health, wasting, cachexia, delayed expansion of the lung and bronchopleural fistula.

An empyema as such may produce pyopneumothorax, rupture into the lungs and involve adjacent structures like pericardium, oesophagus. Brain abscess due to septic embolization is another serious complication. Sudden death may occur due to myocarditis. Many patients are left behind with pleurobronchial fistula or a chronic sinus.

Prognosis in a case shall depend on the underlying condition, response of the patient to treatment and adequacy of line of therapy. Early recognition of the disease and early institution of required antibiotics carries good prognosis. Prognosis is poor in very debilitated patients and those with fulminating infection and bilateral empyema.

PNEUMOTHORAX

Presence of air in the pleural cavity is called pneumothorax. Pneumothorax may be spontaneous (rupture of subpleural tuberculous focus/bullae) traumatic (penetrating injury of chest wall) iatrogenic (introduction of air while aspirating effusion). Pneumothroax has been durther classified into:

1. Closed pneumonothorax where opening in the lung is very small and heals rapidly so the pleura does not communicate with the outside.
2. Open pneumothorax: There is a opening on the surface of the lung which remains patent and air passes in and out of the pleural cavity during both phases of respiration. Pressure in the pleural cavity remains equal to that of outside.
3. Tension pneumothorax. There is a valvular slit on the surface of the lung. Air can enter into the pleural space during inspiration but can not escape during expiration. Thus there is positive pressure in the pleural cavity.

Cause of pneumothorax

1. Rupture of emphysematous bullae or of subpleural tubercular focus.
2. Congenital cystic disease of lung
3. Staphylococcal pneumonia
4. Penetrating injury of chest/fracture of ribs
5. Perforation of bronchus during bronchoscopy
6. Following pleural aspiration
7. Rupture of subdiaphragmatic/subphrenic abscess.
8. Infection of pleural cavity by gas gangrene organisms.

Spontaneous pneumothorax. It is more common in men and commonest causes include rupture of a subpleural emphysematous bullae or rupture of subpleural tubercular focus. While the former is more common in people above the age of 50 years who suffer from chronic bronchitis with or without emphysema, the latter cause is operative at any age more so between the age group of 20 and 40 years. Pulmonary tuberculosis is the commonest cause of pneumothorax in India. Other uncommon causes include congenital cystic disease of lung, staphylococcal pneumonia, penetrating injury of chest, fracture of ribs, accidental perforation of bronchus during bronchoscopy, ulceration of oesophageal growth, subdiaphragmatic pathology, rupture of subphrenic abscess, infection of pleural cavity by gas gangrene organisms and while doing pleural aspirations or biopsy. Sometimes pneumothorax may be produced therapeutically in cases of pulmonary tuberculosis to arrest severe heamoptysis.

Clinical picture. Pneumothorax comes suddenly. Symptoms depend on the amount of air in pleural space and the speed with which it accumulates.

Generally the sudden process starts with a feeling of something snapping inside. There is severe pain, shortness of breath and cough. Patient is restless, cyanosed. Breathing is rapid and shallow. Temperature falls and heart shows severe degree of tachycardia. Blood streaked sputum may be passed. Rapid downhill course with collapse occurs. If not managed, death may occur from asphyxia and cardiac failure in a short time.

Physical signs include patient sitting up in bed, acutely breathless, alae nasi working. The affected side of chest is prominent and bulging. Movements are completely restricted. Heart and trachea are shifted to opposite side. Cardiac dullness may be obliterated if pneumothorax on left side. Percussion note is hyper resonant (tympanitic or drum like). A special diagnostic test is 'Coin test' when a coin placed over pneumothorax cavity is struck by another coin and a metallic note is heard at the back of chest. Auscultation shows amphoric type of bronchial breathing especially in tension and open pneumothorax. Adventitious sounds like clicking sounds synchronous with heart beat may be heard if pneumothorax is on left side.

There may be slight variations in physical signs in various forms of pneumothorax. In closed pneumothorax there are classical signs of bulging of chest. Displacement of trachea and heart. Hyper resonent precrussion note but auscultation shows diminished or absent breath sounds. Coin test is positive.

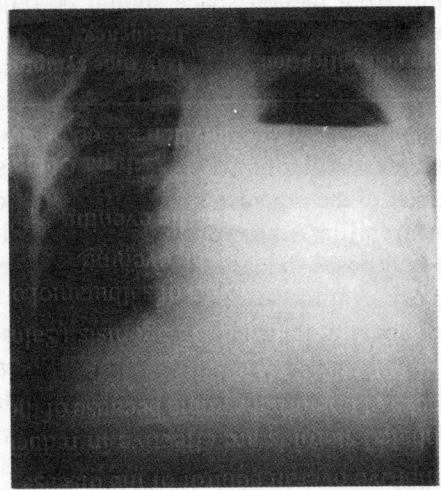

Fig. 5.40. X-ray Chest (PA View) There is fluid and air shadow in left lung hydropneumo thorax.

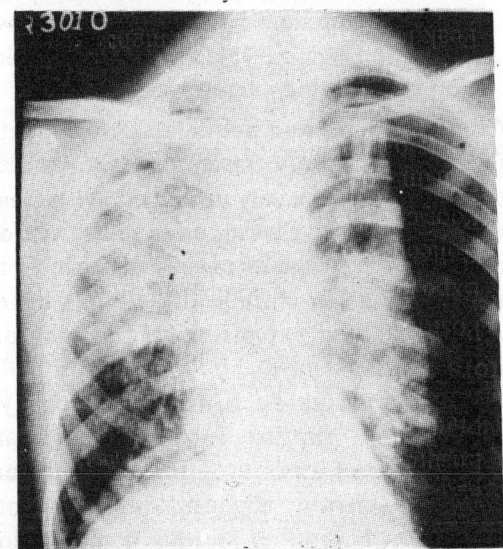

Fig. 5.41. Pneumothorax left lung patient has got extesive tuberculosis both lungs.

In open and tension pneumothorax the signs are as above but in addition cracked pot sound may be heard on percussion and auscultation reveals amphoric type of breathing.

Investigations. Radiological signs are diagnostic. On the affected side there is hyper translucency There is free air in the pleural cavity. Lung markings are absent and lung itself is seen as collapsed with its sharp margin. There is shift of trachea and mediastinum to oposite side.

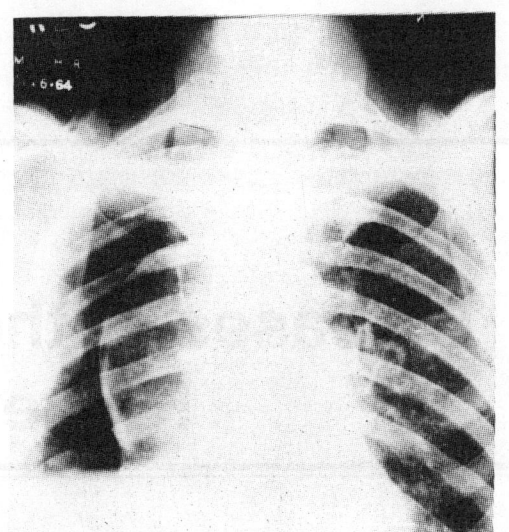

Fig. 5.42. Hydropneumo thorax right side. Shrunken lung on right is seen well.

Complications and sequlae. Severe respiratory embarrassment, cardiac failure and sudden death may occur. Air embolism is another serious complications. Sequlae include permanent collapse of lung, pyopneumothorax and a fistula.

Treatment. In a small closed pneumothorax where symptoms are not marked patient is put to bed rest, along with antibiotics and analgesics. If the air amount is small it will be absorbed in due course. In cases of tension pneumothorax, patient is acutely breathless and condition is desperate. Attempt should be made to let out the air immediately and relieve the distress. This is done by inserting a wide bore needle in the second inter costal space in front and connecting it to rubber tube which is further connected to an underwater seal controlled by pneumothroax apparatus and manometer.

Antibiotics are given to prevent secondary infection. Attempt should be made to find out the underlying pathology and treatment started. In cases where patient fails to improve in a way that vent in the lung does not heal, surgical repair of pleural space may have to be done. Other surgical methods include thoracoplasty and lobectomy.

CHAPTER 6

Diseases of the Kidney

1. Symptomatology in renal diseases
2. Glomerulonephritis
3. Nephrotic syndrome
4. Chronic nephritis
5. Acute renal failure
6. Chronic renal failure
7. Dialysis
8. Renal transplantation
9. Urinary tract infections
10. Renal tuberculosis

Kidney is an important organ in the body which plays a major role in the elimination of waste products and regulates the body fluids. It plays the role of both excretion as well as reabsorption of certain substances such as water, solutes etc. required for metabolism. It also has role in the production of hormones (Renin: Erythropoietin, Prostglandins, Kallikreins) which have both local and systemic effects. Large volume of blood (25% of cardiac output) passes per minute through the glomeruli in kidney. Glomerular filtration defines the exact level of renal function while tubules by their selective reabsorption and excretion of water and other electrolytes keep the body fluids balanced.

SYMPTOMATOLOGY IN RENAL DISEASE

Polyuria. It means increased urinary volume irrespective of frequency of micturition (more than 3000-3500 ml in 24 hours). It may be due to:

1. Inability of the kidney to concentrate urine as in chronic nephritis, diabetes insipidus.
2. Increase in molelcular concentration of glomerular filtrate—diabetes mellitus.
3. Diuresis after administration of a diuretic.
4. Psychological causes like compulsive water drinking.

Oliguria. It means that amount of urine excreted in 24 hours is less than 400 ml. Causes include dehydration, shock, acute nephritis, truma to kidney, reflex inhibition in renal stones, and inadequate intake of fluids. Oliguria and anuria are interrelated conditions and often cases of oliguria may merge into a state of anuria.

Anuria. When urinary output falls below 100 ml in 24 hours it is called anuria but when there is complete failure of formation of urine it is referred to as total or absolute anuria. Causes are:

1. Acute shock, as in peripheral circulatory failure.
2. Acute nephritis, pyelonephritis.
3. Drugs toxicity with drugs like sulfonamides.

4. Severe dehydration, incessant vomiting, diarrhoea.
5. Poisoning with mercury, turpentine, phenol, aluminium phosphide.
6. Thrombosis of renal artery.
7. Bilateral obstruction of ureters by calculi, blood clots or malignancy.
8. Incompatible blood transfusion.
9. Traumatic injury of kidney and ureters.
10. Crush injuries to limbs producing acute tubular necrosis.
11. Severe infections like black water fever, gram negative. Septicaemia; septic abortion.
12. Reflex inhibition of urine by renal colic, renal stones.

Dysuria. Difficulty in passing urine and the process being painful is called dysuria. Causes are lower urinary tract infection, renal stones, malignancy of bladder or urethra.

Frequency of micturition. This is the desire to pass urine more frequently than what a person normally does. Increased frequency of micturition occurs under state of anxiety, stress, urinary tract infection, diabetes and renal malignancy especially of lower urinary tract like urinary bladder. Amount of urine passed by a normal adult varies from person to person and shall depend on number of factors like fluid intake, dehydration and climatic factors. On an average a person's urinary output varies from 600 to 2800 ml in 24 hours. Any increase or decrease shall reflect the state of kidneys and their functioning.

Hematuria. Presence of blood in the urine constitute hematuria. It means bleeding from any part of the urinary tract. When blood is well mixed with the urine its origin is from the kidneys and upper part of ureters. Bleeding from urethra occurs in the first part of urine while that from urinary bladder is in the last part of urine when it is passed. Presence of blood in the urine may give it either a bright coloured or smoky appearance depending on the conversion of haemoglobin into methaemoglobin. Causes of hematuria can be:

1. **Pre-renal.** These include certain systemic conditions where blood passes into the urine such as scurvy, Purpura, bleeding, disorders and haemorrhagic fevers. There is no evidence of renal disease in such people.

2. **Renal.** These include diseases of the kidneys involving kidney, urinary tract and urinary bladder. Common conditions are acute nephritis, chronic nephritis, tuberculosis of the kidney, renal tumours, renal calculus, infarction of the kidney, malignant hypertension, ureteric calculus, papilloma and carcinoma of bladder.

Drugs which alter the colour of urine. Many times a false impression of hematuria may be created in people who are taking certain drugs. Sure way to distinguish it from hematuria is by microscopic examination of urine when red blood cells shall be seen in hematuria. Reddish colour of urine may be seen when certain dyes like methylene blue is used as colouring agent for sweets. Drugs like rhubarb and senna turn the urine reddish brown. Vegetable substance like Beetroot, berries also colour the urine red. Commonly used antitubercular drug Rifampicin discolours urine orange red; Dindevan (Phenindione) oral anticoagulant, phenazopyridine (pyridium) urinary antiseptic also turn urine colour orange red while those taking Nitrofurantoin, Methyldopa, levodopa, metronidazole, their urine turns dark brown on exposure to air. Similarly in those people who are taking vitamin B complex and like substances their urine shall appear deep yellow.

Pyuria. It means pus in the urine. It may come from anywhere in the genitourinary tract like urethra, urinary bladder, kidney or prostate. Frank pus in urine is commonly seen in gonococcal infection. Diagnosis of pus in urine is made by microscopic examination.

Chyluria. Milky colouration of urine is called chyluria. Causes are blocking of thoracic duct by filaria, malignancy and tuberculosis.

Haemoglobinuria. Urine is dark smoky coloured and is as a result of toxic agents producing it. Causes include black water fever, incompatible blood transfusion, drugs like sulfonamides, trimethoprim sulpha methoxazole. Haemogloburia has to be differentiated from hematuria. In the former condition though urine is red coloured but microscopic examination shows no red blood cells.

Paroxysmal haemoglobinuria may occur because the red blod cells in such people are defective and there are polyclonal complement fixing antibodies which react with them in cold to produce lysis. Common causes are Raynaud's disease and syphilis.

Alkaptonuria. It is an inborn error of metabolism and is characterised in early stages by blue discoloration of ears, tendons of hands, brown pigmentary deposits in the sclera and in late stages by kyphosis and a stooping posture. Urine in such patients darkens on standing or immediateley after the addition of an alkali solution. Urine in patients suffering from the disease stains clothes brown.

Porphyrinuria. It is also an inborn error of metabolism where there is defect in the synthesis of prophobilinogen with the result that excess of porphyrins are produced either in the liver or bone marrow and excreted in urine. The urine in such patients turns reddish brown or purple in colour either when passed or after standing for some time. Addition of Ehrlich's aldehyde volume to volume in urine produces a pink colour.

Bilirubin uria. Cases of jaundice especially infective or serum hepatitis exhibit presence of urobilin in urine the urine appearing dark brown while cases of obstructive jaundice have orange yellow colour of urine due to presence of bilirubin.

Characteristics of normal urine. Normal urine is clear and amber coloured with a characteristic aromatic odour which becomes ammonical when decomposition sets in. The quantity of urine secreted in 24 hours varies from 1200-1500 ml and depends on the amount of food eaten, intake of fluids and the fluids lost by sweat, lungs and bowels. In diseases where there is impairment of concentrating ability of kidneys as in diabetes, urine volume increases while as in dehydration where diluting capacity is impaired, amount of urine passed also decreases.

The urine is transparent and clear but at times it becomes cloudy when there are precipitates of phosphates or urates, WBC's, epithelial cells and bacteria. The reaction of urine is acidic pH varying between 4.7 and 10. Urine is more acidic during fasting than during digestion. Proteins in food tends to make it more acidic while fruit and vegetables make it alkaline since organic acids in these substances are converted into alkaline carbonates which are excreted in the urine making it alkaline. Marked alkalinity in fresh urine is indicative of ammonical decomposition in bladder as in chronic cystitis.

Specific gravity of urine is variable ranging from 1.017 to 1.025. Specific gravity is increased when the urine becomes concentrated as in high fevers, dehydration, diabetes mellitus and in renal diseases. A low fixed specific gravity suggests chronic nephritis.

Urine contains number of constituents partly derived from food and partly from the body's catabolism of tissues. Normal constitutes of urine include chlorides, sulphates, calcium, creatinine, purines, ammonia etc.

Nitrogenous constituents. Urea constitutes the major part and its daily excretion ranger from 18-30 g, Increased excretion ococurs in fevers, diabetes while a fall occurs in starvation, liver disease and nephritis. Purine bodies are equally important and uric acid constitutes an important part. Decreased excretion of uric acid occurs in gout.

Creatinine daily excretion ranges from 1-1.5 mg/dl and provides a simple indication of glomerular filtration rate. It is decreased in muscular dystrophy, myasthenia gravis and nephritis. Ammonia excretion normally is in the range of 30-50 meq/24 hrs. daily. Increased excretion indicates acidosis and is characteristically seen in diabetes, repeated vomiting and starvation. Calcium excretion on an average is 7.5 meq/24 hrs. per day and is decreased in cases of tetany.

Non-nitrogenous constituents. These are mainly salts and sodium chloride constitutes an important part. Its daily, excretion ranges from 130-260 meq/24 hours. It is reduced in cases of oedema, less intake and excessive vomiting. Urinary output of chlorides increases in Addison's disease.

Urinary sulphates constitute 1.5 to 3 g per day and their excretion increases in conditions associated with active metabolism. Phosphates are another important constituent.

Abnormal constituents:

Albumin. Normally urine does not contain any albumin or only in traces. Presence of albumin in urine may be physiological or pathological. Physiological causes include after heavy exercise and orthostatic proteinuria a benign condition when albumin is present in urine passed in upright posture but absent in the urine passed on getting out of bed but is again maximum in early hours of morning disappearing by evening. Amount of proteins in the food shall influence it. Orthostatic albuminuria is important to diagnose since it is a benign condition. If urine passed on first rising in the morning is albumin free, then albuminuria in other specimens is innocent.

Other causes of albuminuria are acute fevers, congestive heart failure, toxaemia of pregnancy, post epilepsy, diseases of kidney or genitourinary tract (Acute nephritis, nephrotic syndrome, malignant hypertension, diabetic glomerulosclerosis, renal amyloidosis, renal tuberculosis, conditions of urinary tract associated with hematuria or pus in urine).

Albuminuria is diagnosed by heating the urine when a precipitate is formed. Cases of multiple myeloma show a protein called Bence Jone's Protein which appears in urine when heated at 40 to 55°C but disappears on boiling the urine. Massive albuminuria in urine is diagnostic of nephrotic syndrome. In such cases quantitative estimation of 24 hours specimen for albumin is made. Proteinuria above 3.5 g in 24 hours is pathological. Since albumin in urine is hardly there but its appearance in urine labelled as microalbuminuria is an early indicator of diabetic glomerular disease.

Glucose. Presence of glucose in urine is suggestive of diabetes mellitus. Glycosuria in the presence of normal blood sugar levels is labelled as renal glycosuria and is as result of lowering of renal threshold. Common cause is glycosuria during pregnancy. Other causes of glycosuria are endocrinal (hyperthyroidism acromegaly), cerebral haemorrhage, intracranial injury, and after myocardial infarction for a short period.

Ketone bodies. Presence of acetone in urine occurs during starvation, diabetes mellitus, cyclical vomiting, eclampsia of pregnancy and patients taking limited quantity of carbohydrates. Ketonuria signifies appearance in urine of diacetic acid and its products acetone and beta-oxybutyric acid. Presence of acetone bodies in diabetes signifies approaching coma and require urgent management.

Microscopic examination. It is an important part of urine examination and gives valuable information. An acidic urine may show uric acid crystals (Prism like in appearance) amorphous urates (yellowish or colouorless granules) calcium oxalate crystals (envelope crystals), cystine and fat globules while an alkaline urine shall show presence of phosphates, calcium carbonate and ammonia. Most of the times these crystals are of no significance except in certain disease like renal stones, gout when there is excess of uric acid crystals in urine.

A centrifuged specimen of urine may show erythrocytes (conditions producing hematuria) leucocytes (infection in the urinary tract, after catheterisation) and casts.

Casts are cylinderical structures secreted by the kidney tubules as a result of coagulation of proteins. Presence of casts indicate renal disease. Casts may be cellular (leucocytic red cell casts and epithelial) and non-cellular casts (hyaline, granular, waxy and fatty). Cellular casts indicate acute inflammation of the kidney such as pyelonephritis (leucocytic), chronic glomerulonephritis (red cell casts) nephrosis, toxins (epithelial). Of the non cellular casts hyaline and granular casts are found in glomerulonephritis, and Nephrotic syndrome, while waxy casts are found in advanced stages of glomerulonephritis and amyloid disease.

Gram staining of urinary deposit is done for identification of urinary organisms. A mid stream specimen of urine for this purpose should always be taken. Urine culture should always be done before instituting antibiotics in cases of urinary tract infection so as to establish the type of organism (common are E. coli, staphylococci, Proteus vulgaris, streptococci) and its sensitivity to drugs.

Tests of renal function. Renal functions can be assessed by biochemical tests, radiological investigations and other tests including renal biopsy.

Biochemical tests. Estimations of blood urea (normal values 30-40 mg/dl) and blood urea nitrogen (15-20 mg/dl) along with serum creatinine levels (normal 0.8-1.5 mg/dl) are indicative of glomerular filtration function. Normal kidney has great reserve and these levels do not go up until more than 50 per cent of the kidney GFR (glomerular filtration rate) is reduced. Estimation of serum electrolytes (sodium and potassium), plasma bicarbonate and pH tell us about tubular function, and their capacity of reabsorption. Similarly uric acid levels go up in renal failure while serum calcium levels are low. When secondary hyperparathyrodism develops, serum calcium levels rise.

Radiological investigations:

1. **Plain X-ray abdomen.** It shall tell us about the presence of any calculi in the urinary tract as well as any calcification in the kidneys. Sometimes an idea about the size of two kidneys can be made on X-ray.
2. **Intravenous pyelography.** It is an important diagnostic test and useful for outlining the kidneys for the size, presence of any calculi, renal function and anatomical abnormalities (calyceal clubbing, abnormal dilatation or filling defects). Sometimes rapid sequence and high dose infusion urography are done to better visualise the kidney.

Retrograde cystourethrography is indicated for study of bladder and lower part of urinary tract. Micturiting cystourography means instillation of contrast material into bladder and vesicoureteric reflux studied. This investigation is important where disturbed bladder functions are suspected.

3. **Ultrasonography.** It is a simple non-invasive test and is used for study of the size of kidney, presence or absence of any kidney mass, obstruction in the urinary tract and study of bladder and prostate size.
4. **CT scan.** It is more advanced technique for study of renal size, masses, glands and tumours in the abdomen.
5. **Renal arteriography.** This is indicated in cases of renal artery stenosis, young hypertensives and to study the extent of renal tumours.
6. **Renal scintigraphy.** These are advanced investigations available in limited centres and

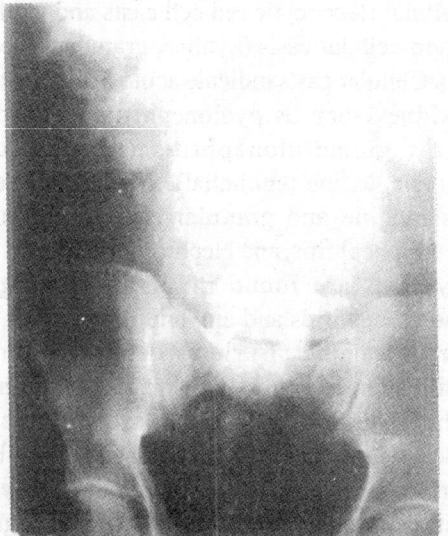

Fig. 6.1. Plain Xray Abdomen: Renal stones left kidey. There was poor functioning of left kidney.

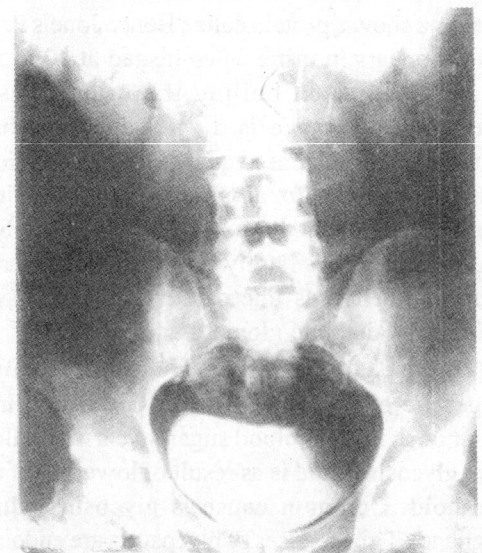

Fig, 6.2. Intravenous Pyelogram (IVP) Normal I.V.P. both the kidney showing normal function.

involve dynamic scintigraphy and static renal scintigraphy. Dynamic studies are useful for studying renal blood flow in cases of renal artery stenosis, severity of obstruction in the kidney and urinary tract as well as for visualizing of kidneys (ectopic kidneys or pseudotumours of the kidney).

Renal biopsy. In cases where diagnosis is not well established, an estimate can be made by study of renal tissue obtained by a punch biopsy needle. Histological examination of tissue not only establishes the diagnosis but also tells the progress of the disease and effect of treatment. Renal biopsy is indicated in cases of nephrotic syndrome, systemic diseases involving the kidney, amyloid disease of kidney and cases with unexplained proteinuria. Renal biopsy has its own drawbacks. It is contraindicated in patients with single kidney, haemorrhagic disorders and hypertension. Complications include massive hematuria, introduction of infection and formation of perirenal haematoma.

GLOMERULONEPHRITIS

Involvement of glomeruli in the kidney either by a process of inflammation or immunologically mediated injury or part of generalized systemic diseases (systemic lupus erythematosus, polyarteritis nodosa, diabetes) constitute glomerulonephritis. Glomerulonephritis may be primary or secondary when it is as a result of various types of systemic diseases. Glomerulonephritis may be classified per clincial, etiological and morphologic norms.

1. Clinical

a. Acute nephritic syndrome
b. Subacute nephritis or nephrotic syndrome
c. Chronic nephritis
d. Chronic renal failure

2. Morphologic based on histological examination

a. Minimal change disease
b. Membranous glomerulonephritis
c. Focal segmental glomerulosclerosis
d. Membranoproliferative glomerulonephritis

3. Etiologic

a. Primary glomerulonephritis
b. Secondary glomerulonephritis due to systemic diseases
c. Hereditory disorders (Alport's syndrome, Fabry's disease) producing glomerulonephritis.

Acute nephritis. Also labelled as type I nephritis as per Ellis classification and is characterised by abrupt onset of hematuria, proteinuria, salt and water retention, hypertension and sometimes with renal failure.

A number of conditions produce acute nephritis ranging from bacterial, viral, collagen disordes to miscllaneous groups like goodpasture's syndrome, infective endocarditis, hypersensitivity angitis. But the commonest cause is post streptococcal infection. The disease is more common in young children and adolescents but may occur at any age.

Aetiology. It follows infection with beta-haemolytic streptococcus Lancfield group A usually type 4 and 12 though other strains are occasionally involved. Usually the infection is either in the throat or skin and interval between streptococcal infection and onset of disease is variable ranging from a few days to more than a month but on an average it is 2-3 weeks. It is usual for the child or young adult to be either at school or work before the onset of disease which may come acutely.

Aetiologically it is considered to be immune response to one or more of the streptococcal coenzymes including antistreptolysin O and antistreptokinase. Immune basis is suggested since the latent period of 10-20 days between the basic infection in throat and development of glomerulonephritis. Another mechanism is autoimmune mechanism when local cellular reaction of the hypersensitivity type mediated by lymphoid cells without the production of circulating antibodies and failure of the host to clear immune complexes from circulation will result in damage to the glomeruli.

Pathology. The kidneys usually are enlarged in size and swollen though sometimes they are normal in size. There may be small punctate haemorrhages on the surface. There is increase in cellularity of the glomeruli with proliferation of endothelial cells and polymorphs. Tubules may also show red cells and leucocytes. Since it is an immune complex disease there is deposition of granular pattern of immune complexes, fibrin and fibrinogen, as seen by electron microscopy and immunoflourescence techniques. The association of HLA types support the Hypothesis of altered immune response. In patients with rapidly progressive disease, epitheloid crescent formation with vas cular necrosis is common while in the slowly progressive disease damaged glomeruli may become organised and disappear leaving behind extensive interstitial fibrosis with involvement of vessels. The end result is extensive disease with a small contracted kidney.

Causes of acute glomerulonephritis

1. Infectious diseases
   i. Streptococcal glomerulonephritis
   ii. Non-streptococcal glomerulonephritis
      a. Bacterial. Infective endocarditis, ty-phoid fever, pneumococcal pneumonia, staphylococcal and meningococcal infection, syphilis
      b. Viral. Hepatits B, infectious monoucleosis, mumps, measles, coxsackie and echo virus
      c. Parasites, malaria
2. Multisystem disease. Systemic lupus erythematosus, Henoch-Schonlein purpura, vasculitis, Goodpasture's syndrome.
3. Primary glomerular disease. Mesangio-capillary glomerulonephritis, mesangial proliferative glomerulonephritis.
4. Miscellaneous. Guillain-Barre syndrome, serum sickness, DPT vaccine.

Clinical picture. The onset is usually acute coming about 2-3 weeks after an acute attack of sore throat or tonsillitis. The patient who is usually a child or a young adult has symptoms of pain in the back, puffiness of face, oedema over legs and feet, headache and decrease in quantity of urine. Oedema first appears on the face and then gradually spreads all over the body. In some the disease may have an insidious course and patient has only headache, vomiting and abdominal pain. In those with more acute course the patient may pass into complications like acute left heart failure, hypertensive encephalopathy and renal failure.

The amount of urine passed is greatly reduced. It is dark coloured, smoky or reddish brown. The urine is loaded with albumin and contains blood. Physical signs include oedema over the face and legs and feet. There is tachycardia and blood pressure levels are raised. Sometimes haemorrhages in the retina may be seen.

Investigations. Urine examination is the most important investigation. On naked eye examination urine may be dark or bright red or smoky. There is proteinuria. Microscopic examination shows blood and epithelial casts. Later on granular and hyaline casts appear. Urine culture is sterile. Blood urea and creatinine levels may be elevated. The antistreptolysin O titre is significantly elevated indicative of recent streptococcal infection. Serum complement levels (C3 & C4) are reduced. Renal imaging is normal, Kidney biopsy is not indicated until and unless there is doubt about the diagnosis.

In case where congestive failure is present, X-ray heart will show cardiomegaly and pulmonary oedema.

Investigation in acute nephritis

Urine. Dark or smoky on naked eye, albumin present. M/E red blood cells and epithelial casts. Later granular and hyaline casts.
Urine culture. Sterile
Blood urea. May be raised
Serum creatinine. May be raised
Antistreptolysin 0 titre. Elevated in post streptococcal glomerulonephritis.
Serum complement (C3 and C4). Level reduced
Creatinine clearance. Reduced
Renal imaging. Normal
X-ray heart. Cardiomegaly
Renal biopsy. Not indicated

Complications. A case of acute nephritis may develop various complications depending on the severity of the disease process. Various complications are:

1. Acute left heart failure especially in those with marked rise in blood pressure levels.
2. Hypertensive encephalopathy with convulsions, headache, vomiting in those with progressive disease.
3. Renal failure may develop when the disease is active and present in severe forms.

Diagnosis of acute nephritis characteristically is made by triad of scanty urine containing RBCs. Hypertension and oedema especially puffiness over the face. It may have to be differentiated from cases of angioneurotic oedema and nephrotic syndrome. Urine examination shall differentiate the two conditions while in former urine is normal and in the latter condition it shows massive albuminuria.

Management.

1. Rest in bed till acute symptoms improve.
2. Restrict dietary proteins. Fluids to be taken as per requirement. Strict restriction is not necessary if urinary output is good. On an average not more than 1000 ml of fluids per day (half strength milk, tea, glucose etc) is permitted. Calories in diet is met by including easily digestible semi solid or liquid diet containing carbohydrates and fats.
3. Monitor daily fluid intake, urinary output and weight.
4. For hypertension a mild anti hypertensive drug be administered.
5. For eradication of any persistent streptococcal infection. Injection Penicillin 50,000-100,000 units intramuscularly 6 hourly or Cap. Ampicillin (250 mg 6 hourly) or Capsule Amoxycillin (250 mg 8 hourly) may be given.
6. Treatment of complications like hypertensive encephalopathy, pulmonary oedema, impending renal failure, has to be carried on usual lines. In patients with progressive renal failure, dialysis may have to be employed.
7. In majority of cases of acute glomerulonephritis disease is self limiting and complete recovery takes place with careful management.

Prognosis and course. Prognosis in cases of acute nephritis is good. More than 80 to 90 per cent of patients recover completely. As the activity of disease ceases, urinary output increases and urinary abnormalities disappear. In a very small percentage of cases, disease may adopt a rapid down hill course. It may be in the form of irreversible glomerular changes leading to progressive renal failure. Development of hypertensive encephalopathy, pulmonary oedema are unfavourable signs. Prognosis is judged to some extent by the acuteness of onset and duration of symptoms like oedema and albuminuria. Longer these features more chances of patient going towards chronic nephritis.

Acute post-streptococcal glomerulonephritis (PSGN). It is a prototype of acute glomerulonephritis and follows streptococcal infection of the throat or skin by group AB-haemolytic streptococci generally type 1,2,4,12. These strains of streptococci which are nephrogoenic have M. protein in their cell wall which triggers an antigenic reaction. Because of variations in the nephrogenicity of group A streptococci strains, attack rates also vary and in some, asymptomatic episodes of PSGN may exceed symptomatic one.

M protein gives a type specific immunity which lasts for a long time and confers protection from further attacks of PSGN. PSGN is common amongst children and is related to poor hygine socioeconomic factors and over crowding which make these children more vulnerable to infection. Cold climate and damp atmosphere further aggravates the problem.

Following a sore throat, the disease manifests in one to two weeks while it is longer with skin infection. Clinically PSGN resembles acute nephritis more or less.

Diagnosis of the condition is made by history of a recent streptococcal throat or skin infection.

Confirmation is done by:

1. Demonstration of group AB-hemolytic streptococcus of nephrogenic M. protein type in throat or skin.
2. Immune response to one or more of the streptococcal exo enzymes (Antistreptolysin O-

ASO, antistreptokinase-ASK, anti-deoxyribonuclease B-ADNase-B).

3. Presence of anaemia. Raised levels of erthrocyte sedimentation rate (ESR).
4. Mild hypoalbuminaemia
5. Urine shows proteinuria which is non-selective and contains raised levels of fibrin-degradation products and C3 protein.
6. Transient cryoimmunoglobulinemia and positive tests for circulating immune complexes.
7. Plain X-ray abdomen and ultrasonography may reval enlarged kidneys.
8. Chest X-ray may show enlarged heart.
9. Renal biopsy may reveal diffuse endocapillary proliferative glomerulonephritis. There is infiltration of glomeruli with polymorphs and monocytes. By immunofluorescence microscopy granular deposits of IgG are seen in peripheral capillary loops and mesangium accompanied by C3.

The prognosis of PSGN is very good in children and young adults though it is less favourable in elder age group.

Treatment. Consists of bed rest, antibiotics, low salt and low protein diet with fluid control. For oedema, diuretics are to be employed while hypertension shall require specific drugs depending on the severity of hypertension.

Cases who develop renal failure, severe oliguria and hyperkalemia shall require dialysis.

Non-streptococcal acute post infectious Glomerulonephritis. This is a condition where number of organisms like viruses, parasites and bacteria other than group A-B haemolytic. Streptococci are responsible for causing acute glomerulonephritis. The clinical picture is like that of PSGN. Diagnosis is based on the presence of bacteriological or serological findings of diseases (typhoid, malaria, endocarditis, hepatitis B) which are capable of producing AGN. There is important role of circulating immune complexes associated with depression of C4, C3 and Clq and elevated levels of rheumatoid factor and circulating cryoimmunoglobulins.

Treatment of non-streptococcal glomerulonephritis mainly is directed towards control of infection. Prognsis in such a case shall be governed by the severity of disease responsible for causing AGN. Occasionally a patient may pass into rapidly progressive form of glomerulonephritis (RPGN).

Rapidly progressive glomerulonephritis (RPGN). Most cases of acute glomerulonephritis recover but a very small percentage of cases have a rapidly progressive downhill course which may take few weeks to even a few months to develop.

Clinically there is development of renal failure which may develop as a renal complication of an acute or subacute infectious disease or a multisystem disease or as a primary or idiopathic glomerular disease. Patient has features of renal failure like nausea, vomiting, weakness, oliguria and abdominal pain. Symptoms of arthritis, skin rash, neuropathy and encephalopathy are seen in patients of multisystem disease who have RPGN. Urine shows proteinuria, red cells casts and fibrin degeneration products.

Pathology. Extensive extracapillary (crescentic) glomerulonephritis is the pathological lesion and the extent and degree of glomerular involvement is variable and in majority of patients more than 75 per cent of glomeruli are involved.

Since it is an immune complex mediated disease, granular deposits of immunoglobulins shall be seen by immunofluorescence microscopy in majority of patients while in others there may be no immunoglobulins and their pathogenesis may not be explainable. But the disease as such has an acute onset and a rapidly progressive course.

Treatment and course. Cases of RPGN have a progressive downhill course and intensive treatment has to be instituted. Supportive and conservative treatment has limited role in the management of the disease. The principle of treatment are:

1. **Corticosteroids.** These may be given in the form of intermittent therapy (Methyl prednisolone 500 mg intravenously six hourly) or continous therapy (oral prednisolone 60 mg per day). These have given variable results but

do have benefit in suppressing immune response.

2. **Cytotoxic durgs.** Drugs like Azathioprine or Cyclophosphamide when combined with steroids have yielded beneficial results.

3. **Anticogulants.** Heparin or oral anticoagulants like warfarin sodium along with anti thrombotic agents (Dipyridamole) are of benefit in the prevention of coagulation process responsible for formation of crescents. Anticoagulants are to be employed with caution in cases of advanced renal failure.

4. **Plasmaphresis.** Intensiye plasma exchange (two to four litres of plasma) either daily or three times a week may be employed to remove antigen-antibody complexes. Beneficial results with plasmaphresis are more when it is combined with steroids and cytotoxic durgs.

5. **Dialysis.** In patients not responding to above therapy and where renal failure is progressive dialysis is done and repeated on weekly or twice weekly basis.

Causes of rapidly progressive glomerulonephritis (RPGN)

1. *Infectious diseases*
   i. Post-streptococcal glomerulonephritis
   ii. Infective endocarditis
   iii. Hepatitis B infection

2. *Multisystem disease*
   i. Systemic lupus erythematosus
   ii. Henoch-Schonlein purpura
   iii. Goodpasture syndrome
   iv. Rhematoid arthritis with vasculitis

3. *Primary glomerular disease*
   i. Idiopathic
   ii. Membranous glomerulonephritis
   iii. Mesangiocapillary glomerulonephritis

---

6. **Renal transplantation.** Where despite aggressive efforts no improvement takes place renal transplantation is considered though RPGN may recur even after renal transplantation.

Prognosis. Cases of RPG generally do not have good prognosis. It is poor in patients with crescent formation in 75 per cent or more of glomeruli, those with oliguria and severe reduction in GFR (less than 5 ml/min) and those with anti-GBM (antiglomerular basement membrane) antibody mediated response.

Most cases of RPGN have to be on maintainence with regular dialysis at frequent intervals till they go for renal transplantation.

Progress of the disease is monitored by renal biopsy.

NEPHROTIC SYNDROME

It is a clinical state which is characterized by generalized oedema, massive albuminuria, hypoproteinaemia and hypercholesterolemia. A number of diverse conditions are responsible for it and it is unusual to obtain a previous history suggestive of acute nephritis. Albuminuria may precede the appearance of oedema by months or even years and it is development of oedema which draws attention to the illness. This may be precipitated by an inter current infection.

Aetiology:

1. Acute glomerulonephritis
2. Minimal change glomerulonephritis and all types of glomerulonephritis (membranous, membroproliferative, focal and segmental).
3. Systemic illnesses (diabetic glomerulosclerosis, collagen disorders e.g. systemic lupus erythematosus).
4. Renal amyloidosis
5. Drugs (gold salts, penicillamine, mercurials, antiepileptic drugs like dilantin sodium, tridione).
6. Allergens, bee stings, poison ivy.
7. Neoplastic illnesses (mutliple myeloma, Hodgkin's disease, lymphomas).
8. Renal vein thrombosis.

Pathology. The kidney is largeand pale. It might be oedematous. The pattern in kidney of cortex and medulla is disturbed and there may be fatty changes in the interstitial tissue and tubules. Depending on the stage and severity of disease, it has been histologically classified into minimal change disease and membranous glomerulonephritis. Two other forms producing nephrotic syndrome are focal glomerulosclerosis and membroproliferative glomerulonephritis. Diagnosing these forms of nephropathy is important since their management and prognosis to a large extent shall be governed by the underlying pathology.

Minimal change disease is the most common form of nephrotic syndrome where the glomeruli have normal appearance under light microsoocope but diffuse loss of epithelial foot processes (blunted or effaced) is seen under electron microscope. In membranous glomerulonephritis, there is diffuse thickening of the basement membrane and under electron microscope there are abnormalities in epithelial cells (Spike and Dome pattern). To start with tubules, interstitium and blood vessels are normal but with the progress of disease, the glomeruli become sclerosed and finally become completely hyalinized. By fluroscence microscopy, granular deposition of immunoglobulins and complement along glomerular basement membrane is seen.

In membrano proliferative glomerulonephritis there is thickening of basment membrane and cellular proliferation while in focal segmental glomerulosclerosis only some of the glomeruli are involved and with progress of disease there is sclerosis and hyalinization of some tufts within the glomerulus especially in the juxtamedullary glomeruli. Progressively areas of tubular atrophy and complete sclerosis of glomeruli may be seen.

Clinical picture. The disease presents an insidious onset. Albuminuria may precede the classical picture for sometime. In most cases there is gradual or rapid onset of generalized oedema with puffiness of eyelids. Patient is pale, anaemic and complains of loss of appetite, malaise, and generalized weakness. Abdomen may be swollen because of ascites. Abdominal wall is oedematous. As of oedema, skin is stretched and tense. There may be pleural effusion and because of it patient may complain of breathlessness. In addition to loss of appetite there may be diarrhoea. Patient is liable to suffer from recurrent chest infections as well as of skin.

Amount of urine passed in 24 hours is reduced. Physical examination reveals a generalized oedematous person. There may be tachycardia but blood pressure levels are normal. Pitting oedema over legs and feet, abdominal wall and lower eye lids can be demonstrated. Eye lids are puffy. Where oedema is severe, ascites and pleural effusion can be seen. Kidneys generally are not palpable.

Investigations:

1. Urine specific gravity is normal. It contains large amount of albumin. 24 hours urinary albumin estimation shows it to be more than 3.5 g/day. Microscopically urine shows granular and hyaline casts and no RBCs.
2. There is fall in plasma proteins and decrease in albumin content, Albumin globulin ratio is altered and is less than one (normal albumin globulin ratio 1.6 to 1).
3. Blood cholesterol levels go up ranging from 300-600 mg%.
4. Blood urea levels usually are normal except in patients with massive oedema and oliguria.
5. Renal biopsy is performed to make a histological diagnosis. It is important for assessing line of treatment as well as prognosis of the disease.

Investigations in nephrotic syndrome

1. **Urine.** Specific gravity normal. Massive albuminuria. M/E granular and hyaline casts. No RBCs.
2. **24 hours urinary proteins.** More than 3-5 g/day
3. **Plasma proteins.** Fall in plasma proteins (Hypoproteinaemia). Decrease in albumin content (hypoalbuminaemia). Albumin globulin ration altered (less than 1).
4. **Blood urea.** Usually normal
5. **Blood cholesterol.** Hypercholesterolemia
6. **Serum complement levels.** Usually reduced in immune complex glomerulonephritis.
7. **Serum electrophoresis.** Reduced albumin with increase in alpha and beta globuline fractions.
8. **Renal biopsy.** Helpful in making a histological diagnosis.

Complications. Cases of nephrotic syndrome may develop pulmonary and cerebral oedema in cases with massive oedema. These patients are more susceptible to bacterial infections of the lungs, skin and peritoneum.

Diagnosis of nephrotic syndrome is not difficult especially when there is massive generalized anasarca with albuminuria, hypoproteinaemia and hypercholesterolemia. A simple urine test for albuminuria shall clinch the diagnosis.

Course and prognosis. Complete recovery in cases of nephrotic syndrome is not possible. Under treatment patient improves, oedema subsides and patient may remain symptom free for a number of years. Albuminuria may persist and these patients are exposed to intercurrent infections. Exaceberation of symptoms may take place. A large number of patients after a number of years pass into stage of chronic nephritis, the disease running a steadily progressive course. Renal failure, malignant hypertension, congestive failure and inter current infections are the usual cause of death.

Management:

1. Restrict sodium in diet. A high protein diet consisting of at least 80-100 g of first class proteins is to be given daily.

2. Diuretics should be given initially daily and subsequently on alternate day. Frusemide (40 mg) or a combination Lasride (Frusemide 40 mg + Amiloride 5 mg) or Aldactide (Spironolactone 25 mg + Hydrofumethiazide 25 mg) are the commonly used diuretics employed. Where oedema is massive injection Frusemide (40 mg intramuscularly or intravenously) daily is given for a few days. Monitoring of electrolytes must be done regularly and especially serum potassium levels.

3. In intractable cases some benefit is achieved by infusion of human serum albumin.

4. Where patient is not responding to conventional therapy (high protein diet, diuretics) and renal biopsy shows minimal change glomerular disease, prednisolone 60 mg per day given for a period of 6-8 weeks may be helpful.

Many patients may have recurrence and require repeat steroid therapy.

In cases where there is resistance to steroids and no improvement takes place cyclophosphamide (endoxan) 2-3 mg/kg body weight daily orally is given for 6-8 weeks. Where patient progresses towards end stage renal failure a combined course of steroids with either Azathioprine or cyclophosphamide is given to halt further deterioration. In majority of cases remission is induced.

5. Care should be taken to prevent infection and early treatment with adequate antibiotics should be instituted.

6. When and whatever complications develop, they should be appropriately managed.

Minimal change glomerulonephritis. It is the commonest form of nephrotic syndrome in children though uncommon in adults. It is often referred to as lupoid nephrosis and because of little or no change in the glomeruli is termed as minimal change disease.

Electron microscopy shows effacement of epithelial foot processes while there are irregular and non-specific deposits of immunoglobulins and complement components (IgM and C3) on immunofluorescence microscopy. Clinically patient presents with overt form of nephrotic syndrome. Proteinuria is highly selective consisting mainly of albumin and minimal amount of high molecular weight plasma proteins (IgG, alpha 2, macroglobulin or C3). Microscopic hematuria may be present. Serum levels of complement components are normal.

Genetic predisposition to the disease is indicated due to high prevalence of HLA-B$_{12}$ in association with allergic diathesis in patients with this disease.

Spontaneous remissions and relapses may occur. Proteinuria decreases and may become nil. Intercurrent infections may occur. Acute renal failure is unknown and occurs rarely.

Treatment. It is symptomatic. Corticosteroids are beneficial and help to induce remission. These may be given either daily or on alternate day.

Prednisolone (60 mg/m2 surface area in children: one to 1.5 mg/kg body weight in adults) given daily or on alternate days is effective way of treating these patients. Best regimen is to give prednisolone daily for 4 weeks followed by alternate day therapy (35 to 40 mg/m2 in children and 1 mg/kg body weight in adults) for next four weeks.

Majority of patients with minimal change respond to steroids with complete remission. This is more so in children. Steroids should be tapered slowly and small doses (5-10 mg prednisolone) may have to be continued for next four to 6 months.

In a patient who is steroid dependent or one with multiple relapses combination with cytotoxic drugs (Cyclophosphamide 2-3 mg/kg body weight per day) or (chlorambucil 0.1 to 0.2 mg/kg body weight perday) for eight to ten weeks shall be useful in preventing further relapses.

Cytotoxic drugs have adverse effects on bone marrow, so careful monitoring be done and their use reserved for patients with threatening serious complications or failure of steroid therapy. Long term prognosis in patients with minimal change is good.

Mesangial proliferative glomerulonephritis. In this there is mild to moderate but diffuse increase in the glomeruler capillary bed. There is uniform involvement of glomeruli with proliferation of mesangial cells and increase in the mesangial areas. By immunoflourescence microscopy a variety of deposits (IgA, IgM and C3) in the mesangium are seen.

Patients with this type of histological picture generally represent multisystem diseases (SLE, Henoch schonlein purpura) involving kidney and producing picture of nephrotic syndrome.

These patients have to be managed with steroids but in some proteinuria may persist and they may progress to renal insufficiency.

Membranous glomerulonephritis. Here there is diffuse involvement of glomeruli and there are deposits of IgG in the capillary wall. With advance in disease process these deposits join together and produce thickening of capillary wall. The increased amounts of basement membrane may give the

appearance of spikes. There is no proliferation of either capillary endothelial or mesangial cells. Mesangial sclerosis may occur in late stages. Membranous glomerulonephritis accounts for a fair percentage of cases of idiopathic nephrotic syndrome in adults but may also develop in association with diseases like SLE, Malaria, Malignancy and Exposure to heavy metals like gold.

Causes of nephrotic syndrome

1. **Primary glomerular disease**
   a. Minimal change disease
   b. Mesangioproliferative glomerulonephritis
   c. Membranous glomerulonephritis
   d. Mesangiocapillary glomerulonephritis
   e. Focal and segmental proliferative glomerulonehphitis
2. **Secondary to other diseases**
   a. Infections
      1. Post-streptococcal glomerulonephritis
      2. Malaria
      3. Endocarditis
      4. Hepatitis B
      5. Infectious mononucleosis
      6. Leprosy, syphilis
   b. Drugs
      1. Dilantin
      2. Tridione
      3. Gold, mercury
      4. Captopril
      5. Penicillamine
      6. Antitoxins
      7. Antivenoms
3. **Neoplasma**
   a. Hodgkin's disease
   b. Leukaemia
   c. Lymphoma
4. **Systemic disorders**
   a. SLE (systemic lupus erythematosus)
   b. Henoch-Schonlein purpura
   c. Vasculitis
   d. Sarcoidosis
   e. Goodpasture's syndorme
   f. Diabetes mellitus
   g. Amyloidosis
5. **Miscellaneous**
   a. Sickle cell disease
   b. Alport's sydrome
   c. Toxaemia of pregnancy
   d. Renovascular hypertension

Spontaneous remissions may occur in children. Steroids either orally or parenterally and given either daily or on alternate days do benefit such patients. In those with progressive renal disease, combination of steroids with cyclophosphamide is administered.

Cases of idiopathic membranous glomerulo-nephritis who have no raised levels of blood pressure, creatinine, cholesterol and where urinary proteins are low (less than 1 g/day) conservative approach to the patient is recommended.

Other forms of glomerulonephritis. These include mesangiocapillary or membrano-proliferative (Type I and Type II), focal and segmental proliferative glomerulonephirits.

In these forms of nephrotic syndrome, patient has hematuria, proteinuria and oliguria. Diagnosis is made by renal biopsy and electron microscopy.

Treatment is symptomatic. Patients with progressive renal disease shall require steroids with antimetabolites.

Prognosis is going to be variable. While it is good in cases of mesangial and focal and segmental proliferative glomerulonephitis it is not so good in cases of mesangiocapillary or membroproliferative forms of glomerulonephritis.

CHRONIC NEPHRITIS

It is a disease of adult life and generally occurs between the age of 25-40 years and may be continuation of acute nephritis which developed some years ago and though clinical symptoms improved but the initial process progressed steadily. Majority of patients of chronic nephritis present with hypertension, headache, weakness and pallor. In some renal failure may be the presenting feature.

Pathology. By the time chronic glomerulonephritis is detected, the changes in glomeruli are so advanced that it is difficult to assess the nature of original lesion. Kidneys are small and contracted surface red brown and diffusely granular. This is as a result of destruction of nephrons and development of interstitial fibrosis associated with atrophy and replacement of many of the tubules. The small and medium sized arteries are narrowed. The renal damage which earns the name of 'end stage kidneys' is a combination of original nephritis and subsequent development of hypertension.

Clinical Picture. Chronic nephritis develops insidiously and is first suspected in the presence of hypertension, albuminuria or renal failure. Hypertension is the dominant feature and may give rise to headache which may be distressing. Epistaxis, visual disturbances (due to retinal changes) cerebral haemorrhage and hypertensive encephalopathy. Uraemia may be the presenting picture in some cases.

Patient is pale, anaemic, emaciated and has peculiar waxy pallor of skin. There may be loss of appetite, nausea, vomiting and diarrhoea. Oedema generally is not present but sometimes it may be present in slight form. Polyuria and nocturia are present. In the presence of hypertension, heart size is enlarged and there may be systolic murmur in the mitral area. Fundus examination shows papilloedema, exudates and haemorrhages.

Investigations:

1. Urine shows albuminuria. Low fixed specific gravity (between 1.008-1.012) is characteristic. Microscopically there are epithelial and coarsely granular casts, occasional RBCs.
2. Blood urea levels are increased and so are serum creatinine levels which are last to rise. Serum proteins are either low or normal. Serum cholesterol is within normal limits.
3. Plain X-ray abdomen shows no abnormality.
4. Ultrasound of abdomen-shows size of kidneys to be reduced.
5. Intravenous pyelography shows poor functioning of the kidneys which are small and contracted.
6. Renal biopsy shows gross changes of chronic glomerulonephritis.

Course of the disease and prognosis. Once chronic nephritis develops it follows a progressively relentless, downhill course. The rate at which the disease progresses is extremely variable. Some come with malignant hypertension with its associated complications like congestive heart failure, hyper-

Table showing differences in clinical profile of various forms of nephritis

	Acute nephritis	*Subacute nephritis /nephrotic syndrome*	*Chronic nephritis*
Onset	Acute	Insidious	Insidious. May present acutely with renal failure or hypertensive encephalopathy.
History	History of sore throat or skin infection in previus weeks may be available.	History suggestive of acute nephritis may or may not be available	History of acute or subacute nephritis may be available. Generally none.
Clinical features	Puffiness of face. Minimal Oedema. Pallor Hypertension. Heart may be slightly enlarged Minimal ascites. Fundus shows narrowing of vessels. Minimal changes.	Generalised anasarca. Skin Waxy Pallor. Blood pressure levels normal. Heart size normal. Massive ascites. Fundus normal.	Pallor. No oedema. Hypertension present. Cardiac enlargement present. No ascites. Fundus Albuminic retinopathy(papilloedema, exudates, haemorrhages).
Urine	Quantity reduced (oliguria) Urine smoky and dark coloured. Specific gravity may be raised or normal albuminuria + M/E RBCs. epithelial, blood and hyaline casts.	Normal or quantity reduced Urine clear. Specific gravity normal. Massive albuminuria M/E granular fatty and hyaline casts.	Polyuria, Specific gravity low and fixed (below 1.012) albumin in traces. M/E occasional RBCs hyaline and coarsely granular casts.
Blood chemistry	Blood urea may be raised. Serum proteins, cholesterol levels are normal.	Blood urea normal. proteins are reduced. Albumin/globulin ratio less than one. Hypercholesterolemia (Cholesterol levels between 300-800 mg%)	Serum Blood urea and creatinine levels are inceased. Serum proteins and cholesterol levels are normal.
Ultrasonography I/V pyelography	Kidney size normal. –	Kidney size enlarged.	Kidneys small and contracted. Kidney functioning markedly impaired.

tensive encephalopathy, cerebral haemorrhage while others present with progressive renal failure.

Some patients remain in compensated stage of renal insufficiency for a long time and it may be either an intercurrent infection or acute exaggeration of the disease that breakdown of renal functions develops. On an average survival is 5-10 years between the onset of first symptoms and death.

Treatment:

1. Rest in bed if acute exaggeration of symptoms.
2. Avoid any infection and it should be promptly treated.
3. Diet. Unnecessary restriction in diet is not desirable. Normal intake of salt is permitted.

Minimum 25 g of proteins in diet daily must be given. Adequate amount of carbohydrates be taken. Many patients may have loss of appetite. So preferably give a diet, which is nutritious and palatable.

4. In patients who are having nausea vomiting, and are unable to take food, intravenous glucose 10% should be given, at least 1000 ml perday to maintain hydration and nutrition. For nausea, Injection Metoclopramide/Stemetil as and when required.

5. Anabolic hormones to prevent protein catabolism in body. Injection Nandrolone phenylprop (25 mg/ml) be given twice a week.

6. Hypertension should be treated with antihypertensive drugs.

7. Any complication developing has to be managed accordingly.

8. In patients with progressive renal failure, renal dialysis done at frequent intervals may alter course of disease.

9. In some cases depending on the stage of disease process. Renal transplantation may be considered.

ACUTE RENAL FAILURE

Functional impairment of kidney characterised by reduction in glomerular filtration rate developing acutely over a period of days or weeks is called acute renal failure (ARF). Causes can be renal, pre-renal or post renal.

Pre-renal causes. These mainly include causes which produce sudden reduction in renal blood flow which results in reduced glomerular filtration rate and decreased excretion of solutes.

1. Causes include condition where there is loss of body fluids. Such as acute dehydration, vomiting, diarrhoea, haemorrhage.

2. Conditions where blood supply to kidneys is effected and it is unable to excrete waste products such as in shock, Septicemia, peripheral circulatory failure, prolonged hypotension, congestive failure.

Renal causes. These include conditions which produce severe functional changes due to acute structural damage of the kidneys because of intrinsic involvement. The various diseases in this group are acute glomerulonephritis, collagen disorders (disseminated lupus erythematosus, polyarteritis nodosa) diabetic glomerulosclerosis, malignant hypertension, eclampsia, acute tubular necrosis following shock, poisoning with heavy metals such as mercury, lead, Endogenous substances such as porphyrins, acute cortical necrosis following abortion, and extensive surgery with inadequate blood replacement.

Causes of acute renal failure

1. *Prerenal.* Acute dehydration, vomiting, diarrhoea, haemorrhage, shock, septicaemia, hypovolaemia, peripheral circulatory failure, hypotension, congestive heart failure.

2. *Renal.* Acute glomerulonephritis, collagen disorders, diabetic glomerulosclerosis. Malignant hypertension, acute tubular necrosis, acute cortical necrosis. Rapidly progressive glomerulonephritis (RPG).

3. *Postrenal.* Bilateral or unilateral obstruction of urinary tract at any site.

Post renal causes. These include diseases leading to obstruction of urinary tract (bilateral pelvic or ureteric obstruction or unilateral obstruction to a single functioning kidney).

Of all the various causes acute tubular necrosis, obstructive uropathy and glomerulonephritis are the most important one.

Course of acute renal failure

1. Oliguric phase
2. Diuretic phase
3. Postdiuretic or recovery phase

Clinical features. These are of the underlying disease. Acute renal failure can present in three phases.

Oliguric phase. This is the initial phase and often remains unrecognized for some time. The amount of urine passed decreases and even comes down to less than 100 ml in 24 hours. There is reduction in renal blood flow whereas glomerular filtration rate falls drastically. Urine is concentrated containing debris of necrosed tubular cells and breakdown products. There is retention of body's waste products. Blood urea, creatinine, phosphates and potassium levels go up. Rise in potassium levels may cause cardiac arrest. Anaemia develops due to bone marrow depression and haemolysis.

Because of loss of regulatory functions, sodium along with water is retained. Breathing becomes acidotic. Hypertension and oedema develops. Fluid over load may cause rise in jugular venous pressure, breathlessness and pulmonary oedema.

As blood urea levels go up patient complains of nausea, vomiting and gradual clouding of consciousness. Rise in potassium levels (hyperkalemia) and fall in calcium levels produce restlessness, parasthesia and cardiac irregularities. Patients in oliguric phase are more prone to get infections. Oliguric phase may last for 2-3 weeks and if recovery does not take place, prognosis becomes poor.

Diuretic phase. The onset of this phase heralds increase in the urinary output along with renal blood flow and glomerular filtration rate. Because of inadequate tubular functioning uncontrolled loss of water and electrolytes occur leading to hyponatremia, hypokalemia and dehydration. Patient now passes large volume of urine and at the height of diuretic phase daily urine volume may even go up to 4-6 litres per day. Patient does have a sense of well being. Nausea and vomiting cease. Appetite improves, Blood urea levels start coming down. The duration of diuretic phase is roughly as that of oliguric phase. Within a period of 2-3 weeks, the urine volume decreases and urinary concentration increases.

Post-diuretic phase. This stage develops gradually following diuretic phase. Renal functions almost improve completely. Renal blood flow, glomerular filtration rate and tubular functions return. This stage is variable and it may last from few months to a year. Though recoveory is substantial but some degree of renal impairment may persist.

Diagnosis of acute renal failure can be made if one is aware of the condition. This should be suspected in all conditions (pre renal, renal and post renal) where patient presents with oliguria and evidence of azotemia. Confirmation of diagnosis is made by urine examination, Biochemical tests (blood urea, serum creatinine, electrolytes), and ultrasonography of abdomen.

Treatment:

1. First confirm whether acute renal failure has developed and oliguria is not due to urinary obstruction. For this catheterize the bladder. If there is any obstruction in the urinary tract it should be relieved by cystography and even by nephrostomy.

2. In cases with pre renal failure, attempt should be made to correct the fluid balance, and induce urinary flow. This may be done by judicious administration of intravenous fluids and giving intravenous Frusemide.

3. Once oliguric phase has developed, total daily intake of fluids is limited to 500 ml plus the amount of urine passed in the last 24 hours as well as that lost by perspiration. Maintain daily fluid input and output chart. Overhydration must not be permitted. Sodium intake is restricted. Monitor potassium levels serially as well as by electrocardiographic control.

   Withdrawl of potassium from food and drinks is advised. Potassium levels are lowered by intravenous infusion of 20% glucose with soluble insulin (one unit of insulin for every 2 gm of glucose). On an average 500-1000 ml of glucose solution containing insulin is administered in 24 hours. Administration of sodium bicarbonate corrects acidosis (100 ml of 20% sodium bicarbonate solution intravenously).

4. Since the amount of fluids to be given is limited, problem of nutrition rises. Diet should contain high calorie carbohydrates (glucose water, soft cooked sweetened rice, mashed potatoes, boiled vegetables). Proteins are restricted but as the condition improves, little amount is permitted (15-20 g per day).

5. Anabolic hormone (durabolin) given on alternate days reduces the rate of protein catabolism.

6. For vomiting control it by metoclopromide, or prochlorperazine.

7. If there is any infections it should be treated. Dosage of antibiotics has to be less than the usual. All nephrotoxic drugs must be avoided. Some advise prophylactic use of antibiotics.

8. If the disease progresses and there is no improvement evidenced by progressive renal failure, vomiting, cerebral irritation, blood urea levels exceed 400 mg. Serum potassium levels exceed 7 meq/l, indications for dialysis

are there and either peritoneal or haemodialysis be undertaken.

9. For patients in diuretic phase, liberal intake of fluids, sodium and potassium is permitted. Diet is advised to be as normal as possible. Proteins in diet are allowed. Monitor patient for any signs of dehydration, electrolyte imbalance (hypotension, weakness, irritability, restlessness).

Prognosis. *Prognosis of a case of acute renal failure shall depend on:*

1. Underlying condition responsible for it.
2. Presence of complications.
3. Intercurrent infections.
4. Response to treatment.

Progressive rise in blood urea, disturbances in electrolytes and non-responsiveness to treatment carry poor prognosis.

CHRONIC RENAL FAILURE

Persistent impairment of tubular and glomerular function of gradual onset so that kidneys are unable to maintain their normal physiological functions constitutes chronic renal failure. It consists of three stages. First or initial stage where there is reduction of renal reserve and the second stage of impaired tubular concentrating power characterized by polyuria, increased frequency of urination and thirst. In the final stage there is failure of glomerular function and now as biochemical alterations take place, symptoms of renal failure manifest.

Aetiology. A number of conditions are known to produce chronic renal failure. Main diseases shall be:

1. Chronic glomerulonephritis
2. Chronic pyelonephritis
3. Diabetic nephrosclerosis (K.W. syndrome)
4. Collagen disorders (polyarteritis nodosa, disseminated lupus erythematosus).
5. Obstruction of the urinary tract (bilateral renal calculi, ureteric obstruction, prostatic obstruction).

6. Polycystic kidneys
7. Amyloid disease of kidney
8. Radiation nephropathy.
9. Multiple myeloma

Causes of chronic renal failure

1. *Renal.* Chronic glomerulonephritis, chronic pyelonephritis, diabetic nephrosclerosis (KW syndrome). Polycystic disease of kidney, obstruction of urinary tract (renal calculi, ureteric or prostatic obstruction), amyloid disease of kidney, radiation nephropathy.
2. *Systemic diseases.* Malignant hypertension, collagen disorders (disseminated lupus erythematosus, Polyarteritis nodosa) Multiple myeloma.

Clinical features. Cases of chronic renal failure may remain asymptomatic for a long time and it is often either an intercurrent infection or exaceberation of the disease process or some complications which draw attention to the patients illness. Symptoms are varied and involve all the major systems of body.

Patient has got marked weakness, lethargy and restlessness. There is anorexia, nausea and vomiting. Sleep rhythm is disturbed. Nausea, retching is most marked in the early hours of morning. Patient develops revulsion towards food. Dehydration is invariably present.

Neurological features include headache, lassitude, neuropathy, muscular weakness. In those with severe degree of hypertension, convulsions, muscular twitchings, irritability and in late stages of renal failure, loss of consciousness even leading to coma. Hypertension is invariably present in chronic renal failure. Patient may develop hypertensive heart failure, myocarditis or pericarditis. Uraemic pericarditis is often a terminal event.

Patient has acidotic breathing (Kussumaul). Repeated chest infections are common. Uraemic lung develops soon. Skin has a yellowish brown pigmentation and patient complains of intractable itching. Because of disturbances in calcium metabolism (osteomalacia, osteoporosis, renal osteodystrophy) and development of secondary hyperparathyroidism, patient has aches and pains in the bones. Initially there is osteoporosis because of poor absorption of calcium and phosphate retention but later on as a result of excess parathyroid hormone activity, osteósoclerosis may develop.

Cases of chronic renal failure suffer from anaemia (reduced erythropoitein production and bone marrow depression) which is normocytic normochronic. Bleeding tendency is often present and patient may bleed from various sources.

Menstrual irregularities in women (amenorrhoea, infertility) are common while men may complain of impotence. Physical examaination reveals generally an ill looking person, anaemic, pale. Skin is sallow with a peculiar earthy colour. Tongue is brown, dry and furred. Breath has a peculiar ammoniuremic smell (uraemic fetor). Hiccough is present. Breathing is acidotic (Kussumaul breathing). Hypertension is invariably present. Signs of uraemic pericarditis may be present. In advanced stage coma is present. Physical signs shall be governed to a large extent by the underlying disease.

Biochemical abnormalities. Cases of chronic renal failure show biochemical abnormalities when renal function has deteriorated to less than 35 per cent of the normal. There is impaired ability to eliminate hydrogen ions which results in systemic acidosis with resultant fall in plasma pH and bicarbonate levels. There is failure to adjust to changes in sodium and potassium with the result that a persistent negative sodium balance occurs while there is tendency for potassium retention whose levels go up. There is little or no calcium absorbed from the gut, urinary excretion of calcium falls to low levels. Thus patients with chronic renal failure develop osteomalacia, osteitis fibrosa and osteosclerosis. There is wide spread decalcification of bone so a rise in plasma alkaline. Phosphatase levels occurs. Hypocalcaemia producing tetany is often present.

The blood urea and creatinine levels rise due to diminished glomnerular filtration. Rise in uric acid, phenol derivatives, nitrogenous metabolites and urochromogen (responsible for dirty yellow pigmentation of skin) takes place. Anaemia develops due to bone marrow depression, reduced erythropoietin production, haemolysis and haemorrhage.

Investigations:

1. Urine. Specific gravity is low (less than 1.012) and fixed. Albuminuria is present. Microscopically there are RBCs and granular casts.
2. Blood urea, serum creatinine, serum uric acid, alkaline phosphatase levels are increased while serum calcium and bicarbonate levels are low.
3. Ultrasonography may reveal a small sized contracted kidney.
4. Intravenous pyelography (double contrast) is helpful in assessing functioning of the kidney.
5. Renal biopsy is helpful especially when a precise histological diagnosis is required.

Management. The aim is to delay the progression of renal failure and main thought is to correct water and electrolyte disturbances, prevent endogenous breakdown of protein and retention of its end products as well as controlling blood pressure levels and improving the quality of life.

Diet. Adequate caloric intake (2500 calories) by encouraging patient to consume high caloric carbohydrate foods such as sweetened rice, sugars, sweetened biscuits, cornflour, bread etc. Restriction of dietary proteins (15-18 g per day) is esential to reduce the rate of production of nitrogenous waste products. High carbohydrate diet gives energy and so it is essential that patient takes adequate amount of calories.

Fluids and electrolytes. Patients in chronic renal failure have to maintain balance in their salt and water intake. Fluid intake should be sufficient so that patient passes at least 2-2.5 litres of urine per day. Over hyration as well as dehydration must be prevented. Salt intake has to be restricted in the presence of oedema, hypertension and congestive cardiac failure.

Intake of potassium has to be restricted. Hyperkalaemia is encountered and should be treated as early as possible. Levels of potassium are lowered by intravenous glucose infusions with insulin in drip. This causes withdrawal of potassium from the cells, the effect lasting upto 6-8 hours. If patient has acidotic breathing and bicarbonate levels are less than 15 meq/litre, I/V sodium bicarbonate is administered.

Anaemia. Anaemia in chronic renal failure requires fresh blood transfusions. It is better to use packed cells. Role of human recombinant, erythropoietin in raising haemoglobin levels has its own importance. Use of anabolic hormones is also helpful.

Renal bone disease. There is hypocalcaemia along with features of hyperparathyroidism. Calcium orally is given to act as phosphate binder from the gut. Large doses of vitamin D or D3 are given to help in the absorption of calcium from the gut. Careful monitoring of calcium levels must be done to detect hypercalcaemia. Hyperphosphatemia is controlled by advising diet low in phosphorus as well as oral aluminum hydroxide which shall bind dietary phosphates in the gut.

Hypertension. Control of hypertension is essential since it shall worsen the renal failure as well as produce various complications. Angiotensin converting enzyme (ACE) inhibitors are the one which are preferred for treating renal hypertension. If congestive heart failure, then digoxin along with diuretics be prescribed.

Treatment of complications:

1. Nausea, vomiting are common complications encountered. Symptomatic relief is obtained by use of Metoclorpramide or Prochlo-perazine.
2. Infections if any must be promptly treated. Dosage of drugs which are excreted by the kidneys must be at lower levels. Nephrotoxic drugs must be avoided.
3. Further deterioration of chronic renal failure can be prevented by controlling hypertension, congestive failure, Urinary tract infection or urinary obstruction must be managed correctly and treatment should be directed towards the primary renal disease producing chronic renal failure.

End stage renal failure. When the renal disease worsens and there is no help from conservative approach as well as drug therapy, this is stage of end stage renal failure and now only approaches available are either regular dialysis at frequent intervals or reanal transplantation.

DIALYSIS

It is a temporary measure to correct clinical and chemical disturbances in body due to renal failure. In this blood flows in such a way that it interacts with fluid of specific chemical composition across a semipermeable membrane of specific pore size thus allowing diffusion of chemical constituents of blood. By this method toxic products and metabolites normally eliminated by the kidney can be removed from blood. *There are two types of dialysis:*

1. Peritoneal dialysis
2. Haemodialysis.

In peritoneal dialysis, peritoneum acts as a natural semi permeable membrane, while abdominal cavity serves as a chamber for dialysis where toxic products like urea, creatinine, potassium, uric acid diffuse from the capillary bed to the peritoneal fluid. Peritoneal dialysis may be either continuous or intermittent. Through a special catheter, dialysis, fluid is introduced into the abdomen, retained for 30 minutes and then siphoned off. About twenty such cycles are repeated in each session. Efficiency of peritoneal dialysis depends on various factors like dialysate volume, its flow rate, dwell time, peritoneal blood flow and the effective surface area of the peritoneal membrane.

Haemodialysis requires the use of hemodialyser or artificial kidney and blood is perfused through a thin film made of cellulose acting as a semi permeable membrane. For haemodialysis a fistula is created, blood drawn from an artery and after passing through a dialyser is returned to the patients vein by another canula. As a result of diffusion of blood and dialysis fluid, the blood chemistry is brought to normal levels. For haemodialysis usually two to three sittings per week are required.

Indications for dialysis:

1. Acute renal failure or acute on chronic renal failure.
2. Failure of conservative treatment in chronic renal failure.
3. Persistent nausea, vomiting, drowsiness and stupor.
4. Deterioration of general condition despite on treatment.
5. Blood urea levels more than 200 mg %. Serum potassium more than 6.0 mEq/litre. Plasma bicarbonate levels less than 12 mEq/L.
6. Anuria not responding to treatment.
7. To prepare patient of chronic renal failure for renal transplantation.
8. Maintenance dialysis for end stage renal failure.

Complications of dialysis. Though dialysis is comparatively a safe procedure yet a number of complications may develop.

1. Infection or sepsis at the site of shunt which may also get blocked. Thrombosis, aneurysm formation may also occur.
2. High incidences of septicaemia, hepatitis and septic embolisation associated with shunt and fistula infection. Blood loss may be there.
3. Dialysis disequilibrium syndrome due to rapid correction of biochemical abnormalities in plasma causing cerebral oedema characterised by headache, vomiting and occasional fits. Depression and altered self image are common.
4. Hypertension after dialysis may be made worse by saline overload. Similarly congestive failure may be precipitated in patients with ischaemic and hypertensive heart disease. Pericarditis occurs in small percentage of cases.
5. Heparin which is used during hemodialysis may produce complications such as subdural haematoma and bleeding at various sites.
6. Peripheral neuropathy and psychiatric problems may arise on long term dialysis.

In sum total dialysis does improve longevity in patients of chronic renal failure ranging from 5-20 years. Deaths in most of the cases are due to cardiovascular diseases.

RENAL TRANSPLANTATION

It is the form of treatment in cases of end stage renal failure where a healthy kidney obtained from a living person or cadaver is transplanted into the patient. The blood group of the donor (ABO) and HLA antigens are the one whose tissue compatibility is matched before a transplant is proposed.

Transplantation is usually restricted to patients between the ages of 15 and 50 years but any age is considered provided the tissue compatibility is there and there are no major contraindications. Better results are obtained when a kidney is obtained from a close relative. Rejection of the transplant is a major hazard. Patient has to be on long term immunosuppression (use of prednisolone and azathioprine). Cyclosporine A is now replacing Azathioprine.

The major complications of renal transplantation are:

1. Rejection
2. Drug toxicity and infections.

Rejection of a grafted kidney may be acute, hyper acute or chronic. Early diagnosis of rejection is essential. Patient gets fever, oliguria, swelling and tenderness over allograft. Rising levels of serum creatinine and decreased creatinine clearance are biochemical parameters of rejection. In cases where process of rejection of graft can not be reversed, attempt should be made to save the patient. After irreversibility of graft rejection is confirmed, graft is taken out and patient put on maintenance dialysis while waiting for another graft.

Since patients are on long term immunosuppressive drugs, there are chances of systemic infection developing. Rejection of graft basically takes place during the first six months. Cases with chronic rejection develop slow deterioration of renal failure. Overall renal transplantation is successful in about 75 per cent of patients with end stage renal failure. Survival after transplantation is variable. It is five year survival in more than 90 per cent of cases where donor is identical twin while it isfive years survival in more than 70 per cent of cases where live donor is from patients family. Lowest survival when donor is from a cadaver i.e. two years in 50 per cent and 40 per cent at four years.

A successful renal transplant not only improves survival but also quality of life of a patient of renal failure.

URINARY TRACT INFECTION

Urinary tract infections are quite common, more so in women as compared to men. They may be either acute or chronic. Recurrent urinary tract infections produce lot of morbidity.

Pyelitis is inflammation of the pelvis of the kidney and when the kidney is involved it is called pyelonephritis. When infection becomes chronic not only there is inflammation of pelvis of kidney and its calyces, there is fibrosis and destruction of renal parenchyma leaving behind a scarred kidney.

Aetiology. A variety of organisms may cause urinary tract infection, most common being E.coli, proteus, streptococci, staphylococci, klebsella, pseudomonas aeruginosa and enterobactariae.

In most of the cases the infection is via the blood stream. Other modes of infection are direct spread of infection from the bowel, or ascending infection from the lower parts of urinary tract. This is because the periurethral area is heavily infested with bacteria and the bacteria may be transferred by periurethral lymphatics from lower parts such as bladder, prostate, epididymis etc. Spread of infection is more in females because of short urethra. Procedures like catheterization, cystography will facilitate the spread of infection. Another mode of infection can be spread of infection from one kidney to other, and infection occurring secondary to inflammation of appendix, gall bladder etc. because of poor host defence mechanism.

Predisposing factors:

1. Women are more prone to suffer from urinary tract infection because of short urethra, presence of bacteria in the periurethral area.
2. Lack of personal hygiene especially of genitalia, bacteria may gain entry to the urethral meatus from ano rectal region and then ascend through the urethra.
3. Persons with congenital anomalies of the genitourinary tract, renal, ureteric or vesicular calculi, polycystic kidneys, hydronephrosis, pregnancy and obstructive lesions in the lower urinary tract. Poor bladder emptying predispose to urinary tract infection.
4. Diabetics are more liable to get urinary tract infection, the incidence being higher in such people.
5. Urinary tract infection may be precipitated by vesicoureteric reflux where urine from bladder regurgitates via the ureter, and infects kidneys during the act of micturition.
6. Host defence mechanism against bacteria as well as local protective factors such as urinary flow, evacuation of bladder and urinary pH as well as prostatic secretions in men have also a role to play.

Clinical features. An isolated attack of urinary tract infection is quite common especially in women but it is the recurrent urinary tract infections which requires serious consideration. It is equally important to know that the patient does not have any congenital structural abnormalities of urinary tract, obstruction or any major renal disease coexisting. The clinical picture differs as to which part of urinary tract is predominantly involved.

Pain is the most important sign. It may be mild, constant or intense and colicky. Increased frequency of micturition and urgency are other common symptoms. Dysuria is also present in some.

In general symptoms patient may get fever coming with rigors and chills, malaise, loss of appetite and vomiting. In patients with chronic infection there are periods of acute exaceberation in addition to malaise, low grade fever, and ill health. Physical signs shall vary according to the stage at which the patient is seen. In acute cases, there is fever, tachycardia and tenderness on deep palpation in renal region. Cases with chronic urinary tract infection may have full fledged picture of chronic pyelonephritis (nocturia, polyuria, hypertension and bone pains) and even of renal failure.

Investigations:

1. Urine. A mid stream specimen is taken for examination. A heavily infected urine may look hazy to naked eye. It may have a fishy smell in E. coli infection and ammonical in proteus infection. Reaction of urine usually is acidic. Albumin is present in traces. Microscopic examination will show clumps of pus cells. Urine should be cultured for type of organisms. Colony count done and sensitivity of the organism to various drugs.
2. Plain X-ray abdomen for renal/bladder/ureteric calculi.
3. Intravenous pyelography for any congenital anomalies, calculi.
4. Ultrasonography for renal size, calculi and any other abnormality.

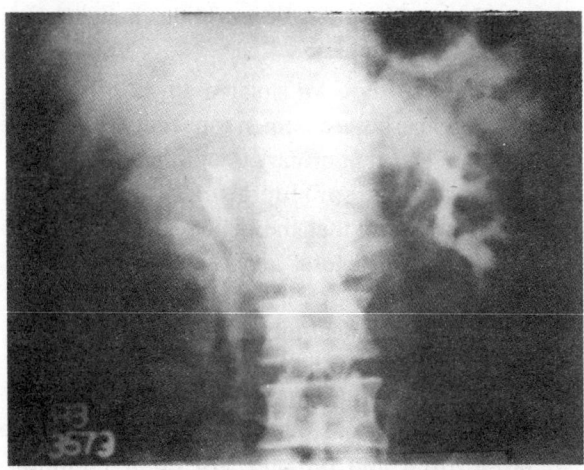

Fig. 6.3. Intravenous pyelogram showing congenital anomaly of left kidney in the form of bifid pelvis. Such patients are more liable to suffer from urinary tract infections.

Diagnosis of urinary tract infection is made in the presence of urinary symptoms, fever, toxaemia and malaise. Further confirmation by urine examination (simple and urine culture) and other relevant investigations (Plain X-ray abdomen, excretion urography and ultrasonography).

Treatment:

1. For a single attack of urinary tract infection, administration of drugs depending on the sensitivity of the organism. Most of the organisms are sensitive to Norfloxacin, Amoxycillin, Nitrofurantoin, Trimethoprim, Aminoglycosides like gentamicin and Amikacin.
2. Patient should be advised to take large quantities of fluids, and not to withold urine when urge comes so that the urinary tract is flushed out.
3. For pain, antispasmodics are to be given.
4. In patients who get recurrent urinary tract infection or do not respond to treatment, detailed investigations be done and treatment instituted accordingly.
5. In patients with impaired renal function, having urinary tract infection dosage of drugs has to be curtailed and so also nephrotoxic drugs like Gentamicin, Amikacin etc.

SYMPTOMS OF URINARY TRACT INFECTION

1. Dysuria
2. Increased Frequency & Urgency
3. Nocturia
4. Constitutional symptoms - fever, malaise, loin pain, ill health

---

FACTORS PREDISPOSING TO URINARY TRACT INFECTION

1. Advancing age
2. Pregnancy
3. Catheterisation/Instrumentation
4. Urethritis - sexually transmitted diseases
5. Vaginal infections in women
6. Pyelonephritis
7. Diabetes
8. Renal calculi
9. Bladder stones
10. Prostatitis

RENAL TUBERCULOSIS

It is an uncommon form of extrapulmonary tuberculosis and presents with varied spectrum. It is caused usually due to reactivation of a focus formed secondary to a primary pulmonary lesion. It is a disease common in the age group of 30-40 years and more common in females as compared to males.

Atieopathology: In early stage the disease is confined to one kidney. The infection is haematogenous being carried from a tuberculous focus in the body. Infection may also reach the kidney via lymphatics of the ureter. Again infection from one kidney to the other takes places by para aortic lymphatic system. There is often a long latent period between the initial pulmonary infection and clinical appearance of renal tuberculosis.

The initial lesion is a tubercle either single or multiple in the cortex or the pyramids of the kidney. There is caseation, inflammatory reaction and spread of the lesion resulting in deposition of tubercles. Complete destruction of one or more pyramids may take place and either one or more calyces or pelvis may be involved. This whole process leads to hydro or pyonephrosis. This infection may remain confined to one kidney for long periods or may spread along the urinary tracts involving ureter, bladder or genitals.

Clinical features

Increased frequency of micturition is the earliest symptom and may be the only symptom. Gradually the frequency increases and it is now more both during day time and at night. As the disease progresses, cystitis develops and there is urgency and painful micturition.

Urine may show no abnormality except for a trace of albumin. With the presence of pus it becomes opalescent but without any organisms. This urine is acid in reaction and is sterile on culture.

In small percentage of cases hematuria may be the first symptom. There is often dull pain in the lumbar region, constitutional symptoms in the form of low grade pyrexia and lassitute may be present. On examination a tuberculous kidney is not palpable though it is oedematous and friable and is more likely to be damaged by trauma. Sometimes when the kidney is enlarged it is hard, irregular and tender. Ureters are thickened and there is tenderness along its course. In male patients involvement of prostate, seminal vesicles and epididymas may take place. These should be examined for any thickening or nodules due to tuberculous involvement. These are further assessed by abdominal and rectal examination.

Investigations

Urine examination for presence of pus cells. Urine culture is generally sterile. 24 hrs urine sample is used for culture for acid fast bacilli. It is generally positive in 72% of cases while guinea pig inoculation results demonstrate higher degree of positive results (94%).

Plain X-ray abdomen. It may show calcification in kidney especially if the lesion is healing. Specks of calcification may be scattered in various parts of kidney.

Intravenous pyelography. It may show hydronephrosis. A normal urogram does not exclude urinary tuberculosis. The bladder may show ulceration and spasm of the bladder. There is loss of natural curves of the ureter due to ureteric fibrosis.

Retrograde pyelography. If renal function is poor this test is required to demonstrate. Renal pathology.

Cystoscopy. It is an important diagnositic test. Ureteric orifices are paler due to oedema and are earliest sign of bladder involvement. Tuberculous ulcers may be seen in the bladder. As disease progresses ureters may show shortening and displacement (Golf Hole ureter) and the capacity of the bladder decreases. A cystoscopic biopsy from the bladder may be taken to confirm the diagnosis.

X-ray chest. It may show a tuberculous focus in the lungs.

Management. Drug therapy is on the same lines as in case of tuberculosis anywhere in the body. General measures include good nourishing diet and adequate rest. A course of isonex & rifampacin + Ethambutol + Pyrazinamide for 3 months followed by INH + rifampacin for 9 months is given. Rifampacin has the advantage of being excreted in high concentration in urine after ingestion so it is of extra advantage in the treatment of renal tuberculosis. For patients who develop ureteric obstruction oral prednisolone in dose of 30mg / day for 6 weeks is advocated. It is followed by maintenance treatment for 10-12 weeks. If conservative treatment fails then obstruction is relieved by surgery. Sometimes construction surgery

may be required for a small contracted bladder. Follow up of patient is done in the form of urine culture and excretory urography.

Course and prognosis. Renal tuberculosis is more resistant to treatment than tuberculosis elsewhere in the body. The disease runs an uncertain course and may run for a few years.

Diseases of the Blood and Lymphatic System

INTRODUCTION

Blood constitutes major part of the body and total volume in an adult ranges from 6000-7000 ml. Blood consists of secretions as well as products of the blood forming organs. The three major constituents of blood are red blood cells white cells and the platelets. Plasma is the liquid component of blood in which these are suspended.

Formation of blood starts in the third week of intrauterine life and by second month blood cells are formed in liver and spleen. The process of erythropoiesis by 5th month is taken over by the bone marrow and after birth erythropoiesis occurs in the marrow of both long and flat bones. As the child grows there is a progressive shrinkage of marrow in long bones to be replaced by fat so that in adult life, process of erythropoiesis is in the ends of long bones (Femur: *Humerus*) and flat bones like ribs, sternum and vertebrae. The process of erythropoiesis is mainly controlled by erythropoietin, a glycoproteid hormone, produced primarily in the kidneys. The stimulus to produce erythropoietin is tissue anoxia. Erythropoietin acts on stem cells resulting in their multiplication. Thyroxine and androgens stimulate its production while female hormone oestrogen suppresses it.

The Red Blood Cell is derived from premature cell called proerythroblast which is a large cell with basophilic cytoplasm a finely reticulated nucleus containing nucleoli but with no haemoglobin. Further division results in early normoblast, a small cell with dense basophilic cytoplasm. As haemoglobin synthesis starts within them, the cell becomes polychromatic. Complete maturation of normoblasts is only reached when the cells are fully haemoglobinized and have a pyknotic nucleus. A mature erythrocyte looses its nucleus and its formation is complete.

The red blood cell is a non-nucleatid biconcave disc with a mean diameter of 7.2 microns (range 6.7 to 7.7 μ). Its shape and size is adapted to carriage of haemoglobin and supply of oxygen to the tissues. In healthy adults only mature RBCs appear in the peripheral blood. Presence of nucleated red cells indicates excessive or abnormal blood formation. The red blood cells normally are uniform in shape but in cases of anaemia certain variability in their size occurs. This is called Anisocytosis and indicates excessive activity of bone marrow Poikilocytosis indicates abnormalities in the shape of red blood cells. Normal life span of red blood cells is 120 days. As red cells age, they become malformed and get disintegrated into fragments which are engulfed by phagocytic cells of reticuloendothelial system. These malformed cells are put into circulation in great number in cases of anaemia.

Microcytosis. The average diameter of red cells is reduced and small sized cells are seen. This is characteristically seen in Iron deficiency anaemia.

Macrocytosis. The size of cell is larger than normal and is seen in megaloblastic anaemia.

Hypochromia. Red cells contain less than normal amount of haemoglobin and look pale. Seen in iron deficiency anaemia.

Normochromia. Where the red cells contain normal haemoglobin.

Haemoglobin. Red cells contain haemoglobin which is a complex molecule consisting of haem moiety and the protein called globin. Haemoglobin is formed in the bone marrow in the maturing red cells and helps in carrying oxygen to the tissues. Foetal haemoglobin (HbF) consists of two alpha and two gamma chains. After birth the synthesis of gamma chains stops and at the end of six months adult haemoglobin (HbA) is formed consisting only of two alpha chains. Persistence of foetal haemoglobin in adult life produces condition called Haemoglobinopathy.

The production of red blood cells and synthesis of haemoglobin require a number of substances mainly iron, vitamin B_{12}, folic acid, ascorbic acid, pyridoxine and riboflavin. In addition trace elements like zinc, copper, cobalt and hormones (Androgens, thyroxine) are other requirements for process of erythropoiesis.

White blood cells (leucocytes). White blod cells broadly may be divided into granular, lymphocyte and monocyte series. Their primary function in the body is to act as a defence mechanism against invasion by bacteria and other similar objects. The process involved is mainly phagocytosis and antibody formation.

The granular series mainly consists of neutrophils, eosinophils and basophils. They are derived from primitive cell myeloblast which passes into the stage of promyelocyte, myelocyte and metamyelocyte. Neutrophls, eosinophils and basophils arise from their respective myelocytes. After release from bone marrow granulocytes circulate in the peripheral blood for varying time ranging upto 10 hours before phagocytosis takes place. Metamyelocytes and neutrophils are found normally in peripheral blood but the presence of myeloblasts or myelocytes in the peripheral blood in the absence of severe infection indicates a disease of the bone marrow (Leukaemia).

Normal white cell count ranges from 4000-7500 per cmm with neutrophils comprising 66%, eosinophils 2.5%, basophils 0.5 per cent, lymphocytes 24 per cent and monocytes 7%. Leucocytosis normally occurs during late stage of pregnancy for a week to 10 days after delivery and after excercise while pathological conditions producing leucocytosis (12,000-30,000) include severe infections, septicaemia, haemorrhage or trauma, acute conditions like diabetic coma, uraemia, poisoning and malignant diseases where growth of tumour is taking place rapidly.

Polymorph or neutrophil leucocytosis. In severe fulminating infections and toxaemias where there is leucocytosis it is predominantly of neutrophils. Polymorph leucocytosis occurs in tissue necrosis, acute haemorrhage, haemolysis, severe infections metabolic disorders such as diabetic coma, acidosis. In patients with poor resistance rise in neutrophil count takes place without any increase in total white cell count and it indicates poor prognosis. In severe infections such as pneumonia, a few myelocytes may be present in peripheral blood.

Eosinophils. Eosinophils are cells with two- or

three-lobed nucleus with coarse eosinophilic granules in the cytoplasm. Eosinophils have quality of phagocytosing certain substance as immune complexes, mast cell granules etc but this activity is less than that of neutrophils.

Eosinophils are usually increased in infestations by parasites, hydatid disease, tropical eosinophilia, Loeffler's sydrome, allergic states (asthma, hay fever) and cases of drug sensitivity. Eosinophil count normally varies from 2 to three per cent. When eosinophil count rises, total white cell count does not rise. Rare conditions where eosinophilia occurs are collagen disorders and eosinophilic leukaemia.

Normal haematological values

1. Haemoglobin: men 13-15 g/dl, women 11.5-14 g/dl.
2. Red blood cells: men 5-6 million per cmm, women 4.5-5.5 million per cmm.
3. PCV: men 40-54%, women 35-48%.
4. Reticulocytes 0.2-2.5%
5. ESR: males 0-10 mm 1st hour westergren, females 0-20 mm 1st hour westergren
6. Total white cells 5000-10,000 per cumm

Neutrophils (polymorphs)	60-70%
Lymphocytes	25-35%
Monocytes	2-8%
Eosinophils	1-4%
Basophilis	0-1%

7. Platelets 2,50,000-3,50,000 per cumm.
8. Bleeding time 2-5 minutes.
9. Clotting time 4-10 minutes.
10. Prothrombin time 12-14 secs.

Basophils. They form not more than 0.5 to 1 per cent of the total white cell count. Basophilis have pale cytoplasm a bilobed nucleus and coarse basophilic granules. These cells are moderately increased in chronic myeloid leukaemia, polycythaemia vera, myxoedema, ulcerative colitis and some exanthematous fevers.

Monocytes. They are derived from primitive cell, Monoblast which is derived from reticulum cells in the spleen. Monocyte has a characteristic notched or kidney shaped nucleus and has a cloudy blue, faintly reticular cytoplasm. Their main function is phagocytosis and they may function as tissue macrophages. Normal blood count is 3-5%. Monocytes are increased during and after crisis in acute infections like typhoid, brucellosis, active tuberculosis, infective endocarditis, hodgkin's disease and monocytic Leukaemia.

Lymphocytes. These are derived from the primitive cell lymphoblast. They are formed in the bone marrow, thymus and endothelial cells lining lymphoid tissue throughout the body. Lymphocytes are either small or large. Large lymphocytes are less mature than the small and have a moderately dense nucleus with clear basophilic cytoplasm. They form 5 to 10% of the total white cell count. Small lymphocyte is round with deeply staining nucleus and very little basophilic cytoplasm. Count range from 20 to 25 per cent. Peripheral blood contains both small and large lymphocytes. Lymphocytes along with plasma cells constitute immunocytes and they play a major role in body's immune response.

Leucopenia. It means reduction in the total white cell count to below 4000 per cmm. Leucopenia occurs in typhoid fever, influenza, measles and undulant fever. Depression of bone marrow produces leucopenia and this is seen in aplastic anaemia and leucopenic leukaemia. Oral lesions in the mouth like cancrum oris, vincent's angina and ulcerative lesions do not develop till the patients immunity is low and there is depression of white blood cells.

ANAEMIA

Fall in haemoglobin levels below the normal standard values at that age and sex constitutes anaemia. Alterations in haemoglobin values lead to changes in plasma volume, erythrocyte count as well as packed cell volume. Anaemias may be classified either on erythrocyte morphology or on their etiopathogenesis.

(a) Classification of anaemia according to erythrocyte morphology

Microcytic hypochromic anaemia. Iron deficiency, haemoglobinopathies.

Macrocytic normochromic anaemia. Vitamin B_{12}, folate deficiency.

Macrocytic hypochromic anaemia (Dimorphic anaemia). Combined iron and vitamin B_{12}, folic acid.

Normocytic normochromic anaemia. Sudden loss of blood, chronic infections, myelophthistic anaemia.

b. Based on the etiopathogenesis the following classification is more complete:

1. Anaemia of diminished erythropoiesis

   a. Iron-deficiency anaemia
   b. Megaloblastic anaemia due to vitamin 12 deficiency, pernicious anaemia.
   c. Aplastic anaemia
   d. Myelophthisic anaemia

2. Increased blood loss anaemia. Acute blood loss or chronic blood loss.

3. Increased rate of red cell destruction. Haemolytic anaemias like hereditary, spherocytosis, sickle cell anaemia, glucose-6-phosphate dehydrogenase deficiency, autoimmune haemolytic anaemia, haemolytic disease of the new born (erythroblastosis fetalis).

General features in a case of anaemia. Most cases with anaemia irrespective of the cause suffer from fatigue, generalized weakness and tiredness, disinclination to work, breathlessness, palpitation and in late stages go into congestive failure. Some cases of anaemia may remain asymptomatic if their haemoglobin levels are coming down slowly, since it allows for haemodynamic compensation and oxygen carrying capacity of blood. But when blood loss occurs rapidly and body is not able to adjust, symptoms appear quickly.

Fall of haemoglobin results in reduction in oxygen carying capacity of blood and most of the symptoms in anaemia are due to this. Cardiac output rises. There is fatty infiltration in liver leading to hepatomegaly. Patient complains of loss of appetite, abdominal distension. Tachycardia is invariably present. In late stages signs of congestive heart failure appear. There is ankle oedema, cardiomegaly, systolic flow murmurs. Patient shows marked pallor, changes in nails koilonychia and hair, loss of mental alertness and parasthesia over limbs. Various signs specific to the different type of anaemia (Jaundice in haemolytic anaemia, leg ulcers in sickle cell anaemia) will be seen.

Clinical features of anaemia

Symptoms
1. Fatigue. Generalized weakness, disinclination to work, tiredness.
2. Palpitation, dysponea on exertion, congestive heart failure.
3. Anorexia, weight loss, abdominal distension.
4. Headache, giddiness, loss of mental alertness, tingling and parasthesia in limbs.

Physical signs
1. Pallor
2. Tachycardia, water hammer pulse
3. Ankle oedema
4. Cardiomegaly
5. Changes in nails (koilonychia) and hair
6. Systolic Flow murmurs across aortic and pulmonary valves.

Investigations. Any patient with anaemia should be investigated for the type and cause of the disorder by careful history, physical examination and relevant investigations.

History. *A detailed history should be taken and various factors considered:*

   1. Dietary and socioeconomic history.
   2. Worm infestations in iron-deficiency anaemia.
   3. History of bleeding piles, menorrhagia, chronic peptic ulcer, acute blood loss due to trauma, surgery, haematemesis, malaena.
   4. Malabsorption, steatorrhoea in megaloblastic anaemia.
   5. Spells of jaundice in haemolytic anaemia.
   6. History of drug intake like chloramphenicol etc. in aplastic or hypoplastic anaemia.
   7. Occupation like lead workers where chronic lead poisoning is responsible for producing chronic anaemia.
   8. History of any prolonged fever (malaria), chronic debilitating illness (tuberculosis, renal failure) malignancy.

Physical examination:

1. Pallor. Sallow colour in iron-deficiency anaemia due to hook worm infestation, waxy whiteness in acute blood loss, lemon-yellow colour of skin in haemolytic jaundice, earthy colour in anaemia due to chronic renal failure.
2. Facial pigmentation in anaemia due to malnutrition.
3. Nails. Koilonychia in iron-deficiency anaemia.
4. Tongue. Pallor and pigmentation in iron-deficiency anaemia. Glossitis and atrophy of papillae in megaloblastic anaemia.
5. Mouth. Angular stomatitis in iron and megaloblastic anaemia.
6. Necrotic and ulcerative lesions with bleeding in aplastic anaemia.
7. Splenomegaly in chronic anaemia due to malaria, haemolytic anaemia, iron-deficiency anaemia.
8. Hepatomegaly in iron and megaloblastic anaemia.
9. Chronic leg ulcers in haemolytic anaemia.
10. Peripheral neuropathy in megaloblastic anaemia.

Investigations. *Every case of anaemia should have the following investigations to detect the degree and cause of anaemia:*

1. Haemoglobin
2. Red blood cell count, P.C.V. Mean corpuscular volume and MCHC. Total and differential white cell count.
3. Peripheral blood film for type of anaemia (microcytic macrocytic) and shape of RBCs (poikilocytosis, anisocytosis) and presence of any abnormal cells.
4. Erythrocyte fragility test, bleeding time and clotting time in haemolytic anaemia.
5. Blood platelets.
6. Reticulocyte count raised in chronic haemolytic anaemia.
7. Bone marrow examination may be done when the cause of anaemia requires further investigations especially to detect the type of eryth-

ropoiesis (megaloblastic or normoblastic), cellularities of the bone marrow (aplastic anaemia) and its infiltration by malignant cells and presence of any abnormal cells (myeloma cells).

Further tests in addition to haematological investigations include:

1. Stools for parasites. Test for presence of occult blood in stools may be done in patients suspected of chronic blood loss.
2. Urine for albumin (renal disease), bile salts pigments and urobilinogen (haemolytic anaemia).
3. Gastric analysis: Histamine fast achlorhydria in pernicious anaemia, megaloblastic anaemia.
4. Studies for detecting steatorrhoea and malabsorption states (D-xylose test, fat balance study, Ba meal study of gastrointestinal tract, jejunal biopsy).
5. Ba meal study of stomach and duodenum for detecting oesophageal webs, malignancy, oesophageal varices, gastric and duodenal ulcer.
6. X-ray chest for evidence of tuberculosis or malignancy. X-ray skull (hair on end appearances in Cooley's thalassemia and sickle cell anaemia) for osteolytic and osteosclerotic lesions (multiple myloma, secondary deposits).
7. Blood chemistry: Serum proteins (total and differential) for hypoproteinaemia. Blood urea and serum creatinine levels for renal pathology.
8. Schilling test for vitamin B_{12} absorption in pernicious megaloblastic, and dimorphic anaemias. Here a small dose of radioactive B_{12} is given by mouth, followed later by a large dose of non-radioactive vitamin dose—the so-called flushing dose. In normal subjects radioactive B_{12} is excreted in the urine during the next 24 hours while in pernicious anaemia, little or no radioactive vitamin B_{12} is excreted in the urine.
9. Estimation of serum folic acid levels in blood. Figlu test is done to assess folic acid deficiency. 15 g of histidine hydrochloride is given by mouth and the urine in which it is excreted

is collected over the next eight hours. Normal excretion is 1-17 mg while in folate deficiency it is markedly increased (more than 17 mg).

Management of a case of anaemia. *It is based on:*

1. Establish the cause of anaemia and it should be treated like eradication of parasites, treatment of infections, menorrhagia, piles and any source of chronic blood loss.
2. Adequate nourishing diet containing all the nutrients (proteins, carbohydrate, vitamins, minerals).
3. Proper physical and mental rest.
4. Use of medication as per requirements of type of anaemia. When haemoglobin levels are low (below 5 gm/dl). Blood transfusions are indicated and preferably packed cells. Presence of congestive failure requires treatment with diuretics.

IRON DEFICIENCY ANAEMIA (MICROCYTIC HYPOCHROMIC ANAEMIA)

This is the commonest type of anaemia which is widely prevalent in all groups of people. It is equally common in women in the reproductive period of their life since there is loss of iron during mensturation and increased demands during pregnancy and lactation. Moreover the intake of iron containing foods is less in women as compared to men.

Causes of iron deficiency anaemia

1. Poor intake of food (due to poor economics, malignancy GI tract, anorexia nervosa).
2. Chronic blood loss. Piles, hookworm infestation, excessive menstrual loss (menorrhagia), repeated pregnancies abortions, bleeding peptic ulcer.
3. Decreased absorption of iron. Hypochlorhydria, achlorhydria, surgery of stomach (partial or complete gastrectomy).

Causes. Nutritional inadequacy because of poor socioeconomic conditions is the commonest cause. Dietary sources of iron include eggs, dry fruits, liver, meat, green vegetables and fresh fruits and there is deficient intake of these in the diet of most of people.

Blood loss. Chronic blood loss due to Hook worm infestation, piles, menstrual loss, repeated pregnancies. Heavy hookworm infestation especially with ankylostoma duodenale is an important cause of iron deficiency anaemia. Peptic ulcer is another common cause. An adult male looses 0.5-1.5 mg of iron daily in sweat and urine while in a female menstrual loss of blood is 10.5 mg/period. During pregnancy an extra 600-750 mg of iron is required. Repeated pregnancies put extra burden on the mother and unless these are met with, the woman is likely to deplete her body stores of iron.

Gastric acidity. Gastric acidity helps to keep iron in ferrous state and thus in its absorption. Presence of achlorhydria which is common in iron deficiency anaemia diminishes the absorption of iron. It is a vicious circle whether achlorhydria causes anaemia or anaemia leads to achlorhydria.

Absorption of iron. It takes place in upper part of small intestines. Iron is absorbed in ferrous form and this process is facilitated by gastric acidity, ascorbic acid while formation of insoluble complexes with phytate or phosphates decreases its absorption.

Body normally maintains a balance between iron loss and absorption. Thus when there is iron deficiency, this loss is made up from body's iron stores. When this equilibrium gets disturbed anaemia develops though this may take some time. Total body iron ranges from 4-5 g and it is made of a circulating red cell mass, ferritin, myoglobin, haem enzymes and plasma iron. Iron is stored in the tissues as ferritin and serum levels of it reflect iron stores of the individual. Normal values of serum ferritin range from 40-340 ug/litre in males and 15-148 ug/litre in females. About 20-40 mg of iron per day obtained from red blood cell, breakdown is utilised for haemoglobin synthesis. Thus two thirds of total body iron circulates in the body as haemoglobin. Iron deficiency anaemia develops when the amount of iron available for haemaglobin synthesis is inadequate. Normal levels of iron are maintained in a normal healthy person but when these levels reach low levels (Serum ferritin less than 12 µg/litre)iron deficiency anaemia manifests.

Clinical features. Cases of iron deficiency anaemia may remain asymptomatic for a long time. Onset is gradual and patient generally complains of tiredness, weakness, lethargy, palpitation and breathlessness especially marked on exertion. There is loss of appetite, epigastric discomfort, sense of distension, retching and vomiting after meals. These symptoms are due to associated gastritis. A feeling of food sticking in the throat and progressive dysphagia may develop. This is due to formation of webs at the crico pharyngeal junction (Plummer-Vinson syndrome—anaemia glossitis, dysphagia, koilonychia, cricoid webs).

Physical signs in a case of iron deficiency anaemia are classical. There is generalized pallor, sallow face, brittle grey hair, nails brittle, hollow and depressed having typically spoon shaped appearances (koilonychia). Tongue is pale, papillae are atrophied and a bald tongue may result. Glossitis, and angular stomatitis are present in majority of cases. Splenomegaly is present in small percentage of cases. Liver may also become palpable. Other signs of nutritional deficiency may also be present. As disease progresses oedema over dependent parts appears and signs of congestive heart failure develop.

Because of presence of achlochydria though it is not histamine fast, loss of appetite, dyspepsia and constipation may be present.

Investigations:

1. Blood. Haemoglobin levels are reduced and often red blood cell count is little below normal. Peripheral blood film shows hypochromia, microcytosis, poikilocytosis and anisocytosis. White cells and platelets are normal. Presence of eosinophilia points to helminthic infection. Reticulocytes are within normal limits or mildly increased (2-3 per cent). An occasional normoblast may be seen.

2. Serum iron levels are low and generally below 80 µg/dl (normal 80-120 µg/dl). Serum ferritin levels are important index of stored iron in the body. In iron-deficiency states these fall below 12 µg/litre.

3. Bone marrow shows erythroid hyperplasia with absence of stainable iron.

Clinical features of iron deficiency anaemia

1. **Tiredness, weakness, lethargy, loss of appetite, abdominal distension, epigastric discomfort, palpitation, breathlessness on exertion.**
2. **Pallor, sallow complexion, angular stomatitis, flattening (platynychia) or spoon shaped nails (koilonychia).**
3. **Tongue pale, papillae atrophied (bald tongue), glossitis, hepatosplenomegaly.**
4. **Dysphagia, cricoid webs (Pulmmer-Vinson syndrome)**

Complications and sequlae. Cases of anaemia are more prone to infections since their immunity is low and even a mild illness may take a more serious turn. Cases of Plummer-Vinson syndrome are known to develop carcinoma of the hypopharynx in a number of years.

Diagnosis of iron deficiency anaemia is based on clinical history, physical findings and laboratory investigations.

Treatment. Basically it is aimed at correcting the anaemia and treating the cause responsible for it.

Aim should be to provide good nourishing diet with supplementation by foods rich in iron (meat, liver, green vegetables, fresh fruits).

Medical treatment consists in administering Ferrous sulphate orally (300 mg tablet) three times a day after meals. Other iron salts such as Ferrous fumerate (200 mg). Elemental iron (Ferrous glycine sulph) 50 mg and ferrous gluconate (200 mg) also can be given three times a day. Ferrous sulphate is an effective drug and levels of haemoglobin start rising quickly (1 per cent per day). Side effects include nausea, vomiting, diarrhoea and constipation. To reduce side effects the drug should be given after food.

In cases where anaemia is very severe (haemoglobin less than 3 g/dl) fresh blood transfusion or better packed cells are administered.

Where patient is unable to tolerate oral iron and there is emergent need to administer iron, injectable iron in the form of iron dextran and iron sorbitol citric acid complex are commonly employed. Iron sorbitol cit. acid complex equivalent to 75 mg elemental rion per 1.5 ml in the dose of 1.5 mg/kg body weight is given deep intramuscularly in gluteal region daily as long as haemoglobin levels do not reach proper levels.

Intravenous infusion of total dose of iron dextran dissolved in 5% glucose or normal saline given slowly is employed. Although a satisfactory response is obtained but intravenous iron has got major side effects like anaphylactic shock, chest pain, respiratory distress, circulatory collapse and even death.

Use of intravenous iron is now discarded. Intramuscular iron produces local reactions at the site of injection and side effects include headache, fever, arthralgia, tachycardia and circulatory collapse. There is also danger of developing sarcoma at the site of injection after 5-10 years. Response to iron therapy should be monitored by estimating haemoglobin levels and reticulocyte count which levels shall start rising after therapy is started.

Prognosis. If a patient of iron deficiency anaemia is treated adequately prognosis is good. Improvement in the condition of the patient must be maintained by iron supplements continued for a period of six months to one year. This assumes significance in young women, pregnant and lactating women, young infants and children as well men in prime of their youth.

MACROCYTIC ANAEMIA

It is a common nutritional anaemia seen in our country and is characterised by large size of red blood cells which are fully haemoglobinized. A large number of persons suffer from associated iron deficiency. Result is dimorphic anaemia where macrocytes are hypochromic. Commonest cause of macrocytic anaemia is deficiency of folic acid and vitamin B_{12}. Impaired DNA synthesis due to absence of these vitamins results in megaloblastosis. Cell division is effected but with an increased ratio of RNA to DNA, synthesis of cytoplasm develops normally, the cells grow more in between mitotic cycles and assume bigger shape.

Macrocytic anaemias are almost synonymus with megaloblastic anaemias and are often associated with iron deficiency (dimorphic). Bone marrow generally shows megalobastic erythropoiesis and sometimes normoblastic erythropoiesis.

Megaloblastic anaemia. Most megaloblastic anaemias are due to folic acid or vitamin B_{12} deficiency and often as a result of both of these. Most of the morphological changes in the red blood cells are reflection of intracellular biochemical abnormalities which interfere with DNA synthesis which itself are due to deficiency of folic acid and or vitamin B_{12}. Megaloblastic anaemia results from a number of causes which include defective dietary intake, defective absorption, increased loss of these vitamins or increased body requirement or the presence of antagonists acting singly or in combination.

Megaloblastic anaemia due to folate deficiency. Folates are widely prevalent in many food stuffs which form part of our daily diet and these are green leafy vegetables, fruits, grains and animal products. Folates are heat labile and the folate content of the diet is influenced by the method of cooking. Prolonged cooking results in loss varying from 50 to 90 per cent. A normal adult has sufficient body stores to prevent the development of folate deficiency anaemia for four to five months even in the absence of dietary folates. The daily requirement of folic acid in an adult is 50-100 µg. It is sufficient to maintain state of equilibirum. Requirement are increased manifold during periods of rapid growth, pregnancy and in the presence of infections.

Because of the wide distribution of folates in food, dietary deficiency of folic acid does not occur unless there is some complicating factor or food intake is very poor. A great percentage of children with protein caloric malnutrition may present with folate deficiency megaloblastic anaemia. Dietary deficiency of folic acid plays important part in the pathogenesis of this condition.

Folate deficiency. Folate is absorbed maximally in the upper part of small intestines. Assimilation of adequate amount of folic acid is dependent to a large extent on the nature of diet and its means of preparation. Folate malabsorption may occur in cases where there is extensive resection of the upper part of small intestines, in malabsorption syndrome, tropical sprue, and uncommonly due to congenital causes.

Commonest cause of increased folate requirement and of folate deficiency megaloblastic anaemia is pregnancy since large amount of folate are needed by the growing foetus. Other conditions which put increased demands of folate include chronic infections, cirrhosis liver, rheumatoid arthritis, skin and neoplastic diseases. Patients with chronic alcoholism frequently have a folate responsive megaloblastic anaemia. This is partly due to decreased folate intake but factors like inteferance with folate absorption and its metabolism also play their role. Chronic use of drugs like amethopterin (methotrexate) pyrimethamine, anticonvulsants like barbiturates, diphenylhydantoin sodium and primidone also produce relative deficiency of folate and are associated with folat responsive megaloblastic anaemia.

Megaloblastic anaemia due to vitamin B$_{12}$ deficiency. Vitamin B$_{12}$ is an important vitamin which affects DNA synthesis by a secondary effect on folate metabolism.

The daily requirements of vitamin B$_{12}$ are not much and an adult may require not more than 0.1 to 1 µg/day. Body stores of the vitamin vary in extent according to average dietary intake. All naturally occurring vitamin B$_{12}$ is ultimately derived from bacterial synthesis. Vitamin B$_{12}$ taken with the diet is liberated by the digestive processes and combines with the intrinsic factor secreted by the gastric parietal cells and this vitamin passes down the intestines and is absorbed in the lower part of small intestines.

Deficiency of vitamin B$_{12}$ can be due to various causes and produces megaloblastic anaemia.

Deficiency of vitamin B$_{12}$. Deficiency of vitamin B$_{12}$ occurs in children born of vitamin B$_{12}$ deficient mothers. Infants who are breast fed by such mothers and receive no other nutritional supplement are likely to suffer from its deficiency. Older children and adults commonly do not have deficiency of vitamin B$_{12}$, since normally it is met from dietary sources except in few cases where diet is poor or the vitamin B$_{12}$ is not being absorbed or its requirements are more.

Any factor which leads to defective secretion of intrinsic factor shall also produce vitamin B$_{12}$ malabsorption. This includes cases of chronic gastritis and partial or total gastrectomy where there is defective secretion of intrinsic factor either because of disease or removal of parietal cells leading to intrinsic factor deficiency.

Vitamin B$_{12}$ malabsorption occurs in patients with lesions of the small intestines as in cases of blind or stagnant loop of small intestines where stasis of intestinal content or their contamination interferes with its absorption. This occurs in cases of intestinal diverticula, gastrojejunostomy and intestinal strictures. Extensive resection of ileum where vitamin B$_{12}$ is primarily absorbed will produce deficiency of the vitamin. But still the commonest cause of vitamin B$_{12}$ deficiency is malabsorption syndrome and tropical sprue.

Further where there are increased demands of vitamin in periods of rapid growth and pregnancy deficiency of the vitamin may occur in persons who already have low stores of it in their body. Infestation with fish tape worm (diphylobothrium latum) will also interfere with vitamin B$_{12}$ absorption and cause megaloblastic anaemia. This worm infestation is more common in Scandinavin countries and not seen in India.

Clinical picture. Cases with mild deficiency of folic acid and vitamin B$_{12}$ may have no symptoms. It is only patients with moderate to severe deficiency who have symptoms in the form of generalized weakness, lethargy, malaise, anorexia, weight loss, glossitis, irritability, diarrhoea or constipation, lack of concentration, hyperpigmentation of skin and symptoms of nervous system involvement in the form of neurologic pains and dementia.

Physical examination shows pallor, a beefy tongue, glossitis, dark pigmentation over the hands, feet, face and exposed surfaces of body, and a mild degree of hepatosplenomegaly. Neurological involvement predominantly with vitamin B_{12} deficiency include peripheral neuropathy and optic neuritis. Involvement of posterior and lateral columns of the spinal cord results in picture of subacute combined degeneration of the cord.

Causes of folic acid deficiency

1. Deficient intake of folate due to poverty, ignorance.
2. Protein caloric malnutriton—kwashiorkor
3. Folate malabsorption:
   a. Congenital defect
   b. Intestinal resection
   c. Tropical sprue
   d. Coeliac disease
4. Increased folate requirements
   a. Pregnancy
   b. Chronic infections
5. Folate antagonists:
   a. Alcohol
   b. Anticonvulsant drugs
   c. Oral contraceptives

Investigations:

Peripheral blood. Haemoglobin levels are reduced while MCHC is normal. MCV is increased. Red blood cells are larger than normal (Macrocytes) and have full complement of haemoglobin uniformily. Some red cells may show punctate basophilia. Nucelar material present in erythrocytes goes by the name of Howel-Jolly bodies and Cabot's rings.

There is anisocytosis and poikilcytosis, while blood cell count is reduced (neutropenia) with hypersegmentation of the polymorphonuclear cells. Platelet count is reduced (thrombocytopenia)

Bone marrow. There is alteration in the morphology of red blood cells which appear nucleated. Bone marrow is hyperplastic with erythyroid hyperplasia. All stages of megaloblastosis

ranging from most abnormal to early changes may be seen. In addition white cells also show changes in the form of delayed maturation, the presence of giant metamyelocytes and hypersegmented polymorphs. In the presence of associated severe iron deficiency, the megaloblastic changes in the bone marrow may be absent or delayed and appear only after start of iron therapy.

Causes of vitamin B_{12} deficiency

1. Deficient vitamin B_{12} intake.
   a. Children breast fed by vitamin B_{12} deficient mothers
   b. Poor diet due to poverty, ignorance.
2. Defective absorption due to intrinsic factor deficiency.
   a. Chronic gastritis
   b. Gastrectomy—total or partial
   c. Pernicious anaemia.
3. Defective absorption due to small intestine disorders.
   a. Fish tapeworm infestation
   b. Blind loop syndrome
   c. Ileal resection
   d. Tropical sprue
   e. Congenital B_{12} malabsorption
4. Increased vitamin B_{12} requirements.
   a. Pregnancy

Biochemical investigations:

1. Serum folate levels: Levels of serum folate and red cell folate are considerably diminished and are usually below 3 ng/ml (normal 6-20 ng/ml) in serum and 100 ng/ml in red blood cells (normal 160-650 ng/ml).
2. Serum vitamin B_{12} level: Levels below 80 pg/ml indicate deficiency of the vitamin (normal above 155 pg/ml).

   In a patient with megaloblastic anaemia, a low serum vitamin B_{12} level with normal folate levels indicates vitamin B_{12} deficiency and vice versa.
3. Tests of absorption.
   Serum levels. After an oral dose of vitamin B_{12}, serum levels rise after 2 hours to reach plateau levels by 8 hours.

a. Schilling test. A small dose of radioactive vitamin B_{12} is given by mouth followed later by a large dose of non-radioactive vitamin dose—the so called flushing dose. In normal persons the radioactive vitamin B_{12} is excreted in the urine during the next 24 hours while in cases of pernicious anaemia little or no radioactive vitamin B_2 is excreted in the urine.

b. *Figlu test.* This is test of folic acid absorption and there is correlation between this test and serum folic acid activity.

15 g of histidine hydrochloride is given orally and the urine is collected over the next eight hours. Formiminoglutamic acid, an intermediate product in the breakdown of histidine appears in abnormally increased amounts in the urine in folic acid deficiency. Normal output is 1-17 mg and abnormal output is more than 17 mg.

Serum folic acid activity of less than 3 ng/ml means Figlu test positive while activity more than 6 ng/ml indicates a negative Figlu test.

c. Fat balance studies and D-xylose test for exclusion of malabsorption.

4. Barium meal study of gastrointestinal tract for evidence of malabsorption (flocculation and segmentation of small intestines).

5. Jejunal biopsy by crosby capsule to study the state of intestinal villi.

Treatment. Basic approach should be to provide nutritious diet so that dietary deficiencies are corrected.

In case there are treatable causes, treatment should be directed towards correcting that abnormality. In folic acid deficiency, folic acid 5 mg twice a day be given orally while those with vitamin B_{12} deficiency, 1000 ug of vitamin B_{12} (hydroxycobalamin) by intramuscular injection to start with daily followed by on alternate days is sufficient to correct the deficiency.

Hydroxycobalamin is better retained in the body than cyanocobalamin so it is preferable for therapy. In patients who have vitamin B_{12} deficiency in

addition to folic acid deficiency, treatment with folic acid alone shall not only worsen but also precipitate acute neurological disorders. So care should be taken in this regard. In cases of doubt, therapy with both folic acid and vitamin B_{12} be instituted. Patients with permanent absorption defects shall require therapy with these drugs almost life-long.

Pernicious anaemia (Addisonian pernicious anaemia). This term is confined to patients of vitamin B_{12} deficiency anaemia where there is genetically determined failure of intrinsic factor secretion secondary to idiopathic atrophy of the gastric mucosa.

Pernicious anaemia is uncommon amongst Indians, it has a tendency to occur in families. It is found more often in the elderly age group generally in the 5th and 6th decade of life. Both sexes are equally effected.

Patients of pernicious anaemia show increased levels of antibodies directed against parietal cells (in 80-90% of patients) and against intrinsic factor preventing the binding of vitamin B_{12}. These antibodies can be demonstrated in the serum as well as gastric juice. Probably an autoimmune mechanism is responsible for them. Patients with pernicious anaemia may have evidence of other auto immune disorders and in particular a high incidence of thyroid antibodies may be seen. A small group of patients with pernicious anaemia like disorder may have other disorders such as diseases of the thyroid (myxoedema, Hashimoto's disease, thyrotoxicosis) adrenals (Addisons disease) parathyroid and hypogamma globulinaemia.

Because of gastric atrophy there is failure of the stomach to produce intrinsic factor. Vitamin B_{12} is not absorbed from the alimentary tract. Result is pernicious anaemia which is as a result of intrinsic factor deficiency due to gastric atrophy, and lack of vitamin B_{12} absorption caused by autoimmune mechanism.

Patients of pernicious anaemia have higher incidence of carcinoma stomach as compared to other people in the same age group.

Clinical picture. The onset of disease is gradual. Clinical picture is like that of a case of megaloblastic anaemia except that neurological features are more predominant in such cases like dementia, neuropathy, posterolateral column involvement (subacute combined degeneration of the cord). There is often yellowish tinge of the skin and mucous membrane. Evidence of increased blood destruction in the form of splenomegaly and hyperbilirubinaemia and increased deposition of iron in the reticulo-endothelial system may be evident.

Investigations. Peripheral blood film shows macrocytosis, anisocytosis and poikilocytosis. Haemoglobin levels are low. There is leukopenia and thrombocytopenia. Bone marrow shows a megaloblastic reaction. Gastric analysis shows histamine fast achlorhydria. On gastroendoscopy there is picture of thinning of gastric mucosa and atrophy which is confirmed by gastric biopsy. Parietal cell antibodies are present in the serum.

Serum vitamin B_{12} levels are low. Schilling test is positivie. Whole body counting scan after administration of radioactive B_{12} orally is done. A normal result meant retention of 50 per cent or more of 1 ug dose of radioactive vitamin B_{12}.

Diagnosis of pernicious anaemia is based on clinical profile and physical findings (pallor, glossitis, parasthesia of hands and feet, splenomegaly dementia, posterior and lateral column involvement leading to ataxia).

Further confirmation is based on laboratory findings like:

1. Low serum vitamin B_{12} levels
2. Normal or elevated folate levels
3. Gastric atrophy
4. Histamine fast achlorhydria
5. Positive Schilling test.
6. Bone marrow shows a megaloblastic reaction, leukopenia with hypersegmented granulocytes.
7. Parietal cell antibodies in serum.

Treatment:

1. Diet should be nutritious, rich in proteins, iron and vitamins, consisting primarily of fresh fruits, green leafy vegetables, milk, dairy products and meat.

2. If haemoglobin levels are low, less than 5 g/dl, fresh blood transfusions be given.

3. All cases must receive 1000 µg of vitamin B_{12} intramuscularly on alternate days to start with. Response to therapy is observed by keeping a watch on reticulocyte count which rises within two to three days of the first injection of vitamin B_{12}. As improvement takes place injections are switched to weekly intervals.

   Cases of pernicious anaemia where there is intrinsic factor deficiency, the drug will have to be administered life long.

4. Folic acid is not to be given in a case of pernicious anaemia unless there is coexisting folate deficiency (as assessed by serum folate levels) since folic acid when given alone in a case of megaloblastic anaemia may precipitate neurological features.

HAEMOLYTIC ANAEMIAS

Haemolytic anaemia may be defined as anaemia caused predominantly by increase in rate of destruction of red blod cells either by cells of the reticuloendothelial system (intracellular) or within the circulating blood (intravascular). Normal life span of the red cells is 120 days and when it is shortened upto few days only and haemolysis is severe, anaemia develops. The premature destruction of the red cells may result from:

1. An intracorpscular or intrinsic abnormality of the red cells which are deformed and phagocytosed in the spleen while grossly damaged cells are destroyed in the circulation. Intravascular haemolysis is caused by trauma to the red blod cells, by fixation of complement to the red blod cells and decrease in the surface area/volume ratio of the cells.

2. An extracorpscular or extrinsic abnormality where haemolysis results due to aobnormal haemolytic mechanism which may be in the form of immune reaction (autoantibodies), acquired defects in the membrane of cells or

toxic substances acting on the red cells causing haemolysis. Most cases of acquired haemolytic anaemia have intravascular haemolysis while it is mostly extravascular in inherited form.

Clinical picture. Cases of haemolytic anaemia may present either in acute or chronic form. Acute presentation is characterised by haemolytic crisis in the form of high fever, toxaemia, marked prostration, shock and haemoglobinuria. Acute renal failure may develop.

Chronic presentation includes jaundice varying from mild to severe form, mongoloid facies, splenomegaly, chronic leg ulcers and pigment stones in gall bladder.

Investigations. Certain group of investigations are required to establish evidence of haemolysis. *These are:*

1. Serum bilirubin, rise in unconjugated bilirubin levels.
2. Excess urinary urobilinogen
3. Increase in reticulocyte count (about 5 per cent).
4. Peripheral blood film shows spherocytes and nucleated red cells in chronic form while in acute form there is leucocytosis and immature white cells in the peripheral blood. Platelets first fall and then rise above normal levels.
5. Bone marrow shows erythroid hyperplasia.
6. Serum haptoglobins levels (normal 50-150 mg/dl) are lowerd.
7. Serum lactic dehydrogoenase levels (LDH) are incresed more so in intravascular haemolysis.
8. Red cell survival studies by using 51Cr-labelled red cells, show reduced survival time.
9. Osmotic fragility: It is increased.
10. Coombs' test, direct Coombs' test is positive in immune haemolytic anaemias.
11. Detection of abnormal haemoglobins.

Classifications of haemolytic anaemias.
Inherited haemolytic disorders:

a. Red cell membrane defect e.g. hereditary spherocytosis, hereditary elliptocytosis.

b. Hereditary haemoglobinopathies (defect in globin structure) e.g. thalassemia: sickle cell disease. Abnormal haemoglobins like Hb C, D, E disorders. Unstable haemoglobin haemolytic anaemia.

c. Metabolic defects (red cell enzyme deficiencies) e.g. glucose-6-phosphate dehydrogenase deficiency. Deficiency of pyruvate kinase, hexakinase.

Acquired haemolytic anaemia:

1. *Immunologically mediated*
   a. Autoimmune haemolytic anaemia (warm antibody and cold antibody type).
   b. Isoimmune: RH incompatibility (haemolytic disease of the newborn), ABO incompatibility (incompatible blood transfusion).

2. *Non-immune haemolytic anaemia*

   a. Defect in the membrane of red cells. Haemolytic uremic syndrome, paroxysmal nocturnal haemoglobinuria, thrombotic thrombocytopenic purpura, disseminated intravascular coagulation.
   b. Mechanical causes of microangiopathic haemolytic anaemia, implantation of cardiac valve prosthesis, march haemoglobinuria.
   c. Infections like malaria, Clostridium welchii.
   d. Drugs like nitrofurantoin, sulfonamides, methyl dopa, poisons like arsenic and snake venom.
   e. Miscellaneous e.g. extensive burns, severe infections, septicaemia.

Inherited haemolytic anaemia:

Hereditary spherocytosis. It is a common hereditary disorder of red cell membrane defect and is charctrised by increased fragility of the red cells, variable degree of jaundice, anaemia, splenomegaly and the presence of spherocytes in peripheral blood. It is an autosomal dominant disorder though in small percentage of cases, neither of the parents is affected.

Pathogenesis. Though exact defect is not clear, yet it is generally accepted that the primary abnormality in such cases resides in the proteins that form the skeleton of the red cell membrane. Most of the erythrocytes have reduced membrane stability and because of this are exposed to stresses in circulation. Reduction in the surface area and membrane substance forces the cells to assume a spherical shape. These cells are unable to maintain their normal biconcave shape. Spleen plays important role in the destruction of these defective cells.

Clinical features. The clinical spectrum of the disease is variable. Many cases remain asymptomatic and the condition is diagnosed on routine examination of blood. Some cases may present with jaundice at birth while in others the features of the disease are delayed and manifest only late in life in the second and third decades of life. Presentation of the disease is in the form of anaemia, jaundice and splenomegaly. Anaemia is usually mild but is severe in cases presenting at early stage of life. Periodic exaceberations due to haemolysis occur.

Jaundice again varies from mild to moderate levels. Many suffer from recurrent episodes of jaundice.

When severe crisis develops in such cases there may be haemolytic, aplastic and megaloblastic crisis. This type of crisis is generally after intercurrent infections particularly with parvo virus. Gall stones generally pigment type may develop as a result of chronic bilirubinaemia due to haemolysis.

Chronic leg ulcers is an important complication. Splenomegaly of moderate degree is usually present but it may increase in size, become painful and tender during crisis.

Investigations. Anaemia is mild. Haemoglobin levels range upto 10 g/dl. Peripheral blood film shows spherocytosis. There is gross irregularity in the size of the cells. There is polychromasia. Red cell count is between 3-4 million per cumm. MCV and MCH are usually normal but MCHC is often slightly increased. Reticulocyte count is raised (10-25 per cent).

Electrophoresis reveals presence of only adult haemoglobin. There is no foetal haemoglobin. Osmotic fragility of the red blood cells is increased. Coomb's test is negative. In haemolytic crisis large number of normoblasts appear in the peripheral blood and there is often polymorphonuclear leucocytosis.

Diagnosis of hereditary spherocytosis is based on presence of anaemia, recurrent attacks of jaundice or long standing jaundice, splenomegaly and presence of spherocytosis in the peripheral blood. Often other members of the family are affected.

Demonstration of autohaemolysis and its correction by addition of glucose indicates that it is a red cell membrane defect and favours hereditary spherocytosis.

Complications. Haemolytic crisis is a major complication. It varies in severity lasting from a few days to a week or so. This is often brought about by some infection. There is malaise, anaemia, nausea, vomiting, fever coming with chills and rise in bilirubin levels. There is often pain in abdomen, increase in depth of jaundice, spleen enlarges in size, and becomes tender. Urine becomes dark coloured.

Treatment. Splenectomy is the treatment of choice in all patients with symptoms. Even in those patients who have no symptoms still splenectomy is advised because of risk of developing severe aplastic crisis.

In children splenectomy is better postponed till the age of 7-10 years because of risk of developing severe infections. Only when anaemia is severe and requires repeated transfusions, it is advised in young children. In such children prophylactic antibiotics (penicillin) may have to be given for long periods.

After splenectomy, though spherocytes persist in blood but there is cessation of haemolysis, jaundice disappears and the haemoglobin levels start rising. Relapse following splenectomy is rare.

Hereditary elliptocytosis. It is another form of hereditary disorder which is characterised by presence of large number of red cells which are elliptical in shape. It is inherited as autosomal dominant disorder. It is common in both males and females. Clinical pifcture is just like that of hereditary spherocytosis but of mild form. Haemolysis is present but not severe and may remain unnoticed for a long time. Only few patients require

PLATE XIII

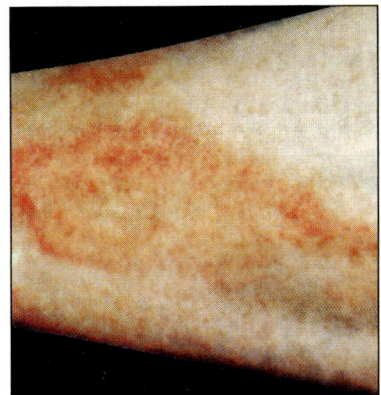

Necrobiosis lipoidica

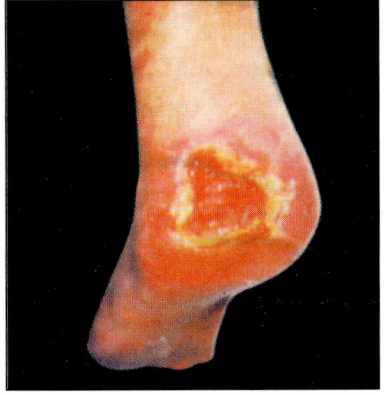

Neuropathic ulcer

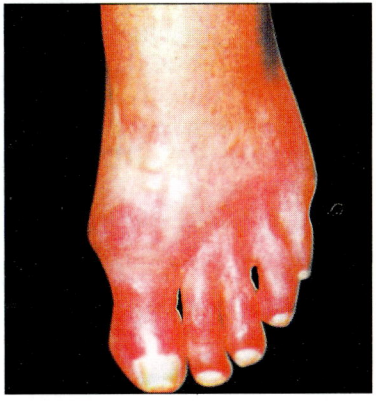

Peripheral vascular disease

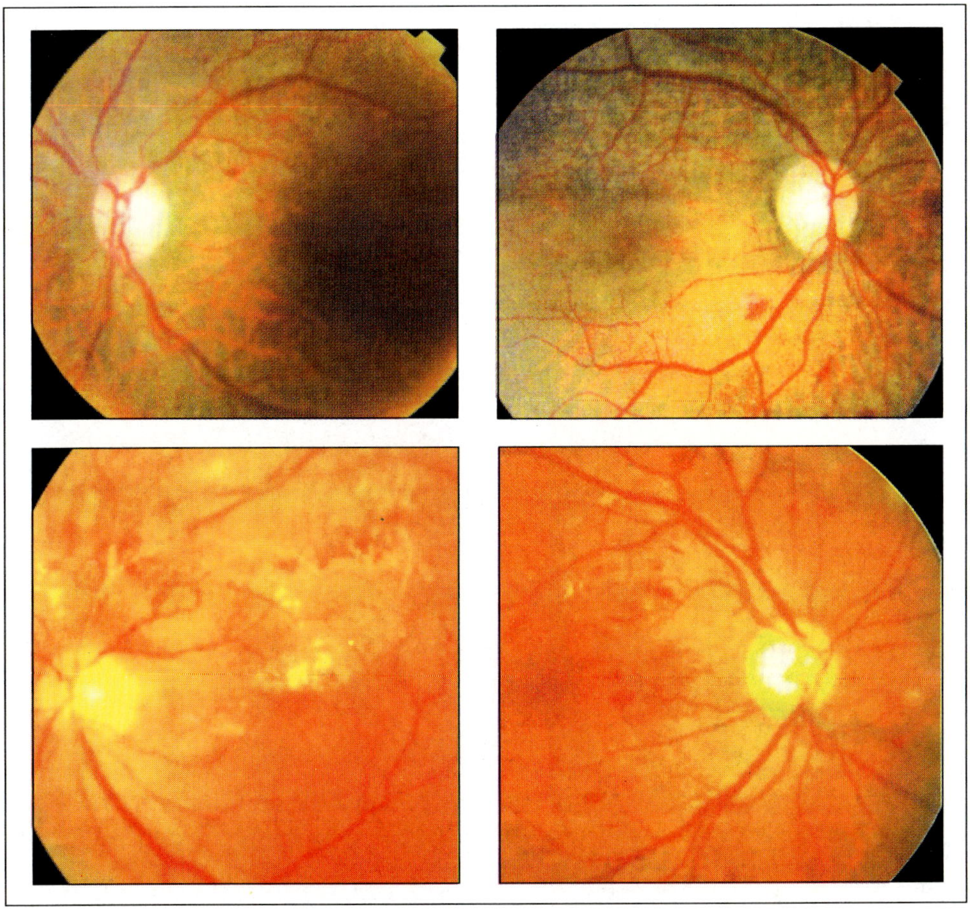

Different stages of diabetic retinopathy

PLATE XIV

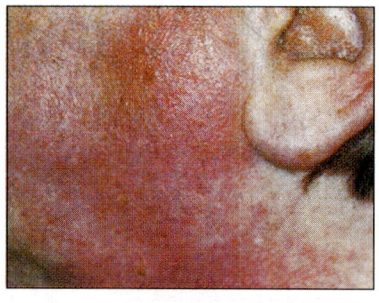

Erysipelas

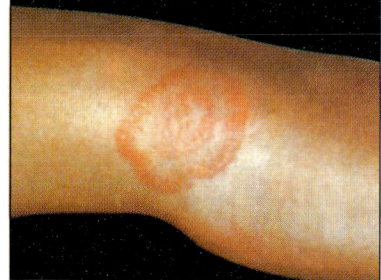

Granuloma annulare

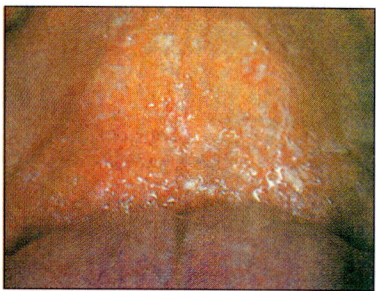

Oral candida

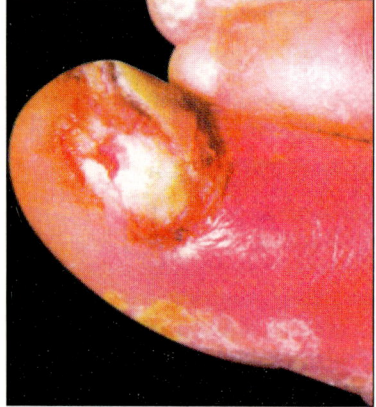

Gangrene of toe

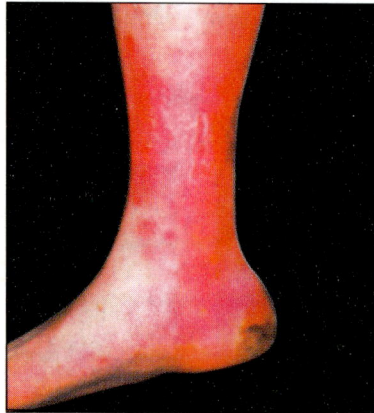

Cellulitis

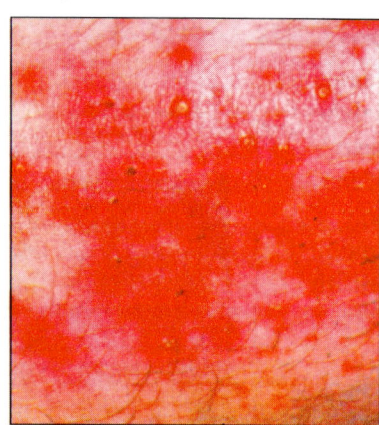

Folliculitis

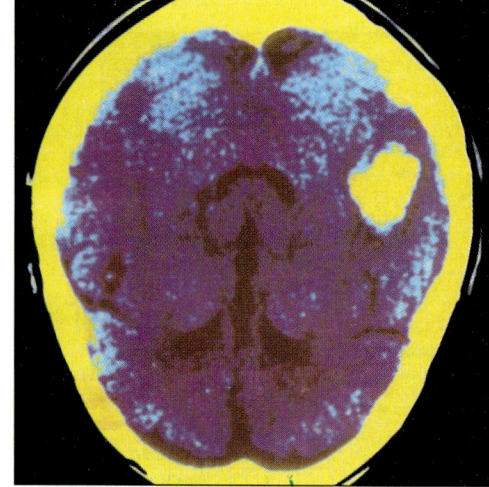

Cerebral haemorrhage

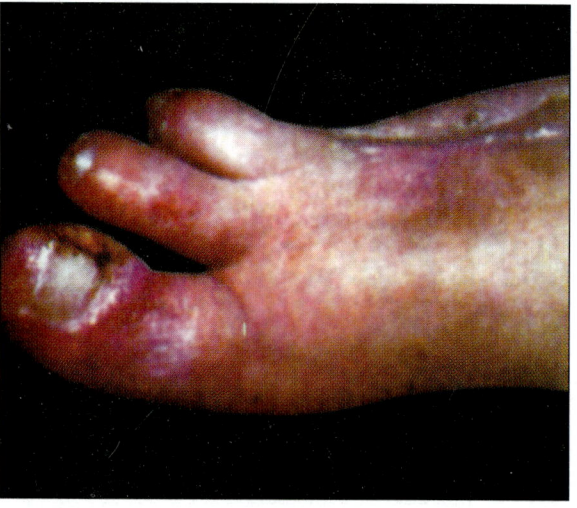

Diabetic foot

splenectomy if the condition worsens.

Hereditary enzymopathies. These are a form of non-spherocytic congenital haemolytic anaemias and include pyruvate kinase (PK) deficiency. Haemolytic anaemia, glucose-6-phospate dehydrogenase deficiency and hexokinase, glutathione deficiency anaemias.

Glucose-6-phosphate dehydrogenase (G-6-PD) deficiency. Deficiency of G-6-PD is common condition which affects people all over the world. It is sex-linked disorder being carried on the X-chromosome. It affects males though females carry the defect showing slightly lower enzyme levels.

G-6-PD deficiency may vary in intensity depending on enzyme activity. Thus where it is below 10 per cent, picture is that of chronic haemolysis while in those where functional activity of enzyme is less than 60 per cent, haemolysis occurs only after exposure to certain drugs which include analgesics (Acetylsalicylic acid, phenacetin) antimalarials, antibacterials (Sulfonamides, Nitrofurantoin, furazolidone, chloramphenicol) probenecid, P-amino-salicylic acid, quinidine, vitamin K.

Ingestion of Fava beans also produces haemolysis in such patients.

Clinical picture is variable. It may be in the form of chronic haemolytic anaemia or acute haemolysis induced by ingestion of certain drugs and exposure to acute infections. In majority of cases the disease is self limiting but in some it may be very acute, with progressive picture of anaemia, acute intravascular haemolysis, jaundice and haemoglobinuria. Rarely neonatal jaundice may be due to G-6-PD deficiency.

Investigations. These shall vary during the acute attack and in between the attack. During an attack blood film shows irregularly contracted cells (Bite and Blister cells). Heinz bodies. Reticulocytes are increased. Evidence of haemolysis is present. G-6-PD enzyme levels can be assayed and found to be reduced. There is also haemoglobinuria.

Treatment. Most cases have mild symptoms and withdrawal of the cause (stoppage of offending drug and treatment of infection) limits the disease. In cases with severe anaemia. Blood transfusions may be given. Splenectomy is not required nor is of much use. Patient should be told of the disease and warned about use of offending drugs.

Hereditary haemoglobinopathies. These are a group of clinical disorders where there is impairment of synthesis of normal adult haemoglobin due to genetically determined abnormalities. The haemoglobin in normal individuals is made up of Alpha and Beta chains. During fetal life HbF is the main haemoglobin which is suppressed within the first six months of life and there is very little haemoglobin F produced after this period, it being completely replaced by adult haemoglobin. Failure on this account results in both qualitative and quantitative abnormalities. The qualitative haemoglinopathies are characterised by production of haemoglobin molecules where there are physical and chemical alterations resulting in structural abnormality producing reduced red cell survival. These express themselves as haemoglobinopathy disease e.g. Hb-S, Hb-C, D, E, J, K and H. The qualitative haemoglobinopathies result due to defective production of either alpha or beta chains components of the adult haemoglobin and produce disorders like thalassemia and sickle cell disease.

Sickle cell disease. It is the commonest of haemoglobinopathy which results from mutation in the gene coding for the beta globulin chain that causes formation of haemoglobin S which is much less soluble than normal haemoglobin. When it is reduced due to lowered oxygen tension; the cells which contain it become markedly distorted assuming a sickle or characteristic crescent shape. Hb-S results from a single aminoacid substitution in the globin chain (valine for glutamine at the sixth position of beta chain). Hb-S is inherited as mendelian dominant and occurs predominantly among negroes or blacks. It has also been seen in people of Greece, Turkey, Middle East and tribal population of Assam, Andhra Pradesh and many others parts of India.

Sickle cell disease constitutes a number of diseases, depending on its genetic variations and these include Sickle cell anaemia (Homozygous S-

S) Sickle cell trait (Heterozygous A-S) haemoglobin S-thalassaemia, Haemoglobin S-C and S-D disease.

Sickle cell anaemia. It represents the homozygous state for haemoglobin-S. Cells which sickle have a shortened life span and trivial events may induce sufficient hypoxia to trigger a sickling crisis. Sickle cells are easily destroyed and this results in haemolytic anaemia. Factors like dehydration, sweating, fever, infections or use of diuretics provoke sickling. Because of increased viscosity of Hb-S, slowing of circulation with occlusion of microcirculation and because of rigidity and log jamming of sickled cells thrombosis in small vessels results with necrosis of tissue involved as well as a number of systems especially vascular in body also get involved.

Clinical features. These are variable and do not become apparent before 6 months of age since replacement of Hb-F by Hb-S does not take place by this age. Common symptoms are anaemia, fatigue, malaise, weakness and irritability. Anaemia generally is not very severe but growth is retarded with delay in skeletal maturation. Cases of sickle cell anaemia are of slender built, underweight and have greenish yellow icterus. Liver is moderately enlarged. The course of the disease is often punctuated by episodes of crisis which consist of painful episodes of abdominal or bone and joint pains. Abdominal pain is accompanied by constitutional symptoms like fever, toxaemia and worsening of haemolysis and anaemia. There is nausea, vomiting and attack may simulate an acute abdomen. Occlusion of cerebral vessels manifests in the form of headache, convulsions, psychic changes and even hemiplegia.

An "aplastic crisis" due to temporary cessation of bone marrow activity may come suddenly. Splenomegaly is common in children and often becomes painful. With repeated infections following thrombosis of splenic vessels, the spleen may shrink and eventually become atrophic converting into a fibrous streak. This process is called auto splenectomy and an adult case may be left with a small fibrotic impalpable spleen. Hepatomegaly may result due to infarcts. Liver becomes tender and

enzymes levels rise. Crisis in patients of sickle cell anaemia is usually triggered by infection to which these patients are highly susceptible because of impaired splenic function and failure of alternate defence pathway.

Cardiac involvement in the form of cardiomegaly, pulmonary hypertension and presence of cardiac murmurs is generally seen. Chronic leg ulcers either single or multiple are common. Gall stones, and chronic cholecystitis are seen and often cause colicky pain. Renal involvement presents with hematuria, acute nephritis and even uncommonly as nephrotic syndrome. Skeletal symptoms are bone pains, arthralgia and salmonella osteomyelitis. Blindness may result due to retinal involvement.

Investigations. Anaemia moderate to severe (Hb 6 to 9 gm/dl) is present. Exaceberation of haemolytic process causes fall in haemoglobin levels. It is usually normochromic normocytic type.

Peripheral blood film shows sickle shaped erythrocytes with poikilocytosis. A few nucleated red cells may be seen. Reticulocyte count is increased. Platelet count is either normal or moderately increased. A positive sickling test with sodium metabisulfite, a reducing substance is seen.

Tests for sickle cell anaemia

1. Haemoglobin levels low. anaemia normochromic normocytic.
2. Peripheral blood film shows sickle shaped cells with poikilocytosis, target cells.
3. Rise in reticulocyte count.
4. Platelet count is either normal or moderately increased.
5. Positive sickling test.
6. Bone marrow shows erythroid hyperplasia with normal normoblasts.
7. Confirmation by demonstration of Hb-S.

Serum bilirubin levels are increased moderately. Final confirmation of diagnosis depends on demonstration of Hb-S on electrophoresis.

Prenatal diagnosis of sickle cell anaemia can be made by analysing DNA in fetal cells obtained by aminocentesis. Bone marrow shows erythroid hyperplasia with normal normoblasts. X-rays of skeleton show rarefaction while in elderly patients there is sclerosis of long bone with cortical thickening.

Diagnosis of sickle cell anaemia is based on clinical picture of chronic haemolytic anaemia often accompanied by episodes of crisis and demonstration of sickling phenomenon and Hb-S on electrophoresis.

Course. It is variable, prognosis generally is not good. Many children do not reach adult age often dying of fulminating infection, aplastic crisis meningitis and neurological complications.

Treatment. It is supportive and aim is to prevent development of complications by avoiding severe infections, exposure to cold and stress. Small doses of folic acid daily (5 mg) are beneficial. Intercurrent infections must be treated promptly. Crisis has to be managed as emergency by intravenous fluids, oxygen, antibiotics and analgesics.

Blood transfusion is indicated when anaemia becomes severe. In patients with recurrent episodes of crisis, exchange transfusions are used. Drugs like nitrates, phenothiazines, hyperboric oxygen and corticosteroids have been used for treating sickling crisis but with variable results. ·

Prophylactic measures. These include careful genetic counselling especially when both parents have sickle cell trait. If prenatal diagnosis establishes the diagnosis of foetus suffering from the disease the pregnancy should be terminated.

THALASSAEMIA

Thalassaemia represents a group of genetic disorders of haemoglobin synthesis where there are quantitative abnormalities of globin chain synthesis. The disease may manifest in varying degrees of severity depending on the amount of HbA2 and HbF present.

According to descending order of severity thalassaemia is classified into thalassaemia major, thalassaemia intermedia, and thalassaemia minor. Thalassaemia is inherited as an autosomal condominant condition. The heterozygous form (thalassaemia minor or thalassaemia trait) is generally asymptomatic and anaemia is either mild or absent while homozygous form (thalassaemia major) is associted with severe degree of haemolytic anaemia.

Beta thalassaemia major (Cooley's anaemia). It is one of the commonest form of haemolytic anaemia which is present during the first year of life after birth. Two factors contribute to the pathogenesis of anaemia in such patients. One is reduced synthesis of beta globulin leading to inadequate Hb-A formation and secondly the haemolytic component which is not due to lack of beta-globulin but due to relative excess of alpha chains. These alpha chains form insoluble aggregates that precipitate within the erythrocytes damaging the cell membrane and render red cells more liable to be phagocytosed. There is hyperactivity of the bone marrow and massive erythropoiesis invades the bony cortex. Splenomegaly and hepatomegaly are as a result of marked extramedullary haemopoiesis as well as reticuloendothelial hyperplasia.

The disease manifests itself as fetal haemoglobin is being replaced by adult haemoglobin.

Clinical features. Child with thalassaemia fails to develop normally and his/her growth is retarded almost from birth. Because of excessive extramedullary haemopoiesis, gross hepatomegaly leading to protuberant abdomen develops. Bone growth is impaired and skeletal deformities develop. A peculiar thalassaemia facies (prominent malar bones, depression of nasal bridge, frontoparietal bossing) appears. Child becomes more susceptible to intercurrent infections. Anaemia progresses and if not treated by repeated transfusions child may not be able to survive.

Investigations. Haemoglobin level is low (3-5 g/dl). Blood film shows hypochromic microcytic picture with presence of anisocytosis poikilocytosis, target cells and normoblasts. Blood count is generally normal. Platelet count is within normal limits.

Bone marrow is hypercellular with marked erythroid hyperplasia. Osmotic fragility of red cells is decreased. X-ray skull shows 'hair on end' appearances. There is thinning and widening of metacarpal shaft. Blood electrophoresis shows severe reduction or absence of Hb-A and increased levels of Hb-F.

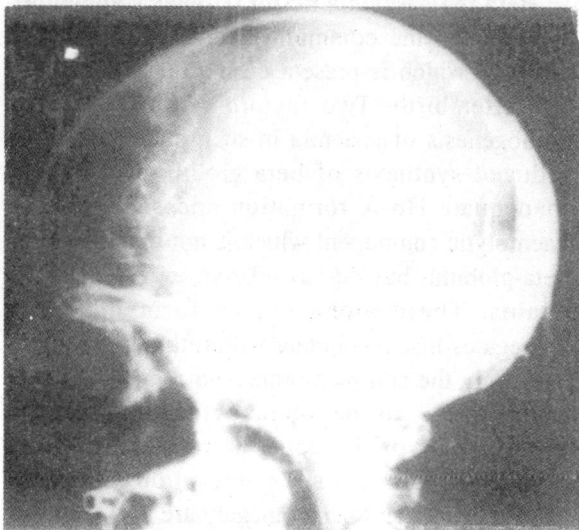

Fig. 7.1. X-ray skull showing "Hair on end" appearances in case of cooley's anaemia.

Clinical features of Cooley's anaemia (B-thalassaemia major).

1. Retarded growth, failure to grow
2. Serve anaemia
3. Protuberant abdomen
4. Gross hepatomegaly
5. Thalassaemia facies (prominent malar bones, depression of nasal bridge, frontoparietal bossing)
6. Increased susceptibility to intercurrent infections.

Diagnosis. Thalassaemia is diagnosed in a child with severe anaemia with history of failure to thrive retarded growth, hepato splenomegaly and typical facies. Further confirmation is made by blood picture, radiological tests and electrophoresis of blood (reduction or absence of HbA and increased levels even upto 80-90% of fetal haemoglobin).

Treatment. Main stay of treatment in a case of thalassaemia is repeated blood transfusions. An attempt should be made to keep haemoglobin levels above 10.0 g/dl. Generally a transfusion of fresh blood is required almost every 4-6 weeks. One of the major side effect of repeated transfusions is iron over load which may damage liver, pancreas and myocardium. Cardiac failure as a result of secondary haemochromatosis is a significant cause of death in these chlldren as they reach adolescence.

Diagnostic features of Cooley's anaemia

1. Low levels of haemoglobin
2. Blood film shows hypochromic microcytic picture with anisocytosis, poikilocytosis, target cells, basophilic stippling and normoblasts.
3. Blood count normal
4. Platelet count within normal limits
5. Increased reticulocyte count
6. Bone marrow hypercellular with marked erythroid hyperplasia
7. Decreased osmotic fragility of red cells
8. X-ray skull shows 'Hair-on-end' appearances
9. Thinning and widening of metacarpal shafts
10. Severe reduction or absence of Hb-A
11. Increased levels of Hb-F

Iron overload is corrected by use of iron-chelating agent—Desferioxamine. Dose is 0.5-1 g/daily or by overnight subcutaneous infusion several times a week. Total dose is dependent on age and weight of child and is further assessed by monitoring serum ferritin levels. Condition of the lens in eye must be observed regularly, since reversible cataract may occur with desferioxamine treatment. Other side effects include abdominal pain, loose motions, muscle cramps and fever. Vitamin C given in heavy doses also helps to increase iron chelation.

In children where requirement of repeated blood transfusions increase, splenectomy is considered but there is danger of intercurrent infections.

Course. Unless treated properaly by repeated and adequate blood transfusions, the course of disease is downhill. Even haemosiderosis develops later on despite treatment. Many children survive to adolescence but many succumb to intercurrent infections, cardiac failure, diabetes and cirrhosis of liver.

Acquired haemolytic anaemias. It constitutes a group of haemolytic anaemias which are as a result of development of acquired extracorpscular haemolytic mechanism. These anaemias may be immune (destruction of red cells by auto antibodies; allo-antibodies: haemolytic disease of newborn), non-immune (acquired membrane defects of red blood cells: microangiopathic haemolytic anaemia) or other miscellaneous causes where toxic substances act and disrupt red cells causing haemolysis (malaria, arsenic, clostridium welchii infection).

Immune haemolytic anaemia. Here autoantibodies develop against the red blood cells and haemolysis results from their increased destruction. Antibodies attach themselves to the red cells. These autoimmune haemolytic anaemias are divided into 'warm' or 'cold types' depending on which temperature the antibody binds itself to the red cell. When it agglutinates the red cell at body temperature (37°C) it is called warm antibody or at lower temperature (cold antibody). Whatever the cause of antibody formation, diagnosis of these anaemias depends on the demonstration of anti red cell antibodies.

Warm autoimmune haemolytic anaemia. It is characterised by presence of IgG antibodies and rarely IgA. These are active at body temperature. Most of the cases are idiopathic and in primary form cause of antibody formation is not known. Approximately 25 per cent of the cases of this type of anaemia are due to secondary causes which include systemic lupus erythematosus, lymphomas, hodgkins disease and drugs. Clinical picture consists of short episodes of anaemia, jaundice and splenomegaly. In secondary form features of underlying disease are present. Many patients go on to chronic form of the disease while in some acute massive haemolysis with profound fall in haemoglobin levels occurs.

Diagnosis is based on presence of haemolysis. Haemoglobin levels are low. Blood film shows anisocytosis, poikilocytosis and spherocytosis. Direct coombs test is strongly positive. Rarely platelets may be reduced due to development of

antibodies against them (autoimmune thrombo-cytopenia—Evan's syndrome).

Cold autoimmune haemolytic anaemia. It is characterized by the presence of IgM antibodies which have enhanced activity at low temperatures. Haemolysis occurs intravascularly or in distal body parts. It may be primary (idiopathic) or secondary due to infections (infectious mononucleosis, mycoplasma pneumoniae) or in association with myeloproliferative disorders (lymphomas). Paroxysmal cold haemoglobinuria occurs in persons exposed to severe cold when sudden haemolysis with haemoglobinuria occurs. Chronic cold agglutinin syndrome occurs in elderly patients. In addition Raynaud's phenomenon may occur due to aggluination of red cells in the capillaries of hands and feet leading to acrocynosis and even gangrene in extreme cases. Blood picture is that of anaemia. Peripheral blood shows almost the same picture as in warm type. Here red cells agglutinate in the cold or below room temperature.

Serum antibodies to IgM are demonstrable. Direct antiglobulin test is positive.

Treatment. Where the cause is not known, if anaemia is severe blood transfusions are given. Majority of cases require steroids (prednisolone 40-60 mg/day). Once remission is obtained the drug is tapered off and patient kept on maintenance dosage.

If response to steroids is poor, splenectomy may be required. Before planning splenectomy use of immunosuppressive drugs like Azathioprine (2-3 mg/kg body weight) or cyclophosphamide (1-2 mg/kg body weight) are employed and are found effective. In secondary form of these haemolytic anaemias underlying disorder should be managed. In case of cold type of autoimmune haemolytic anaemia exposure to cold and extremes of temperature be avoided. Blood transfusions are often required. Treatment with steroids and splenectomy in such patients is less effective.

Remission and improvement in all these cases is considered satisfactory if haemaglobin levels of above 10 gm/dl can be achieved and maintained.

Haemolytic disease of the newborn (erythro-blastosis fetalis). It is an isoimmune haemolytic anaemia of the new born caused by Rh or ABO blood group incompatibility between mother and foetus. IgG antibodies pass from the maternal circulation into the foetus via placenta and destroy the fetal red cells causing haemolysis and child is born with jaundice on the first day of life.

Pathogenesis. When an Rh negative mother carries an Rh positive foetus, immunization of the mother by blood group antigens on fetal red cells takes place. There is passage of antibodies from mother through placenta to the foetus. There is risk of fetal red cells reaching maternal circulation during the last weeks of pregnancy and during labour.

Of the various antigens included in the Rh system, D antigen is the major cause of Rh incompatibility. Rh positive cells are those wnich bear D Antiigen while those lacking it are all Rh negative. A number of Factors influence the immune response to Rh positive fetal red cells. These include:

1. ABO incompatibility which protects mother Rh immunization because of fetal red cells coated by isohaemagglutinins.
2. Dose of immunizing antigen. Thus haemolytic disease develops only when mother has experienced a significant transplacental bleed and lastly.
3. Prior sensitization of mother due to previously Rh incompatible blood transfusions. Initial exposure to Rh antigen evokes formation of IgM antibodies which are relatively harmless, since they can not cross the placenta. That is why in the first pregnancy, Rh. disease is uncommon. During subsequent pregnancies there is brisk IgG antibody response which cross the placenta and cause haemolysis.

Clinical picture. It depends on the severity of the disease process. In mild form there is only moderate haemolytic anaemia and jaundice. In moderate and severe form of disease where unconjugated bilirubin levels rise, bile pigment deposition occurs in basal ganglia. There is not only jaundice present within 24 hours of birth, but apathy, poor feeding, high pitched cry, cerebral irritation and convulsions (Kernicterus). As the child grows there is mental retardation, cerebral palsy, cranial

nerve palsies, and extra pyramidal signs. Anaemia may progress and lead to congestive heart failure.

In very severe forms of the disease, erythroblastosis fetalis develops. Infant may be stillborn or it dies soon after birith. There is gross generalised oedema, anaemia and hepatosplenomegaly.

Investigations. Amniotic fluid obtained by amniocentesis shows high levels of bilirubin. Mothers blood shows the presence of antibodies by indirect Coombs' test. A sample of blood obtained from cord or baby shows positive direct Coombs' test, raised bilirubin levels, anaemia, reticulocytosis and large number of erythroblasts.

Management. A mild case of haemolytic anaemia in the new born requires phototherapy. This may be in the form of fluorescent light which converts bilirubin to water soluble biliverdin which is excreted by the kidneys. Phenobarbitone also is employed since it induces liver enzymes to conjugate bilirubin and thus helps in its excretion.

Prenatal management. If antibody titre is low, the pregnancy is allowed to continue. But if there is risk of hydrops fetalis or still birth induction of labour after 33 weeks is done followed by postnatal exchange transfusions. Sometimes the baby is treated with intrauterine intraperitoneal transfusions before 33 weeks and then labour induced.

Post natal management. It includes correction of anaemia and hyperbilirubinaemia. When serum levels of unconjugated bilirubin exceed 20 mg/dl in full term babies or 15 mg/dl in pre term babies, exchange transfusion is advised. It is generally done by Rh negative group O blood.

Prevention. All Rh negative mothers susceptible to immunization should be given Anti-D gamma globulin (500 IU) intramuscularly within 48 hours of delivery or abortion.

BLOOD COAGULATION

Blood coagulatin is a complex process which involves number of enzymatic reactions. When bleeding occurs small amounts of thrombin are formed, which is insufficient for the formation of a fibrin clot. But this produces rapid generation of thromboplastin which quickly completes conversion of prothrombin to thrombin and converts soluble plasma fibrinogen to fibrin clot.

This whole process involves a number of factors which are either enzyme precursors (Factors IX, X, XI, XII and thrombin) or cofactor (V and VII).

The various factors involved in the process of coagulation are:

Factor I   *Fibrinogen.* It is mainly synthesized in the liver and is completely utilized during clotting. Thrombin by its action splits a glutamic acid containing peptide fraction (fibrin monomer) from fibrinogen, leaving it to form fibrin fibres in the form of a fragile polymer. Factors XIII to factor XIIIa are activated to enzymatically convert fibrin monomers to stable fibrin polymers and fibrin clot.

Factor II   *Prothrombin.* During the process of clotting prothrombin which is normally present in plasma is converted to thrombin which converts fibrinogen to fibrin.

Factor III *Tissue thromboplastin.* It appears during the process of trauma or shock. Thrombin appears in plasma during the process of coagulation and is derived from plasma prothrombin, playing important part in its various reactions. It activates factor XIII, VIII and factor V, causes aggregation of platelets and releases contractile protein from platelets causing clot retraction.

Factor IV   *Calcium.* It does not play significant role in the process of coagulation.

Factor V   *Proaccelerin labile factor.* It is essential for the action of tissue thromboplastin along with Factor VII, Factor X and calcium (Factor IV)

Factor VII *Stable factor—Proconvertin.* Iit is essential for the conversion of prothrombin to thrombin in the presence of tissue thromboplastin, Factor V, X and Factor IV.

Factor VIII *Antihaemophilic globulin AHG.* An important factor essential for the intrinsic generation of thromboplastin.

Factor IX   *Christmas factor PTC.* Essential for the intrinsic generation of thromboplastin. The amount of thromboplastin formed and not its rate of formation is influenced by this factor.

Factor X   *Stuart-Prower factor.* This factor is essential for the conversion of prothrombin into thrombin in the presence of Factors V, VII, calcium and thromboplastin. It is also essentially required for the generation of intrinsic thromboplastin.

Factor XI   *Plasma thromboplastin antecedent, PTA.* This factor is required for the generation of intrinsic thromboplastin but not for the activation of tissue thromboplastin.

Factor XII *Hageman factor.* It is required for normal generation of intrinsic thromboplastin.

Factor XIII *Fibrin stabilising factor, Fibrinase.* This factor is essential for polymerization of fibrin monomers into insoluble polymerized fibrin.

In addition apart from Factor XIII, the enzymes taking part are serine proteases and hydrolyse peptide bonds.

Process of clotting. Normal process of clotting is controlled through extrinsic pathway where after injury tissue factor released from damaged cells along with factor VII and IV activate Factor X. In the intrinsic pathway prekallikrein (PK) is converted to Kallikrein by factor XII which itself has been activated by contact with the damaged surface. This in itself activiates fibrinolytic pathway which along with Factors IX, VIII, IV activates Factor X.

Common pathway in the process of clotting is the role of activated Factor X which converts prothrombin to thrombin which releases fibrinopeptides A and B from fibrinogen to form insoluble fibrin.

Factors like II, VII, IX and X are produced in the liver and are vitamin K dependent. So the presence of this vitamin is essential for making them functional. Coagulation is confined to the site of injury by removal of activated coagulation factors while process of fibrinolysis helps to restore vessel patency.

Tests of coagulation disorders. These mainly include testing for clotting time (normal 5-7 minutes). Prothrombin time (normal 16-18 seconds), partial thromboplastin time (normal 30-50 seconds), thrombin time (10-20 seconds) and clot retraction time (55-65 per cent of the total quantity of blood).

Prothrombin time (PT) partial thrombop!astin time (PTTK) and thrombin time (TT) are prolonged in patients with coagulation disorders. Clot retraction time is important when platelet function is grossly deranged.

Coagulation disorders. These are both acquired and hereditary. Acquired clotting disorders are usually associated with deficieny of multiple clotting factors and are often associated with a severe clotting defect.

Disseminated intravascular coagulation (DIC)

Causes

1. Severe infection (malaria, typhoid)
2. Septicaemia
3. Snake bite
4. Disseminated malignant process
5. Haemolytic uraemic syndrome
6. Abruption placentae

Clinical features

1. Bleeding from mucous surfaces
2. Epistaxis
3. Haemorrahage from various sites
4. Platelet count low
5. Prothrombin time prolonged
6. Thrombin time prolonged
7. Partial thromboplastin time prolonged
8. Reduced plasma fibrinogen levels
9. High levels of fibrinogen degradation products (FDP)

Deficiency of vitamin K either due to inadequate stores or its poor absorption due to diseases of liver and gall bladder produces severe coagulation defect. Liver is an important site of synthesis of several coagulation factors. Extensive liver damage not only affects the synthesis of these factors but also effects platelet and fibrinogen metabolism.

Disseminated intravascular coagulation (DIC) is another acquired coagulation defect characterised by wide spread haemorrhage and bleeding from various sources like mouth, nose and mucous surfaces as well as skin. Causes of DIC include severe liver disease, malaria, typhoid, snake bite, septicaemia and disseminated malignant pathology. In addition to prolonged PT, PTTK and TT, plasma fibrinogen levels are reduced and high levels of fibrinogen degradation products are found. Treatment of the condition is of the underlying disease. For bleeding transfusion of platelets or fresh blood is indicated. Role of heparin in DIC is controversial.

Inherited coagulation disorders. These are identified by deficiency of each of the coagulation factor and occur singly. Commonest of these disorders is haemophilia transmitted as an X-linked recessive disorder. Common inherited disorders in this group include Haemophilia, Christmas disease and von Willebrands disease.

Haemophilia. It is the most common inherited disorder which affects males though transmitted by females. It is an X-linked recessive disorder caused by deficiency of factor VIII procoagulant protein or factor VIIIC. Deficiency of this factor leads to classic case of haemophilia (Haemophilia A). It along with vonWillebrands factors (vWF) though synthesised separately, join together to form a common factor which promotes clotting as well as platelet vessel wall interaction.

Clinical presentation in cases of haemophilia include spontaneous bleed from very early life. There is frequent history of epistaxis, bleed from mouth, lips, gums, gastrointestinal tract and hematuria. Recurrent bleeds are common. Severe bleed follows even after minor injury. Bleeding in joints (Haemarthrosis) is commonly seen. Knee joints are most commonly involved. Acute attack may last for few days to few weeks. Incomplete recoveory may leave behind crippling deformity.

Laboratory investigations show a prolonged clotting time and PTTK while bleeding time and prothrombin time are normal. Immunoassay of factor VIII procoagulant (Factor VIIIc) show reduced levels while that of factor VIII vWF are normal.

Treatment is by fresh blood transfusion, when bleed is massive. In addition factor VIII concentrate or cryoprecipitate are employed. Use of these products carries risk of infecting the patient with hepatitis B and AIDS virus.

Each unit of factor VIII which is normally present in 1 ml of normal plasma, will raise the plasma level of the recipient by 2 per cent per kilogram of body weight. An uncomplicated case of haemophilia can be treated with an infusion of cryoprecipitate to raise level of Factor VIII to 15 to 20 per cent.

An haemophilic will require treatment especially before a dental procedure. Such a patient is managed by intravenous infusions of either cryoprecipitate or factor VIII combined with e-aminocaproic acid (4 to 6 gm four times daily).

Prognosis in a case of haemophilia shall depend on the extent of disease and episodes of bleed as to how frequent and how massive. Most patients of haemophilia get infected either with AIDS or hepatitis B due to repeated transfusions.

Christmas disease (Haemophilia B, Factor IX deficiency). This disorder is clinically indistinguishable from haemophilia A. It mainly involves males inherited as X-linked recessive trait. Disease may present without any symptoms or features of bleed from various sources.

Investigations show prolonged coagulation time while bleeding time is normal. Immunossay shows factor IX deficiency.

Treatment is by fresh blood transfusion and factor IX concentrates. Complications include hepatitis, AIDS and increased hypercoagulability.

von Willebrand's disease (vWD). It is caused by deficiency of second component of factor VIII (von Willebrand's factor—vWF) whose important function is to facilitate the adhesion of platelets to subendothelial tissue, it itself playing a crucial role in coagulation. It is transmitted as an autosomal dominant disorder.

Clinical features of the disease include spontaneous bleed from mucous membranes, and excessive bleed from various sources. Epistaxis and menorrhagia are quite common. Clinical presentation as compared to haemophilia is less severe and often mild.

Investigations show prolonged bleeding time while prothrombin time is normal. Platelet count is within normal levels. Immunoassay shows levels of both factor VIII-C and VIII-vWF to be reduced. Ristocetin aggregation test shows defective platelet aggregation. In other words patients from this disease suffer from a compound defect involving both platelet function and coagulation pathway.

Treatment is by fresh blood transfusions and factor VIII concentrates in severe cases. Mild cases may require no treatment.

BLEEDING DISORDERS

These disorders are characterized by easy bruising and excessive bleeding into the skin and other tissues by trauma. The process of bleeding and co-agulation are interlinked and a number of factors play their role in both of them. Thus bleeding is dependent on elasticity of the vessel wall, platelet deficiency or dysfunction as well as derangement of clotting mechanism.

Elasticity of the vessel wall helps in closing any wound by its intrinsic contractile strength. This aspect of the vessel wall is involved in conditions like vitamin C deficiency, septicaemia and hypersensitivity reactions. Platelets play their part by adhering and aggregating at the site of endothelial damage. Platelets may be blamed for bleeding when their function is impaired as in uraemia or their number is reduced either due to diminished production or increased destruction. An haemorrhagic diathesis purely on the basis of vascular fragility is characterised by spontaneous appearance of petechiae and ecchymosis in the skin and mucous membranes. Minor injury or trauma may play role in this. This group includes Hereditary haemorrhagic telengiectasis, connective tissue disorders (Ehlers-Danlos syndrome, Marfan's syndrome SLE) senile purpura. Purpura due to steroids, sulphonamides and severe infections (septicaemia, meningococcal infections).

Laboratory investigations show normal platelet count, bleeding and clotting times. Very occasionally in some cases bleeding time may be prolonged.

Platelet disorders. Platelets are round flat discs and every healthy individual has a constant platelet count within fairly narrow limits. The normal platelet life in peripheral blood is 8-11 days. Upto twenty per cent of the platelets are normally destroyed in the circulation within 3-5 days.

Platelets contain a number of factors (Factor 1-Factor 4) which accelerate the conversion of prothrombin to thrombin (Factor I) and conversion of fibrinogen to fibrin by thrombin (Factor 2). Factor 3 acts along with factors VIII and IX to form factor X while factor 4 acts as an antiheparin agent. They act as mechanical plug when small vessels are damaged, play an essential part in thrombin generation as well as release factors needed for blood coagulation and clot retention.

Normal platelet count in an adult ranges from 140000 to 340000 per cumm. When the platelet count falls below 100000 cmm it is generally considered to constitute thrombocytopenia. At this count mild bleeding tendency may be seen but spontaneous bleeding does not become evident till the count falls below 20000 cmm. Bleeding following trauma may occur when count is in the range of 20000 to 50000 cmm.

Thrombocytopenia may occur because of reduced production in the bone marrow or excessive destruction of platelets or impaired production of platelets in the bone marrow with various forms of diseases, leading to marrow failure or injury. These diseases include aplastic anaemia, marrow infiltration by malignant or paramalignant disorders (Leukaemia, myeloma, myelofibrosis, lymphomas) dyshemopoietic states(Megaloblastic anaemia)and

drugs like cotrimoxazole which lead to inhibition of megakaryocytes.

Increased destruction of platelets or their excessive consumption in peripheral blood occurs in immune disorders (idiopathic thrombocytopenic purpura, secondary immune mechanisms like SLE, viral infections) Drugs (quinine, sulfonamides, chloramphenicol, carbimazole, phenyl butazone). Haemolytic uraemic syndrome and hyper splenism. Drug induced thrombocytopenia is sometimes considered immunologically induced while non-immunological causes include disseminated intravascular coagulation (DIC) thrombotic thrombocytopenic purpura, prosthetic heart valves and massive transfusion of stored blood (dilutional loss).

Causes of thrombocytopenia

Diminished or impaired production of platelets.

1. Aplastic anaemia.
2. Infiltration of bone marrow (myeloma, myelofibrosis, lymphoma, disseminated malignancy, leukaemia).
3. Reduction or absence of megakaryocytes (Pernicious anaemia, megaloblastic anaemia)
4. Physical agents like radiation, X-rays, severe burns.
5. Chemical and drugs like sulphonamides, cotrimoxazole, arsenic, nitrogen mustard.
6. Heavy metals
7. Biological agents like snake bite, spider bite.

Excessive Destruction of Platelets.

1. Immune mechanism:
   a. Primary. Idiopathic thrombocytopenic purpura
   b. Secondary. Viral infections, connective tissue disorders (SLE) lymphomas, chronic lymphatic leukaemia, drugs (Quinine, Quinidine, sulphonamides, chloramphenicol, carbimazole pheyl butazone).
2. Non-immune mechanisms: Disseminated intravascular coagulation (DIC), prosthetic heart valves, thrombotic thrombocytopenic syndrome.
3. Hypersplenism
4. Massive transfusion of stored blood
5. Disseminated intravascular haemolysis.

Whatever be the cause, thrombocytopenia is characterised by Petechiae and bleeding from small vessels. Ecchymosis in the skin, bleed from various mucous sites including gastrointestinal and urinary tract is common. Females suffer from severe degree of menorrhagia. Bleed in central nervous system is a major hazard.

Idiopathic thrombocytopenic purpura. It is one of the commonest bleeding disorder which is due to an autoimmune mechanism. An antiplatelet antibody IgG reacts with the cell surface glycoprotein making these sensitized platelets more vulnerable to be sequestrated by the reticuloendothelial system including liver, spleen and bone marrow. Spleen plays major role in the pathogenesis of this condition in being major site of production of antiplatelet antibodies and in destruction of IgG coated platelets.

Clinical features of acute idiopathic thrombocytopenic purpura

1. Commonly seen in children
2. Follows an acute viral illness
3. Onset sudden, generally occurs 2-3 weeks of viral illness
4. Purpuric spots
5. Epistaxis
6. Self-limiting disease
7. Fall in platelet count
8. Bone marrow may be normal but increase in number of megakaryocytes

---

Acute form of the disease is commonly seen in children following a viral infection while chronic form is seen in adult women. Platelet antibodies are present in great percentage of such patients.

Clinical features. Idiopathic thrombocytopenic purpura commonly involves young women though both sexes are involved but its incidence in females is four times to that of men. These patients suffer from petechiae, and purpuric spots especially over the legs and arms. Disease pursues a chronic slow course. Severe haemorrhage occurs when platelet count is less than 20,000 cmm. Epistaxis is common. Majority of females present with menorrhagia and intermenstrual bleeding.

Physical examination reveals purpuric spots over various parts of body. When there is little bruise haematoma may develop. Retinal bleed or bleed in central nervous system may produce serious complications. Spleen is generally not palpable.

Investigations. Most important abnormality is fall in platelet count which generally is less than 50,000 cmm. Bleeding time is prolonged but whole blood clotting time is normal. Hess test is positive.

Bone marrow may appear normal but usually reveals increased number of megakaryocytes many of which have only a single nucleus and do not show any budding activity. Antiplatelet antibodies can be demonstrated by direct or indirect tests.

Clinical features of chronic idiopathic thrombocytopenic purpura

1. Commonly involves adults mostly women of child-bearing age.
2. Four times more common in women as compared to men
3. Petechiae and purpuric spots over legs and arms
4. Bleeding into mucous membranes
5. Chronic slow course
6. In females history of menorrhagia and intermenstrual bleeding
7. Platelet count reduced (less than 50,000 cmm)
8. Bleeding time prolonged
9. Clotting time normal
10. Hess capillary test positive
11. Bone marrow shows increased number of megakaryocytes
12. Antiplatelet antibodies present.

Treatment. Acute form of the disease especially in children remits spontaneously. In moderate to severe from, treatment is by steroids (prednisolone 2 mg/kg daily) along with platelet transfusion. In chronic form of ITP, treatment of choice is steroids (40-60 mg of prednisolone per day in divided doses). In majority of patients response is good. Patient may have to be kept on maintenance dose of steroids for sometime. In patients with severe form platelet tranfusions along with intravenous immuno-globulins (1 g/kg) are employed.

In cases where response is poor and relapses occur more frequently, splenectomy is considered. Splenectomy is contraindicated in young children because of the risk of developing infection which generally is very severe. In others results after splenectomy in majority of the patients are good. Some may require maintenance with small doses of steroids. Response to splenectomy is assessed by return of platelet count to normal which usually occurs in a period of few weeks.

In patients not responding to splenectomy, immunosuppressive drugs are employed.

Cyclophosphamide in a dose of 1-2 mg/kg or Azathioprine in a dose of 1-4 mg/kg body weight along with corticosteroids (40-60 mg/day) is the regimen generally followed. Injection Vincristine in a dose of 1 mg/m^2 given once a week may be required to induce remission in a severe case of ITP.

Intravenous infusion of large dose of gamma globulin in a dose of 0.4 ml/kg is effective in arresting severe haemorrhage and preparing the patient for any surgery.

Thrombotic thrombocytopenic purpura. It is an uncommon condition characterised by wide spread microthrombi in small vessels of all major organs. Manifestations of the condition consist of ischaemia in various organs including kidney and brain. There is also haemolytic anaemia because of fragmentation of red cells. Though the cause is not known but it has been considered to be due to immunologically mediated endothelial injury.

Anaphylactoid purpura (Henoch-Schonlein syndrome). The disease is characterised by a purpuric rash, colic and gastrointestinal lesions.

It is an immune complex disorder caused by type III hypersensitivity reaction. It is common in children and young adults. It is related to allergic conditions such as angioneurotic oedema, erythema multiforme, serum sickness. In some increased sensitivity to food and drugs is seen.

Clinically a case of anaphylactoid purpura presents with general bodily disturbances such as headache, malaise fever, and loss of appetite. A purpuric rash appears on the limbs, and buttocks often symmetrically. The lesions may be small, urticarial blotchy which later become dusky red. In severe cases lesions may become extensive, irregular and sometimes pemphigoid lesions may appear. Abdominal symptoms in the form of colic are common. Joint pains may occur though joints are seldom swollen. There is often bilious vomiting and diarrhoea with blood in stools.

Renal involvement may take place in the form of acute glomerulonephritis. Hematuria may be the first sign. Spleen may become enlarged. Some cases may have haematemesis, malaena and even picture simulating peritonitis.

Investigations show haemoglobin levels reduced. There is mild leucocytosis. Platelets are normal or only slightly diminished. Bleeding time and coagulation time are normal. Tests of platelet and capillary function are normal.

Treatment. In majority treatment is symptomatic. Steroids in the form of prednisolone (40-60 mg/day in divided doses) are employed for short periods and are beneficial. When the disease is severe, immunosuppressive drugs like Azathioprine and cyclophosphamide are employed with good results. In addition to the above supportive treatment is to be given as per the individuals complaints. Most of the cases recover completely and prognosis in majority is good.

AGRANULOCYTOSIS

Fall in neutrophil count is called neutropenia but when the fall is severe, almost to pathological levels it is called agranulocytosis. A number of conditions are responsible for it and these range from immunological mechanisms to drugs, chemicals and radiations. It may be manifestation of generalized bone marrow failure. Drug induced agranulocytosis is probably the commonest.

Aetiology. Agranulocytosis may result due to various causes. These are:

1. Agranulocytosis as part of a syndrome of pancytopenia.
2. Depression as part of syndrome of aplastic anaemia.

3. Bone marrow damage due to X-ray iradiation, infections (disseminated tuberculosis, septicaemia) poisoning with benzene, gold and insecticides.

4. Obliteration of bone marrow due to myelofibrosis, malignancy myeloma, lymphoma, leukaemia, sarcoma.

5. Immune antibodies due to drug sensitivity. The drugs in this group include amidopyrine, chlorpromazine, hydantoin, sulfonamides, chloramphenicol, phenothiazines.

6. Neutropenia due to other immune reactions as in primary atypical pneumonia. Infectious mononucleosis. Infections like viral hepatitis, measles, diseases like disseminated lupus erythematosus and felty's syndrome.

7. Deficiency of vitamin B_{12} and folate.

8. Endocrinal causes like hypopituitarism, hypoadrenalism.

9. Agranulocytosis due to drugs. This is a very important cause and may be related to dosage of drugs as well as sensitivity reaction. The main drugs in this are:

   a. Anticancer drugs (mercaptopurine, cyclophosphamide, busulphan, methotrexate, nitrogen mustard etc).

   b. Anti-inflammatory drugs (phenylbutazone, amidopyrine, gold compounds, indomethacin).

   c. Phenothiazines and tranquilizers (chlorpromazine, prochlorperazine, promazine, meprobamate).

   d. Sulfonamides, co-trimoxazole

   e. Antithyroid drugs (carbimazole, methyl and propylthiouracil, potassium perchlorate).

   f. Antidiabetic drugs (tolbutamide, chlorpropamide).

   g. Antihistaminics (chlorpheniramine).

   h. Anti-epileptic drugs (phenytoin, troxidone, primidone, barbiturates).

   i. Antimicrobial agents (chloramphenicol, streptomycin, Isoniazid, thiacetazone).

   j. Diuretics (acetazolamide, mercurial diuretics).

   k. Miscellaneous drugs like procainamide, phenindione, quinine etc.

Pathogenesis. Various mechanisms play their role in the pathogenesis of agranulocytosis. In the case of drugs in many it occurs as an idiosyncratic reaction while in others immunological mechanisms play an important role. Production of antinutrophil antibodies and production of T8+ cells which act as suppressor of granulocytic precursors in the bone marrow are other markers towards pathogenesis of the conditions.

Bone marrow is hypocellular. It contains its normal complement of megakaryocytes. Erythropoiesis is normal. But there is marked reduction in the granulocytic precursors and granular leucocytes and myelocytes are absent. In early stages small islands of dying myeloblasts are seen but in later stages these disappear leaving behind in the marrow accumulation of lymphocytes. In case of drugs neutropenia may occur after first exposure or after intermittent or prolonged exposure. So a number of factors, have their role.

Clinical features. Earliest manifestations of agranulocytosis may be in the form of sore throat or pain there. There may be fever going upto 103°F, sometimes coming with rigors and chills, body aches and pain, and extreme degree of prostration. In large number of cases ulcero membranous lesions appear on throat, tonsils, gums, tongue and genitalia. These are often covered with greyish black exudate and may become gangrenous. Lymph glands generally cervical group are enlarged and in some there is generalized lymphadenopathy. Liver and spleen may be enlarged. Jaundice may appear. As disease progresses, severe toxaemia develops and patient may go into shock.

Diagnosis of agranulocytosis is based on clinical history, physical examination and investigations.

Laboratory investigations show gross neutropenia, white count is generally below 2,000 cmm. Reduction in cell count mainly affects granulocytes. Peripheral blood film may show almost or complete absence of neutrophils and whatever leucocytes are present are mostly lymphocytes. Erythrocytes and platelet count is normal. There are no primitive white cells. Bone marrow is hypocellular and there is depletion of myeloid elements.

Course and prognosis. Most cases of agranulocytosis get intercurrent infections. Prognosis in majority is poor especially in agranulocytosis due to drugs. Shock, severe toxaemia, infections and haemorrhage from ulcerative lesions generally kills these people. If the diagnosis is made early and offending drug removed, prognosis may become good. Reduction in neutrophil count bears relationship to the severity of the disease.

Treatment. First step is to remove the cause which can be identified like drugs etc.

Secondly infection must be controlled. Patient be put in isolation ward and barrier nursing done. Antibacterial drugs like Penicillin 5 mega units I/M or I/V every 4 hourly or Ciprofloxacin 500 mg I/V 4 hourly be started immediately. In addition Injection Metrogyl 500 mg every 6 hourly to take care of anaerobic infection. At the same time blood culture and sensitivity be carried out and appropirate antibiotics substituted. Anabolic steroids are also given (Injection Nandrolone phenyl prop 25 mg I/M twice a week) and are useful. In cases where toxaemia is severe, corticosteroids are employed (Injection Dexamethasone 4 mg I/v 6 hourly).

Granulocyte transfusions are given to tide over the crisis. This is given daily for 5-7 days. Side effects include allergic reactions and transmission of hepatitis and AIDS. Human granulocyte colony stimulating factor (Filgrastim-neupogen 1 ml ampoule contains 30 million IU) obtained by recombined DNA-technology reduces the duration of neutropenia associated with use of anti cancer drugs. Drug is employed by S/C or I/V route. Side effects include hypotension and disturbances in levels of uric acid and liver enzymes.

Molgrastim (Leukine) is another recombinant preparation of human granulocyte/macrophage stimulating factor (GH-CSF). Its administration stimulates myelopoiesis. The drug is well tolerated and is used in patients of Hodgkin's disease, non-Hodgkin's lymphoma who are undergoing bone marrow transplantation with high dose chemotherapy and have got granulocytopenia/ agranulocytosis.

APLASTIC ANAEMIA

Failure to produce formed elements of blood due to aplasia of the bone marrow resulting in pancytopenia is called aplastic anaemia.

Aplastic anaemia is an uncommon condition and primary form is very rare. Whatever cases of aplastic anaemia are seen are secondary to toxic effects of drugs, infections and chemicals.

Etiology. In a great number of case, aplastic anaemia is seen without any apparent provocating cause and this is termed idiopathic.

Of the congenital cause, Fanconi's anaemia is the most common type which is inherited as autosomal recessive disease usually seen in children. There are often other associated congenital anomalies. Patients with this disoder who survive are at greater risk of developing leukaemia and other forms of malignancies.

Concept of immune mediated aplastic anaemia following immunosuppressive preparation of bone marrow grafting points to concept of an antibody or a cellular autoimmune process. This factor operates in a case of thymoma. But the commonest cause is the incrimination of certain drugs and chemical agents which produce aplastic anaemia. Bone marrow depression is usually related to the dose and duration of administration of the drug. But in some cases it may be either a sensitivity or idiosyncratic reaction.

Severe infections like disseminated tuberculosis, HIV, Infective hepatitis (type A and Non-A and B) Epstein bar virus infection and use of anti cancer drugs are other important causes. Aplastic anaemia has also been seen in cases of pregnancy, chronic renal failure, hypothyroidism, addisons disease, and paroxysmal nocturnal haemoglobinuria.

Pathogenesis. Since there is suppression of bone marrow function, the proliferation and differentiation of stem cells is effected leading to a hypocellular marrow, thrombocytopenia and agranulocytosis.

A number of mechanisms are incriminated in the pathogenesis of aplastic anaemia. These are (i) defective or deficient haematopoietic stem cells (ii) immune mechanism suppressing bone marrow and (iii) thirdly a defect in the microenvironment in which the stem cells are functioning with inability to support their normal cell function.

The bone marrow is hypocellular with increase in fat cells. All types of cells including mega-karyocytes, myeloid series and erythroblasts are reduced and even may be absent leading to thrombocytopenia, agranulocytosis and anaemia.

Table showing causes of aplastic anaemia

1. Idiopathic
2. Congenital (Fanconi's anaemia)
3. Autoimmune (thymoma)
4. Secondary to
   a. Drugs (anti-cancer drugs, chloramphenicol, sulfonamides, phenylbutazone, gold, antidiabetics, antithyroid drugs, antiepileptic drugs, anti histamine (chlorpheniramine) organic arsenicals, psychotropic agents (chlorpromazine, promazine).
   b. Chemicals like benzene, and its derivaties insecticides, dyes.
   c. Physical agents like ionizing irradiation.
   d. Infections like viral infections (hepatitis A and non-A, non-B hepatitis), Epstein-Bar virus infection, HIV (human immunodeficiency virus) measles and disseminated tuberculosis.
5. Infiltration of bone marrow in myelofibrosis, hematological malignancies (Hodgkin's and non-Hodgkin's lymphoma), myelodysplastic syndromes, myeloma, carcinoma, acute leukaemia.
6. Systemic disorders such as chronic renal failure, hypothyroidism, addison's disease, systemic lupus erythematosus.
7. Pregnancy
8. Hypersplenism.
9. Paroxysmal nocturnal haemoglobinuria.

Clinical picture. The disease presents with a slow insidious course but in some cases presentation may be acute. There is anaemia, pallor, generalized weakness and progressive dyspnoea. Thrombocytopenia manifests in the form of petechiae, ecchymosis, bleeding from gums and various sources. Granulocytopenia presents with frequent infections, fever coming with chills, and prostration. As the disease progresses person starts having a downhill course. Spleen is not enlarged.

Blood picture. Haemoglobin is reduced (3-5 g/dl). Total white cell count is markedly reduced. Erythrocytes, granulocytes and platelets are reduced. Reticulocytes may be absent. Bone marrow aspirate may be dry. When available it shows aplasia or hypoplasia, depletion of haematopoietic cells with presence of fat cells.

Course. The disease follows a downhill course in majority of cases. Severe cases have grave prognosis. Early response to therapy is a favourable sign. Course of the disease is to some extent effected by infections, bleeding and complications.

Diagnosis of aplastic anaemia is dependent on clinical picture, blood and bone marrow examination. Presence of splenomegaly or lymphadenopathy goes against diagnosis of aplastic anaemia. It may have to be differentiated from a case of acute leukaemia, myelodysplastic disorders, haemolytic anaemia with aplastic crisis, lymphomas etc.

Treatment. Depending on the degree of aplasia, treatment shall be guided. It consists of withdrawal of the offending agent.

Supportive therapy consists in isolating the patient and doing barrier nursing. Care should be taken to prevent any infection involving the patient. Prophylactic antibiotics (Injection Penicillin 5 million units I/M or I/V 6 hourly) are employed in severely ill patients.

Fresh blood transfusions preferably of packed cells are given at frequent intervals. Care be taken that blood is free of hepatitis and HIV infection. Stimulation of marrow is done by use of semisynthetic androgens (Oxymethalone 2-3 mg/kg body weight per day) for at least 3 months.

Corticosteroids (60 mg prednisolone per day) are also employed in some cases and are also useful.

Bone marrow transplantation is definitive form of treatment in all cases of aplastic anaemia where response to supportive therapy is poor. This process is more successful in younger group of patients. Complications include infection and graft versus host disease (GVHD). Use of immunosuppressant drugs like cyclosporin A can prevent this complication. Injections of recombinant colony stimulating factors are also useful in some cases.

Ideally a case of aplastic anaemia is best treated in addition to supportive therapy with bone marrow transplantation provided facilities are available at that centre. Splenectomy has no role in the treatment of aplastic anaemia.

The most important signs to assess the improvement is to regularly monitor neutrophil, reticulocyte and platelet cell count. Rise in the cell count and if maintained means that the patient is responding to treatment.

LEUKAEMIAS

These are a group of malignant disorders of the blood forming (Haematopoietic) cells, characterised by proliferation of the immature cells in the bone marrow resulting in interferance with normal process of haemopoiesis. Not only there is suppression of normal tissue but also of immune mechanism. The abnormal cells spill over into the peripheral blood and also infiltrate several organs in the body.

The exact cause of leukaemias is not known though a number of factors ranging from genetics to environmental factors are incriminated.

Leukaemias are widely prevalent all over the world. They are broadly classified into acute and chronic leukaemias. Whereas acute lymphoid leukaemia is primarily a disease of childhood and young adults. Acute myeloid leukaemia occurs in all age groups though mainly in adults. Chronic forms of leukaemia are seen in middle aged adults while chronic lymphoid leukaemia is predominantly seen in elderly people. Both sexes i.e. men and women are effected though incidence is more in men as compared to women.

Aetiology. It is not known in majority of patients though a number of factors having their role in their causation can be considered.

Aetiology of leukaemias

1. Genetic (familial, identical twins, congenital disorders)
2. Environmental factors (atomic radiation, pollution)
3. Ionizing radiations
4. Viral (retroviruses (RNA) DNA viruses)
5. Chemical (alkylating agents, cytotoxic drugs).

---

a. Genetic factors have important role as evidenced by increased incidence of leukaemia in identical twins and in certain families. A variety of congenital disorders with chromosomal abnormalities like Down's syndrome, Klinefelter and Fanconi's syndrome have not only increased risk but have also higher incidence of developing leukaemias especially acute.

Philadelphia chromosome (Ph) is found in precursors of white cells erythrocytes and platelets in almost all cases of chronic myeloid leukaemia. Similarly many chromosomal translocations or deletions have been found in cases of acute leukaemias.

b. Environmental factors also have an important role. People exposed to ionizing radiation either as a result of occupation or radiation therapy run the risk of developing leukaemias. In survivors of atomic bomb and nuclear radiations the incidence of leukaemias is higher. Chemicals like Benzene, Alkylating agents and other cytotoxic drugs lead to increased incidence especially of acute myeloid leukaemia.

c. Viral aetiology of leukaemias is considered in some cases. Retroviruses (RNA) and DNA viruses (Epstein-Barr virus) may induce leukaemia while a Human T cell leukaemia has been found to be due to HTLV virus.

d. Presence of leukaemia and other related disorders in close relations and families is a

PLATE XV

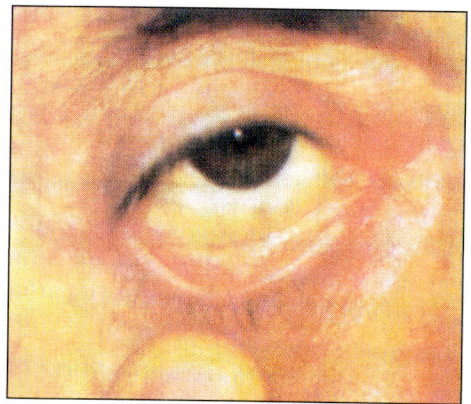

Anaemia. Conjunctiva and sclera in eyes are important sites to look for.

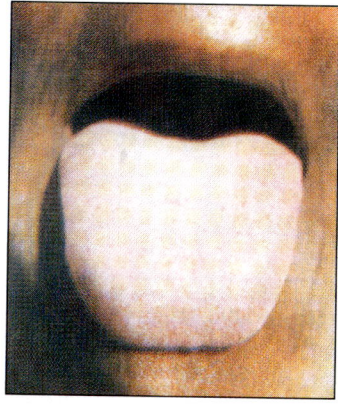

Anaemia. Tongue is pale in a case of iron deficiency anaemia.

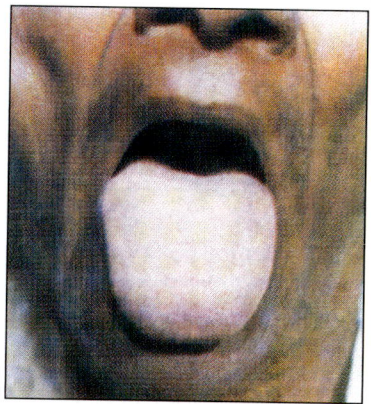

Macrocytic anaemia. Tongue is pigmented.

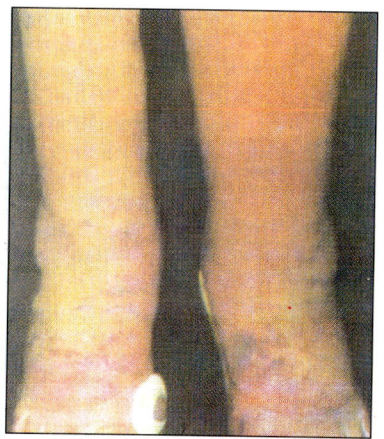

Coagulation disorder. Recurrent thrombophlebitis due to clotting factor V.

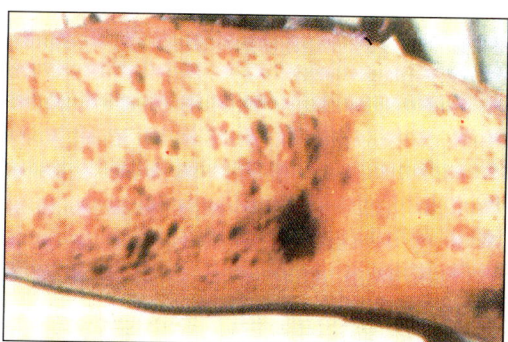

Leukaemia. Purpura and bruising associated with low platelet count in a case of leukaemia.

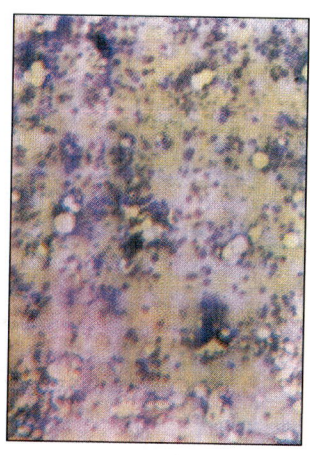

Aplastic anaemia. Bone marrow showing hypocellular fatty picture.

LYMPHADENOPATHY

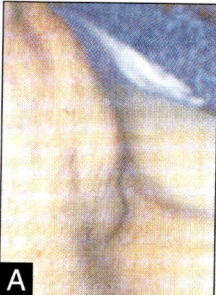

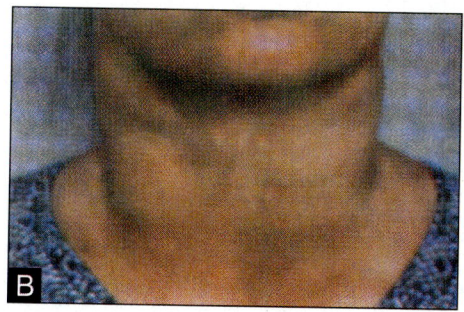

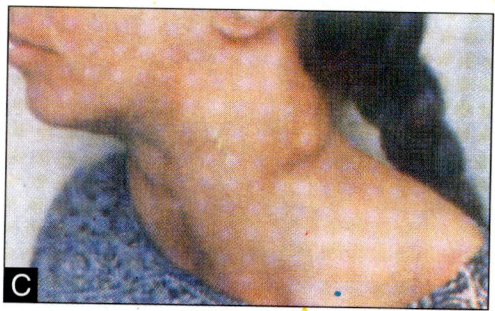

(A) Hodgkin's lymphoma. (B & C) Hodgkin's disease. There is pyramid type swelling in the neck.

PLATE XVI

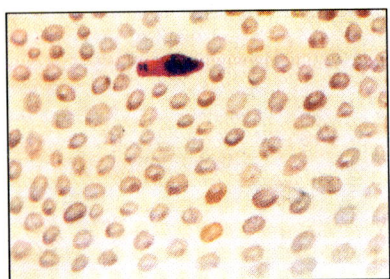

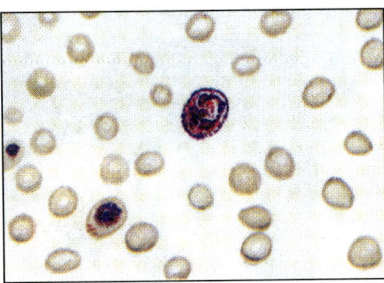

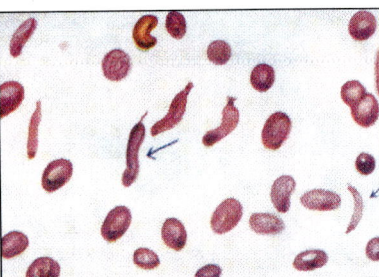

Iron deficiency anaemia (peripheral film). Red cells are small and poorly stained (microcytic hypochromic). There is irregularity in shape (poikilocytosis) and size (anisocytosis) of cells.

Macrocytic anaemia (peripheral blood) Red cells are large in size (macrocytic) and more deeply stained (hyperchromic). There is also anisocytosis and poikilocytosis.

Haemolytic anaemia. Sickle cell anaemia (peripheral blood film). Observe peculiar shape (sickle cells) of red blood cells

LEUKAEMIAS

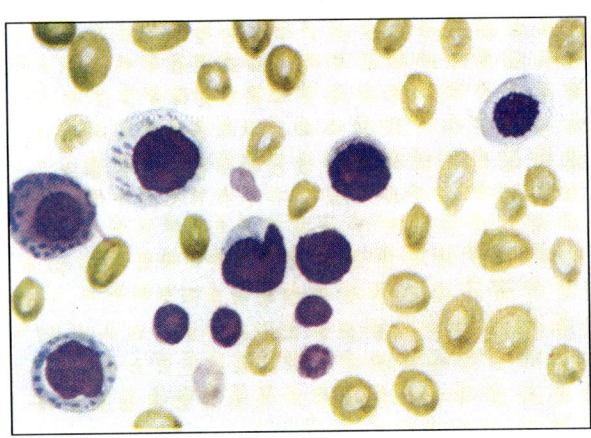

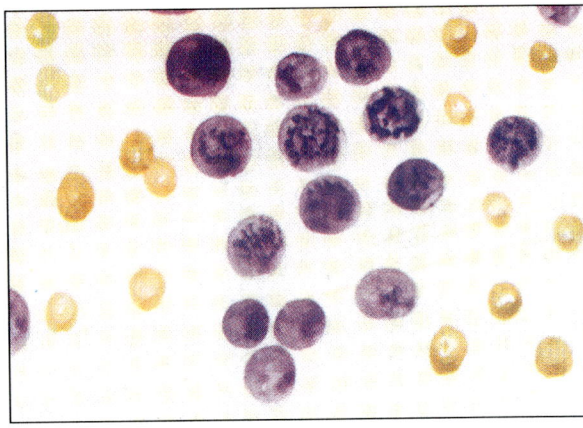

Acute myeloblastic leukaemia (peripheral blood). There is presence of myeloblasts.

Acute lymphoblastic leukaemia (peripheral blood). Lymphoblasts are seen.

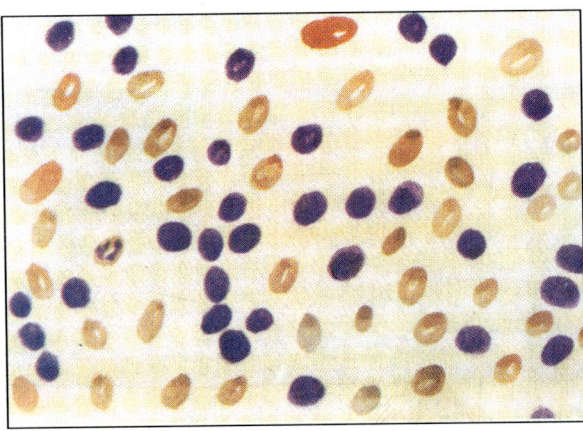

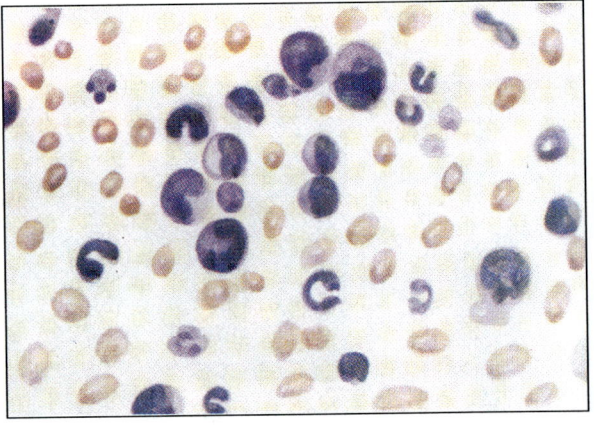

Chronic lymphocytic leukaemia (peripheral blood). White cell count is increased and there is increase in number of small lymphocytes. Red cells show some anisocytosis and poikilocytosis.

Chronic granulocytic (myeloid) leukaemia (peripheral blood). There is increase in the number of granulocytes. A few immature cells are also seen.

pointer to not only enviornmental factors but also genetic. There is also high incidence of leukaemias in immunodeficiency states.

Classification. Classically luekaemia is classified on the basis of cell type and its morphology. There are two types of leukaemias:

1. Acute type (acute lymphoblastic leukaemia (ALL) and acute myelogenous leukaemia (AML)
2. Chronic (chronic lymphatic leukaemia (CLL) and chronic myeloid leukaemia (CML).

Acute leukaemia has very immature cells called blast cells and follows a rapidly downhill and fatal course if not treated. As compared to this cases of chronic leukaemia initially are associated with well differentiated mature cells and follow a rather less serious course.

Pathophysiology. In acute leukaemias there is replacement of normal marrow by proliferating blast cells which do not go into normal maturation. There is defect in maturation beyond myeloblast or promyelocyte level in acute myeloid leukaemia and the lymphoblasts levels in acute lymphoid leukaemia. Since there is accumulation and proliferation of leukaemia cells in the bone marrow, a loss of mature myeloid elements such as granulocytes, platelets and red cells occurs. Result of proliferation leads to circulation of these cells in the peripheral blood as well as infiltration into other organs. Leukaemic transformation of cells may occur at various levels when differentiation is taking place. This process involves alterations in DNA synthesis of cells.

In contrast to acute leukaemias, chronic leukaemias can not be grouped under one stage, since they lack the common clinical and morphological features.

It is now well accepted that chronic myeloid leukaemia, polycythemia vera and myeloid metaplasia result form committed proliferation of multipotent myeloid stem cells. If there is dominence of erythrocyte precursors, it is called polycythemia vera while dominance of granulocyte series of cells manifests as chronic myeloid leukaemia. As compared to chronic myeloid leukaemia, lymphoproliferative disorders include chonic lymphoid leukaemia and hairy cell leukaemia representing proliferation of lymphoid cells of B-cell lineage.

While acute leukaemias are mainly dominated by a picture of anaemia, infections and haemorrhage due to bone marrow failure resulting in neutropenia and thrombocytopenia cases of chronic leukaemia do not have any bone marrow failure in early stages and it is the proliferation of mature cells, splenomegaly and lymphadenopathy which predominates the clinical picture.

Acute leukaemias. In acute leukaemia there is accumulation of blast cells due to failure of maturation into functional end cells. As the blasts cells accumulate in the bone marrow, it becomes hypercellular and there is marked reduction in normal haematopoietic activity. The result is depression of normal activity of red cells, white cells and platelets. Subsequent clinical picture is dependent on the bone marrow activity and proliferation of the abnormal cells.

In very early stages it may not be possible to differentiate between the two leukaemias but leukaemic transformation effects the differentiation of haematopoietic stem cells. When lymphoid series are involved it gives rise to acute lymphoid leukaemia whereas transformation of myeloid progenitor cells results in acute myeloid leukaemia.

Acute lymphoid leukaemia is further classified in terms of different immunologic phenotypes and different antigenic markers on the surface of the leukaemic blast cells while in acute myeloid leukaemia classification is based on the morphology and cytochemistry of blast cells.

Clinical picture. The onset is generally acute and rather short and stormy. The dominant clinical features are because of depression of bone marrow function. There is rapidly developing anaemia, pallor, easy fatiguability, fever, repeated bouts of infections, sore throat, ulceration in the mouth, petechial spots on the palate, bleeding from gums which are hypertrophied and bleeding from various other mucous surfaces. There is often hepatosplenomegaly, lymphadenopathy and aches and pains all over the body. Because of infiltration of leukaemic cells in various organs of the body, symptoms are referred to these structures. Thus involvement of bones may simulate a picture of rheumatic or rhematoid arthritis. Bony tenderness is invariably present.

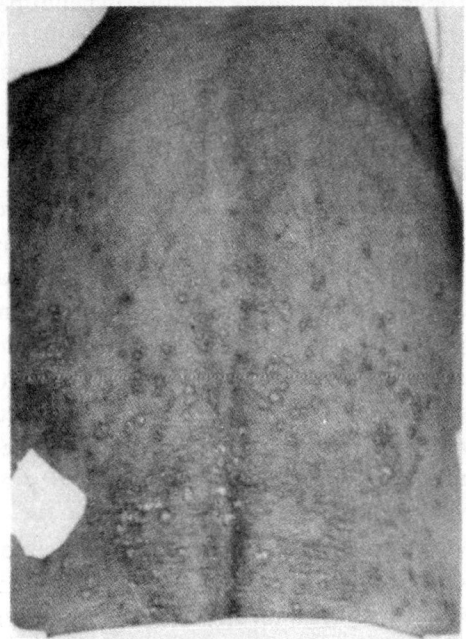

Fig. 7.2. Leukaemic deposits in skin.

In the early stages of acute leukaemia, it is difficult to distinguish between the two leukaemias and cytochemical status and analysis of antigens of both cells is required.

Neurological involvement produces headache, vomiting, signs of raised intracranial tension, cranial nerve involvement, seizures and meningitis. Further neurological features shall depend on where infiltration of leukaemic cells is. Rarely leukaemic infiltration may involve the retina producing haemorrhages (Leukaemic retinopathy).

Generally the patient is a child or a young adult though cases of acute lymphoid leukaemia are also seen in elderly. There is pallor, severe degree of anaemia, petechial haemorrhages over the palate. Gums are hypertrophied and bleeding. Bleeding may be present at various sites. Lymph glands are enlarged. Hepatosplenomegaly is seen in about 50 to 70 per cent of cases.

Investigations:

Blood picture. Haemoglobin is reduced. Anaemia is normocytic normochromic. Total leucocyte count ranges between 50,000 to 100,000 cells per cmm. Immature white cells (Blast cells) are present in the film. They may range from small number to even 80-90 per cent of the total. Platelet count is reduced.

Lymphoblasts and myeloblasts may be differentiated by sudan black staining (negative in lymphoblasts, positive in myeloblasts) PAS staining (Coarsely positive in lymphoblasts finely positive in myeloblasts) Terminal Deoxytransferase (TdT) is positive in acute lymphoid leukaemia and generally negative in acute myeloid leukaemia. Lymphoblasts have one to two nuclei as compared to myeloblasts which have between 2-5 nuclei. While immature cells in these cases (ALL) are generally lymphocytes and non-granular with negative peroxidase staining the cells in acute

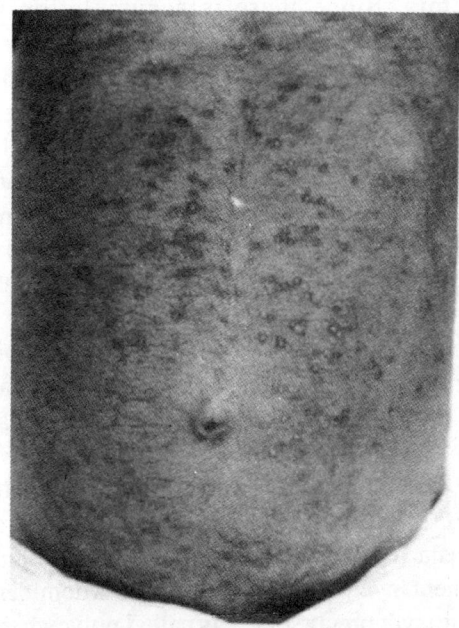

Fig. 7.3. Leukaemic deposits seen on abdomen and back.

myeloid leakaemia are promyelocytes myelocytes and neutrophils with positive peroxidase staining.

Bone marrow shows a hypercellular reaction with blast cells forming from 60 to 90 per cent of all the cells. *X-ray chest* is helpful in detecting lesions in the lungs and presence of any mediastinal mass.

French-American-British (FAB) classification of acute myeloblastic leukaemias

FAB class-ification	Common name	Morphologic
M1	Acute myelocytic leukaemia	Myeloblasts predominate
M2	Acute myeloblastic with differentiation	Myeloblasts and promyelocytes predominate
M3	Acute promyelocytic leukaemia	Promyelocytes predominate
M4	Acute myelomonocytic leukaemia	Myelocytes and monocytes predominate
M5	Acute monocytic leukaemia	Promonocytes dominate (undifferentiated and differentiated)
M6	Erythroleukaemia	Multinucleated erythroblasts predominate
M7	Acute mega karyocytic leukaemia	Undifferentiated blasts cells and cytoplasmic blasts.

Course and prognosis. Prognosis in all cases of acute leukaemias depends on the number of blast cells. Total leucocyte count, age of the patient (age below 2 years or above 60 years). Phenotype of leukaemic cells, central nervous system involvement and presence of metabolic abnormalities. All these portend grave prognosis.

Laboratory findings of acute leukaemias

1. Haemoglobin levels are reduced.
2. Anaemia normocytic normochromic
3. White cell count—markedly increased
4. Immature white cells (blast cells) ranging upto 80-90%

5. Platelet count reduced
6. Reticulocyte count raised
7. Bone marrow shows hypercellular reaction with blast cells forming 60-90%. Increase in megakaryocytes. Auer rods in the cytoplasm of blast cells of myeloblastic leukaemia.
8. Sudan black staining (negative in lymphoblasts, positive in myeloblasts)
9. PAS staining (coarsely positive in Lymphoblasts, finely positive in myeloblasts)
10. Peroxidase staining (negative in lymhoblasts, positive in myeloblasts)
11. Terminal deoxytransferase (TdT) positive in lymhoid leukaemia, negative in myeloid leukaemia.

Classification of acute lymphoblastic leukaemia (ALL)

Subtypes	Cell markers
L1 Small uniform cells with scanty cytoplasm (C-ALL).	Blast cells posses T cell markers
L2 More uniform type with more abundant cytoplasm (NULL-ALL)	Blasts cells have surface immunoglobulins Mature B cells
L3 Heterogenous cells which are large and have characteristic vacuolation (T-ALL)	Blast cells do not possess surface Ig or T cell antigens (Non-T Non-B group)
L4 Burkitt's type of cells (B-ALL)	Lymphoblasts are negative for T cells, B cell and acute lymphoblastic leukaemia (CALLA) antigens.

Principle of treatment of acute leukaemia:

Supportive therapy

1. Adequate levels of haemoglobin should be maintained by transfusion of fresh blood and preferably packed red blood cells.
2. Patients of acute leukaemia are more prone to suffer from intercurrent infections. It is important to not only treat the infection but attempts should be made to prevent them. Barrier nursing must be done in all seriously ill

patients. Fever may be either due to bacterial, fungal infections and should be suspected when a patient is running unexplained fever.

3. Adequate nutrition and maintenance of proper hydration by intravenous fluids where required.

Therapy of acute lymphoblastic leukaemia (ALL). Acute lymphoid leukaemia mainly occurs in first two decades as well as in elderly age group. Clinically there is anaemia, fever, bleeding from various sources, lymphadenopathy and occasional case presenting with neurological involvement. Total leucocyte count varies from 20,000 to above with lymphoblasts forming upto 90 per cent of the cells in peripheral blood and bone marrow. *Treatment consists of four phases:*

1. Induction of remission.
2. Consolidation therapy.
3. Cranial prophylaxis
4. Maintenance therapy
5. Management of relapse.

Induction of remission. It is induced by combination of vincristine, daunorubicin or L-asparginase and prednisolone given in repeated doses. Complete remission is obtained in a period of 4 weeks in 90 per cent of children. Vincristine (Oncovin) is a rapidly-acting drug useful for inducing remission but not good for maintenance therapy. Dose is 1-1.5 mg/m^2 intravenously in drip to be given at weekly intervals.

L-Asparaginase is another drug but clinical response to it is disappoiting. Though remission is induced, it is short lasting. The drug is now used only when other drugs have failed to induce remission.

Dose 50-200 Ku/kg I/V daily for 2-4 weeks.

Daunorubicin is antitumour antibiotic which is highly effective in acute leukaemia. Its major side effects are cardiotoxicity (Arrhythmias, hypotension), Marrow depression, stomatitis and G.I. symptoms.

Dose 30-60 mg/m^2 BSA (Body surface area) I.V. daily for 3 days and is repeated weekly.

Predinisolone is given in dose of 60 mg/day. It induces remission rapidly but relapses occur after variable intervals.

Drug treatment of acute lymphoblastic leukaemia (ALL)

1. Induction of remission. Combination of vincristine, daunorubicin or L-asparginase and prednisolone.
2. Complete remission in 4 weeks in 90% of cases.
3. Conslidation phase. Repeat the drugs used for inducing remission. On an average one to two courses required.
4. Cranial prophylaxis. Methotrexate intrathecally. Plus prednisolone orally.
5. Maintenance phase. Methotrexate, 6-mercaptopurine.
   This treatment is given for 2-3 years.

Consolidation phase. Once remission has been obtained there are likely to be undetectable leukaemic cells. Further eradication of these cells is by repeating the same drugs used for induction of remission and on an average one to two doses are required.

Cranial prophylaxis. Since there are high chances of central nervous system involvement in acute lymphoblastic leukaemia prophylactic use of methotrexate intrathecally and orally combined with steroids is employed. It is highly effective in maintaining remission (dose 2.5 to 15 mg/day or 50 mg intrathecally). Cranial irradiation is employed in some cases but they produce considerable damage to neurological functions.

Maintenance therapy. Once remission has been obtained and maintained, maintenance therapy is given for a period of two years. Methotrexate (2.5 mg) and 6-Mercaptopurine (1.5 mg/kg/day) are the drugs employed.

Relapse. Even when the child is on maintenance therapy relapse may occur. In such cases remission is induced by high doses of drugs, total body irradiation and bone marrow transplantation. Central nervous system relapse is not common but if it occurs intrathecal methotrexate with steroids followed by cranial and spinal irradiation.

Prognosis. *It depends on number of factors. Poor prognostic signs are:*

1. Total leucocyte count in the range of 40,000 and above.
2. Blast cells (60-90%).
3. Extremes of age (below 2 years and above 60 years).
4. Platelet count. Less than 100,000/cmm.
5. Central nervous system involvement.
6. Splenomegaly, hepatomegay and lymphadenopathy especially mediastinal.
7. Presence of complications
8. Presence of T or B cell markers.

Prognosis is good in children who go into remission and maintain it. Absence of complications, central nervous system involvement, organomegaly, age group between 2-10 years are favourable prognostic signs.

Acute myeloid leukaemia. The clinical picture of acute myeloid leukaemia is similar to that of acute lymphoid leukaemia in that there is fever, progressive anaemia pallor, ulceration in the mouth and petechial haemorrhage from various sites. Spleen usually is not palpable. Blood picture shows typical immature cells of myeloid series (myeloblasts, myelocytes). Blood count is usually between 20,000 to 50,000 cell per cmm. Abnormal cells generally constitute 90 per cent of the white cell count.

For *induction of remission* the two most important drugs are Cytarabine and daunorubicin which induce remission in 60-80 per cent of cases.

Cytarabine inhibits DNA synthesis as well its repair. Its main role is in induction of remission in myeloid form. Dose 1.5-3 mg/kg intravenously by continuous infusion twice a day for 5-10 days. If residual leukaemia is present 2-4 weeks after chemotherapy the repeat course of the two drugs is given.

Consolidation phase is continued by repeating one to three phases of the cycle. Phase of remission continues varying from periods ranging upto two years. In patients control is maintained by giving lower doses of the two drugs. Long term maintenance therapy is not much effective. Central nervous system involvement occurs in only few cases and prophylactic treatment of this complication does not benefit much. When relapse occurs, after inducing remission use of ablative therapy supported by allogenic or autologus bone marrow transplantation is advised. This is often followed by graft versus host disease associated with high degree of mortality.

Drug treatment of acute myeloid/myeloblastic leukaemia

1. Induction of remission. Cytarabine, daunorubicin. Remission in 60-80 per cent of cases.
2. Consolidation phase. Repeat cycle of drugs used for inducing remission, consolidation phase ranges upto 2 years.
3. Cranial prophylaxis. Not required since cranial involvement only in few cases.
4. Maintenance phase. Generally maintenance therapy is not required since intensive treatment in remission and conlidation phase sufficient to give relief. If relapse occurs, use of ablative therapy supported by allogenic or autologus bone marrow transplantation.

Differential diagnosis of acute myeloid leukaemia. Acute myeloid leukaemia may have to be differentiated from other haematological conditions. This includes cases of myelodysplastic syndrome where anaemia is normocytic normochromic. Bone marrow is hypercellular and is infiltrated with leukaemic blast cells. This disease occurs in elderly people. Chemotherapy is not effective and supportive therapy including blood transfusion and antibiotics are given. Patients of acute promyelocytic leukaemia often present with picture like that of AML but with excessive bleeding. Spontaneous haemorrhages are common due to DIC.

There is production of fibrin, platelet aggregation and fibrinogen depletion. Promyelocytes are seen in large numbers. Treatment is by platelet transfusion. Subsequently these cases require chemotherapy. Heparin plus E-amino caproic acid is indicated in patients with excessive fibrinolysis.

Prognosis in acute myeloid leukaemia. Patients

with complex chromosomal abnormalities have poor prognosis. Patient in elderly age group do not have complete remission and also tolerate intensive therapy poorly.

Factors like white cell, platelet count, LDH levels and presence of complications also determine prognosis. Patients of promyelocytic leukaemia who achieve remission have better prognosis as compared to patients with monocytic or myelomonocytic leukaemia.

Chronic leukaemias. *There are two mains forms of chronic leukaemias:*

1. Chronic myeloid leukaemia (CML) and its variants
2. Chronic lymphatic leukaemia (CLL) and its variants.

Chronic myeloid leukaemia. It is the commonest form of chronic leukaemia commonly involving adults generally in the fourth and fifth decades and equally common in both sexes. The disease runs a chronic mild course with vague symptoms of ill health, anaemia, loss of weight and a sense of dragging in the left side of abdomen due to gross splenomegaly. Lymphadenopathy is rare in this group.

Pathophysiology. Cases of chronic myeloid leukaemia have excessive production and proliferation of granulocytes and their precursors both in the peripheral blood and bone marrow. Over 95 per cent of cases of chronic myeloid leukaemia show a chromosomal abnormality called Philadelphia chromosome present in the myeloid, erythroid and megakaryocyte cells. Total leucocyte count is grossly raised often going upto 250,000/cmm. During the course of chronic phase of the disease patient may pass into a more malignant phase of the disease called blast crisis. Earlier on the bone marrow showed hyperplasia in the form of increase in myeloid cells (Myelocytes, metamyelocytes and neutrophils) but passage into blast phase results in increase in number of blast cells and promyelocytes. This phase is characterised by rise in leucocytes, thrombocytopenia or thrombocytosis. All organs show infiltration by myelocytes. Spleen gets enlarged progressively.

There may be development of lymphadenopathy or extramedullary tumours.

Clinical picture. Majority of cases of chronic myeloid leukaemia present insidiously with vague complaints. There is sense of discomfort in the abdomen due to splenic enlargement. There is often low grade fever, weight loss, progressive pallor and exertional dysponea due to anaemia. Physical examination generally reveals presence of anaemia, bony tenderness and a large spleen. Hepatomegaly may be present.

Laboratory investigations. Haemoglobin is low. White cell count is raised (60,000 to 150,000 cells/cmm). Peripheral blood film shows a normocytic normochromic picture with abundance of neutrophils, myelocytes and metamyelocytes including blast cells and a few basophils, lymphocytes and monocytes. Platelet count may be normal or elevated.

Bone marrow shows a hypercellular reaction with increase in premature and primitive cells of granulocyte series. There is presence of philadelphia chromosome which is diagnostic of chronic myeloid leukaemia. Leucocyte alkaline. Phosphatase level is markedly reduced. Serum vitamin B_{12} and B_{12} binding capacity are elevated and return toward normal with treatment of the disease.

Clinical features of chronic myeloid leukaemia

1. Insidious presentation (weakness, ill health, tiredness, loss of appetite).
2. Low grade fever. Night sweats, weight loss
3. Pallor, palpitation, breathlessness on exertion
4. Sense of discomfort in abdomen
5. Aches and pains in bones
6. Anaemia, pallor, bony tenderness
7. Easy bruising
8. Splenomegaly (90% of cases)
9. Hepatomegaly

Serum proteins and lactie dehydrogenase (LDH) levels are elevated. Serum uric acid levels are increased due to increased cell turnover and are often elevated prior to therapy. Basal metabolic rate is also increased and produces picture of sweating, fever and loss of weight.

Laboratory findings of chronic myeloid leukaemia

1. Haemoglobin low
2. Peripheral blood film shows normocytic normochromic picture with abundance of neutrophils, myelocytes, metamyelocytes, promelocytes, myeloblasts and few bosophils, lymphocytes, monocytes and nucleated red cells.
3. White cell count markedly elevated (60,000 to 1,50,000/cmm).
4. Platelet count may be normal or elevated.
5. Bone marrow. Hypercellular reaction with premature and primitive cells.
6. Philadelphia chromosome present
7. Leucocyte alkaline phosphatase level markedly reduced
8. Serum vitamin B_{12} and B_{12} binding capacity elevated.
9. Serum proteins, uric acid, and LDH (lactic dehydrogenase levels) elevated.

Complications. Recurrent infections, progressive anaemia and haemorrhagic tendencies are important complications. Splenic infarcts, deep vein thrombosis and priapism may occur due to increased thrombotic tendencies. An attack of gout may be precipitated while patient is on therapy due to raised levels of uric acid. Blast crisis is the most serious complication and is characterised by anaemia, infection and lymph node enlargement. Patient of chronic myeloid leukaemia follows a downhill course. Extramedullary growths consisting of blast cells develop in bones, lymph nodes and even skin. Peripheral blood and bone marrow consists predominantly of blast cells. Myeloid blast crisis resembles that of acute myeloid leukaemia and is brought about by proliferation of a genetically altered clone, Auer rods are not seen.

Diagnosis. A case of chronic myeloid leukaemia is diagnosed with characteristic clinical findings, peripheral blood film, bone marrow picture, biochemical changes and presence of philadelphia chromosome. Atypical cases have to be differentiated from leukemoid reactions associated with infections and neoplasms. Here Philadelphia chromosome is absent, Leukocyte alkaline phosphatase (LAP) levels are elevated.

Myelofibrosis is another condition to be differentiated from chronic myeloid leukaemia where there is gross splenomegaly, leucoerythroblastic blood picture and bone marrow tap which is dry and biopsy reveals fibrosis.

Treatment. A number of drugs like busulfan (myleran), cyclophosphamide, melphalan and hydroxyurea have been used in the treatment of chronic myeloid leukaemia. But the drug of choice is *busulfan*. It is an alkylating agent which is cell specific for myeloid element.

Dose is 2-5 mg per day orally (0.06 mg/kg/day). The dose is adjusted by monitoring the total cell count every week which starts falling after 2-3 weeks. The dose at this stage is reduced till the count goes to 10,000 or below. Patients response is observed with cell count falling to normal levels and reduction in size of spleen. But a true remission does not occur since proliferating granulocytic mass is only reduced and immature cells disappear from the peripheral blood.

Busulfan is again started when blood count starts rising. With passage of time patient may become unresponsive to the drug. Adverse effects include bone marrow depression, pulmonary or retroperitoneal fibrosis and skin pigmentation resembling that of Addison's disease.

Hydroxyurea is another drug. It block the conversion of ribonucleotides to deoxyribonucleotides by interfering with DNA synthesis. It is an effective drug. Dose is 0.5-1 g/day orally. Fall in white cell count is slow and steady. Major side effect is myelosuppression.

Both the above drugs have no effect on philadelphia chromosome. Treatment with interferon has been shown to reduce the number of Philadelphia chromosome positive cells.

Despite the above treatment the survival in cases of chronic myeloid leukaemia has not improved. Allogenic bone marrow transplant is beneficial if employed in patients below the age of 50 years. Splenectomy has little place in the management, since it neither prolongs survival or delays the onset of blast crisis. Splenic irradiation (total radiation 800-1000 rads given in divided doses) does bring about clinical and haematological relief. The blast phase of the disease is generally refractory to treatment. The same regimen as in acute myeloid leukaemia is employed. Hydroxyurea may be given in addition to other therapy (Vincristine + Prednisolone) to arrest proliferative aspect of the disease.

Prognosis. The disease pursues a progressive downhill course though slowly. Medical therapy does not bring cure though it does improve clinical and blood picture. Acceleration of the disease is reflected by unresponsiveness to chemotherapy, increased cell count with large proportion of immature cells, and thrombocytosis. Blast crisis means poor prognosis and survival on an average is between 4-5 years. Cases with negative Philadelphia chromosome (atypical myeloid leukaemia) have poor prognosis and usually die within one year.

Variants of chronic myeloid leukaemia. These are eosinophilic leukaemia (Eosinophilic count above 100,000 cmm) with immature eosinophilic myelocytes. Chronic basophilic leukaemia (gross increase in basophils) chronic monocytic leukaemia (monocytes increased) and chronic myelomonocytic leukaemia. In all these cases clinical picture resembles that of chronic myeloid leukaemia except that cell morphology is different.

Chronic lymphatic leukaemia (CLL) and its variants. Chronic lymphatic leukaemia is not as common as chronic myeloid leukaemia. It occurs generally in middle aged and above individuals and mainly is seen in people with genetic predisposition. The disease is characterised by the presence of excessive number of lymphocytes both in peripheral blood, bone marrow and tissues.

Pathology. Chronic lymphoid leukaemia is neoplastic disorder of B cells who have monoclonal surface immunoglobulins (IgM and IgD) present on the surface though in reduced amounts. The disorder itself is characterised by accumulation of long-lived non-functional B-lymphocytes that infiltrate the bone marrow, blood, lymph nodes and other tissues. It is a form of neoplasm which arises from clone of immunocytes. Reticuloendothelial system shows varying degree of infiltration. Bone marrow is gradually replaced by these cells leading to hyperplasia of the fat cells. Aetiologically genetic predisposition plays main role while environmental factors have no role to play.

Clinical features. Onset is insidious and most often the patient of Chronic lymphatic. Leukaemia is asymptomatic. Symptoms include easy fatiguability, lethargy, loss of weight and appetite. There is increased susceptibility to infections. Physical examination reveals anaemia, generalized lymphadenopathy and moderate enlargement of liver and spleen. Cutaneous lesions in the form of nodules or diffuse infiltration may be seen.

Clinical picture of chronic lymphatic leukaemia

1. Commonly patients are asymptomatic
2. Symptoms include easy fatiguability, lethargy, loss of weight, anorexia, palpitation, dysponea.
3. Increased susceptibility to infections
4. Physical examination shows pallor, anaemia, generalized lymphadenopathy, cutaneous lesions in the form of nodules. Moderate enlargement of liver and spleen.
5. Haemoglobin low, anaemia normocytic normochromic, Total white cell count raised (100,000-200,000/cmm). Platelet count normal.
6. Peripheral blood film shows small lymphocytes (90-95%), only small percentage are large lymphocytes. Smudge cells or basket cells often seen.
7. Bone marrow: Almost complete replacement by lymphocytes, abnormal proliferation of cells.
8. Hypogamma globulinaemia present.
9. Serum folate levels reduced.

Laboratory investigations. Anaemia is present and is of normocytic normochromic type. Peripheral blood shows rise in leucocyte count (100,000-200,000/cmm) containing mostly small mature looking lymphocytes. Only a small percentage of cells are large lymphocytes. SMUDGE cells or basket cells are often seen. Platelet count is normal. Bone marrow examination shows almost complete replacement by lymphocytes. Hypogammaglobulinaemia is present. This increases susceptibility of patient to infections.

Staging. RAI system of staging is considered important for evaluating prognosis in cases of chronic lymphatic leukaemia. This has been further modified.

Rai staging system in chronic lymphatic leukaemia

Stage O   Lymphocytes 150,000 or more in peripheral blood and 40% or more in bone marrow. No enlargement of lymph glands, liver or spleen, Haemoglobin above 11 gm/dl.

Stage I   Stage O + enlarged lymph glands

Stage II   Stage O + enlarged liver and spleen. Lymph glands enlarged.

Stage III As in stage II but haemoglobin less than 11 gm/dl.

Stage IV   As in stage III but with platelet count reduced (<100 × 10⁹/L).

Prognosis. Disease follows a slow and progressive course. Patient in stage I and II have better prognosis as compared to those in stage III and stage IV. Acute lymphoblastic crisis when occurs is terminal. Many patients with uncomplicated disease live for a number of year while those with intercurrent infections often follow a rapid deterioration in health, death occurring within few years.

Treatment. For stage O, no treatment required. In stage I, II if patient symptomatic drug threapy. For stage III & IV, drug threapy plus blood transfusion and radiothreapy. In addition to supportive therapy, chlorambucil is the drug of choice. It is a slow acting alkylating agent especially active on lymphoid tissue. Dose is 0.5 to 0.1 mg/kg body weight per day to start with and continued till the leucocyte count becomes normal. Side effects include neutropenia, pulmonary fibrosis, hepatotoxicity and seizures. Corticosteroids are often combined with chlorambacil in the dose of 60 mg per day. Other drugs which are employed in resistant cases are cyclophosphamide and vincristine.

Radiotherapy in the form of splenic irradiation (300-1000 rods in divided doses) is mainly employed in resistant cases. Other indication for it is in cases with mediastinal compression due to lymphatic enlargement.

Leucophoresis is another mode of treatment. Since these patients are liable to suffer from fulminating infections prophylactic antibiotics are employed in severe form of chronic lymphoid leukaemia. Splenectomy has limited role and is employed when it is massively enlarged.

Hairy cell leukaemia. It is a rare form of leukaemia and is a variant of chronic lymphoid leukaemia. Total leucocyte count is either normal or raised. Spleen is enlarged grossly and blood shows characteristic, Hairy type of lymphocyts with pancytopenia. Treatment is by alpha interferon and 2-Deoxycoformycin along with corticosteroids. Splenectomy is also advised in some cases.

SPLEEN AND ITS DISORDERS

Spleen lying in the left hypochondrium behind 9th, 10th and 11th ribs moves freely with respiration. It is smooth and uniform with a characteristic notch and sharp edge. Normally it is not palpable and to become palpable it must enlarge to about twice its normal size. Though spleen plays an important part in phagocytising dead cells as well as acting as a reservoir of formed elements of blood yet it is not essential to life since the tissues found in it are also present in other parts of the body. Spleen consists of a capsule, trabeculae and a lobule with largest collection of lymphocytes in the white pulp while red pulp consists of reticuloendothelial cells. Normally spleen weighs between 120-200 gm. In massive splenomegaly spleen may weigh more than 1000 gm.

Functions of spleen:

1. It is an important reservoir of blood and its formed elements which are released into circulation in conditions of stress.
2. Old red cells which have been damaged by

hypoxia, low glucose and pH and are present in sinuses of red pulp are phagocytised along with other circulating matter like antibody (IgG) coated cells and bacteria.

3. Immunological functions in the form of production of antibodies, antitoxins and agglutinins to circulating antigens.
4. The cells of reticuloendothelial system play an important part in the storage of lipids, haemoglobin and iron.
5. Normal adult spleen looses its haematopoiesis function which is present during foetal life. But when there is impairment of normal bone marrow activity during periods of severe haematological stress, pleuripotential stem cells (CFU-S and BFU-E) proliferate and extramedullary haemopoiesis takes place. This happens in severe haemolytic anaemia, thalassaemia and osteosclerosis.
6. Generation of humoral factors which control haemopoiesis.

Splenomegaly. A clinically palpable spleen is called splenomegaly and it may be mildly enlarged (weight upto 500 gms) moderately enlarged (500 to 1000 gm) to massive splenomegaly (weight over 1000 gm). Enlargement of spleen clinically is descrribed in terms of finger breadths or inches below the costal margin. An enlarged spleen has to be differentiated from:

1. Enlarged left kidney (hydronephrosis, tumour and a normally displaced kidney);
2. Tumours of the splenic flexure of colon;
3. Tabes mesenterica or omental mass;
4. An enlarged left lobe of liver;
5. Carcinoma of body of stomach;
6. Pancreatic tumour.

While looking for an enlarged spleen one has to consider its (i) shape (deranged in growths of spleen), (ii) consistency (soft in typhoid fever, septicaemia, firm in cirrhosis of liver and portal hypertension and hard in chronic malaria), (iii) tenderness (typhoid splenic infarct) and a splenic rub (splenic infarction in subacute bacterial endocardi-

tis). Splenic enlargement may be looked into either on its size or due to its aetiology.

Mild splenomegaly in acute splenitis, splenic congestion, acute febrile conditions, septicaemia, typhoid, SLE.

Moderate splenomegaly in chronic congestive splenomegaly (portal hypertension) thalassaemia, hereditary spherocytosis, autoimmune haemolytic anaemia, amyloidosis, tuberculosis, sarcoidosis, Niemann picks disease.

Massive splenomegaly. Chronic myeloid leukaemia, chronic malaria, kala-azar, lymphomas, Banti's disease. Gaucher's disease, hairy cell leukaemia and myeloid metaplasia with myelofibrosis.

Above is a broad classification of splenomegaly as per its size. Let us look at aetiological causes of splenomegaly.

Causes of various grades of splenomegaly

Mild splneomegaly. Acute splenitis, congestive heart failure, typhoid, acute malaria, SLE infective endocarditis.
Moderate splenomegaly. Portal hypertension, thalassaemia, hereditary spherocytosis, autoimmune haemolytic anaemia, tuberculosis, sarcoidosis, idiopathic thrombocytopenic purpura, Niemann pick's disease.
Massive splenomegaly. Chronic myeloid leukaemia, chronic malaria, kala azar, myelofibrosis, hairy cell leukaemia, Banti's disease (Tropical splenomegaly) myeloid metaplasia, Gaucher's disease, hepatic vein obstruction (Budd-Chiari syndrome).

---

1. Infections

a. *Acute.* Typhoid fever, septicaemia, infectious mononucleosis, subacute bacterial endocarditis, typhus. Spleen is soft.
b. *Chronic.* Malaria, kala-azar, disseminated tuberculosis, schistosmiasis, brucellosis and syphilis. Spleen is firm in consistency.

2. Congestive splenomegaly. Portal hypertension, chronic congestive heart failure, hepatic or portal vein thrombosis, polycythaemia vera.

3. **Reticuloendothelial disease.** Haemolytic anaemia, megaloblastic anaemia, thalassaemia, haemoglobinopathies, thrombocytopenic purpura.

4. **Haemotological** neoplasia lymphoma, lymphatic leukaemia, lymphosarcoma, myelofibrosis, multiple myeloma and myeloproliferative disorders.

5. **Haemolytic process.** Sickle cell anaemia, hereditary spherocytosis, acquired erythroblastosis foetalis, paroxysmal nocturnal haemoglobinuria.

6. **Granulomatous disorders.** Felty's syndrome, sarcoidosis, systemic lupus erythematosus.

7. **Miscellaneous.** Lipoid storage disease, primary amyloidosis, tropical splenomegaly (Banti's syndrome), tumours of spleen (haemangioma, fibroma), histiocytosis X.

Spleen in malaria. In chronic forms of malaria where the person has been having repeated infection spread over a period of months to year, the spleen is very much enlarged. The capsule gets thickened and often there are adhesions which bind it to the diaphragm. The adhesions may become calcified later on. Consistency of the spleen is hard but this spleen is liable to rupture with any blunt trauma to abdomen.

Spleen in kala azar. Spleen along with liver is enlarged in kala azar caused by Leishmania donovani. Spleen to start with is soft, pulpy and friable but as the disease progresses, the capsule gets thickened. There may be perisplenitis and splenic infarcts may occur. Spleen now becomes fibrous and hard. Thus an enlarged hard spleen reaching very large dimensions with irregular, remittant fever, anaemia, dark pigmentation of the skin and an enlarged liver are the features seen in cases of kala azar.

Tropical splenomegaly. This is characterised by gross enlargement of spleen. Capsule of spleen is normal but there is hyperplasia of lymphoid follicles and kupffer cells, dilatation of blod sinuses, generalised fibrosis of the reticulum and trabeculae. Liver shows variable changes. Gradually a picture of portal hypertension develops dominated by massive splenomegaly which is smooth and of firm consistency. Average weight of spleen is about 900-1000 g but in some cases it may go upto 3000 g. Anaemia along with features of hypersplenism are common findings in addition to that of portal hypertension.

Chronic myeloid leukaemia. It is characterized by the massive size of the spleen which occupies greater part of left side of abdomen. It often reaches to the iliac crests below and in the middle line to the umbilicus. Spleen in chronic myeloid leukaemia forms a hard smooth tumour with rounded edges and characterstic notches. It is not tender, Sudden enlargement in size may occur due to haemorrhage or infarction in the organ. Liver is also enlarged. Lymph glands are not palpable. Diagnosis of chronic myeloid leukaemia is based on blood picture and bony tenderness.

As compared to chronic myeloid leukaemia spleen in chronic lymphatic leukaemia is not much enlarged.

Portal cirrhosis. In about 80 per cent of the cases spleen is enlarged. It is firm to hard in consistency. If rapid enlargement takes place there may be pain or discomfort in the left hypochondrium. Spleen enlargement in portal cirrhosis is not very massive. Liver is enlarged in early stages but later on it becomes small, shrunken with irregular surface. Ascites may be present. Features of portal hypertension in the form of spider naevi, palmar erythema testicular atrophy, gynaecomastia and bleeding at various sites are commonly present.

Lipoid storage disorders. There are rare lysosomal disorders due to inborn error of metabolism inherited in autosomal recessive manner (Gaucher's disease) characterised by slowly progressive splenomegaly as the first sign. It may become enormous in size. Later on liver also enlarges followed by lymph glands. Niemann picks disease another rare disorder characterised by accumulation of sphingomyelin in reticuloendothelial system has also characteristic enlargement of liver and spleen as well as of lymph glands. The disease usually is seen within first six months of life. Child has massive hepatosplemegaly and mental retardation.

Hypersplenism. This is characterzied by splenomegaly either moderate or massive with presence of anaémia, leukopenia and thrombocytopenia. Hypersplenism may be primary where no cause is available or secondary as in cases of portal hypertension, Felty's syndrome, lymphomas, tropical splenomegaly, haemolytic anaemia and other conditions where spleen is overactive (malaria, kala azar, myeloproliferative disorders). Patient with hypersplenism has anaemia which is either hypochromic or normocytic normochromic. There is pancytopenia and haemolysis due to excessive destruction of red cells, as a result of splenic sequestration. Bone marrow shows a hyperactive, hypercellular picture.

Treatment in primary case of hypersplenism is by splenectomy. Clinical improvement as well as in blood picture occurs promptly. For secondary causes of hypersplenism treatment is of the underlying condition.

LYMPHADENOPATHY

Lymph glands constitute important part of lymphatic system which consists of lymphatic vessels, thoracic duct and collections of lymphoid tissue scattered all over the body. Lymph glands act as filters to the lymphatic fluid which flow through them.

Enlargement of lymph glands can be either acute or chronic. It may be localised or generalized.

Acute lymphadenopathy. It occurs in any acute infectious process. The glands become enlarged, tender and are fixed. Skin overlying the glands is warm and brawny. There is often focus of infection in the area which is drained by the gland. Causes include acute infection, septicaemia, measles, diphtheria, scarlet fever and glandular fever (infectious mononucleosis). In glandular fever, lymphadenopathy is generalized but may be confined to cervical region. Glands are moderately enlarged, and slightly tender. There is often acute onset with chills, sore throat and fever. Diagnosis is made by rise in white cell count with predominant mononuclear cells. Paul Bunnel test is positive. Disease is self limiting and recovery takes place in a period of one to two weeks.

Chronic lymphadenopathy. A number of diseases ranging from tuberculosis to neoplastic conditions constitute this group.

Inflamantory:

Tuberculosis. It is the commonest cause of lymphadenopathy and involves mostly children and young adults. Primary tuberculous infection is in the mediastinal and mesenteric glands. Involvement of cervical glands is equally common but less commonly axillary and inguinal glands are enlarged. The cervical glands may be enlarged on one or both sides of the neck. Pain is generally not present. Initially when the nodes enlarge they are elastic and there is no matting. Further on the glands became adherent to each other (matting) which is a characteristic feature of tubercular glands. Later on caseation takes place and often the gland ruptures forming a chronic sinus discharging greenish thick pus. Tubercular lymphadenopathy is associated with evening rise of temperature, night sweating, loss of weight and appetite and often there is evidence of tuberculosis in lungs or elsewhere in the body.

Syphilis. It is a disease of young adults. There is often history of contact available. In the primary form the glands are discrete, hard, painless and shotty without any tendency towards suppuration. while in secondary stage there is generalized lymphadenopathy especially of posterior cervical and epitrochlear group of glands. There is associated pink macular rash over the trunk, limbs along with mucous patches. The rash appears almost 4-8 weeks after the primary sore and fades in few weeks leaving almost no residuae. Papular rash follows almost closely the macular rash. Diagnosis of syphilis is made by positive Wasserman reaction.

Filariasis. It generally involves inguinal group of glands. Lymphangitis is associated with rigors, high temperature and enlarged glands in the groin which are tender and painful. The axillary, epitrochlear and cervical glands may become enlarged. Enlargement of deep seated glands (iliac, retroperitoneal, lumbar, mesenteric and thoracic) may also occur. Living or dead calcified microfilariae may be found in these glands. Lymphangitis asociated with lymphangiectasis produces acute inflammation and tenderness of the spermatic cord and scrotum. Lower limbs are frequently involved next to scrotum. Elephantiasis results.

Diagnosis is made by eosinophilia in blood, a positive intradermal test, demonstration of microfilariae drawn from blood at night and gland biopsy for the presence of filarae.

Lymphogranuloma inguinalae. It is a sexually transmitted disease characterised by a small herpetiform lesion on the genitalia or perianal region. The onset is generally insidious with slight stiffness in the groin. General symptoms include fever, headache, joint pains and rashes. Bilateral glandular involvement occurs in groin region. To start with pain is absent. The glands are hard to touch and only slightly tender. Lymph nodes later on fuse and suppuration takes place with rupture forming tiny fistulae. Diagnosis is made by Frei' intradermal test and histology of material obtained from gland.

Disseminated lupus erythematosus. A connective tissue disorder which may have acute, subacute or chronic forms. The disease is characterised by erythematous lesions on the trunk, extremities and butterfly like pigmentation over face. There are joint pains, pleurisy, pericarditis and endocarditis. Spleen is often enlarged and there is generalized lymphadenopathy which is mainly confined to superficial group of glands. Glands are firm, non-tender and subside as clinical picture improves.

Blood diseases:

Acute lymphatic leukaemia. seen in young children and adults comes acutely. There is pallor, enlargement of superficial lymph glands especially in the neck. Glands are discrete and non-tender. Purpuric haemorrhages, hepatosplenomegaly, stomatitis are other features. Blood picture confirms the diagnosis.

Chronic lymphatic leukaemia. Disease of elderly age group. It may be present for months or years before a diagnosis is made. Swelling of glands is usually the first symptom. Often enlargement of tonsils and spleen may be seen along with. A typical case has all the superficial lymph glands enlarged. The enlargement is moderate. Glands are not hard and do not alter in consistency during the course of disease. They are freely mobile, non-tender and not adherent to one another.

There is often history of fever, skin lesions and haemorrhages in mucous surfaces. Diagnosis is made by blood picture (raised total leucocyte count with predominant small lymphocytes) sternal picture and sometimes by gland biopsy.

Hodgkin's disease. It is disease characterized by painless enlargement of glands in the cervical region, situated in the anterior or posterior triangles of neck. Commencing from there other group of glands in the axillary, inguinal abdominal or mediastinal areas get involved. The enlarged glands are discrete and have a rubbery consistency. These are mobile with little tendency towards matting or softening. In advanced cases a pyramidal swelling with its base at the clavicle level may appear in the neck. Pressure symptoms in the surrounding stractures develop. Enlargement of spleen is there but gross enlargement is uncommon. Liver is often involved. Patient runs a typical fever called Pel-Ebstein type (fever takes 3 days to rise, remains remitted for 3 days, comes down in next 3 days; then after an afebrile period of 9 days, the same cycle of fever is repeated). Diagnosis of Hodgkin's disease rests on presence of eosinophils and Dorothy Reid giant cells. Biopsy of the lymph node, X-ray chest and CT scan is done to assess the extent of disease.

Neoplasms:

Lymphosarcoma. It is a highly malignant condition seen in young adults, characterised by enlargement of cervical group of glands. The glands rapidly progress losing their normal shape and form a big, large firm mass, movable to start with and later become fixed to the underlying structures. They are hard and often painful. They may sometimes burst.

Infiltration into the skin is not common though skin overlying glands becomes stretched and shiny. Diagnosis is by gland biopsy and histological examination.

Secondary carcinoma. Glandular enlargement due to secondaries from malignancy anywhere in the body is equally common. Glands in such cases are hard, painless, non-tender and fixed. As the glands enlarge in size, they become painful and in some cases ulceration may take place. Diagnosis is made by locating the primary lesion and by gland biopsy.

Miscellaneous:

AIDS and HIV infection. An individual may remain symptom free for months or years after getting the infection. Presentation of the disease is heralded by weight loss, fever which is intermittent, and generalized. Lymphadenopathy. Glands are discrete, non-tender and do not suppurate. Diagnosis by detecting antibodies to HIV by ELISA test.

Sarcoidosis. It is a multisystem granulomatous disorder seen in third and fourth decades. Characteristic features are bilateral hilar lymphadenopathy which is often asymptomatic. There is low grade fever, fatigue and weight loss. Generalised lymphadenopathy occurs only in small percentage of cases. Diagnosis is by Kveim test, Angiotensin converting enzyme estimation. X-ray chest to demonstrate hilar lymphadenopathy and transbronchial biopsy.

Investigation of a case of lymphadenopathy:

History. It is important to enquire about history of fever (low grade evening rise in temperature in tubercular lymphadenopathy, Pel-Esbstein's type in Hodgkin's disease, fever coming with rigors and chills in filariasis) weight loss (malignancy AIDS) bleeding tendencies (leukaemia, lymphomas). Acute lymphadenitis comes on acutely and often there is history of acute infection, septicaemia. History of contact is useful in cases of STD (syphilis, lymphogranuloma venereum, AIDS).

Age. Tubercular lymphadenitis is seen in young children and adults while malignancy mainly is seen in elderly or mididle aged individuals.

Physical examination. It includes general physical examination for evidence of anaemia, weight loss and presence of any systemic disease. In local examination, look for the number of glands involved, site, character, presence of any sinus. Palpate for local temperature, tenderness, consistency (soft, hard, stony hard) mobility (whether adherent to underlying structures or skin) and whether glands are matted to each other (tuberculosis). Neighbouring structures should be examined for any involvement. In some diseases like Hodgkins pressure symptoms are often seen. One should also look for primary focus like any inflammatory pathology or malignant disease.

In case of cervical node enlargement, careful examination of throat, pharynx, tonsils be made. Glands in the supraclavicular region (Virchow's glands) are enlarged in cases of carcinoma stomach, testes and lungs. Abdominal glands may be enlarged in tuberculosis, lymphomas. Enlargement of liver and spleen should be looked for in cases of leukaemia. One should look for any signs suggestive of syphilitic stigmata in case of enlargement of occipital and epitrochlear group of glands.

Investigations. *These include general as well as specific:*

Blood. Total and differential white cells count shall help in diagnosis of leukaemia, infectious mononucleosis. Blood test is equally useful in case of filariasis, W.R. and STS test in syphilitic adenopathy. Paul Bunnel test for infectious mononueleosis, FREI test for lymphogranuloma, ELISA for AIDS and HIV infection. KVEIM test for sarcoidosis. In tubercular lymhadenopathy, tuberculin test and guinea pig inoculation are often required to confirm the diagnosis.

X-ray chest. For mediastinal lymphadenopathy (sarcoidosis) any malignancy or tubercular lesion. Plain X-ray abdomen for any calcification (Tubercular lymphadenopathy).

CT scan of abdomen for evidence of any malignancy.

Gland biopsy. It is the most reliable diagnostic aid. Gland biopsy of superficially placed glands is done. It may be in the form of FNAC or a gland removed surgically and histology studied.

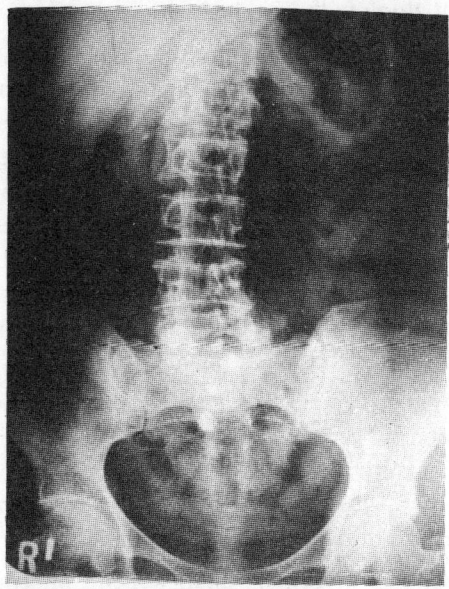

Fig. 7.4. Plain X-ray abdomen showing calcified glands. Cause tubercular lymphadenopathy.

ORAL MANIFESTATIONS OF HAEMATOLOGICAL DISORDERS

Oral cavity to a large extent reflects the state of health of an individual. A number of disorders present with tell tale signs in the oral cavity. The common haematological disorders in this connection shall be:

1. Anaemia/deficiency states.
2. All forms of leukaemia.
3. Thrombocytopenic purpura
4. Neutropenia/agranulocytosis/aplastic anaemia
5. Haematological malignancies.

Anaemia/deficiency states. Iron deficiency anaemia is characterised by atrophy of oral mucosa as well as of tongue papillae. Tongue looks pale and bald. Occasionally pigmentation is present. There is redness and soreness present. Vitamin deficiencies are notorious for oral lesion. Vitamin A deficiency leads to imperfect enamel formation of teeth. while vitamin K deficiency produces bleeding in oral cavity especially from gums due to prothrombin deficiency. More significant changes are seen due to deficiency of vitamin Bcomplex group.

Riboflavin (vitamin B2) deficiency presents with dermatitis of seborrhoeic type affecting skin of nose and round about the mouth. There is glossitis which starts with loss of fur in patches from the dorsum of the tongue. It later on becomes smooth fissured and painful. Colour of the tongue is magenta, very often riboflavin deficiency occurs along with nicotinic acid deficiency.

Nicotinic acid deficiency leads to glossitis and stomatitis. Tongue is hypersensitive to hot and spicy food. It is fissured, beefy red and an angry looking fiery tongue. Aphthous ulcers are commonly seen.

Pyridoxine deficiency results in cheilosis and glossitis while vitamin C deficiency results in spongy, haemorrhagic gums which are not only swollen but bleed readily. There may be bleed in the oral cavity. Bacterial contamination especially with Vincent's spirochetes and anerobic organisms is quite common.

Megaloblastic anaemias produce glossitis with a glazed raw tongue accompanied by painful burning sensation. There is pigmentation in the oral cavity but no petechial or bleeding spots.

Leukaemias. All forms of leukaemia produce lesions in oral cavity. In acute leukaemia there are purpuric and haemorrhagic spots in the oral cavity including palate. Gums are swollen and bleed easily. Acute monocytic leukaemia effects the oral cavity in more malignant form. There are petechiae, bleeding and marked swelling of the gums with ulceration. Cases of chronic leukaemia may have sometimes petechiae or haemorrhages in the oral cavity as first lesion. There is often associated anaemia and nutritional deficiencies present which manifest in oral cavity. In chronic lymphatic leukaemia there is often enlargement of tonsils.

Thrombocytopenic purpura. There is bleeding from gums and purpuric spots on the palate ranging from pin point to pin head are present. There is also presence of ecchymosis and large purple areas over skin. Haemorrhage may occur from any of the mucosae like nose and mouth. Slightest injury or trauma in the oral cavity gives rise to bleeding. It is equally important when dental procedures are being carried out. Bleeding may not be controlled easily since bleeding time is greatly prolonged.

Haemophilia. Cases of haemophilia may bleed from gums, lips and tongue. A minor scratch may produce bleeding and some patients may not be able to use a tooth brush for cleaning of their teeth because the gums may be swollen and bleed readily even while doing brushing.

Neutropenia/agranulocytosis. Ulcers may occur in the oral cavity which is a common site of involvement in cases of agranulocytosis. Common sites in the oral cavity are gums, lips, tongue, tonsils and throat. Ulcers are superficial covered with greyish black exudate. These often become secondarily infected. The surrounding area is often inflamed red and necrotic. The lesions tend to extend to the surrounding structures. There is foul smell emanating from the mouth. Gums are swollen, spongy, ulcerated and bleed readily. Features of toxaemia in the form of fever, malaise are present. Lymph nodes get enlarged and severe degree of prostration may develop.

Aplastic anaemia. It is slow in onset and the symptoms are due to pancytopenia. There is anaemia, bleeding from the gums which may be swollen and are spongy. They may bleed readily on touch. Petechial spots are present on the palate and haemorrhages may be seen in oral cavity. There are features of bleeding from nose, gastric or intestinal tract. Ulceration in the mouth and pharynx may be present along with lymphadenitis.

Haematological malignancies. There constitute a varied group of diseases including lymphomas. Lymphoma involves gingiva, palate, tongue and tonsillar area. There are elevated ulcerated areas in the oral cavity. These proliferate rapidly giving the appearance of a traumatic inflammatory lesion. Tonsils and cervical lymph nodes get enlarged. The disease follows a down hill course. Lymphomas are malignant tumours of lymphoreticular system and are classified on basis of histology.

Diagnosis. Since oral manifestations are just a reflection of various haematological disorders, so they just mirror the disease which is lurking somewhere else but presence of these signs should alert one to think of various disorders.

Diagnosis invariably shall depend on clinical picture of the patient as a whole (local as well as systemic) along with tests (total and differential leucocyte count, Peripheral blood film, bleeding time and clotting time, platelet and reticulocyte count), gland biopsy and other relevant investigations.

Treatment. It consists of treating the underlying condition and maintaining good oral hygiene and prevention of secondary infection. Any patient coming with bleeding gums or bleeding spots in the oral cavity must be investigated thoroughly and cause looked into.

CHAPTER 8

Diseases of the Endocrine Glands

1. Pituitary and its disorders
2. Thyroid gland and its disorders

3. Disorders of parathyroid glands
4. Adrenal gland and its disorders

Ductless glands are important structures in the body whose secretions in the blood have a direct or indirect effect on metabolic processes, maintenance of cellular constancy of body, Body growth process of reproduction and secretion of hormones in the body which act as chemical messengers. In fact endocrines glands are important controlling authority in body for maintaining various functions of the body and any disease involving them puts the whole body system into disarray.

PITUITARY AND ITS DISORDERS

Pituitary. It is a small gland ococupying sella turcica and consists of two lobes—anterior and posterior. Anterior pituitary is the main constituent which controls the activities of many of the other endocrine glands through its secretions. Anterior pituitary directly or indirectly controls the process of growth, sexual development, thyroid and adrenocortical functions by means of its hormones, i.e. adrenocorticotrophic hormone (ACTH), follicle stimulating hormone (FSH),

thyroid stimulating hormone (TSH), growth hormone (GH) and prolactin (PRL).

Post-pituitary mainly secretes anti diuretic hormone (ADH) which increases the reabsorption of water by its effect on distal convoluted and collecting tubules of the kidney. Oxytocin the other hormone enhances uterine contractions. Pituitary may be involved by tumours, inflammations and trauma. Syndromes associated with hyperpituitarism are gigantism, acromegaly, cushings syndrome while in cases with hypopituitrism the main disease is simmond's disease and involvement of hypothalamo hypophysial system leads to diabetes insipidus, a disease characterised by great excretion of large quantities of very dilute urine.

GIGANTISM

This is a disorder seen in early childhood and is caused commonly by excessive production of growth hormone as a result of hyperplasia of eosinophilic cells of the anterior pituitary. Gigantism develops because of excessive and rapid growth before fusion of bony epiphyses.

Hormones of pituitary

Anterior pituitary

1. Adrenocorticotrophic hormone (ACTH)
2. Thyroid stimulating hormone (TSH)
3. Growth hormone (GH)
4. Prolactin (PRL)
5. Follicle-stimulating hormone (FSH)
6. Gonadotrophins
7. Melanocyte-stimulating hormone (MSH)

Posterior pituitary

1. Antidiuretic hormone (ADH)

Clinical features. There is abnormal growth more in linear form of the bones of the extremities with resultant strength of a giant by the age of ten to fifteen years. There is disproportion in various parts of the body. Height of lower part of body exceeds that of the upper part. There is muscular hypertrophy and sexual precocity. Growth continues till the adult age when epiphysis fuse and then it may do so now at a lower rate. Though all the bones of body are effected but since the long bones are more effected their growth gives a giant appearance. Abnormal growth may diminish after epiphyseal closure but if abnormal stimulus persists, changes of acromegaly may supervene. A deep seated headache may be an early symptom though signs of raised intracranial tension or pressure on optic chiasma are less common. The pituitary fossa may or may not be enlarged. Cranial air sinuses, viscera are enlarged. Exostosis may develop at the site of insertion of muscles. Diabetes may develop as sugar tolerance is decreased. Gonads and genitalia atrophy. Body hair become sparse. Body metabolism declines. Temperature is low. Intercurrent infections are common.

Diagnosis. Strikingly abnormal growth in infancy is sufficient to make a diagnosis of gigantism. Radiological examination will show abnormal ossification of bones, density of bones increased and exostosis at bone ends. In the regressive stage of gigantism when features of myxoedema or addison's disease appear, diagnosis may be difficult and investigations are required to clinch the basic diagnosis.

Treatment. It may be surgical or medical. Surgery is indicated if a pituitary tumour is suspected. Irradiation of pituitary by implantation of radon seeds may be tried. Where surgery can not be planned, bromocriptine is used and it may help in regression of physical abnormalities in a fair percentage of cases.

Prognosis in a case of gigantism is not good. Patient may die from intercurrent infections or may pass into a stage of hypopituitarism.

ACROMEGALY

It is a disease characterized by excessive growth of the bones and other parts (jaws, hands and feet) seen in adult life generally in the age group of 20-40 years in both sexes.

Major symptoms in a case of acromegaly

1. Typical appearance both of body and face.
2. Excessive growth of body.
3. Enlargement of hands and feet.
4. Voice coarse and husky
5. Face enlarged and elongated. Lower jaw prominent with teeth widely spaced (proganthic jaw).
6. Tongue enlarged (macroglossia), lips thick.
7. Brownish pigmentation of face. Skin coarse and greasy.
8. Spine may show lordosis, kyphosis and scoliosis.
9. Excessive sweating, body hair growth increased.
10. Headache, visual disturbance, polyuria/polydypsia.

Acromegaly is the result of excessive secretion of growth hormone (GH) and insulin-like growth factor-I (IGF-I) produced mainly by an adenoma of the acidophilic cells of anterior pituitary as compared to gigantism where it is hyperplasia of eosinophilic cells. Most of these adenomas are slow growing and, because of this, it may be difficult to identify the disease in its initial stages. Acromegaly may occasionally occur as a result of hypersecretion of growth hormone-releasing hormone (GHRH) from the hypothalamus or from an ectopic source.

Clinical features. Disease has an insidious onset with a prolonged course marked by remissions. There is increase in soft tissues and generalized thickening of the bones especially of the hands and feet which become coarse and thick spade like. Face becomes elongated because of growth of lower jaw and enlargement of facial bones. Lips, nose and ears enlarge with lips becoming thick. Jaw is prominent and gives a typical appearance of proganthic jaw with widely separated teeth. Tongue enlarges and so does larynx. Speech become hoarse or husky. Skin is thick, coarse and greasy. Areas of brownish pigmentation especially on face may appear. Spine shows changes in the form of kyphosis, scoliosis and even lordosis.

Various organs in the body are effected. Heart may enlarge, congestive failure develops. Conduction defects in the form of heart blocks develop. Lungs also enlarge along with thoracic cavity, breathlessness may develop.

In females amenorrhoea and in men impotence develops. Features of insulin resistant diabetes develop in form of polyuria and polydypsia. Because of adrenal cortical overactivity, excessive hair growth takes place. In some cases because of over production of thyrotrophic hormone (TSH) goiter may develop. Basal metabolic rate is increased. If optic chiasma is being involved patient may develop visual deterioration. Headache, tiredness, joint pains and weakness are other common features.

Investigations:

1. Blood chemistry: Glucose levels are increased. Glucose tolerance test is abnormal.
2. X-ray skull: Enlargement of sella turcica and sinuses (lateral view).
3. X-ray hands shows 'tufting' of terminal phalanges.
4. X-ray long bones: Broadening of epiphysis and exostosis at site of muscle insertion.
5. X-ray chest shows cardiomegaly.
6. CT scan and MRI give better visualisation of the pituitary tumours.
7. There may be hypercalcaemia

8. MRI is useful to identify the size of the pituitary tumour. In 75% of the cases there is macroadenoma while in 25% of cases there is microadenoma.
9. There may be excess of prolactin in body due to co-secretion with GH or due to stalk compression.

Treatment

It is aimed at stabilizing or decreasing pituitary tumour as well as decreasing levels of growth harmone (GH). Treatment consists of surgery. Radiotherapy and drugs.

1. Surgery. Transphenoidal surgery for removal of pituitary tumour is the treatment of choice. It is rapid and effective with cure rates of upto 90% in micro adenomas and 48% for macroadenomas. It is followed by radiotherapy. This line of treatment is advocated when there are symptoms of compression. Following surgery GH levels fall (GH < 5 m u/L). Development of hypopituitism follows surgery in 10-20% of cases.
2. Radiotherapy. It is indicated in cases of medical or surgical treatment failure. Irradiation of pituitary is done by implantation of radon seeds (ytrium) into pituitary. Side-effects include optic nerve damage and neuropsychiatric disturbances. It may take several years for GH to normalize following radiotherapy. Adjunctive medical treatment may have to be given. External radiotherapy is employed in some cases though it takes much longer time to be effective.

Medical. It consists of use of somatostatin analogues such as lanreotide SR, lanreotide autogel, octreotide lar, dopamine agonists (bromocriptine, cabergaline) and new drug pegavisomant.

These drugs are used as primary therapy when the tumour is not causing mass effects. Patients may be complete responders with suppression of GH to < 5 m u/l in 50% of cases. In cases where response is partial, GH is reduced but not to normal levels.

Dopamine agonist (Bromocriptine) is usually given to shrink the size of the tumour before radiotherapy. It is not as effective as somatostatin analogues but may be of use when there is co-existent prolactin secretion. The drug is usually given in elderly patients. Dose 20-60 mg/day. The effects of the drug are erratic and tumour shrinkage may not be usually achieved.

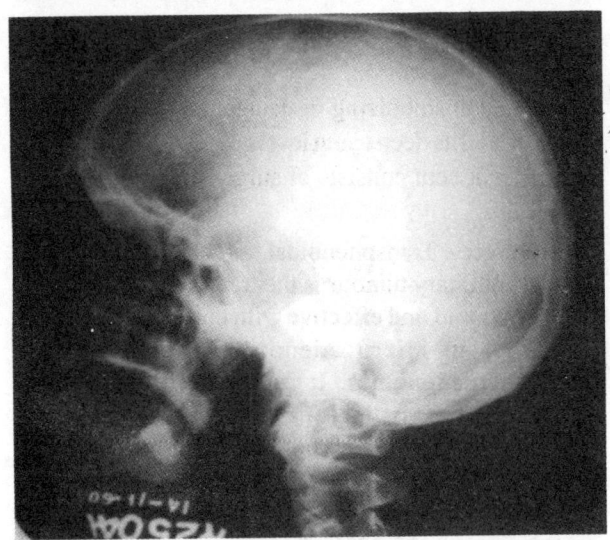

Fig. 8.1. X-ray skull in a case of pituitary tumour. There is widening of pituitary fossa. Clinoid processes are destroyed.

Somatostatin analogue (octreotide) is better drug and causes lowering of GH levels as well as tumour regression. Dose 50-100 µg administered subcutaneously 8 hrly. The acute response of GH following injection of octreotide can be used to predict the long term response. Side effects include steatorrhoea and increased incidence of cholelithiasis.

PEGAVISOMANT is a new drug which acts as a growth hormone antagonist. It reduce IGF-I levels to normal in over 90% of cases and also improves the symptoms of disease.

Assessment of cure in a patient should be done by regular check on GH. Curve or OG-TT and once a cure has been achieved, medical treatment may be gradually with drawn.

Course and prognosis. Prognosis shall depend on the extent of disease. Survival ranging from 10-15 years is in uncomplicated cases. Most cases die of intercurrent infections or congestive heart failure.

CUSHING'S SYNDROME

It is a clinical entity in which patient has got moon-shaped face, buffalo type obesity, purplish striae on the abdomen and other parts of body, hypertension, osteoporosis and tendency to diabetes mellitus. Earlier on cushings was considered to be associated with basophilic adenoma of anterior pituitary but subsequently hyperplasia of the adrenal cortex or a thymic carcinoma were also added as aetiological factors. Cushing like picture also develops after administration of corticosteroids in therapeutic doses for long periods. The condition results due to effect of increased amount of circulating adreno-corticotrophic hormone (ACTH).

Clinical features. It is common in age group of 20-35 years, more in females as compared to men. The classical features are obesity which develops rapidly on the face, neck and trunk. Face is rounded having a moon like face.

Skin is thin, bruises easily and there are reddish striae on the abdomen, thighs and shoulders. Hair growth occurs over the face and there are acne. Blood pressure is raised. In addition to change in appearance patient complains of marked weakness, insomnia. Because of osteoporosis pain in the back and other parts of body is common. Deranged carbohydrate metabolism produces, polyuria and polydypsia. Diabetes mellitus invariably develops. Sexual functions are disturbed. Amenorrhoea or oligomenorrhea in women, impotence in men and loss of libido in both sexes are other features.

Diagnosis. The clinical features of obesity, moon shaped facies, Hirsuitism, purple striae, hypertension anddiabetes makes the diagnosis easy. Main thing to decide is whether the disease is due to pituitary basophilic adenoma or an adrenal cortical hyperplasia or it is drug induced due to administration of corticosteroids.

Investigations:

1. Urinary excretion of 11-oxysteroids and 17-ketosteroids is increased. Normal or increase levels of ACTH suggest pituitary cause

of cushing syndrome. Dexamethasone suppression test showing failure of significant plasma cortisol suppression favours adrenal tumour as the cause.

2. Glucose tolerance test suggests diabetes.

3. X-ray chest for evidence of thymic carcinoma (lateral view).

4. X-ray skull for pituitary adenoma is not helpful. since a pituitary basophilic adenoma does not expend and so sella turcica and clinoid processes are normal.

5. X-ray dorsal spine may show collapse of vertebrae producing "fish-spine" appearances.

6. Intravenous pyelography for adenocortical tumour. Perirenal insufflation, tomography, ultrasonogoraphy, CT scan and MRI to detect adrenal hyperplasia.

Treatment. It shall depend on the aetiological factor. When pituitary adenoma is the cause, then treatment mainly is surgical and trans-sphenoidal microadenectomy of pituitary. When adrenal cortical hyperplasia or tumour is suspected bilateral adenalectomy followed by pituitary irradiation. Prior to undertaking surgery, cortisol hypersecretion should be controlled by use of drug Metyrapone (dosage 3 g daily in 3-4 divided doses). Plasma cortisol levels should be monitored. In cases where Cushing's syndrome is produced as a result of excessive use of corticosteroids, withdrawl of the drug shall reverse the symptoms to some extent.

Signs and symptoms in Cushing's syndrome

1. Moon-shaped face.
2. Acne and hair on face.
3. Buffalo type obesity.
4. Purple striae on abdomen, thighs, breasts and shoulders.
5. Aches and pain in body especially back (osteoporosis).
6. Hypertension.
7. Diabetes (polyuria, polydypsia, polyphagia).
8. Sexual function disturbed. Amenorrhoea/oligomenorrhoea in women. Impotance in men. Loss of libido in both sexes.

HYPOPITUITARISM

Deficiency of anterior pituitary hormones due to diseases of anterior pituitary resulting in partial or complete destruction of the gland, produces not only direct effect on body metabolism but also causes secondary failure of other endocrine glands in the body.

Pituitary dwarfism. This is so called because of either congenital deficiency of anterior pituitary hormones or involvement of the glands in early childhood due to either infection, trauma or malignancy. In fact the same causes which may operate in adult life are equally responsible in young adults. Result of this is cessation of growth (dwarfism) sexual development is halted (hypogonadism). Dwarfism or hypogonadism may exist in combination or as separate entities.

Causes of hypopituitirism mainly are:

1. Tumours of the pituitary.
2. Removal of gland by surgery.
3. Granulomatous diseases involving pituitary.
4. Infiltration of pituitary by leukaemia, lymphomas and malignancy.
5. Post-partum haemorrhage leading to infarction and haemorrhage in the pituitary.
6. Tuberculosis.

Clinical features. A pituitary dwarf is normal at birth. Absence or retardation of growth becomes evident by the age of 2 or 3 years. Some degree of obesity is present but the child is intelligent. Body proportions are maintained though the head may look large. Hands and feet are small though abdomen appears protubrant. Due to associated hypogonadism, the sexual organs in male children are small. In girls lack of sexual development is not seen till the child reaches puberty. Secondary sexual characters do not develop. Bones are thin and epiphyseal closure is delayed.

Diagnosis is made by clinical features of retarded growth. Basal GH levels have no value. Its secretion by insulin induced hypoglycemia may help to confirm the dignosis. There is no response in patients with pituitary dwarfism. X-rays of long bones shall show delay in the epiphyseal fusion. X-ray of skull may show a widened sella turcica. Pituitary dwarf is to be differentiated from all those disease which produce retardation of growth like protein, caloric malnutrition, malabsorption syndrome, Turner's syndrome skeletal disorders (achondroplasia), endocrine disorders (cretinism, Frohlich's syndrome), rickets, congenital cyanotic heart diseases etc.

Causes of hypopiuitarism

1. Tumours of pituitary
2. Removal of gland by surgery
3. Head injury
4. Radiotherapy
5. Post-partum necrosis (haemorrhage/ infarction of pituitary)
6. Granulomatous diseases (tuberculosis/ sarcoidosis)
7. Infiltration of pituitary by leukaemia, lymphoma, malignancy.
8. Autoimmune

Treatment. It shall depend on the underlying cause. When there is deficiency of growth hormone, treatment of choice is growth hormone 2-3 IU (0.4-0.7 iu/kg/week) twice a week. In addition anabolic hormones are also helpful.

SIMMOND'S DISEASE/ SHEEHAN'S SYNDROME

It is a disease where there is either partial or complete destruction of anterior pituitary occurring in adult life. The condition does not become apparent till more than two third cells of the pituitary are effected. It is more common in women as compared to men. Most commonly it presents in acute form due to necrosis of anterior pituitary as a result of thrombosis of pituitary vessels or infarction following post partum haemorrhage. Other lesions which may produce the condition in subacute or chronic forms include granulomatous lesions, tuberculosis, tumours, damage to the gland during surgery and cystic degeneration of the gland.

Clinical features. In a mild case there may be no clinical signs. In women the first sign is failure of lactation in post partum period. Breasts do not become engorged. Sex urge is lost. Complete loss of hair in axillary and pubic areas occurs. Men need to shave infrequently. Patient complains of generalized weakness and asthenia. Skin assumes a waxy pallor. There is absence of pigmentation on exposure to sun. Absence of sweating and sensitivity to cold is significant. Men with the disease have testicular atrophy, loss of secondary sexual characters, diminished or loss of sex urge and there may be absence of spermatogenesis. Premature senility may develop. As the disease progresses other endocrine glands including thyroid also get involved leading to manifestations of their involvement. Pulse and heart rate slow down.

Investigations:

1. Haemoglobin levels are decreased. Hypochromic or normochromic type of anaemia is present.
2. Blood sugar levels are low and less than normal.
3. Basal metabolic rate is decreased.
4. Serum cholesterol levels are raised.
5. Insulin tolerance test: In this a small dose of insulin (0.03 units/kg body weight) is injected after 12 hours of fasting. There is abnormal sensitivity to insulin and hypoglycaemic unresponsiveness.
6. X-ray skull (lateral view) may show empty sella turcica. Clinoid processes are effected. There may be calcification.

Diagnosis. A diagnosis of simmond's or sheehan's disease is based on clinical features and investigations (low blood sugar, low BMR, empty sella turcica). If patient is a female and there is history of post partum haemorrhage diagnosis is easier. Differential diagnosis is from cases of addison's disease, anorexia nervosa and myxoedema.

Treatment. The main aim is replacement of hormones. A number of hormones require replacement. Cortisone is given in a dase of 12.5-25 mg daily. In males Injection Testosterone 25 mg I/M on alternate days or 250-500 mg by implantation method every 3-4 weeks. In females cyclical oestrogen/progesterone therapy is employed. For thyroid, start with small doses either thyroid extract (30 mg) or thyroxine (0.1-0.2 mg) daily. Gradually increase the dose. High doses may preceipitate pituitary crisis. Once patient is maintained on cortison, ACTH is also added (50 mg once a week). Gonadotrophin replacement in the form of short courses of FSH and LH followed by human chorionic gonadotrophin (HCG) are helpful in inducing ovulation.

Prognosis. With adequate treatment, results are good and so is the prognosis. Success of therapy means a sense of well being and improvement in sexual functions.

DIABETES INSIPIDUS

It is a disease in which there is passage of large quantities of dilute urine along with increased thirst. Aetiologically it results due to damage or lesions of the hypothalmohypophysial system either as a result of inflammation, tumour (primary or metastatic) or trauma (head injury, fracture skull). Main abnormality is deficiency of antidiuretic hormone of the post pituitary. When it results due to unresponissiveness of distal convoluted tubules of kidney to ADH it is called Nephrogenic diabetes insipidus.

Causes of diabetes insipidus

1. Neoplasms of hypothalmohypophysial system or pituitary (craniopharyngioma, adenoma, secondaries)
2. Head injury, fracture skull
3. Surgery
4. Inflammation
5. Vascular

Clinical features. Disease has a gradual onset and is characterised by increased thirst and passage of large quantities of a very dilute urine. Patient is dehydrated and fluid intake is unable to cope with the diuresis. Temperature is subnormal. There is restlessness, lack of sleep, micturition may take place every half an hour. Because of excessive water intake sometimes signs of water intoxication

(nausea, vomiting, headache and chills) may develop.

Clinical features of diabetes insipidus

1. Increased thirst
2. Passage of large quantities of dilute urine
3. Signs of dehydration
4. Subnormal temperature
5. Restlessness, lack of sleep
6. Pale coloured urine with low specific gravity

Diagnosis. It is based on clinical features. Patient passes a very dilute urine with very low specific gravity. There is absence of albumin or glucose from urine. A urine concentration test where patient is deprived of fluids for 10-12 hours still does not show any rise in specific gravity (below 1010). X-ray skull may show widening of sella turcica in case of pituitary tumour. CT skull and MRI are helpful. Blood sugar and glucose tolerance curve are normal. Vasopressin test helps in differentiating cranial diabetes insipidus from nephrogenic diabetes insipidus. Diabetes insipidus has to be differentiated from diabetes mellitus, psychogenic causes and chronic nephritis.

Treatment. It shall be of the underlying cause. For symptomatic relief:

1. Nasal insufflation of post pituitary extract (10-20 ugm two to three times a day).
2. Injection Pitressin tartate in oil 5 units (1 cc) I/M daily for a fortnight and then on alternate days. Monitoring of patients daily urinary output and specific gravity is essential to assess the progress.

Prognosis. It shall depend on the underlying cause.

THYROID GLAND AND ITS DISORDERS

Thyroid gland controls body's metabolism and its secretions are controlled by thyroid stimulating hormone (TSH) of the anterior pituitary which in return stimulates the receptors in thyroid to increase synthesis of T3 and T4 producing their increased plasma levels. Thyroid hormone controls body's metabolic rate, physical and mental development and is essential for proper growth. In addition it controls intracellular and extracellular fluid balance, iodine, protein, cabohydrate, cholesterol levels and calcium and phosphorus metabolism. Abnormalities of thyroid function result in cretinism, myxoedema (hypothyroidism) thyrotoxicosis (hyperthyroidism) and goitre (thyroid enlargement without endocrine disturbances).

GOITRE

It is enlargement of thyroid which is non-inflammatory non-neoplastic and without any endocrinal disturbances. Goitre generally is observed as a diffuse enlargement of the gland (simple or non-toxic). It may be sporadic or endemic.

Endemic goitre is a public health problem and is observed in areas where there is iodine deficiency in the water and vegetables. Daily intake of iodine in foods is also very low and generally is less than 50 mg per day. Poor diet, economics and social customs of people in these areas accounts for high incidence of goitre. Common areas in India where goitre is endemic include Himalayan range, Himachal, Rajasthan, Madhya Pradesh, Haryana, Tamil Nadu and hilly areas of Uttar Pradesh.

Sporadic goitre. This goitre occurs more in women as compared to men and is common at puberty and pregnancy. Exact cause is not known. But possible causes include increased demand for thyroid hormone and iodine at these periods of life. Since the thyroid in such persons is unable to meet the increased demands or unable to utilize the iodine available in the diet because of some infective, genetic and metabolic factors, result is goitre. Goitre may also result due to exogenous goitrogens like drugs (PAS, chlorpropamide, sulphonylureas, serpina, phenyl, butazone, lithium) foods (cabbage, turnips, soyabean, tapioca), Defective hormone synthesis (dyshormonogenesis) is another cause.

Pathology. Goitre is the result of relative lack of iodine which occurs during periods like pregnancy, Adolescence and menarche where there is increased demand for thyroid hormone. Result is that there is hyperplasia of the thyroid due to compensation for thyroid hormone insufficiency. When the stress is over or iodine from diet is available increased demand for thyroid hormone ceases, the gland hyperinvolutes and excessive formation of colloid occurs resulting in a diffuse colloid goitre. Thyroid in such case functions normally. The process of hyperplasia and involution in a case of colloid goitre may not take place uniformly and nodules may form later on especially in cases with long standing goitre. Result is nodular goitre where nodules may join together due to degenerative changes, haemorrhage, rupture of small nodules to form large fibrosed nodules which are inactive (non-toxic nodular goitre).

Clinical features. Simple goitre mainly is a cosmetic problem. Generally it is a uniformly enlarged thyroid but nodules may be seen in some. If goitre become large enough it may produce pressure symptoms on trachea and oesophagus resulting in respiratory difficulty and dysphagia. Examination shall show a uniformly enlarged thyroid. Its shape, mobility be observed. Sometimes an enlarged gland may extend going into retrosternal space when its lower margin can not be reached.

A colloid goitre may undergo toxic changes and more so in nodular form. At this period signs of thyrotoxicosis may develop. A bruite may be heard over thyroid. A few patients with sporadic goitre may also pass into hypothyroidism.

Investigations:

1. X-ray chest and X-rays thoracic inlet for restrosternal thyroid.
2. Thyroid function tests are normal (radioactive iodine uptake and PBI). Plasma T4 is normal but T3 may be high.
3. Thyroid scan when nodular form of goitre is suspected or retrosternal goitre.

Treatment:

1. Goitre developing at time of puberty or adolescene in the presence of normal thyroid

function tests does not require any treatment. Where resolution of goitre does not take place spontaneously. Combined treatment with iodine (Lugol's iodine 5-10 minims in milk) and thyroxine (0.1 mg/day) may bring good response. The gland may start shrinking in 3-4 months time. Treatment has to be continued for 1-2 years. This treatment has its own hazards as the thyroid state is normal and there is danger of inducing thyrotoxicosis.

2. For prevention of goitre in endemic areas adequate intake of iodine in the form of iodised salt should be advocted, Diet should also be improved.

THYROTOXICOSIS

Over activity of thyroid gland resulting in increased liberation of thyroid hormone produces a picture of excessive thyroid activity called thyrotoxicosis which exists in two forms.

1. Primary
2. Secondary.

Primary thyrotoxicosis or Graves' disease. It is a disease which generally effects people between the ages of eighteen and forty years, more common in women as compared to men. The exact cause of thyrotoxocosis is not known. It is considered to be an autoimmune disorder in which thyroid stimulating autoantibodies (LATS) stimulate production of thyroid hormone. The thyroid enlarges diffusely with epithelial hyperplasia, lymphocytic infiltration with increased vascularity, Colloid in the acini becomes scanty. Genetic studies show the linkage of Graves' disease with HLA B8, DR3 and DR4.

Clinical features. The clinical picture of a case of thyrotoxicosis has basically four components.

a. Thyrotoxic component where there is over activity of the thyroid. There is loss of weight, intolerance to heat, palpitation, tachycardia and tremors. Patient complains of excessive sweating, increased appetite, diarrhoea, restlessness and lack of sleep.

Effects of thyrotoxicosis

1. General. Irritability, nervousness, fatigue, heat intolerance, weight loss.
2. Skin. Warm and moist. Hyperhidrosis.
3. Eyes. Exophthalmos, chemosis, opthalmoplegia
4. Cardiovascular. Tachycardia, atrial fibrillation, angina pectoris, increased pulse pressure, congestive heart failure, dyspnoea.
5. Neuromuscular. Tremors of hands, myopathy, weakness of proximal muscles, periodic paralysis.
6. GI tract. Increased appetite, diarrhoea, tremors of tongue.
7. Hematopoietic. Anaemia
8. Reproductive. Irregular menses, decreased fertility, micturition disturbances.
9. Neurological. Anxiety, restlessness, emotional lability, shortness of temper.

---

b. Thyrocardiac component. Palpitation and tachycardia are the main symptoms. Thyroid is warm and pulsatile. An arterial thrill may be present and a bruite heard. Systolic hypertension with wide pulse pressure and good bounding pulse are present. Cardiac arrhythmias especially atrial fibrillation, atrial tachycardia and later on congestive failure may develop.

c. Ophthalmic component consists of widened palpeberal fissue, deficient convergence on looking at a near object and failure to wrinkle forehead on looking upwards. Eyes are prominent (exophthalmos) with a staring look, infrequent blinking and lid lag. Eye signs indicate sympathetic overactivity. Exophthalmos may precede appearance of thyrotoxicosis or appear concurrently. These signs usually subside after treatment of thyrotoxicosis. Proptosis of eyes with chemosis, corneal ulceration periorbital oedema may develop in malignant form of exophthalmos.

d. Other manifestations include pressure effects on trachea and oesophagus when the gland is massively enlarged. Thyrotoxic patients may develop myopathy in late stage. Skin in most cases is soft and moist. Sometimes deposits of myxoedematous tissue may occur over the dorsum of legs and feet. These are called localized or pretibial myxoedma and are discrete, itchy well demarcated orange peel like having a nodular appearance. Pretibial myxoedma is due to non responsiveness of tissues locally to thyroid hormones.

Diagnosis. A case of thyrotoxicosis with classical signs (exophthalmos, tremors, tachycardia, thyroid enlargement) and symptoms (sweating, intolerance to heat, restlessness, increased appetite, diarrhoea, weight loss, palpitation) is not difficult to diagnose. Difficulty arises in a case of occult thyrotoxicosis. Differential diagnosis is from tuberculosis, diabetes and malignancy. Anxiety states especially in young women also require special attention since they are often mistaken for thyrotoxicosis. In anxiety states the hands are cold and moist while in thyrotoxicosis they are warm and also moist.

Investigations:

1. Basal metabolic rate (BMR) is raised (normal ± 10%).
2. Blood chemistry shows cholesterol levels to be decreased. Blood sugar may be normal or raised. Glucose tolerance curve shows decreased tolerance. Serum calcium and phosphorus levels are decreased. while creatinine levels are raised.
3. Radioactive iodine uptake: In thyrotoxicosis it is upto 75% (24 hours uptake in normal subjects is 20-25%). Protein (PBI) bound iodine (range 3-20 μm/100 ml), T3 and T4 levels are increased while levels of TSH are low.

Secondary thyrotoxicosis (Toxic nodular goitre). It develops in a person who has already got a colloid goitre or a nodular goitre. Clinical picture shall vary according to the age of the patient and state of the gland. The symptoms mainly pertain to heart and other components of the clinical picture are less prominent, Ophthalmic component is often absent or incospicous. Palpitation, loss of weight, a warm skin and preference for cold weather are common features. Cardiac complaints include tachycardia, palpitation and there may be signs of congestive failure. Multiple premature beats, paroxysmal tachycardias, atrial fibrillation are often present. Biochemical findings in secondary thyrotoxicosis are the same as in primary thyrotoxicosis. Radio active iodine uptake shall be increased while thyroid scan will show hot or cold areas depending on the activity of the thyroid nodule.

Treatment. *Treatment of thyrotoxicosis can be divided into:*

1. General
2. Drug therapy
3. Surgery
4. Radio-iodine treatment

General:

1. Rest both physical and mental.
2. Maintain nutrition of the patient by giving nutritious diet.
3. For anxiety patient be sedated by alprazolam (0.25-0.5 mg) twice a day.
4. Most patient of thyrotoxicosis are apprehensive because of increased sympathetic activity. Use of beta-blockers (Propranolol 40-80 mg twice a day) is helpful. Care should be taken in cases with bronchial asthma or congestive heart failure.

Anti-thyroid drugs. These form the main line of treatment in every case of thyrotoxicosis. These drugs act by blocking the synthesis of thyroid hormone. Carbimazole (Neomercazole) is the commonly used drug. Dose is 30 mg per day to start with. Adjustment of doses is made when thyrotoxicosis comes under control and then patient is kept on maintenance dose (10-20 mg per day). Drug is to be stopped when patient complains of sore throat, fever or rash. Side effects include bone marrow depression, mouth ulcers, rashes, fever and liver damage. The drug as a whole is safe, less toxic and does not increase vascularity of thyroid.

In cases with toxicity developing due to carbimazole, propyl thiouracil 100-150 mg 8 hourly is substituted. Thiouracil compounds take longer time to induce remission and are more toxic. Use of antithyroid drugs should be monitored by regular checks on toxicity and improvement in general condition.

Potassium per chlorate. It is an effective antithyroid drug. Dose is 800 mg per day to start with and is to be reduced with the improvement in patients condition.

Iodides. They act by blocking the release of preformed thyroid homone from the gland (release of T3,T4 and uptake of iodide). With daily administration the peak effect is seen in 10-15 days. When given along with thiourea compound it decreases not only the vascularity of the gland but also prevents increase in its size. Iodides are mainly indicted for preparing the patient for thyroidectomy and during thyroid crisis. Dosage of Lugols iodine is 3-5 minims of the drug in an ounce of milk daily. Saturated solution of potassium iodide (50 mg) may be substituted for Lugols iodine.

Surgery. Surgery in the form of subtotal thyroidectomy is performed. Its main indications are:

1. Severe form of thyrotoxicosis not responding to medical treatment.
2. Toxic nodular goitre.
3. Recurrence after adequate medical treatment.
4. Sensitivity or serious toxic reactions to antithyroid drugs.
5. Poor patient compliance to drugs and quick results are desired.
6. Pressure symptoms.

Commonly performed surgery is subtotal thyroidectomy. Prior to surgery antithyroid drugs are given to make the patient euthyroid. Iodine (potassium iodide 50-100 mg per day) is given 10-14 days before surgery to reduce vascularity of the gland.

Advantages of surgery are cure in high percentage of patients in a short time. Side effects include damage to recurrent laryngeal nerve and parathyroid glands. Hypothyroidism may follow in small percentage of cases.

Radioactive Iodine. It is another method employed in treatment of thyrotoxicosis. *Main indications are:*

1. Cases of thyrotoxicosis not tolerating antithyroid compounds.
2. Recurrent thyrotoxicosis after surgery.
3. Poor surgical risks.
4. Thyrotoxicosis complicated with cardiac complications.

Radioactive iodine treatment is convenient, highly effective and is acceptable to most of the patients. Radioactive iodine (1_{131}) is employed and thyroid is irradiated (7000 rods). Average effective dose is 8-10 millicuries. The treatment is contraindicated in patients below the age of 50 years, because of the danger of developing malignancy, and pregnant women as well as women of child bearing age. Disadvantages include development of hypothyroidism, late development of carcinoma and irreversibility of the process. In very ill patients of thyrotoxicosis, radio iodine may precipitate thyrotoxic crisis. Complications include acute thyroiditis, aggravation of eye signs, acute tracheitis and oesophagitis.

Thyrotoxic crises (Thyroid storm). This is development of extreme degree of hypermetabolism in a patient of thyrotoxicosis. It follows if thyrodectomy has been undertaken in an improperly controlled patient or in the presence of an acute infection or injury. Thyrotoxic crisis can also be worsened by radio iodine treatment.

Clinical features are hyperpyrexia, tachycardia, irritability, restlessness. Acute degree of psychotic behaviour, nausea, vomiting and diarrhoea may further worsen peripheral vascular collapse. Thyroid storm is an acute medical emergency and early suspicion and management is important.

Main principles of treatment are:

1. Supportive measures like sponging to bring down the temperature. Intravenous fluids (glucose and glucose saline) and O_2 administration.
2. Antibiotics for treatment of infection. Injection Hydrocortisone 100 mg I/V 6 hourly for management of shock.
3. Iodides preferably intravenously (sodium iodide IG by intravenous infusion). Saturated

solution of potassium iodide 300-500 mg orally till condition improves.

4. As there is excess of adrenergic sympathetic activity. Injection Propranolol (5-10 mg I/V) be given. This dose can be repeated every 4-6 hours.

5. As patient is generally restless Injection Diazepam 5-10 mg intramuscularly, to be repeated after 6 hours. Where restlessness is extreme the drug can be given intravenously but watch be kept on respiration since diazepam can cause respiratory depression.

6. If a patient in thyrotoxic crisis develops congestive heart failure then digitalis, diuretics have to be administered.

7. Antithyroid drugs (Propylthiouracil/ carbimazole) are also to be administered though their benefit may not be immediate.

Prognosis. Thyrotoxic crisis is a serious emergency and carries poor prognosis. Best is to prevent the condition from developing by taking adequate precautions.

HYPOTHYROIDISM

Inadequate release of thyroid hormone and its defective synthesis give rise to clinical condition of hypothyroidism which may be either primary or secondary.

Primary hypothyroidism results from diseases of thyroid like congenital defect, autoimmune disorders, following surgery of thyroid, after radio iodine treatment, use of anti thyroid drugs, iodine deficiency, drugs like iodide, PAS, phenylbutazone, chronic thyroiditis and idiopathic group.

Secondary hypothyroidism follows diseases effecting hypothalmo pituitary axis. Thyroid in such cases is intrinsically normal but is deprived of stimulation of TSH. This occurs in cases of hypopituitarism. Hypothyroidism following involvement of hypothalamus is not very common.

Forms of hypothyroidism:

1. Cretinism

2. Juvenile myxoedema
3. Adult myxoedema.

Primary hypothyroidism is commonly associated with circulating anti thyroid antibodies, substantiating the theory of auto immune disorders. Congenital absence of thyroid hormone leads to condition called cretinism. When thyroid insufficiency develops after birth it is called juvenile myxoedema and when this deficiency occurs in adult life it is called myxoedema.

Causes of primary hypothyroidism

1. Congenital deficiency
2. Autoimmune
3. Chronic thyroiditis (Hashimoto's disease)
4. Antithyroid drugs
5. Following subtotal thyroidectomy
6. Radio-iodine treatment
7. Drugs (PAS, iodides, phenylbutazone lithium)
8. Iodine deficiency
9. Dyshormogenesis

Cretinism. Cretinism may be either endemic or sporadice. Endemic cretinism is seen in places where endemic goitre is present. Sporadic cretinism occurs in children where thyroid is congenitally absent or the mother has been given high doses of antithyroid drugs.

Clinical picture. The onset of cretinism is insidious because the mothers milk contains thyroid hormone, so its appearance is delayed in breast fed children. A cretin has retarded physical and mental growth. Child is obese, with pads of fat in the supraclavicular region, coarse features, limbs which are stumpy, thick lips and tongue, protuberant abdomen, small eyes, coarse hair, dry skin and temperature which is subnormal. Intelligence is very poor and child may not be able to perform normal functions as per his age. A cretin is more of an imbecile, whose all round development remains retarded. Lethargy and constipation are other features. Intercurrent infections are common and may kill the patient.

Investigations show high levels of cholesterol in blood, ECG is helpful in making a diagnosis.

Estimation of T3,T4 and TSH levels are diagnostic.

Treatment is both prophylactic and curative. In areas where endemic goitre is prevalent pregnant women must be given potassium iodide (50-60 mg) daily. Curative treatment means giving thyroid extract or eltroxin (0.05 mg) and this has to be continued all life. Close monitoring of the patient is required.

Juvenile myxoedema. It differs from cretinism in that thyroid insufficiency occurs in early infancy. Clinical features in young children resemble to some degree the features of cretin while in those where disease develops in later years it resembles adult form of myxoedema. Growth of the child is retarded and stature is less than normal. Skin is dry, sallow, hair scanty and coarse, Teeth development is retarded.

Investigations like BMR (low) serum cholesterol (raised levels), ECG (poor voltage graph, generalized T waves inversion) and T3, T4, TSH estimation help in confirming diagnosis.

Treatment is by thyroid extract or eltroxin to be given throughout life.

Prognosis shall depend on the reponse of the patient and the delay in institution of treatment after onset of symptoms.

MYXOEDEMA

When thyroid functions fail during adult life it result is adult myxoedema which usually appears insidiously and often so insidiously that it is difficult to pin point when its onset took place. Commonest cause of primary form of myxoedema is autoimmune reaction while secondary form results from thyroid disorders such as chronic thyroiditis (Hashimoto's disease) endemic goitre, following surgery of thyroid, radio iodine treatment, of thyrotoxicosis, radiation, and prolonged use of drugs like PAS, Potassium thiocynate, phenylbutazone. All these conditions damage the gland leading to atrophy of secreting tissue. Panhypopituitarism following post partum haemorrhage results in features of myxoedema though may be temporary.

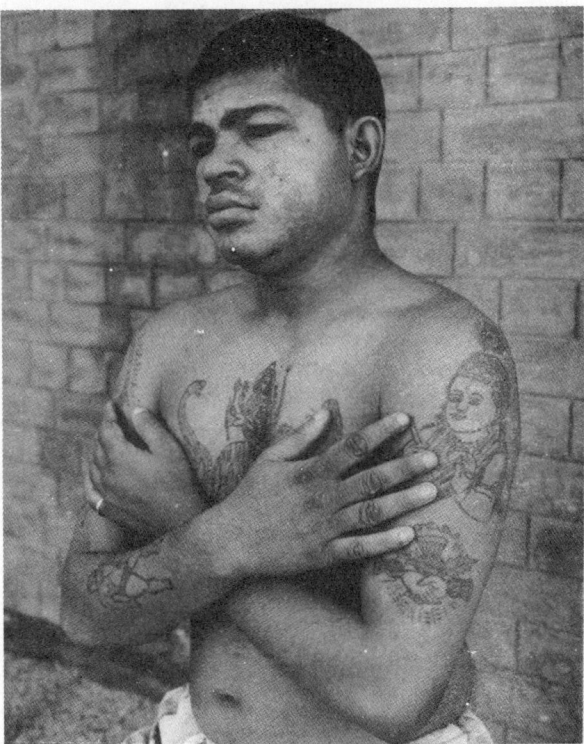

Fig. 8.1. A case of Myxoedema.

Clinical Features. It is a disease of middle age, affecting women more as compared to men. There is total slowing of all body functions. Lethargy, somnolence, and coarse features, like thick tongue, slow speech, hoarse and slurred. Thickened lips, weight gain are important features. Hair are coarse, dry and there is loss of hair over outer third of eyebrows. There is no pitting oedema. Constipation, accumulation of adipose tissue and cold intolerance are other features. There may be pain and stiffness of joints. Pulse rate is slow. Bradycardia with pulse rate less than 50 per minute is common. Mental functions are slowed. Movements are slow. Patient takes longer time to think and answer. Features of parasthesia, muscle cramps and muscular hypertrophy may be present. Tendon reflexes are diminished and relaxation phase especially observed in ankle jerk is delayed.

Cardiovascular complications include cardiomegaly, due to myxoedematous infiltration, anginal pain, pericardial effusion and hypertension. Constipation is often intractable. Myxoedematous involvement of middle ear may produce deafness. Young women may show oligomenorrhoea, amenorrhoea, menorrhagia and infertility. Sex urge is reduced in both sexes. Anaemia is generally of macrocytic type but may be normocytic or hypochromic.

Clinical manifestations of hypothroidism

1. Cold intolerance
2. Thickening and dryness of skin and hair
3. Swelling of hands and face
4. Change in shape of face
5. Thick lips
6. Non-pitting oedema
7. Yellowish discoloration of skin
8. Hoarseness of voice
9. Decrease or loss of sweating
10. Loss of hair on outer third of eyebrows
11. Slow pulse/bradycardia

Patients of myxoedema when exposed to severe cold or infections pass into myxoedema coma chracterised by hypoventilation, hypoglycaemia and confusion going into coma. Death incidence in such cases is very high. In severe foms myxoedema patient may become demented or psychotic. This is called myxoedema madness more common in elderly patients.

Investigations:

1. BMR is low.
2. Serum cholesterol levels raised (more than 300 mg%).
3. Iodine uptake (I_{131}) by thyroid is poor.
4. Serum T3,T4 levels are low while TSH levels are raised in primary myxoedema, TSH levels are low or nomal in myxoedema following Pan hypopituitarism.
5. Creatine phosphokinase levels are increased.
6. Titres of antithyroid and antimicrosomal antibodies are high.
7. Electrocardiogram shows a slow heart rate (less than 50 per minute) poor voltage and generalized flattening or inversion of T waves.

Treatment. Principle of therapy is replacement of deficient thyroid hormones.

Thyroid extract was the most commonly used drug earlier on. Dosage 30-60 mg to start with. It has been almost replaced by Eltroxine (L-thyroxine) which is the most widely used drug (available 0.05 mg and 0.1 mg tablet).

In all cases of myxoedema start with a relatively small dose since sudden changes in metabolic levels may produce undesirable psychological or cardiovascular disturbances espepcially in elderly persons. The drug is cumulative and may take at least a weak to act. Gradually increase the dose at weekly intervals till either desired results are achieved or side effects occur (tachycardia, irritability, restlessness, lack of sleep). It is better to give the drug in morning hours to obviate sleeplessness. The occurrence of angina or congestive failure during therapy may require either decrease in dosage of drug or even its withdrawl.

The maximum effect from a given dosage will not be obtained for at least 7 to 10 days. Dosage has to be adjusted and monitored according to clinical improvement as well in other parameters (serum cholesterol levels, T3,T4 and TSH measurements).

Patients with myxoedema coma should be treated with Tri-iodothyroxine (T3) given intravenously in a dose of 20 µm and repeated 8 hourly along with inj. hydrocortisone (100 mg I/V8 hourly) and intravenous dextrose. Adequate ventilation must be maintained alongwith electrolyte balance and slow warming. Patients vital signs must be monitored and after recovery from acute crisis, thyroid functions be assessed and adequate therapy instituted.

DISORDERS OF PARATHYROID GLAND

Parathyroid hormone secreted by the four parathyroid glands maintains and controls calcium levels in the body by its dual action on bones, the calcium replacement and bone remodelling effect. Its main function is to maintain concentration of calcium in extracellular fluid compartment. Circulating calcium exerts major control on parathyroid hormone

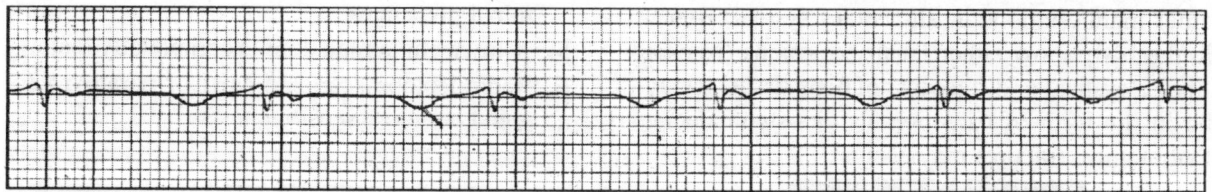

Fig. 8.2. ECG in a case of myxoedema showing poor volgage and bradycardia

secretion and subsequent release. Thus fall in serum calcium levels stimultes the secretion while rise inhibits the hormone release.

Parathyroid hormone by its action on kidneys conserves calcium and eliminates phosphates and bicarbonates while at the same time it maintains balance in resorption of calcium and phosphorus from bones by interplay of vitamin D, renal functions and osteoblastic activity.

Hyperparathyroidism. Increased activity of parathyroid hormone produces clinical picture of hyperparathyroidism which may be primary or secondary.

Primary hyperparathyroidism. It is a disease which effects females more than men in the age group of thirty to fifty. The main cause is a benign adenoma of the parathyroid gland. Malignant tumours can also produce the condition but they seldom reach the stage to produce increased secretion of the hormone.

Clinical features of hyperparathyroidism

1. Aches and pains all over the body.
2. Loss of weight, generalized lethargy, muscular weakness.
3. Loss of appetite, nausea and vomiting.
4. Deformities of bone, shrinkage of spine. Bones show localized lesions (osteitis fibrosa cystica), pathological fractures.
5. Urinary infections, renal stones, nephro-calcinosis, calcification, renal failure.
6. Corneal calcification.

Clinical features. Hyperparathyroidism mainly involves bones and kidneys so the symptoms mainly pertain to these structures. The onset of disease is rather insidious and by the time patient presents he or she has already got decalcification of bones, hypercalaemia, hypophosphatemia and renal damage. Patient generally complains of aches and pains all over the body, loss of weight, lethargy, generalized muscle weakness often accompanied by loss of appetite, nausea and vomiting. Bony swellings may appear at various sites (Jaw, tibia, phalanges) and are painless to start with but later on become tender.

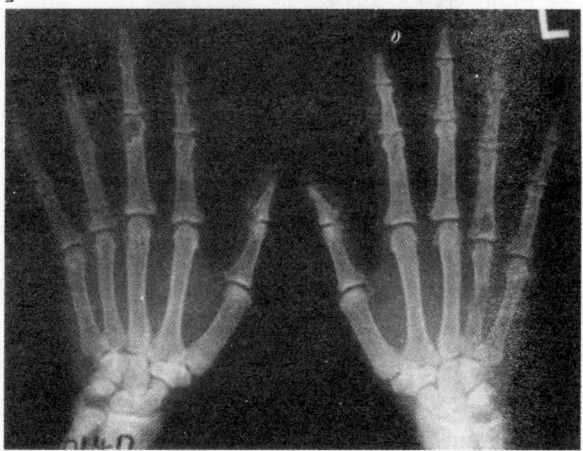

Fig. 8.3. Xray hands show osteolytic lesions in the phalanx.

High levels of calcium reduce excitability of nerves and muscles leading to diminution of muscle tone. Deformities in bones may occur leading to increased curvature and shrinking of spine. Renal involvement with formation of renal stones, calcification of the kidney and predispostion to urinary infections with reduced glomerular filtration rate as well as tubular damage in the end leads to renal failure. Hypercalcaemia also increases gastric secretions and often produce peptic ulceration.

Chronic pancreatitis and pancreatic calcification are other manifestations in alimentary system. Bones in the body show either localised lesions (osteitis fibrosa cystica) or diffuse loss of bony tissue. It may be in the form of osteoporosis or osteomalacia. Pathological fracures may occur.

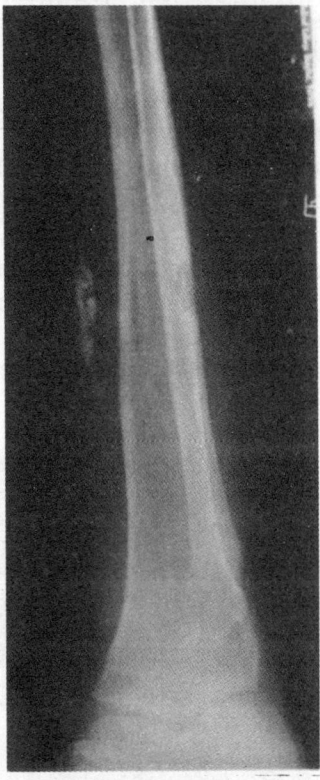

Fig. 8.4. Xray lower limbs shows soft tissue calcification.

Investigations:

1. Serum calcium levels are increased and may reach 20 mg/dl (normal 9 to 11.5 mg/dl) while plasma phosphorus levels are reduced (2 mg per 100 ml or less). Urinary excretion of calcium rises and exceeds 300 mg (normal less than 3 mg/kg body weight). Plasma alkaline phosphatase levels increased (normal 3-13 KA/units).

2. X-rays of long bones show diminished density. Cysts may be seen in bones. Local destructive lesions and subperiosteal erosion of cortical bone are other features.

3. X-ray skull shows multiple areas of mottling (pepper pot skull).

4. X-ray hands shows complete resorption of terminal phalanges.

5. X-ray teeth lamina dura is completelty lost.

6. Radio-isotope scan and MRI of parathyroid gland are more sensitive tests.

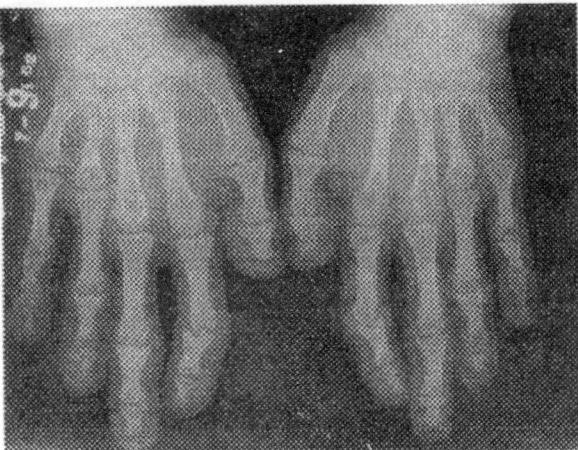

Fig. 8.5. X-ray hand in a case of primary hyperparathyroidism there is subperiostal erosion of middle phalanges of inded and middle fingers.

Diagnosis. Hyperparathyroidism is suspected in a patient with bony pains, pathological fractures, cystic lesions in bones and renal calculi. Confirmation is made by biochemical and radiological investigation.

Treatment. All cases where there is involvement of bone or kidney, surgical intervention in the form of removal of tumour of parathyroid is indicated. Sometimes the tumour is so small that it may be difficult to distinguish it from a normal gland. Usually all the four glands are removed and only a portion of one gland is left behind. Some cases may develop hypocalcaemia in post operative period. If hypocalcaemia persists for long periods then treatment on the line of hypoparathyroidism is indicated. Medical treatment of hyperparathyroidism is not advocated except cases in where surgery is not advised because of poor surgical risk. Here attempts are made to lower calcium levels in blood. Intake of calcium in diet is restricted. Patient is given potassium phosphate 1-2 g daily since it helps in the deposition of calcium in bones.

Prognosis. After successful removal of parathyroid tumour prognisis is good. Serum calcium levels fall and resolution of bony changes takes place.

Secondary hyperparathyroidism. This is a compensatory phenomenon where hyperplasia or hypertrophy of the parathyroid glands takes place due to low levels of calcium in the body. Hypocalcaemia is seen in cases of rickets, osteomalacia, chronic renal failure. In this case, low calcium levels stimulate the glands to secrete more of parathyroid hormone but later on the glands may become autonomous.

Long-standing secondary hyperparathyroidism leads to the development of adenomas in the gland. At this stage plasma calcium and parathyroid hormone levels rise leading to condition called tertiary hyperparathyroidism. In secondary form calcium levels are generally low or normal with serum phosphate levels rising. Since parathyroid activity is there, bony changes shall be just like that in primary form of disease.

Treatment in both these conditions is of underlying cause. Low levels of calcium have to be raised so that they do not act as source of chronic stimulation for secretion of parathyroid hormone. In tertiary form where adenomas have been formed and biochemical abnormalities (raised levels of calcium and parathyroid hormone) are there, surgery(parathyroidectomy) is advised.

Hypoparathyroidism. Hypoparathyroidism means deficiency in secretion of parathormone hormone and is characterized by low levels of serum calcium, hyperphosphatemia and features of neuromuscular irritability as well as tetany. A number of factors are responsible for the causation of this disease. These include accidental removal of parathyroids during surgery on thyroid, involvement of parathyroids due to malignancy, secondaries, irradiation of neck, radio iodine treatment of thyrotoxicosis and occasionally the cause is idiopathic. Uncommonly hypopara-thyridism may be associated with other congenital anomalies and in some it may be an autoimmune disorder.

Causes of hypoparathyroidism

1. Congenital
2. Autoimmune
3. Accidental damage or removal of gland during thyroidectomy.
4. Malignancy of the gland.
5. Destruction of parathyroid gland by irradiation to neck.
6. Secondaries involving the gland.
7. Radio-iodine treatment in thyrotoxicosis
8. Idiopathic.

Clinical features. Clinical picture of hypoparathyroidism is that of hypocalcaemia and its manifestations shall depend on degree and severity of hypocalcemia. Patient has got irritability, parasthesiae in limbs along with stiffness. Tetany is a very predominant symptom and generally shows itself with carpo pedal spasm. Laryngeal spasm produces hoarseness of voice along with spasm of muscles of mastication and facial muscles giving appearance of 'Risus Sardonicus'. Chvostek's sign (a tap over the facial nerve exit in front of external auditary meatus produces contraction of facial muscles) and Trousseu's sign (applying a blood pressure cuff over the arm and keeping pressure exceeding systolic, elicits a carpal spasm) when present are quite diagnostic.

Clinical signs

1. Trousseau's sign
2. Chvostek's sign
3. Risus sardonicus.

In addition to tetany, patient has psychotic disturbances (dementia, delusions, hallucinations). Skin is dry, nails brittle and ridged. Fissures form at the angle of mouth. Atrophic glossitis, opacities in optic lens to gross cataract are present. Enamel of the teeth assumes a pitted appearance. Dental roots become short and blunt. Early loss of teeth may occur. Cardiac irregularities may occur. Electro-cardiogram shows a prolonged Q-T interval.

Biochemical changes. Serum calcium levels are low (less than 5 mg per 100 ml) while plasma phosphorus levels are raised (more than 6-7 mg per

100 ml). Levels of parathyroid hormone are either low or even absent.

Diagnosis of hypoparathyrodism is based on clinical picture of tetany and biochemical findings. All those conditions where tetany and low calcium levels are present (osteomalacia, uraemia, steatorrhoea, alkalosis, infantile rickets) have to be differentiated.

Treatment. Basis is to bring serum calcium levels to as normal levels as possible and to treat tetany. For tetany slow intravenous injections of 20 ml of 10% calcium gluconate is given. Its effect is immediate and lasts for 4-6 hours. In acute cases it has to be repeated every 4-6 hours. As the condition improves oral calcium salts are given.

(2) Replacement of parathormone hormone (10-15 units subcutaneously or intramuscularly). There is danger of over dosage by this method. Its therapeutic use is limited. Vitamin D is a better substitute. Oral dose of vitamin D_2 (calciferol) or a related steroid substance (1-alpha OHD3 (1-2 μg) be given daily.

Along with vitamin approximately 1.0 g of elemental calcium is provided in the diet. Diet should contain good amount of calcium but low in phosphorus. Effect of vitamin D may not be seen till a few weeks of therapy. While using vitamin D preparations as well as calcium care should be taken that over treatment does not produce hypercalcaemia and subsequent renal damage. A close watch should be kept on calcium levels.

Clinical picture of Hypoparathyroidism

1. Parasthesia, tingling numbness in limbs. Picture of tetany.
2. Laryngeal spasm.
3. Generalized convulsions.
4. Vomiting and abdominal cramps.
5. Psychotic disuturbances (delusions, dementia, hallucinations)
6. Features of bronchial spasm.
7. Trophic changes in skin.
8. Lenticular opacities in eyes.
9. Dental roots short and blunt. Early loss of teeth.

Prognosis in a case of hypoparathyridism is good depending on the underlying condition. Adequate control of tetany ensures good recovery.

ADRENAL GLANDS AND ITS DISORDERS

The adrenal glands, two in number constitute important part of endocrinal system. They are concerned with the secretion of a number of hormones some of which are responsible for maintaining a number of important body function. Adrenal cortex secretes substances which control electrolytes, carbohydrate and protein metabolism. Further resistance to stress, shock and growth as well as development of sex glands is dependent on it. This mechanism of glucocorticoid secretions is controlled by hypothalamic pituitary axis while mineralocorticoid secretion is mainly controlled by renin-angiotensin system.

Adrenal medulla is responsible for the production of adrenaline and noradrenaline which have their own role to play but this is not so significant as that of adrenal cortex which controls a number of body functions and is essential for life. A number of diseases result due to malfunctioning of the adrenal cortex.

Hyperfunctioning of the adrenal cortex produces hyperplasia of adrenal cortex and raised levels of glucocorticoids. *Cushing's syndrome* is the clinical condition which is also associated with basophilic adenoma of anterior pituitary. Other syndromes associated with over activity of the cortex is congenital adrenal hyperplasia (adrenogenital syndrome) which is charactersed by features of viralization, hirsutism, urogenital abnormalities in females while in male often the syndrome is unrecognised but may produce picture of precocious puberty.

Hypofunctioning of the adrenal cortex produces picture of hypoadrenalism, which may be primary called addison's disease or secondary adrenocortical insufficiency due to disease of Hypothalamus and pituitary.

ADDISON'S DISEASE (PRIMARY ADRENAL CORTICAL INSUFFICIENCY)

It is characterised by hypo-functioning of the adrenal cortex due to diseases involving primarily the gland. It is manifested by brownish pigmentation of the skin and mucous membrane of the mouth, hypotension and disturbances of electrolytes. It is a disease which is more common in men as compared to women and is often seen in the age group of 30-35 years. A number of diseases are responsible for Addison's disease.

Aetiologically these are:

1. Destruction of the adrenal cortex by tuberculosis. It is the commonest cause in more than 80 per cent of cases.
2. Infiltration of gland by secondaries.
3. Post-surgical
4. Severe degree of meningococcal septicaemia (Waterhouse-Friderichsen syndrome)
5. Autoimmune disorder
6. Amyloidosis, haemochromatosis, and vascular lesion are rare causes.

Causes of adrenal insufficiency:
1. Primary
   a. Idiopatic
   b. Autoimmune
   c. Tuberculosis, AIDS, meningococcal septicaemia
   d. Haemorrhage
   e. Secondaries
   f. Surgical removal
   g. Haemochromatosis/amyloidosis
2. Secondary
   a. Hypopituitarism
   b. Suppression of hypothalmopituitary axis by long-term steroids use.

Clinical features. Disease has an insidious onset and patient has generalized weakness, asthenia and apathy. Pigmentation of the skin and mucous membranes is an important feature. It may be in the form of either a dusky brown or bluish black discoloration on lips, gums, inside of cheeks, buccal mucosa, palate and tongue. It occurs on exposed as well as covered areas. Face, neck, genitalia, dorsum of hands forearms and pressure areas of the body have pigmentation. Pigmentation is due to disturbance of tyrosine metabolism which is being converted into melanin. Cutaneous areas of pigmentation may give appearances suggestive of vitilgo. A low blood pressure is characteristic. Faintness and giddiness may result on change of posture. Pulse is of low volume and heart sounds are feeble. Gastrointestinal symptoms include anorexia with nausea and vomiting. Gastric acidity is low. Loss of weight is there. There is wasting, marked weakness (asthenia). Lassitude and apathy which are important complaints.

Apart from these patient presents a picture of poor health. Physical signs include a thin wasted individual with a weak pulse, feeble heart sounds and blood pressure levels low. Pigmentation of the skin and mucosal surfaces especially of oral cavity is invariably present. Temperature may be subnormal.

Clinical features of Addison's disease

1. Marked asthenia and wasting
2. Weight loss
3. Hypotension (low blood pressure)
4. Dusky brown pigmentation of skin (exposed areas) and mucous membranes.
5. Nausea, vomiting, abdominal pain

Investigations:

1. Serum sodium and chloride levels are diminished while serum potassium levels are often raised.
2. Urinary excretion of chlorides is increased.
3. Blood sugar levels are low. Glucose tolerance level is low and flat. Insulin tolerance test shows extreme sensitivity to insulin.
4. Blood urea levels may be raised when there is coexisting renal failure.
5. Urinary excretion of 17-ketosteroids (normal males 10-20 mg, females 8-15 mg/per 24 hours) and 11-oxycorticosteroids (normal 0.1-0.44 mg per 24 hours) is diminished.

6. Basal metabolic rate is low.
7. Plasma cortisol levels are low.
8. No response to ACTH tests. Normally 50 per cent fall in circulating eosinophil count occurs after an injection of ACTH but in cases of Addison's disease the fall is less than 30 per cent.
9. Adrenal antibodies are present in cases where autoimmune mechanism is responsible.
10. X-ray chest for evidence of tuberculosis. Plain X-ray abdomen for calcification in adrenals.
11. CT scan abdomen may be helpful sometimes.

Treatment. Since there is deficiency of glucocorticoids and mineralocorticoids main aim is to replace these hormones. Mild to moderate cases require life long replacement therapy. Initially patient is put on Injection Hydrocortisone sodium succinate 25-100 mg daily and when patient is improving and stabilised, oral medication is switched on (Tablet Cortisone 20 mg in the morning and 10 mg in the evening).

For mineralocorticoids deficiency, fludrocortisone (0.05-0.4 mg daily) orally is to be added but only after administration of cortisone for few days. Deoxycortisterone acetate (DOCA) 2-5 mg given as intramuscular injection is a weak but good substitute.

In addition patient should receive adequate quantity of salt in diet. Diet should be low in potassium. Any intercurrent infection must be promptly treated.

Since in most of the cases aetiology is tuberculosis, treatment is directd towards it. Improvement in patients conditions is assessed by state of well being, rise in blood pressure levels, and monitoring of plasma cortisol levels in blood. Dosage of steroids be adjusted accordingly.

Secondary hypoadrenalism. It results from disorder of hypothalamicpituitary axis (encephalitis, meningitis, injury to base of skull, panhypopituitarism) as well as in patients on long term corticosteroids.

In secondary hypoadrenalism there is suppression of thyroid, adrenals and gonadotrophic functions because of involvement of the axis. Clinically patient has got features of asthenia, generalized weakness and of hypothyroidism. Treatment is by substitution therapy of thyroxine and cortisone.

Acute adrenal insufficiency (Addisonian crisis). Sudden development of adrenal failure leads to Addisonian crisis. It is an acute medical emergency and requires urgent management.

Causes include severe infection, acute gastroenteritis, surgical operations, trauma, septicaemia, sudden withdrawl of steroids.

Clinical features include severe degree of prostration, shock, vomiting and diarrhoea. Patient may pass into coma and death may occur.

Treatment. Aim of treatment should be to raise blood pressure levels. Correct fluid imbalance and prevent hypoglycaemia. 10 per cent glucose saline be administered immediately.

Injection Hydrocortisone Hemi succinate sodium 100 mg be given intravenously stat and repeated every 4-6 hours. Intravenous fluids are to be continued till the conditon improves and patient starts taking orally. Broad spectrum antibiotics be given since infection often is complicating the crisis. By 2nd or 3rd day Injection DOCA (10 mg I/M 6 hourly) is substituted and gradually replaced by oral cortisone (12.5-25 mg daily). Since cases of addisonian crisis have to be given heavy doses of steroids careful watch be kept that pulmonary oedema does not develop.

Prognosis. It shall depend on the underlying cause. Cases of tuberculosis can be managed successfully. As potent cortical extracts are available prognosis is good depending on the underlying disease whether treatable or not. Care about development of crisis must be ensured especially during acute infection, surgical operation or an attack of gastroenteritis.

ALDOSTERONISM

This is a condition where there is excessive secretion of aldosterone from the adrenals. It is either primary or secondary. In primary aldosteronism, there is excessive liberation of aldosterone within the adrenal gland whilein secondary aldosteronism the stimulus is extra-adrenal.

Primary aldosteronism (Conn's syndrome). It is a condition characterized by hypertension and hypokalemia. Because of potassium depletion there is marked weakness and fatigue. Hypertension which is predominantly diastolic is probably due to increased sodium reabsorption and expansion of extra-cellular volume. As a result of impaired concentrating ability of the kidney patient complains of polyuria and polydipsia. Oedema is absent in the absence of congestive failure or renal disease.

Aetiologically there is adrenal adenoma which is usually small and unilateral while in small percentage of cases there is bilateral adrenal hyperplasia. Primary adosteronism is more common in women as compared to men (2:1) in the age group of 30-50 years.

Laboratory investigations. These are dependent on the severity and duration of the disease. Predominant abnormalities are:

(i) Hypokalemia (< 3 mmol/l)

(ii) Hyper natremia

(iii) Elevated Plasma aldosterone levels

(iv) Urinary potassium loss (>30 mEq/day) in contrast to low serum potassium)

(v) Fall in serum Magnesium levels

(vi) Localisation of adenoma by CT/MRI. Radioisotope scanning will diffirentiate adenomas from adrenal hyperplasia.

Diagnosis of Conn's syndrome is made by

(i) Persistent hypokalemia in a non-oedematous patient, who is not on diuretics.

(ii) Diastolic hypertension

(iii) Low plasma rennin levels and increased levels of aldosterone.

Treatment. An adenoma is treated surgically (adrenalectomy). Those with bilateral adrenal hyperplasia, aldosterone antagonist, spironolactone (100-400 mg/day) is given, Other drugs like trimetrone, amiloride may be employed alternatively. If symptoms are not controlled by medical therapy, then surgery is the only alternative.

ADRENAL MEDULLA

Adrenal medulla produces hormonal substance which consists of adrenaline and noradrenaline. It consists of numerous chromaffin cells similar to the sympathetic nerve endings which are important in the storage and secretion of catecholamines.

Adrenal medulla is not essential for life and its hypofunction does not produce any disease. When a tumour arises from chromaffin cells it is called Phaeochromocytoma.

Phaeochromocytoma. It is an adrenal tumour arising from chromoffin cells of the adrenal medulla. It is uncommon and is responsible for 0.1% of cases of hypertension. In great majority (90%) the tumour arises from adrenal medulla while in small percentage (10%) the extra-adrenal growth occurs from sympathetic chain or para gangliomas. Phaeochromocytoma may be a single unilateral lesion in 80% of cases while 10% cases have bilateral lesions. The tumours arise in either sex and are common between the ages of twenty to forty years. Rarely familial phaeochromocytoma is known to occur as an autosomal dominant trait eiter alone or in association with multiple endocrine neoplasia. Such tumours are bilateral.

The tumour generally is benign and small but may attain size of 10 cm. It is highly vascular and releases catecholamines in body which is responsible for the clinical picture and morbidity.

Clinical picture

Classically a case of phaeochromocytoma presents with paroxysms of hypertension while in some it is sustained hypertension especially in a young person. Paroxysms of hypertension lasting from a few minutes to many hours and spread over symptom free interval lasting from weeks to month occur. An attack is associated with pallor, sweating tachycardia, Headache and anxiety. Other symptoms like pain in chest, nausea, vomiting, flushing may be present during the attack. There is fall of body temperature, parasthesiae vasoconstriction of the peripheral vessels with blanching of the fingers and toes.

An attack may be precipitated by foods like cheese, Beer, Wine and drugs like beta-blockers, tricyclic antidepressants, opiates, Histamine, glucagon and ACTH. Besides features of paroxymal hypertension, patient may suffer from orthostatic hypotension, cardiac arrhythmias, weight loss and impaired glucose tolerance.

Investigations

(a) There are increased levels of catecholamines and their metabolites in urine.

(b) Twenty four hours estimation of metanephrine and vamillymandelic Acid (VMA) is helpful in making a diagnosis. Normal value of metanephrine is 1.3 mg/day while upper limit of VMA is 7.0 mg/day.

(c) Blood sugar estimation (Hyperglycaemia).

(d) Plain X-ray abdomen before and after perirenal insufflation to demonstrate adrenal tumour.

(e) Intravenous pyelogram which may reveal displacement of a kidney or distortion of calyces or pelvis.

(f) CT scan, meta-iodine 131-iodobenzyl guanidine (MIBG) is specific and sensitive in identifying the tumour.

(g) Pharmacologic tests (histamine test, Regitine test), postural and cold pressor test, phentolamine test are now obsolete since they are non-specific and are also risky.

Diagnosis. It is based on clinical picture of paroxysmal or sustained hypertension in a young adult. Confirmation is done by biochemical and radiological investigations.

Treatment. Surgical removal of the tumour is the treatment of choice. Preoperatively patient is put on Phenoxybenzamine (10 mg BD) increasing to a total dose of 40-200 mg/day. It is administered for at least 10 to 14 perior to surgery. Alternatively prazosin (a selective alpha antagonist) is given in doses of 1-2 mg TDS. Beta blockes are given only after adequate alpha blockade has been established. If there is tachycardia then Propranolol 10mg there to four times per day is given, Beta Blockers are also helpful in controlling arrhythmias.

Prognosis. Once the tumour has been successfully removed, hypertension levels come down in 70% of the cases. Five year survival is usually more than in 95% of cases. Persistance of hypertension even after surgery is because of irreversible damage caused by catecholamines.

CHAPTER 9

Nutrition and Metabolic Disorders

1. Normal daily requirements of food
2. Balanced diet
3. Vitamins
4. Obesity
5. Protein caloric malnutrition
6. Calcium homeostasis
7. Diabetes mellitus

NORMAL DAILY REQUIREMENTS OF FOOD

Human body is a complex machine. It requires nutrients for its daily wear and tear and for the maintenance of not only the vital functions but also the person's vitality. The normal human body gets its nutrition from the food which consists not only of proteins, carbohydrates, fats but also vitamins and minerals.

The body needs differ from person to person and it is not essential that every individual will require the same amount of nutrition as the other.

Tastes differ from people to people. Some may like the same food while it is disliked by others. Food fads are of common occurrence and no generalization in the field of nutrition can be made. But there is agreement on one point that a certain basic food and nutrition needs of the person must be met with so that the body's needs and vitality does not suffer. Normal human body requires three types of foods.

1. Energy-building foods which are constituted mainly by fats and carbohydrates also called protein sparers. Proteins also produce energy to some extent.
2. Body-building foods which mainly are proteins, minerals and salts.
3. Protective foods which constitute inorganic salts and vitamins. This group also includes proteins and water.

When an individual consumes food it is digested, assimilated and utilized for energy production by a complex process of metabolism. The amount of heat and energy which a food can impart to the body provided it is completely utilised is measured by a unit of heat which is termed as calorie. Caloric value of a food is not an index of its usefulness but every food has to possess a biological value to supply the needs of an individual. Thus 1g of carbohydrate yields 4.1 calories, 1 g fat 9.3 calories and 1 g proteins 4.1 calories.

An average adult at rest requires 2600 calories while in females it is about 2100 calories. Children between 10-15 years 1800-2400 calories. The caloric requirements of a pregnant or nursing mother are proportionally more and go upto 3000 calories per day. It is again of importance to impress that heavy manual work entails a greater intake of calories requirements and these have to be met with by additional food supplements. Daily requirements of food include sufficient quantities of carbohydrates, proteins, fats, vitamins and minerals.

Daily Energy Requirements	
1. Average adult doing normal physical work	2600 Calories
2. Females (housewife)	2100 Calories
3. Pregnant females/ lactating women	3000 calories
4. Agricultural/manual workers	3000-3500 Calories
5. Children (between 10-15 years)	1800-2400 Calories

An ideal balanced diet is one that meets the body requirements both in health and sickness. Perfect nutrition depends on the coordinated constitution of the major essential constituents of food. All the food stuffs should be present in suitable proportions to supply the body growth and nutrition. An ideal diet has to be balanced and should contain not only carbohydrates, proteins and fats but also minerals and vitamins, derived from organic as well as inorganic sources.

An average individual's daily requirement of various food constitutents is as follows:

Organic food	Daily requirements
Proteins	75 to 100 g
Carbohydrates	400 to 500 g
Fats	75 to 100 g
Inorganic foods	
Sodium chloride	4 to 10 g
Phosphates	1.5 g
Calcium	0.8 to 1 g
Iron	15 to 20 mg

Iodine	150 mg
Copper	1.5 mg
Vitamins	
Vitamin A	700 mg
Vitamin D	800-1000 units for adults and 400 units for infants
Vitamin B_1	1.2 mg to 2.5 mg
Vitamin B_2 (Riboflavin)	2.0 mg
Nicotinic acid	10-20 mg
Vitamin C	30-50 mg
Pyridoxine (Vitamin B_6)	1.5 mg

Most of the daily requirements of an individual are met from the food consumed.

Proteins. These are the most important and essential food factors required for the maintenance and repair of body tissues. Dietary proteins are an important source of energy for the human body but less so than carbohydrates or fats.

The major function of proteins is to repair the worn out body tissues and build new ones in addition to producing energy. In this aspect proteins are superior to carbohydrates and fats.

The properties of protein depend on the arrangement of amino acids in its structure. There are about 23 amino acids commonly found in dietary proteins and among these nine are essential for the body and so their presence in the diet is necessary while the rest of the amino acids can be synthesized in the body. Most of the proteins are obtained from animal and vegetable sources. Animal proteins contain all the essential amino acids so they are rated first class while vegetable proteins only contain some of the essential amino acids so they are rated as second class proteins. Exclusion of even one single essential amino acid leads to a negative nitrogen balance. Though the exact role played by them may not be completely understood yet there is hardly a single body process in which the amino acids do not take active part.

Proteins are needed as body builders, are essential for growth and regulation of body processes. If they are insufficient, growth is either slowed or retarded.

That is why proteins in large quantities are required not oly by children but also by adults during period of stress and by women at the time of pregnancy, and lactation.

Proteins:

These are constituted by amino acids, out of which nine are essential for maintaining nitrogen balance. These cannot be synthesized in the body and have to be provided in the diet. These amino acids are tryptophan, histidine, methionine, valine, tyrosine, lysine, leucine, threonine and isoleucine.

Animal proteins contain all essential amino acids while proteins derived from vegetable sources lack one or two of these.

In addition to keeping the vitality, proteins are also necessary for the formation of enzymes, hormones, antibodies and haemoglobin. When we talk of proteins not only it is the quantity but also the quality which is equally essential. Many a time it is not the total diet which is deficient but some essential constituent may rather be lacking. Ideally one should try to achieve a food supply in which at least 10-15 per cent of the energy for an adult is provided by proteins.

Surveys carried out in various parts of the country show that 90 per cent of children of pre-school age (1-5 years) from poor socioeconomic groups are deficient in calories and deficiency of protein in varying degrees was present in 30 per cent of these children. Infants and very young children suffer from marasmus where both proteins and overall food intake is deficient while kwashiorkor is the result of severe protein deficiency. In children suffering from this malady there is not only retardation of growth, weight loss, wasting and swelling of the body but the child is apathetic, skin and hair are unhealthy.

Protein deficiency also leads to deterioration in mental faculties and fatigue, irritability and apathy may develop. Studies in different part of the world have shown that children who survive severe protein malnutrition in early childhood perform less well in intelligence tests. However, some try to explain it on social or psychological influence in which the child was brought up.

Apparently the necessity of proteins for the maintenance of proper physical, mental and emotional health cannot be minimized.

Proteins are derived from two sources, the animal and vegetable. Animal proteins derived from meat of all kinds, poultry, fish, eggs, cheese, milk and milk products, are superior and first class proteins while the vegetable proteins are derived from vegetable sources like pulses, soyabean, beans and nuts etc. A mixed diet containing both animal and vegetable proteins will meet the optimum requirements of the body. Vegetarians, however, can obtain proper quality and quantity of proteins only from vegetable sources.

Milk is nature's beautiful gift to human beings since its regular use produces not only fine physique and good health but also a good source of vitality. It is an ideal food for children and young adults since it is a rich source of essential minerals, lactose, proteins and fats. But in itself milk is not a complete food since it lacks vitamin C and to some extent iron. That is the reason why nutrition supplements have to be given to infants and people who are only on milk diet.

Milk is about 87 per cent water so it is not a concentrated food. Sufficient quantities of milk have to be taken daily. For vegetarians milk protein is the only source of their animal proteins.

For an infant and a child milk is the nearest approach to a complete food. For people who can not take milk due to economic reasons or otherwise, skimmed milk is a good substitute. Though it will lack vitamins and fat yet it will still be an important and rich source of proteins.

Meat, fish and eggs are the most important body building foods. Bulk for bulk more beneficial proteins are derived from them rather than from vegetable sources. Animal food is more of a compact balanced type so it tends to meet the body's requirement not only in proteins but also in vitamins, minerals and fats. Liver and kidney are important sources of vitamin B complex group while brain is a rich source of phosphorus, copper and iron. Fish food is an excellent source of animal proteins while eggs provide everything that is expected of a first rate protein food. Eggs are easily digestible and promote growth especially in young children. They are good source of vitamin A, D, E. Iron and phosphorus. A combination of eggs and milk is an ideal one for maintaining proper development of an individual.

Apparently the advantages of meat and meat products, eggs, fish are there but there are religious sentiments of a greater chunk of our population against them and moreover they may be expensive. So animal proteins from these sources are ideal for those who want them but are not very essential.

In addition to proteins derived from milk vegetarians have an important source of proteins from nuts.

Soyabeans are a very rich source of proteins. Groundnuts are another good source, while pulses, cereals like rice, wheat, maize, jowar and ragi are a fair source. Whole natural rice and oats and pulses like Bengal gram, green gram, peas, beans can be good substitute for meat, fish and eggs.

Ideally the protein should be derived from both animal and vegetable sources to maintain the proper body balance.

Carbohydrates. They form the major and largest component of staple diet consumed by most of our people and thus may meet most of the daily energy requirements. In the diets of poor people, upto 90 per cent of the energy may come from this source. But such an extreme imbalance may not be desirable. Important sources are starch, cereals, beetroot, sugarcane, fruits and seeds.

Generally three kinds of carbohydrates are recognized i.e. sugar, starch and cellulose. Sugars are the concentrated form of carbohydrates and an important source of energy. A large amount of sugar is present in fruits like bananas, mangoes, grapes, dates, apples, apricots and vegetables like sweet potatoes, potatoes, peas etc. Honey and jams are other sources of sugar.

Starches are derived mainly from wheat, rice but are also present in other foods such as seed grains, tuber vegetables, potatoes, sweet potatoes, peas, bananas etc.

Large part of carbohydrates is constituted by the cellulose which forms the outer lining of the walls of cereals, fruits etc. Cellulose and bran are hard substances difficult to digest but are important since they form the bulk of the food stuff. Lack of cellulose in the diet is responsible for a number of ills and that is the reason why there is more stress these days on a wholesome food rather than on purified food. People who are accustomed to take cellulose free food suffer from chronic constipation and its ensuing ills.

Carbohydrates

These comprise polysaccharide (starch) disaccharides (sucrose, lactose, maltose) and mono saccharides (glucose, ribose and fractose) and form main bulk of carbohydrates.

Dietary fibre is a non-starch polysaccharide and is often removed from food during processing. It is non-energy producing.

Fats are a form of concentrated food and act like body fuels. They form a very convenient source of energy. Apart from this fats are important in a way that vitamins like A, D, E and K are taken into the body through them.

Though fats have been considered essential for meeting the body's energy requirements but if taken in excess may prove harmful. Fat intake should not exceed 25 per cent of total calories once a person reaches middle age.

Fats are derived both from animal and vegetable sources and are present both in saturated and unsaturated form. Fats derived from vegetable sources is preferred since it is present in an unsaturated form and does not raise blood cholesterol and lipid levels. So the consensus at present is to use more of vegetable oils like corn oil, sunflower or seed oil. But this does not mean that butter and pure ghee be excluded from the diet. These fats are equally essential especially in the growing period of life when one is leading an active life. One should take equal amounts of saturated, mono unsaturated and polyunsaturated fats. It is misconception that polyunsaturated fats are safe and can be taken freely.

From the above it would be apparent that no single source can meet the body's daily needs and one has to depend on a variety of food stuffs for one's needs and the body's proper growth.

Fats. These mainly comprise:

1. Saturated fats (palmitic acid, myristic acid, stearic acid, lauric acid)
2. Polyunsaturated fats (linoleic acid, arachidonic acid). These are essential fatty acids (EFAs) and are precursors of prostaglandins.
3. Monosaturated fats (oleic acid, elaidic acid)

After having discussed the main body requirements one has to keep in mind the accessory substances present in the food in small quantities that are essential for maintaining the normal functions of the vital organs as well as the biological activity of the body. The body requires them in small amounts for its metabolism, yet it cannot make them for itself in sufficient quantities. Vitamins are not only necessary food substances but very vital for the body with the result that consumption of diet devoid of vitamins taken for long periods can give rise to certain deficiency diseases. At the outset, it must be made clear that vitamins do not supply energy but are simply protective foods, and essential for the body growth and development.

Vitamins are the protective foods and guard us from a number of deficiency diseases. There are two groups of vitamins, the fat-soluble vitamins like vitamin A, D, E and K and water-soluble vitamins mainly constituted by members of vitamin B complex group and vitamin C. A healthy individual ingesting a well-balanced diet must receive adequate amounts of vitamins and vitamin preparations have to be used where prompt relief of hypovitaminosis is desired.

Minerals. In addition to the vitamins the body requires some minerals like iron, calcium, phosphorus, cobalt, iodine etc. Though minerals form a very little part of the body yet they are a very rich source of providing protection to the body and assist in the coordinated working of various body processes. Deficiency of minerals would not only interfere with the normal growth processes in the body but also interfere with the working of essential organs.

OMEGA-3 fatty acids.

These are polyunsaturated fatty acids found almost exclusively in fish and shell fish. OMEGA-3 fatty acids (PUFA) are known as EPA (eicosapentaenoic acid) and DHA (docosahexaenoic acid). EPA is required for the production of prostaglandins. It lowers lipids (decreases total cholesterol and increases HDL) and has an antithrombotic effect and protects against atherosclerosis. DHA also lowers lipids, has antihypertensive and antiinflammatory effect and also improves mental functions in old age.

Eating 200-300 g of oily fish weekly fulfills dietary requirements.

Calcium and phosphorus. Both these minerals are essentially required for the proper growth and development of body bones and teeth. These must be supplied in adequate amounts during the process of body growth so as to ensure the proper bone formation. Deficiency of these causes softening of the bones, stunted growth and bony deformities. These are distributed evenly all over the body, a greater proportion being present in the skeleton and only a small portion is found in body fluids. For the proper utilization of both calcium and phosphorus adequate amounts of vitamin D are essential. So one can suffer from calcium deficiency even when the intake of this mineral is sufficient if phosphorus and vitamin D are not available in adequate amounts. Calcium deficiency leads to rickets, osteomalacia, delayed blood coagulation, poor development of bones and teeth, hyperplasia of parathyroid glands.

Good sources of calcium are eggs, milk, dairy products, cheese, meat, soyabean, carrots, cabbage, potatoes and wheat flour. Average daily requirement in an adult is 1 g and during pregnancy and lactation a mother requires 1.5 g daily.

Phosphorus plays an important part in regulating the various functions of the body including uptake and release of energy. Phosphorus is also said to have a role in the functioning of normal brain power. Deficiency leads to softening of bones, stunted growth, caries of teeth and depression of body vital functions. Daily requirement in diet is 1.5 g.

Common minerals and their sources:

Major minerals	Best source	Deficiency symptoms
Calcium	Milk and milk products	Back and leg pain, osteoporosis osteomalacia
Phosphorus	Meat, poultry, fish and eggs	Poor appetite
Potassium	Vegetables, citrus fruits, soup and yogurt	Lethargy, aches and pains generalized weakness, loss of appetite.
Iron	Meat, fish, poultry, leafy vegetables	Generalized weakness, pallor, lethargy
Iodine	Sea food and iodised salt	Lack of interest, lethargy, constipation, metabolism at low levels

Foods which are rich source of phosphorus are eggs, liver, fish, meat, milk, cheese, brain, cereals, oat meal, pulses, beans, nuts, spinach and whole grain.

Iron. It is needed for the formation of haemoglobin and nuclei of cells. Its deficiency gives rise to anaemia which is probably the most common affliction of people in our country.

Iron is present in animal foods like lean meat, liver, kidney, eggs and others sources are leafy green vegetables, cereals, onions, groundnuts, figs and dried fruits. Milk is a poor source of iron. It is said that cooking in iron vessels increases the iron content of food. Since milk is not a good source of iron so in children on milk diet adequate supplements of iron have to be added. Daily requirement of iron in food is 15-20 mg.

Iodine. It is widely distributed in the soil and water. Its adequate amount in food keeps the thyroid gland working in order and thus keeps the person active and alert. At places where either the soil or water is deficient in iodine, people suffer from swelling of the thyroid gland called goitre. This is a commonly seen condition in the Himalyan region where goitre is endemic.

Iodine as such is well distributed in most of the natural foods but sea-foods are a very rich source. Other common food stuffs are Sardines, cod liver oil, yolk of eggs, spinach, oat meal, milk, cabbage etc. Where iodine is deficient in the soil or water supply iodised salts are being used and they have proved effective in reducing its deficiency. Supplementing table salt with iodine in the form of iodized salt takes care of most of the daily requirements of iodine. Daily requirement is 150 mg.

Copper. This mineral is essential for the utilization of iron in the body and thus tries to combat anaemia. It is present in plenty in most of the natural foods. Rich sources are liver, shell fish, eggs, whole grains, nuts, oat meal and green leafy vegetables. Daily requirement 1.2 mg.

Sodium and potassium. Common salt (sodium chloride) is present in large quantity in the body and its fluids. It also carries to the various parts of the body essential factors. Sodium is retained in the body fluids so its consumption has to be kept slightly on the lower side but in adequate quantities since deficiency of sodium causes listlessness and exhaustion.

Salt has to be taken slightly in excess in summer when it is being lost from the body during excessive perspiration. Persons suffer from heat cramps and even heat stroke may occur if salt is not consumed in adequate quantity.

Most of the food stuffs contain sodium in sufficient amount so as a rule adequate quantity is always available to the body. Processed food, fish meat, corn and wheat flakes are abnormally high in sodium. Soft drinks and even ordinary drinking water contain sodium. Excessive use of salt is undesirable since it leads to retention of fluids as well as raised blood pressure as a long term.

Potassium is also a balancing mineral along with sodium and helps to maintain the equilibrium in the cells and body fluids. Deficiency of potassium leads to marked weakness, listlessness and exhaustion. Rich sources of potassium are tomatoes, citrus fruits, green vegetables and meat soups.

Other minerals. Body also requires a number of other minerals. These are present in adequate amounts in most of the common food stuffs and as a rule their deficiency does not occur.

Flourine in adequate quantities when present in water prevents caries of the teeth. When its concentration exceeds 4 PPm, the bad effects occur. The teeth become mottled and discoloured while bones as well as nervous system are equally affected and flourosis results.

Other minerals like magnesium, zinc, cobalt, sulphur, selenium, etc. also take active part in maintaining various body functions. They are available from milk, green leafy vegetables and cereals.

To sum up, the minerals are essential for the proper functioning of the body and should be taken in adequate quantities in the natural foods.

Water. When we talk of the nutritive values of various food stuffs we tend to forget that water is a very important elixir of life essential for the living processes. A person may live for weeks without food but not without water. Lack of water can kill the person by depriving the body of not only its vital fluids but also of minerals.

Water constitutes 65 per cent of body weight and even bones contain about 20 per cent of water.

Every person must be advised to take as much as possible of fresh sparkling pure water. It is essential since water is being lost in sweat, breath, urine, feaces and also from other body fluids.

An average adult requires at least 2 litre of water per day. Insensible water loss from various sources is about 1000 ml and loss occurs from intracellular and extracellular compartments. Water loss causes dehydration in which there is intense thirst, dryness of the mouth, decrease in urinary output and urine becomes highly concentrated. There is rise in haemoglobin and haematocrit values. When dehydration is severe, there is listlessness, apathy, confusion and hallucinations.

As compared to dehydration, water intoxication may also occur when large quantities of water relative to sodium are taken. Water intoxication occurs only when renal functions are deranged. Clinical features are restlessness, twitchings and convulsions. Subsequently cardiac failure, pulmonary oedema and terminally coma supervenes.

Diet for pregnant and lactating mothers. There are the periods when there are increased demands on the women to supply the needs of the foetus and infant. Diet during this period must be nutritious and contain adequate amounts of proteins, vitamins and minerals especially calcium and iron. Diet should be well balanced and nutritive containing adequate quantities of proteins, carbohydrates, fats and vitamins. A pregnant women shall require atleast 2600 calories and a lactating mother 3000 calories per day. Caloric value of food to a lactating women should be of higher order as the nutritive demands of the infant are mainly to be met through breast milk.

Nutrition and ageing. Ageing is a process of senescence where there is decline of all bodily functions. Elderly people have their own problems regarding nutrition. Loss of teeth makes chewing of food difficult. Similarly digestion may be impaired due to decrease in gastric juices and bile secretions. Though nutritional requirements are qualitatively same as those of younger persons yet since their energy expenditure is less, energy requirements shall be different. But nutrition plays important role in prevention of disease in elderly. Because of ageing process, intake of food may suffer so elderly require special care in this regard. Nutritive, palatable food containing sufficient quantities of easily digestible foods with adequate quantities of proteins, vitamins and calcium must be ensured.

BALANCED DIET

A balanced diet may not be easy to define but broadly a well balanced proportioned diet should contain enough of proteins, carbohydrates, and adequate quantity of vitamins, minerals and fats.

For the proper growth, maintenance and development of our body an ideal combination of the essential nutrients, vitamins and minerals must be aimed at. What type of food a person takes has a bearing on his/her health. An average Indian diet is poor both in quality as well as in quantity in meeting the daily needs. Our diet is mainly dominated by cereals like wheat, rice, maize, bajra etc and proteins especially of animal origin are sadly neglected since most people are vegetarians. Poor diet is partly due to ignorance, social customs and cultural habits and to a large extent may be due to economic reasons. But there are number of rich people who are as ignorant about the importance of balanced nutrition in contrast to the poor person who can not afford the diet. Then there are food faddists who are always selective in choosing the foods they eat. Whenever a diet is devised it must look to the individuals basic needs. The calories should be neither too little nor too much since both way the balance can be tilted and harm the person.

Usually the balanced diet should contain 30 calories/kg optimal body weight. The total calories prescribed should take into account the activity levels of the person whether a sedentary worker or a manual worker. Similarly calorie requirements shall go up in pregnant women and during lactation.

A balanced diet should contain 60-70 per cent carbohydrates of the total calories and protein intake should be approximately 0.8-1 g/kg ideal body weight, usually comprising around 12-18 per cent the total calorie intake. Further protein intake will have to be increased in elderly people, during pregnancy and lactation. Fats should be restricted to around 20-25 per cent of the total calories and should preferably be taken in equal amounts of saturated, monounsaturated and polyunsaturated fats.

Let us look at some of the important ingredients of a balanced diet. Firstly intake of proteins must be adequate and that too of first quality. It is preferable to take proteins derived both from animal and vegetable sources.

Protein in the diet helps in replacing worn out body cells, prevents tissue break down and in this way the aging process. In fact protein in diet is needed for maintaining not only the health and upkeep of every part of the body but also of the vital tissues like hair, skin, muscles and nails. When there is inadequate protein intake the skin ages prematurely, the wrinkles appear and there are signs of what a person would complain of lack of glow. So the first principle of ideal diet is to have enough of proteins daily (atleast 60-80 g perday). Protein quota shall be selected from non-vegetarian diet like eggs, chicken, fish cheese, skimmed milk, Yogurt, curd and eggs. For vegetarians legumes and pulses like grams, soya, bengal gram shall be the ideal source of proteins in addition to cereals like wheat, rice, ragi etc.

Carbohydrates shall be required in adequate quantities to give energy and strength. Many people have the wrong belief that carbohydrates shall make them fat. It is wrong notion. Excess of any constituent of food taken shall prove harmful this way or that way. Fats should be taken in measured quantity and not in excess. Adequate quantities of saturated and unsaturated fats should be taken but at the same time hydrogenated fats like vanaspati be avoided.

Diet should contain as much of fresh fruits and vegetables as possible since a number of vitamins and minerals are destroyed while cooking. Diet must be monitored in such a way that it contains enough of vitamins and minerals.

One should take adequate amount of fresh leafy vegetables, tomatoes, lettuce, cucumber, spinach, amarnath, mint etc. since these are rich sources of calcium, iron, carotene, riboflavin, vitamin C and folic acid. Fresh fruits like oranges, mosambi, melons, guava, amla, papaya are good source of vitamin C and carotene. Vitamin B complex is important for many body needs. Most of the members of this group are present in liver, kidney, whole wheat floor, fresh fruits and green vegetables.

Milk is an ideal food and contains all the proximate principles of a balanced diet. For people who can not afford, skimmed milk is a satisfactory substitute since it will contain all the essential constituents of whole milk except fats and vitamins A and D. Fruits and fresh vegetables provide important nourishment. The sugars of fruits are easy to digest and at the same time the fruit juices help in the elimination of acids formed during digestion. Foods are required for body building, protective functions and for energy. Milk, cheese, eggs, fish, liver pulses, nuts, beans, legumes are all body building, while milk, butter, cheese, ghee, green leafy vegetables, eggs and fresh fruits are protective food.

Causes of nutritional disorders

1. Poor intake
2. Socioeconomic conditions
3. Chronic debilitatng disorders (malignancy, tuberculosis, diabetes).
4. Inadequate absorption of food (malabsorption syndrome, steatorrhoea, helminthic infestation, coeliac disease)
5. Loss of nutrients from body (protein losing enteropathy, blood loss).
6. Excessive energy expenditure (thyrotoxicosis, pregnancy, adolescence).
7. Loss of appetite (anorexia nervosa, chronic hepatitis, malignancy, portal cirrhosis).

Minerals also have an important role in a balanced diet. Iron is essential for giving ruddy glow to skin since its deficiency leads to pallor and anaemia. Animal foods like meat, liver, kidney, eggs and vegetables sources like leafy green vegetables, ground nuts are a good source of iron. Iodine is important in body's metabolism and is well distributed in most of the natural foods, spinach, milk, cabbage, eggs and sea foods. Other minerals like magnesium found in corn, cucumber, onion, apples, peaches and pears while phosphorus (source root vegetables, lentils, citrus fruits, lettuce, egg yolk, fish, lean meat, cheese, butter milk, almonds etc) and calcium (rich source eggs, milk, dairy products, cheese, meat, fish etc) are equally essential for the general bodily health. A balanced diet not only looks after the well being of the person but may have role to play in prevention of certain diseases.

The role of dietary fibre in a balanced diet can not be minimized. Fibre is an important part of foods of plant origin and is present in number of substances. Vegetables like corn, spinach, carrot, radish, turnip, green peas, cauliflower, yam, lady finger, tinda, bittergourd, beans, legumes. Whole wheat flour, oat meal, jowar, bajra, soya beans and fruits like apple, peach, grape fruit mulburry, pomegranate, strawberries, orange, etc are important source of fibre. Fibre is vital for cancer protection and in the diet it delays absorption of sugar and choles-

terol and thus helps in decreasing levels of sugar and cholesterol. Fibre diet is a major factor in determining faecal bulk and greater the daily output, the more dilute the concentration of potentially harmful faecal components is likely to be. By facilitating quicker transit of foods in the G.I. tract it reduces the retention time of faecal matter in the colon and acts as a preventive measure against malignancy.

Cancer of the colon, ovaries, breast, testicles, prostate and lymphomas are more common among people who consume rich diets high in fats. Fats including of animal and vegetable origin act as a facilitating factor in the causation of cancer.

Again consumption of excess non-vegetarian food is not recommended since such people are more likely to suffer from cancer colon as high ammonia concentrations due to such food in the colon is toxic and produces neoplastic changes.

There are no substitutes for fresh fruits and vegetables in a balanced diet. One has to appreciate that concentration of nutrients in foods varies from batch to batch, from one season to the next, in various geographical regions and in the method of preparation. The quantity and potencies of many chemical compounds in vegetables and fruits are often small. So consumption of a variety of fruits and vegetables is essential so that the beneficial effects can be availed.

So while planning a balanced diet, care should be taken that all essential ingredients in diets are adequately incorporated with lot of fresh fruits and vegetables. Fibre diet should be preferred to rich starchy diet.

Food should be palatable, properly cooked and well balanced providing a balance between food intake and energy output.

VITAMINS

Vitamins are the protective foods and guard the human body from a number of deficiency disorders. They are partly synthesised in the human body and small quantities generally adequate to maintain the integrity of body cells is supplied by the food the person takes. There are two groups of vitamins, the fat soluble vitamins like A,D,E, and K and water soluble vitamins mainly constituted by members of vit.B complex group and vit.C.

Vitamin A. It is essential for the proper growth and health of normal skin. It also improves body resistance. Preservation of function of the eyes is to a large extent dependant on this vitamin. Vitamin A aldehyde (retinoaldehyde) is present in the rods (Rhodopsin) and cones (Iodopsin) of the retina and changes undergone by it form the basis of visual excitation. Vitamin A (retinol and retinoic) is involved in the proper maintenance, cell proliferation, differentiation and integrity of epithelial cells. B carotene a dietary precursor of vitamin A in combination with vitamins E and C acts as important antioxidant and has a role in prevention of coronary heart disease, protection against cancer and elevating body's immune system.

Source. Chief sources of vitamin A are milk, butter, ghee, eggs, fish, cod liver oil while vegetable sources contain carotene which is converted in the body into vitamin A. Carotene is mainly found in green vegetables such as spinach, carrots, tomatoes, pumpkins and fruits like mangoes, papaya, peaches etc.

Daily requirements. In adults it is 700 ug/day and in infants it is 300-400 ug/day while growing children shall need 400-600 ug/per day.

Vitamin A deficiency. It shall depend on poor intake of either vitamin A or carotenoids in the diet because of economic reasons while diseases effecting small intestines (malabsorption) liver and biliary tract are the other causes.

Clinical features. Earliest sign of deficiency of vitamin A is in the form of difficulty in reading or sewing at night or finding anything in darkness (night blindness). Conjunctiva becomes dry (xerosis) and small greyish white raised spots (Bitot's spots) appear. Cornea subsequently becomes dry and lustreless and if eye changes do not reverse because of lack of treatment keratomalacia involving the cornea leading to ulceration and blindness may result.

Children with vitamin A deficiency not only have retarded growth but also increased tendency to chest infection. Skin become dry, rough and is often given the name of "TOAD" skin.

Treatment. Main thrust should be on prevention of vitamin A deficiency by giving good nutrition, intake of fresh leafy green vegetables and addition of vitamin A to food stuffs. In those with vitamin A deficiency, vitamin A may be administered orally as retinol 30 mg daily for 3 days. In advanced cases or where absorption is effected vitamin A in dose of 50,000 iμ parenterally for 2-3 days and later on substituted by oral preparations of vitamin A.

Vitamin A toxicity. Over dosage and prolonged use of vitamin A for long periods leads to body aches, anorexia, bone damage, hair loss, benign intracranial hypertension and vomiting. Women who take heavy doses of vitamin A during pregnancy are likely to have infants with birth defects. Excessive intake of food containing carotene may lead to yellowish pigmentation of skin which clears up when the intake of carotene containing foods is stopped.

Vitamin D. It is derived from the food and also manufactured by photactivation of 7-dehydrocholesterol present in the skin under the action of ultraviolet light of the sun. This is the primary source of vitamin D in the body and that is why deficiency of this vitamin occurs in people who are confined indoors and do not move out in the sunlight. Examples are purdah or burqa wearing women or nuns or monks confined to monasteries.

There are two forms of vitamin D, vitamin D_3 formed by activation of dehydrocholesterol present in skin and vitamin D_2 obtained from irradiation of ergosterol which is of plant origin. Both these components of vitamin D are identical except for a change in the configuration of their side chain. Deficient intake or inadequate absorption of vitamin D alongwith defective or inadequate production of it from the skin gives rise to deficiency of the vitamin. Deficiency of this vitamin leads to rickets in children who become stunted in growth, their bones are soft and deformed and they get frontal bossing, bow legs and knock-knees. Lack of dietary intake coupled with lack of sunlight produces osteomalacia in women who are likely to suffer from it because of repeated child births, prolonged breast feeding of the child and poor socioeconomic status and living conditions.

Vitamin D deficiency. It leads to rickets in a growing child and osteomalacia in the adult.

Rickets. It is a disease of poor nutrition in a young child associated not only with inadequate intake of nutritious food but also lack of exposure to sunlight. The chief changes are seen in bone where normal process of proliferation of the cartilage shows abnormality. There is irregular deposition of osteoid and cartilage which remain uncalcified. The affected areas show increased vascularity and the new bone formed is soft with the result that ossification is defective. End result is development of skeletal abnormalities. Bones calcium is reduced. Epiphyseal thickening takes place.

Earliest sign of the disease in a young child is restlessness and irritability. There is no wasting though infant may look flabby. Enlargement and softening of the skull (Cranio tabes) may be seen. Dentition is often delayed and with the progress of the disease changes in various bones of the body become apparent. Appearance of bead like deformity of chest wall along costochondral junction, (Rickety rosary), sternum projects forward (pigeon chest) and a transverse groove from the junction of ribs and cartilages towards axilla (Harrison's sulcus), as well as curving of leg bones (bow-leg) and thickening of the frontal and parietal eminences (bossed head) take place. As the child crawls, deformities of limbs develop leading to deformities of spine (Kyphosis and scoliosis) along with green, stick fractures and pseudofractures.

The teeth show changes in the form of delayed dentition defective enamel and more prone to develop caries. Permanent teeth may also show pitting, groove formation and a softened enamel.

In addition to bony deformities other abnormalities include distended abdomen, chronic diarrhoea, hepatosplenomegaly, recurrent chest infections, tetany or even convulsion and sometimes development of laryngismus stridulus. Often child because of bony deformities may be left with a stunted growth (Rachitic dwarfism).

Diagnosis of rickets is based on clinical presentation of a child with bony deformities and delayed milestones.

Biochemical investigations show raised levels of serum alkaline phosphtase, low serum phosphorus and serum calcium which is generally normal except in a florid case where blood calcium levels are low. Serum 25-hydroxy Vitamin D3 level is low.

X-ray findings of long bones in active rickets show defective mineralization and looser's zones i.e. areas of low density surrounded by sclerotic borders. Trabeculations are prominent and there is subperiostal osteoid formation. X-rays of distal ends of radius and ulna are helpful. There is widening, cuffing and flaying of the ends.

Treatment. Prevention of rickets by a balanced diet and exposure to light is the best line of trreatment. In a fully developed case of rickets parenteral administration of a single intramuscular injection of 600,000 units (15 mg) of calciferol repeated 4-6 weeks later. Simultaneously calcium must be prescribed to avoid initial hypocalcemia following vitamin D administration. Close monitoring of calcium levels in blood are essential to prevent hypercalcaemia from developing.

In mild to moderate forms of rickets oral administration of vitamin D in doses of 1500-5000 iu is beneficial. After improvement in clinical picture as well as by biochemical and radiological parameters, vitamin D in oral dose of 400 units daily is continued to prevent recurrence.

Osteomalacia. It may be called adult rickets since in both there is deficient calcification of osteoid tissue. Osteomalacia commonly occurs in women whose dietary intake of vitamin D is poor, along with lack of exposure to sunlight. The disease often occurs in pregnancy when there is strain on bone forming substances like vitamin D and calcium. There may be a feeling of slight betterment after the delivery of the child but every subsequent pregnancy makes the mother worse till she presents with a full florid picture of osteomalacia.

Pathology. It is identical in both rickets and osteomalacia. In both there is nutritional deficient intake of vitamin D with the result that there is deficiency of calcifying mechanism and the result is inability of the body to convert osteoid tissue into bone. Excess of poorly mineralized osteoid tissue leads to defective bone remodelling. The bones become soft and readily bend. Spontaneous fractures may occur.

Clinical features. Earliest complaint in a patient of osteomalacia is aches and pains more prominent in back and thighs.

Pain is vague in character and is present in various parts of the body. As the bones are soft they easily bend. Marked changes may occur in various bones of the body. Some bones may show prominences while in others there are depressions. Spontaneous fractures may occur presenting with acute localised pain. Teeth are normal. Because of kyphoscoliosis height of the women may be reduced.

In pregnant women because of pelvic deformities, delivery may be via caesarean section. If untreated the disease worsens, cachexia, wasting develop and patient may become bedridden.

Physical signs include an anaemic woman with kyphoscoliosis, shortened height and a typical 'waddling gait'.

Biochemical investigations show plasma phosphorus and serum calcium levels to be low while serum alkaline phosphatase levels are increased. Measurements of bone density by dual energy X-ray absorptometry (Dexa) show low levels. Radiographic appearances of the bones shall show them to be translucent, with increased trabeculations. Characteristic signs are milkman's lines and Looser's zones (Pseudofractures) linear lines of decalcification extending prependicular to the cortex and seen predominantly in pubic bone, ischium, neck of femur, ribs and vertebrae. Vertebrae may show compression. There is widening of intravertebral spaces producing a codfish vertebrae.

Diagnosis of oseomalacia depends on clinical featuress, biochemical changes and typical radiographic signs. Osteomalacia may have to be differentiated from other conditions like hyperparathyroidism (high serum calcium, low plasma phosphorus and increased calcium excretion in the urine), osteoporosis, multiple myeloma, chronic renal failure producing hypophosphatemia and vitamin D resistant rickets.

Clinical profile of rickets

1. Delayed milestones. Child irritable, abdomen distended, muscles flabby.
2. Skeletal abnormalities. Children below the age of one year, skull soft (craniotabes), costochondral junctions enlarged, lower ends of wrists and ankles show beaded appearance.
3. Craniotabes disappears by the age of one year, frontal and parietal bossing. Head enlarges. Closure of anterior fontanelle delayed.
4. Dentition delayed. Teeth show defective enamel. Susceptibility to caries increases, permanent teeth show grooving and pitting.
5. Chest. Pigeon shaped chest. Rickety rosary. Harrisons sulcus.
6. Spine. Kyphoscoliosis.
7. Extremities. Long bones show deformities. Epiphysis are thickened and become promient, knock knees pseudofractures, rachitic dwarfism.
8. Miscellaneous. Hepatosplenomegaly, tetany, convulsions laryngsmus stridulus, recurrent chest infections.

Treatment. It should basically be directed towards giving good nutrition with increase in sunlight exposure. Diet should consist of adequate quantities of milk, eggs, butter, ghee and green leafy vegetables. Cod liver oil is the richest source of vitamin. In severe forms of osteomalacia, oily solution of vitamin D_3 (Alfacalcidol/Arachitol) 300,000 IU (7.5 mg) to 600,000 IU (15 mg) per ml per day is administered. Repeated serum calcium measurements are essential.

In less severe cases oral vitamin D (25,000-50,000 IU) daily in the form of gelatin capsules for 6-8 weeks followed by 400 IU daily. In addition supplements of calcium are to be given.

Source of vitamin D. Rich sources of the vitamin are milk, butter, ghee, egg yolk, cod liver oil and fish liver oil. In addition synthesis of the vitamin takes place from irradiation of skin.

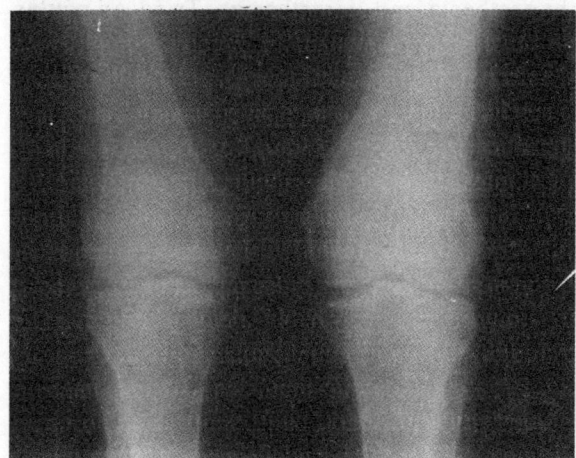

Fig. 9.1. X-ray bones of legs showing marked osteoporosis, decalcification, demineralisation of bones and increased trabeculation.

Hypervitaminosis D. Excessive intake of vitamin D and its prolonged administration results in features of toxicity in the form of hypercalcaemia, nausea, vomiting, muscular weakness, irritability, drowsiness, metastatic calcification, and deterioration of renal functions, leading to renal failure.

Vitamin K. This fat-soluble vitamin is essential for synthesis in the liver of coagulation factors. Deficiency of this vitamin results in bleeding tendencies.

Vitamin K is found in large variety of foods especially green vegetables, pulses, liver, cheese, butter and in human milk though milk as such is a poor source of this vitamin. In addition bacteria present in the intestines synthesise the vitamin so there is adequate supply of this vitamin to the body.

Deficiency of vitamin K occurs in cases of obstructive jaundice, malabsorption states, prolonged use of anticoagulants. Newborn infants may sometimes develop deficiency of the vitamin and this is seen during first few days after birth. Probably it is due to exhaustion of vitamin K acquired in utero, exaggeration of the physiological hypoprothrombinaemia and before the infant's intestines start synthesising the vitamin. This condition can be prevented by giving 5-10 mg of vitamin K to the mother during the last days of pregnancy. Otherwise in an infant with such problem 1 mg of vitamin K shall give relief.

Daily requirement of vitamin K are very minimal and being met from natural sources and synthesises from body. Doses of vitamin K in excess generally do not produce any toxicity except in elderly people where there is increased tendency to thrombotic lesions.

Vitamin E. It is found in the form of tocopherol and related compounds and more than 90% of this vitamin in the human body is in the form of a-tocopherol.

Vitamin E is mainly derived from vegetable oils, wheat germ, egg yolk, soya bean, sunflower, cereals and nuts. Whole grains and a wide variety of green vegetables constitute the other source.

Daily requirement of vitamin E are 15 IU or 15 mg which is mainly met from the diet. Vitamin E has been called anti-stress and anti-sterility vitamin. A number of properties have been ascribed to the vitamin. Its main role is as an antioxidant in conjunction with vitamin C and A. It helps in oxidation of low density lipoproteins (LDL) thus guarding against atherosclerosis. Patients with a recent attack of myocardial infarction have low levels of vitamin E in their blood while those with high levels are relatively at low risk. Other uses of the vitamin include improvement in diabetic state, reduction in anginal attacks, prevention of ageing, slowing the process of senescence, elevating body immune system, protection against cancer of the colon, breast and lungs, reduction in progression of cataract in eyes and degenerative neurological disorders (Parkinson's disease, Alzheimer's disease). Empirically the vitamin has been used in cases of muscular dystrophy, sterility, threatened abortion, habitual miscarriages, improving menstrual disorders and muscle power. But these claims remain unsubstantiated.

Deficiency of this vitamin is suspected to cause haemolytic anaemia in premature and newborn infants. Further a clinical syndrome in children with biliary tract obstruction and a beta-lipoproteinaemia with spinocerebellar degeneration has been ascribed to deficiency of vitamin E.

Normally since there is hardly any deficiency of this vitamin no supplementation is required as diet provides adequate quantities of the vitamin. But as an antioxidant a daily oral dose of vitamin E in conjunction with vitamin C (300 mg) and B carotene is advocated.

Water soluble vitamins. These constitute important group of vitamins which play important part in maintaining body metabolism. Most of the constituents of B complex group occur together both in animal and vegetable foods like liver, kidney, whole wheat floor, legumes, pulses, green leafy vegetables, fresh fruits, yeast etc. Some of these vitamins can also be synthesized in the gut. Important members of this group are thiamine (vitamin B_1) riboflavin, niacin, pyridoxine (vitamin B_6), pantothenic acid, vitamin B_{12} and vitamin C.

Thiamine (vitamin B_1). It is mainly found in whole grains, cereals, pulses, nuts, liver, kidney, pork and eggs. An average adult requires not more than 1 mg per day of the vitamin which is generally available in the daily diet. Deficiency of the vitamin occurs in severe malnutrition, chronic alcoholics and those suffering from chronic debilitating diseases.

Thiamine forms an essential part of two coenzymes important in the oxidative decarboxylation of alpha-ketoacids. Deficiency of the vitamin leads to accumulation of these alpha ketoacids whose toxic effects result in the production of beriberi which mainly targets the heart, peripheral nerves and central nervous system. Beri-beri may be wet where cardiac involvement predominates and dry when there is involvement of central nervous system.

In beri-beri heart is markedly dilated. There is pallor, tachycardia, pulmonary congestion and flabbiness of myocardium. Extremities are warm and pulse is bounding, high volume. Initially there is oedema over dependent parts which extends upwards causing ascites, pleural effusion and later on generalized anasarea. Electrocardiogram may show conduction defects and T wave abnormalities.

Dry beri-beri has involvement of central nervous system. There is calf muscle tenderness, cramps, tingling sensation and numbness in the limbs (hyposthesia and parasthesia). Triad of ocular abnormalities (nystagmus), ataxia, confusion and loss of equilibrium occurs. Psychological disturbances, confusion and even loss of consciousness may occur (Wernicke-Korsakoff syndrome). Patient is unable to rise from a squatting position (squatting test). Peripheral nerve involvement is usually bilateral in nature and is present in the form of wrist and foot drop. Gait is shuffling type. General symptoms include anorexia, nausea and vomiting. Diagnosis of vitamin B_1 deficiency is not difficult if one considers a chronic alcoholic or those with chronic malnutrition. Further confirmation is made

Important signs in nutritional deficiencies:

Nutrient	Signs
Vitamin B_1 (thiamine)	Parasthesia, Tinglings sensations, Calf muscle tenderness, Loss of ankle and knee jerk.
Vitamin B_2 (Riboflavin)	Angular stomatitis, cheilosis, atrophic papillae, magenta tongue.
Nicotinic acid (Niacin)	Pigmentation over exposed surfaces. Pellagra skin. Scarlet and raw tongue, glossitis, dementia.
Vitamin B_6 (Pyridoxine)	Glossitis, peripheral neuropathy.
Vitamin C	Bleeding in mucous surfaces. Spongy and bleeding gums. Painful epiphyseal enlargement, Failure of wound healing.
Vitamin B_{12}	Anorexia. Pallor, parasthesia, loss of position and vibration sense. Optic neuritis, ataxia.
Vitamin A	Dryness of the conjunctiva Xerophthamia, bitot's spots, corneal ulceration, failure to adapt in darkness
Vitamin D	Failure to grow, rickets in children, osteomalacia in adults.
Vitamin K	Bleeding from mucous surfaces, failure of bleeding to stop.

by demonstrating raised levels of blood pyruvate. Another test is measurement of transketolase activity in red cells.

Treatment. Once a diagnosis of beri beri has been made treatment is by parenteral administration of vitamin B_1 (50-100 mg daily), intra-muscularly or intravenously depending on the clinical condition. Prompt recovery occurs in most of the patients.

CLINICAL PROFILE OF BERI-BERI

1. **Wet beri-beri or cardiovascular beri-beri**
   Palpitation, dysponea
   Cardiac enlargement
   Extremities warm
   Good volume bounding pulse
   Anasarca
   Signs of congestive heart failure in late stages

2. **Dry beri-beri or neuritic type**
   Cramps, tingling and numbness in the limbs
   Nystagmus
   Wrist and foot drop
   Ataxia
   Loss of equilibrium
   Wernicke-Korsakoff syndrome
   Hyposthesia and parasthesia
   Confusion
   Inability to arise from squatting position
   Shuffling gait

Once acute crisis is over, patient is maintained on small oral dose (5 mg) daily along with good nourishing diet. Diet should consist of high B complex and protein content like eggs, milk, nuts, and green vegetables. Thamine is safe, has no toxicity and high doses can be given safely. Cases of wet beri beri with cardiac involvement may require in addition digoxin and diuretics if congestive failure is present.

Riboflavin (Vitamin B_2). It is widely distributed in food stuffs like milk, cheese, liver, eggs, meat and leafy vegetables. Riboflavin is an essential component of coenzyme flavins (FMN and FAD) and is involved in a variety of oxidative reactions.

Isolated deficiency of the vitamin is not common though it occurs along with other nutritional deficiencies. Secondary deficiency may occur in those with diffuse intestinal disease, chronic alcoholics and those suffering from chronic debilitating diseases. Riboflavin resists heat and is fairly stable while cooking but sunlight destroys the vitamin. Daily requirement of the vitamin is 2 mg. Deficiency of the vitamin leads to lesions involving the tongue, lips, eyes and skin.

Lip lesions are in the form of angular stomatitis (pallor and redness at angles of lips) followed by painful fissuring at the corners of the mouth (cheilosis). Tongue becomes red inflamed (magenta tongue). There is loss of lingual papillae along with atrophy. Sometimes fungiform papillae may become enlarged producing a pebbled appearance of the tongue which now is painful. A greasing scaling dermatitis may appear on naso labial folds round the mouth, scrotum and vulva. Eyes show corneal vascularization and degenration of the corneal epithelium with opacification of the lens. With severe deficiency, bone marrow becomes hypoplastic. Deficiency of riboflavin is generally along with other nutritional deficiency. Riboflavin content of plasma or of white blood corpusiles can be measured and these indicate level of deficiency.

Treatment of riboflavin deficiency involves total management of deficiency state with good nutritive diet and vitamin B complex group of vitamins. Where riboflavin deficiency predominates daily intake of riboflavin in dose of 5 mg three times a day is sufficient. Riboflavin is comparatively a safe vitamin. No toxicity has been observed with use of large doses of it.

Niacin (Nicotinamide/nicotinic acid) (Vitamin B_7). Niacin constitutes two important components i.e. nicotinamide and nicotinic acid who have equal biological potency. Niacin is required for the formation of coenzymes (NAD and NADP) which participate in a wide variety of redox reactions. Unlike other members of B complex group, nicotinamide can be synthesised in the body from tryptophane.

Dietary sources of the vitamin include cereals, pulses, meat, liver, kidney, fish, groundnuts, milk and green leafy vegetables. Daily requirement of nicotinamide are 10-20 mg per day. Deficiency of this vitamin occurs in maize and jowar eaters. This is because these grains contain niacin in unabsorbable form as well as the content of tryptophan from which the vitamin is synthesised is poor in maize. Lack of protein in diet further worsens the deficiency.

Pellagra. It is clinical condition produced as a result of nicotinic acid/niacin deficiency. It classically occurs in maize and jowar eaters, chronic alcoholics, patients suffering from steatorrhoea, malabsorption syndrome and a rare disorders of inborn error of metabolism—Hartnup disease.

Pellagra literally means rough skin and characteristically has triad of dermatitis, diarrhoea and dementia. Dermitis is usually bilateral present on exposed areas of the body. To start with there is redness, thickening and roughening of the skin followed by scaling and pigmentation of the skin (pellagrous dermatosis). Unexposed parts of the body such as skin folds, knees and elbows may also show such changes.

Patient may have loss of appetite, nausea and vomiting. Diarrhoea is a common feature. Tongue becomes red, swollen and beefy with fissuring. Papillae over the tongue may become atrophic. Glossitis, angular stomatitis and recurrent mouth ulcerations are common.

Clinical profile of pellagra

Alimentary system

Loss of appetite, nausea and vomiting, Diarrhoea
Glossitis and stomatitis. Beefy, angry looking. Fissured tongue. Aphthous ulcers, angular stomatitis.
Skin. Dermatitis on exposed parts (pellagrous dermatitis) like front of neck, hands, feet and ankles.
Skin scaly (crazy pavement) pigmented rough and thickened (hyperkeratotis).

Nervous system.

Irritability, apathy
Loss of power of concentration
Acute psychosis
Delirium
Dementia.

Dementia in the form of apathy, tremors, encephalopathy and acute psychosis may be seen. Advanced cases may show delirium, dementia and acute psychotic disturbances.

Diagnosis of pellagra is based on clinical picture. Treatment initially is by Injection Nicotinamide 50-100 mg I/M daily for a week along with high nutritive diet containing adequate quantity of proteins. After parenteral administration of nicotinic acid, improvement is dramatic. Maintenance dose of 50 mg orally per day be continued.

Over dosages of niacin produces no serious side effects. Whereas nicotiniamide produces no side effects even when taken in large doses, nicotinic acid in a dose of 25 mg produces intense flushing, sensation of heat, headache and itching though this passes off in an hour or so.

Pyridoxine (vitamin B$_6$). It is widely distributed in cereals, yeast, whole grain, wheat grain, pulses, eggs, liverand peanuts. It is present in the form of three compounds, pyridoxine, pyridoxal and pyridoxamine in the foods stuffs and all of these possess vitamin B$_6$ actively. Out of these pyridoxine is the most important, since it is involved in the oxidation of unsaturated fatty acids and amino acids. Daily requirements of the vitamin are 1.25 mg which are mostly met from the diet. Some drugs like isoniazid, hydralazine, oral contraceptives may interact with its metabolic product (pyridoxal phosphate) and produce deficiency of this vitamin.

Clinical features of deficiency of the vitamin include glossitis, dermatitis, cheilosis, angular stomatitis and peripheral neuropathy with symmetrical motor and sensory deficits more marked in the lower extremities. In infants convulsions while in adults, confusion, mental depression, hypochromic anaemia and granulopenia are other features associated with the deficiency. Treatment is by use of pyridoxine 10 mg orally. Concomitant use of pyridoxine with isoniazid prevents development of neuropathy.

Pantothenic acid. It is widely distributed in animal and vegetable foods and hence its deficiency is very rare.Daily requirements are 10 mg. Pantothenic acid forms part of coenzyme A which is concerned with the process of acetylation and functions of the adrenal cortex. Though deficiency of pantothenic acid is not very common yet dermal and hair changes and feeling of burning in the feet and legs (burning feet syndrome) may occur.

Cyanocobalamin (vitamin B$_{12}$). It is an important member of B complex group and is often called a 'Wonder vitamin'. It is synthesized by microorganisms and is mainly found in animal sources such as fish, meat, eggs, yeast and milk. Vegetable sources are deficient in this vitamin.

Daily requirements of the vitramin are 1-2 ug. Liver can store upto 2 mg of the vitamin for several years and it may take at least two years or more before deficiency of the vitamin manifests.

Clinical profile of scurvy

Infants and young children
Irritability, fretfulness,
Increased tendency to cyring,
Loss of appetite and weight,
Delayed milestones,
Pallor,
Gums spongy and bleed readily,
Teeth loose,
Petechiael spots on skin, hard palate,
Joints swollen and painful,
Nose bleeds and haemorrhages in conjunctive,
Delayed wound healing,
Pseudoparalysis of hands,
Scorbutic beading of ribs.

Adults
Spongy gums with loosened teeth,
Haemorrhages in joints, deep tissues,
Painful swelling of joints,
Bleeding at various sites (brain, kidney, GI tract, eyes, skin, soft tissues),
Delayed healing,
Follicular hyperkeratosis.

Deficiency of virtamin B$_{12}$ occurs due to dietary inadequacy especially those on poor vegetarian diet, malabsorption states, disease of ileum (blind loop syndrome), intrinsic factor deficiency (pernicious anaemia) partial or total gastrectomy and long term use of drugs like PAS, neomycin, phenformin which interfere with its absorption. Abnormality in DNA synthesis occurs because of deficiency of this vitamin and results in megaloblastic erythropoiesis. Vitamin B$_{12}$ deficiency produces anorexia, pallor, diarrhoea, red sore tongue, angular stomatitis and megaloblastic anaemia. Neurological lesions include parasthesia, optic neuritis, peripheral neuropathy and subacute combined degeneration of the cord in addition to dementia.

Treatment of vitamin B$_{12}$ deficiency especially in those with megalobastic anaemia is Vitamin B$_{12}$ 1000 ug intramuscularly twice a week for 3-4 weeks. Oral supplements (1-2 ug) are then continued as maintenance therapy.

Folic acid (pteroyl glutamic acid). Folic acid is found in abundance in green vegetables as well animal sources such as liver and kidney. Folic acid is destroyed partially by cooking. It is absorbed in proximal part of small intestines. Human body can store about 6-10 mg of this especially in the liver.

Deficiency of folic acid takes place due to poor nutritive diet especially green vegetables, in malabsorption states, chronic alcoholics, debilitating illnesses and patients on drugs like trimethoprim, hydantoins and oral contraceptives where metabolism of folates is interfered with.

Clinically deficiency of the folic acid takes longer time to develop though body reserves of folate are low as compared to vitamin B$_{12}$. Patients with poor dietary intake and excess utilization of the folic acid may rapidly develop it.

There are features of anaemia, pallor, glossitis, anorexia and generalized weakness. Neuropathy is not present.

Treatment. Oral supplements of 5-10 mg of folic acid daily are sufficient to ward off the deficiency state.

Vitamin C (ascorbic acid). It is abundant in green leafy vegetables, citrus fruits, amla, guavas, germinating pulses, liver, fish, and in potatoes. Milk and milk products contain only small amount of the vitamin. It is water soluble vitamin which is readily absorbed from the intestines and its stores in the body under normal conditions are sufficient for long periods to tide over the negative balance. The vitamin is destroyed by storage and cooking.

Vitamin C is a powerful antioxidant vitamin and has important role to play in the synthesis of normal collagen and maintenance of folate pool and mobility and phagocytic activity of neutrophils and macrophages.

Daily requirements of vitamin C are 30-40 mg per day in an adult. Body stores of the vitamin are small and it is mainly stored in leucocytes, platelets and adrenal glands. Vitamin C deficiency is not very common these days except in severe malnutrition, famine and starvation states.

Major consequences of deficiency of vitamin C are in the form of weakened blood vessels, defective synthesis of osteoid and delayed wound healing. Clinically the picture produced is called **scurvy** seen in children and adults.

Early symptoms include marked weakness, lassitude and apathy. In infancy and childhood, there are bleed from the gums which become spongy. Painful epiphyseal enlargement producing pseudoparalysis of hands leading to painful swollen joints which often mimic arthritis. Nose bleeds and haemorrhages into the conjunctiva, eye balls and brain are present. Subperiosteal haematomas particularly into the ends of long bones, irritability, painful legs and anaemia are other features.

In adults early symptoms are follicular hyperkeratosis with coiled hairs and perifollicular haemorrhages (pink halo). There are haemorrhages in the deep tissues, joints which are swollen. Gums are swollen into large purple flashy masses and bleed readily with loosened teeth. There are petechial spots and ecchymosis in the skin. Intrarticular subperiosteal or intramuscular haemorrhages may cause painful swelling of the joints at the end of extremity. Gum changes may be aggravated by infection. Bleeding may occur at various sites including brain, kidney, eyes. Bleeding in the G.I. tract may produce malaena. Healing of wounds is delayed.

Diagnosis of scurvy is made on clinical picture. There are low levels of vitamin C in blood (normal levels of vitamin C in blood 0.7-1.5 mg/dl). After administration of vitamin C, urinary excretion of vitamin C is measured (saturation test) which is low. Capillary fragility is increased (positive tourniquet test). Bleeding and clotting time are normal.

X-ray of bones show increased density and epiphyseal separation. Lower end of radius and ulna show shadow due to subperiosteal haemorrhage and a sharp dark epiphyseal line, thinning of cortex of diaphysis with lateral spurs at the ends. Sometimes microfractures may be seen.

Treatment. Patient should be nursed carefully. In infants and young children 50-100 mg of vitamin C orally is given daily while in adults 500 mg daily in divided doses. In cases with advanced disease vitamin C can be given parenterally in dose of 500-1000 mg daily. In addition to drug therapy patient must be given adequate amounts of fresh fruits and nourishing diet.

Toxicity of vitamin C. Excessive use of vitamin C produces gastritis, loss of appetite and burning sensation in epigastrium. Stone formation in urinary tract may result due to its prolonged and excessive use.

OBESITY

Obesity is one of the commonest physical abnormality and a serious health hazard found all the world in people of all races and all age groups irrespective of any barriers. It lies in the twilight zone between health and disease and is a potent danger to the health of all irrespective of age and sex.

Obesity indirectly means short life span with all its associated illnesses. How truthful is the expression, "the longer the belt line, the shorter the life line". One can appreciate the truthfullness of this aphorism if one examines the problem of obesity in all its perspectives.

The slow but gradual collection of fat not only hampers activities but inevitably interferes with the adequate functioning of the vital processes. And not only the body suffers, the mind also becomes slow witted, for, "Danity bits make rich the ribs but bankrupt quite the wits". It has been truly said that for every inch the waist measurement exceeds the chest measurement: the person may subtract two years from his life expectancy.

Obese are physically handicapped. Apart from mechanical inefficiency and aesthetic undesirability it is the cause of many degenerative and metabolic diseases with resultant premature death. The handicaps enumerated are too many but it is often that the fat person fails to appreciate the necessity for reduction and seriousness of what to him appears to be nothing but a benign condition.

Studies have shown that at all ages men and women who are overweight have a higher mortality than the average weight individual of that age and sex and the greater the degree of obesity, greater the mortality and morbidity. A rough estimate puts 20 per cent excess weight in the bracket of 25 per cent mortality and 30 per cent over weight carries 45 percent more mortality and morbidity.

With indirect evidence based on life insurance records the seriousness of condition is well established. Life expectancy is shortened and there is greater incidence of hypertension and atherosclerosis, coronary heart disease and diabetes in these people. Obese are a surgical risk and do not stand operations well. They are more liable to develop hernias, varicose veins and gall bladder disease. Accidents are more frequent presumably because obese are slow and clumsy in their movements. They are prone to get arthritis of the back bone, hips and knees due to the strain of putting up with excess weight. Complaints of pains in the knee and back are equally common at a much earlier age and this is not surprising when one takes into view the extra weight these people have to carry. In the course of pregnancy and child birth obesity is a hazard; there being greater frequency of complications, toxaemias and large fat babies. Post operative recovery is delayed. There are greater chances of obese manifesting diabetes at a much earlier age as their pancreas are constantly put to a condition of stress.

As a result of mechanical restrictions due to increased deposition of fat in the abdomen and in the chest wall their respiratory reserve suffers. Obesity itself produces shortness of breath in an otherwise healthy person. A stout person can not breathe as freely as his normal friend. Complaints of palpitation, easy fatiguability, lack of interest in work and

lethargy are equally common in apparently normal obese individuals. The slow and gradual collection of fat not only hampers activities but ultimately interferes with the adequate functioning of the vital processes.

Marked obesity is essentially a repulsive phenomenon. The obese are handicapped socially. They feel unwanted and rejected. Often they feel embarrassed and shun company. Alacricity is lost and the young obese becomes a recluse to save him or herself from the jeerings and taunts of his or her friends.

What is obesity? As a general rule, 10 per cent above the standard weight for that height and age has been considered as over weight and 20 per cent above the standard weight as pathological obesity. This is correlated with age, height, weight and sex of the individual. A correlation between the thickness of subcutaneous tissue and relative weight (as judged from standards for given sex, age and height) has been suggested. Use of skin fold calipers to measure the thickness of body fat provides the easiest and the simplest anthropometric method. Ideal place for measuing skin fold thickness is middle of triceps muscle. Another defination of obesity is body mass index (BMI) greater than 30 or even 27.

But the best criteria of judging obesity is not so much the individuals weight as his or her appearances. The general build and in particular the abdominal girth in relation to chest measurements are perhaps the most reliable guide. When the abdominal measurements exceed that of the unexpanded chest the individual be considered as fat and this should be taken in relation to height, weight standards.

Aetiology. The question is as to what is the cause of obesity? The problem of obesity is complex. It is not only a disease of richer and affluent people but also of poorer sections of society. Poor people are obese because they can not afford protein rich foods and have to depend on starch rich foods while the rich people suffer from the habit of over eating. When intake of calories exceeds expenditure obesity results. The commonest cause of obesity is overeating but sometimes obesity is associated with endocrinal disorders like hypothyroidism, cushings syndrome but then the scenario is different.

There may not only be a disordered appetite control but a number of other factors like heredity, lack of exercise and physical effort. Social and cultural habits and psychological factors may also be playing a part.

Aetiology of obesity
1. Genetic and environmental factors
2. Familial predisposition
3. Food intake
4. Energy expenditure

Factor of genetic predisposition is also important. In obese subjects leptin secreted from fat cells and acting as a feed back mechanism between fat cells and brain, controls fat stores by regulating hunger and satiety. In obese leptin concentration in tissues is 80 per cent than in controls. Further hormones like cholecystokinin, bombesin somatostatin, glucagon and insulin which are responsible for control of appetite have a role to play in the causation of obesity.

The whole thing to start with appears simple yet it is exceedingly complex. Most of the affected persons either are consuming or have consumed food in excess of their requirement at one time or other in their life. Many people ascribe their obesity to an illness when they were fed nutrients food during their period of recovery and they started putting on weight. In a number of times the habit of overeating may have been started in childhood by misguided parents who were doting on their child and showered on him the lavish gifts of chocolates and sweets.

Obesity runs in families and many will just brush off the problem as nothing but familial predisposition. It is true to some extent but on close analysis one would appreciate that indulgence in culinary delights runs in families and no doubt corpulence also gives company. When both parents are obese the chances of children being obese are almost 80 per cent. It is not only the heredity but the food habits of the family which make the child a 'fat so'.

It is rather rare to meet any person who will admit to over eating as a causative factor and many times the physician also postulates some hypothetical disorders of the endocrine glands. Most authorities now agree that endocrine disorders are rarely if ever a cause of pronounced obesity and if at all they exist they are a minor factor and operates only in a few cases. There is an important QUIP in this regard. It says that the only glands which over act in fat people are the salivary glands.

Genes have also a role to play in the causation of obesity and this factor cannot be ignored. The role of genes is very significant as they determine how fat we are. Here the role of hormone called leptin is also being appreciated. Since it closely regulates the body fat and hunger.

Our social and family customs to a large extent dominate our eating habits and people go on gobbling extra foods. One does not appreciate that tongue is a shameless instrument and it eats whatever tasty food it gets. Emotions and psychological disturbances also have a role to play in the causation of obesity. The disturbing emotional experiences and traumas like death of a loved one, break up of a love affair may force a person to take refuge in over eating. Many a fat person feels insecure frustrated and helpless in meeting his/her day to day problems, and this is probably an important factor.

Though uninhibited indulgence in culinary delights constitutes an important cause of obesity, a very small percentage is due to glandular factors. Fuel for the body comes from the food consumed and if the consumed calories are in excess of what is required they are stored in the form of excess fat.

At the same time it is not only the excessive indulgence in food but also lack of its expenditure. Limitations or lack of energy expenditure coupled with good food goes a long way in increasing slothfulness. Extraordinary inactivity and sedentary habits form a very pernicious factor for corupulance.

The affluence of society acquired in the form of more day to day comforts like cars, television and newer gadgets deviate people from physical activity. This happens more as the person reaches middle age; the portliness increases while the lack of physical effort and exercise increases in inverse ratio.

Indian women have a tendency to put weight after marriage because they feel "What the hell, I have got my man: now I can relax and grow fat". Such attitudes go a long way in increasing the waistline. One often finds rich and affluent people boasting of their corpulance as a sign of prosperity.

Some may be eating more since they are getting bored and thus find eating beyond their needs a good way to fill up their leisure hours especially when they have nothing very active to do.

In fact it is a vicious circle. Once obesity is well established, over eating becomes secondary to obesity and lack of physical effort or exercise further worsens the situation.

In sum total obesity is in no way a desirable physical state since it has the baneful effects not only on the body, the psyche but also cuts short the life span. One's waistline is one's life line, so if one takes care of the former, the later shall take care of itself.

How to manage obesity? Managing an obese person basically requires will on the part of the sufferer to reduce as the management is mainly ditetic and there is no short cut to it.

Main aims to be achieved are:

1. Reduction in body weight.
2. Following strict dietary regimens but at the same time maintaining adequate nutrition since too much deprivation of food may make the person listless and tired.
3. Physical activity to be followed so that excess of calories and fats are burnt.

Dietary regimen. Any reducing diet should contain sufficient calories to meet the basal requirements but below the total caloric output. Provision of sufficient quantities of proteins to make for the body wear and tear be made. At least 10-20 per cent of the total calories must come from proteins (vegetarian/non-vegetarian). A carbohydrate content to meet the body needs and prevent acidosis. In addition enough quantity of minerals and vitamins to guard against any resultant deficiency.

The number of calories to be taken per day shall depend on the persons age, sex, occupation and urgency of weight reduction. Thus an obese person should be sparing with fats butter, ghee, cream and strarch foods (Pastries, cakes, pudding, ice cream). Fruits like grapes, bananas, mangoes, dates, figs, dry fruits like nuts, vegetables like potatoes, peas. But at the same time his/her food should consist of lean meat, poultry, fish (boiled/steamed) vegetables such as cabbage, cauliflower, cucumber, spinach, lady finger, lettuce, mushrooms etc. Fresh fruits like oranges, papaya, grape fruit, skimmed milk, tea, curd, non-sweetened mineral water, orange juice etc.

As a principle a person on reducing diet should maintain strict discipline in the choice of foods which he/she takes as well as the amount of calories taken per day. Food should be taken in small morsels, chewed slowly and second helping of any kind be avoided. A desire to reduce weight has to be cultivated. No doubt it requires will power not to indulge in gustatory pleasures.

Exercise. Most of the obese people hardly take any exercise. Habit of regular physical exercise has to be cultivated and sufficient time in the early hours of morning on empty stomach be devoted. One should stretch one's flabby muscles by taking morning and evening walks, Jogging, stretch exercise and taking active part in swimming tennis and other outdoor games.

Massage is of value in tightening up loose and flabby muscles but has no direct slimming effect. Turkish baths or steam or sauna baths serve no valid purpose in weight reduction except some degree of eliminating water and electrolytes. They can not be a substitute for either dietary restrictions or active physical exercises.

Drug therapy. A number of drugs have been advocated or rather misused to reduce weight but these have limitations. Various drugs which have been employed are:

Thyroid. It obtained early favour because obesity at some time was thought to be due to hypothyroidism. It is not advisable to use thyroid extracts in obese people except in those with myxoedema.

Anorexogenic drugs. These drugs came into use since in majority of obese the underlying factor is unrestricted gluttony and these drugs suppress appetite. At the same time patient must be told that he/she must control weight by diet also. The two commonly used drugs as Dexfenfluramine and Fenfluramine.

The drugs are contraindicated in patients with advanced arteriosclerosis, hypertension, hyperthyroidism, glaucoma, agitated state and those with history of drug abuse. Usual dosage is 15 mg with meals to start with and can be increased to 30 mg. But this dose should not be exceeded. A major side effect with these appetite suppressants drugs is the develoment of primary pulmonary hypertension which may sometimes prove fatal.

These anorexogenic drugs decrease the energy intake from main dishes and snacks. They allow better compliance with diet and less preoccuption with the diet even if weight loss is small. But unfortunately even after taking the drug for 3 years, when it is discontinued patient regaines more weight. Phentermine, a drug with less sympathomimetic and stimulant properties than amphetamines, is often combined with Fenfluramine and this combination is one of the commonly used treatment. Fenfluramine with a half life of 20 hours crosses the blood brain barrier and is distributed in almost all body tissues while Phentermine stimulates the hypothalmus to decrease appetite, an effect likely mediated by nor epinephrine and dopamine. The drug is absorbed more slowly and has more clinical effects.

With the combined regimen, recommended dose of feufluramine is 20 mg three times daily before meals. This dosage may be increased weekly by 20 mg per day until it reaches the dose of 40 mg three times a day. It is better to start the drug in a dose of 10 mg three times a day. Phentermine resin (15 mg capsule) is taken once in the morning before breakfast. In some patient dose of the drug may be raised to 30 mg. The combined therapy causes adequate appetite suppression. The drug is contraindicated in patient with advanced arteriosclerosis, hypertension, hyperthyroidism, glaucoma and alcohal abuse.

Side effects of the drug include exaceberation of hypertension, depression of mood, development of pulmonary hypertension (Both reversible and irreversible).

But the main issue with these drugs is that if diet control has not worked and patient has not lost weight these drugs will not work since they act by making people eat less.

It is equally important that patients on long term use of these drugs be assessed for their side effects and safety.

Surgical treatment. In patients with severe form of obesity, certain surgical methods have been devised. These inclued:

1. Wiring of the jaw. Idea is to prevent eating. Only liquids are given. Results are good but patient regains weight once wires are removed.
2. Gastric plication. Here size of stomach is reduced by creating a small pouch as a result of stapling of stomach to abdominal wall. Good results may be achieved.
3. Gastric balloon. A small balloon is placed inside the stomach endoscopically and inflated. Capacity of stomach is reduced. It is of doubtful value.
4. Liposuction. This method is quite popular. Here fat is sucked from specific areas like abdomen, thighs, buttocks. It is comparatively a safe procedure.

To sum up obesity is a social aesthetic and health problem with all its associated shortcomings. Weight reduction can be achieved only when the obese person feels for it and sets his/her mind to achieve it. There are no short cuts to it. Sustained efforts are required and once the aims are achieved, efforts may be worth all the trouble.

PROTEIN CALORIC MALNUTRITION

Protein caloric or energy malnutrition is a disease of third world countries and is wide spread. It is related to the development, economics, social milieu and supply of correct nutritious food. Proteins play a major role in building and repair of body tissues and its deficiency plays havoc with the health of the person suffering from it.

World Health Organisation has defined it as a range of pathological conditions arising from coincident lack of protein and calories in varying proportions occurring most frequently in infants and young children and commonly associated with infections. The two spectrums of the disease are marasmus and kwashiorkor. The oft held view is that marasmus is caused by deficiency of total calories whereas kwashiorkor develops when there is deficiency of quality proteins relative to the total caloric intake. But both the entities are interrelated, overlap, and often a child with marasmus passes into picture of kwashiorkor by excessive loss of proteins especially during periods of infections. Moreover protein energy malnutrition depresses body immune defence mechanism thus making the child more prone to infections.

Marasmus. It is the type of protein caloric malnutrition seen in infants and young children. There is history of poor intake of breast feeds or inadequate supply of milk and other nutrients. This results in lack of development and delay in milestones. The child or infant is wasted, emaciated and there is loss of body fat and muscle with skin hanging loose from extremities. The withered look, a big head compared to rest of the body a slightly protuberant abdomen, pinched nose and sunken eyes gives the appearance of an old man. Hair are sparse and dry. As the disease progresses the child looks apathetic. There are other signs of malnutrition and vitamin deficiencies. Child suffers from recurrent infections. In fact bacterial and parasitic infections plague these children and may sometimes prove fatal. Aetiologically marasmus is due to poor nutrition as a result of poor food availability but marasmus like picture may be produced in coeliae disease. Fibrocystic disease of the pancreas infantile renal acidosis and idiopathic hypercalcaemia.

Kwashiorkor. It is the original name given to malnutrition syndrome first described in indigenous African children. It occurs most commonly in children between the ages of one and four years but also occurs in other age groups.

Kwashiorkor results due to severe malnutrition which started when the child was being breast fed and then went on to period of poor nutrition, bad dietetic habits and recurrent infections.

Clinically a child suffering from it has retarded growth, is apathetic, listless with muscular wasting. Pitting oedema is present. Skin shows excoriated lesions seen over areas of pressure (flaky paint) with marked hyperkeratosis, scaling. Pavement or mosaic appearance on legs,(crazy pavement skin) forearms and chest. Ulceration with bed sores may occur. Hair are sparse, thin, lustreless and brownish red in colour. There may be alternate bands of pigmentation (yellowish or reddish) and depigmentation of hair producing a peculiar picture (Flag sign). Abdomen is protubrant. Hepatomegaly may be present. There may be other signs of vitamin deficiencies and of other nutrients. The features of a case of kwashiorkor are typical in a child of protein malnutrition. In most of the cases there is generalized oedema with fluid present in abdomen (ascites) and abdominal wall. Gastrointestinal disorders like diarrhoea and poor digestion are present. The child may pass loose ill formed stools containing undigested food particles. In some patients when steatorrhoea is present stools are foul swelling. Signs of various vitamin deficiencies in the form of stomatitis, cheilosis, xeropthalmia, photophobia are common. There is iron deficiency anaemia.

Clinical manifestations of kwashiorkor

1. Retarded growth, failure to grow.
2. Child is thin, wasted, generalize oedema.
3. Child apathetic, irritable, lying listless.
4. Skin shows excoriated lesions with marked hyperkeratosis, scaling, desquamation, ulceration (crazy pavement skin)
5. Hair, thin sparse, lustreless, brownish red in colour. Changes in hair colour (yellowish or reddish) with patches of depigmentaion.
6. Mouth, angular stomatitis, cheilosis, bald tongue.
7. GI tract, diarrhoea, loose ill-formed stools, loss of appetite, abdomen protuberant, hepatomegaly.
8. Vitamin defeciencies especially of Vit. A (xerophthalmia, night blindness), Vit. K (ecchymosis, petechiae) and Vit. B complex group.

Investigations. Haemoglobin levels are low and there is picture of normocytic normochromic anaemia. Blood proteins are markedly reduced. Serum albumin is low. Serum cholesterol and blood urea levels are diminished or low. Renal plasma flow is diminished and produces impairment of renal function.

Blood sugar levels are low while serum sodium is increased and there is fall in serum potassium levels. X-ray chest may show evidence of pulmonary tuberculosis. Liver biopsy shows fatty infiltration of liver.

Pathology. Mainly liver, gastrointestinal tract are involved in kwashiorkor. Liver shows fatty changes. Mucosa of small intestines is atrophic and there is loss of microvilli. Anaemia is of normocytic normochromic type but when there is superadded helminthic infestation blood picture may turn to that of iron deficiency type. Bone marrow shows erythroid hypoplasia and a disturbed erythroid myeloid ratio. Since immune response in these patients is depressed and impaired they are more prone to get infections. There may be marked atrophy of thymus and number of T cells in peripheral blood may be reduced.

Prognosis. It shall depend on the severity of the disease process. Presence of intercurrent infections, hypoglycaemia, myocarditis, cardiac failure, marked wasting, fluid and electrolyte imbalance portend poor prognosis. In untreated cases mortality ranges from 40-50 per cent.

Diagnosis of kwashiorkor is made by the presence of clinical features like oedema, skin and hair changes and presence of various deficiencies. Confirmation is made by laboratory investigations. Liver biopsy will help in differentiating it from cirrhosis.

Treatment. The basic approach to treatment is to supply food of high caloric value with good amount of proteins in diet. Frequent small feeds are given throughout the day. Diet should be high in proteins (3-6 g/kg of high class proteins daily). Skimmed milk with milk proteins is a suitable diet. For non-vegetarians, fish and eggs in good quantity are to be given while to vegetarians a mixture of whole wheat, bengal gram, ground nut and jaggrey

is given. Anorexia is sometimes a very distressing symptom. In such patients tube feeding may have to be given.

Fats have to be given in sufficient quantities to meet the caloric needs. Supportive treatment in the form of vitamins especially A and D should be added in the form of cod liver oil and vegetable extracts. In severe form of disease blood transfusion or plasma be given. Diarrhoea when present is generally resistant to conventional line of treatment and shall only improve when proteins are given.

If intercurrent infections are present they be treated appropriately. Many children with protein caloric malnutrition have in addition helminthic infestation. This should be diligently treated. As treatment starts having effect, recovery starts and initial response is disappearance of oedema over a period of two to three weeks. Appetite improves and child starts taking food normally as well takes interest in his/her surroundings.

Once recovery takes place it must be maintained with adequate intake of proteins and good nutrition. Protein caloric malnutrition is preventable. It starts in infancy when infant must be properly breastfed and not weaned early. Subsequently additional food supplements be given and in early childood proper protein balance be maintained.

CALCIUM HOMEOSTASIS

Calcium forms an integral part of the body and is an essential constituent of the bones. It plays important role in maintaining various cellular functions of the body like bone formation, blood coagulation, cardiac contractility and neuromuscular activity.

Body's main external source of calcium is mainly from food, Milk and its products. Cheese, leafy green vegetables, eggs, fish and cereals are rich source of calcium. An adult person requires 500-600 mg/day of calcium which is normally met from the diet. During childhood and adolescence the requirements shall vary being more in the growing years of life. The requirements of calcium increase substantially during pregnancy and lactation going upto 1200-1400 mg/day.

An adult body contains 1.2 to 1.4 kg of calcium, ninety per cent of which is present in the bones in the form of calcium salts chiefly as hydroxyapatite. The extracellular calcium is present mainly in the plasma and its level normally varies between 9-11 mg/dl. Plasma calcium is present in three forms i.e. ionic (65% of total calcium) protein bound and combined with other organic acids.

Absorption of calcium primarily takes place from distal part of small intestines though absorption also takes place from the proximal part. Vitamin D enhances intestinal absorption via its active metabolites $(1,25(OH_2)D_3)$ while it is interfered in intestines by excess of phosphates oxalates (derived from vegetables) and phytates (derived from cereals). Fats as such do not interfere with its absorption except in cases of steatorrhoea or malabsorption syndrome when precipitation of calcium by fatty acids takes place. Further its absorption is interfered with due to lack of vitamin D and parathyroid hormone.

Calcium is mainly excreted in faeces, urine and sweat. More than ninety per cent of calcium filtered by the kidneys is reabsorbed from the proximal tubules while the rest is absorbed under the influence of vitamin D and parathyroid hormone. Calcitonin inhibits tubular reabsorption and increases its excretion.

Calcium homeostasis is mainly controlled by vitamin D, parathyroid hormone and calcitonin. Vitamin D helps to conserve body calcium by enhancing its intestinal absorption and renal tubular reabsorption. It also mobilises calcium from the bones by the process of resorption.

The role of parathyroid hormone in calcium homeostasis can not be minimized. By stimulating osteoclastic activity in bones, it accelerates osteolysis and brings calcium to extracellular fluid. It not only increases osteoclastic resorption of bone but also increases intestinal absorption of calcium, synthesis of vitamin D metabolites $(1,25(OH_2)D_3)$ tubular reabsorption of calcium and renal loss of phosphates. This effect of parathyroid hormone is influenced by vitamin D and adequacy of renal functions.

The exact role of calcitonin which is produced by thyroid C cells, in this regard is not well defined. Its actions are generally opposite to parathyroid hormone though it promotes calcium deposition by osteoblasts. Its secretion as such is controlled to some extent by calcium levels in blood. High levels of calcium in the blod is a stimulus for calcitonin secretion. Thyroid hormone (T3-T4) also causes increased bone turn over. Lack of the hormone plays a negative role and delays bone growth.

Calcium is essential for bone formation and teeth, its deficiency leads to defectivie and delayed dentition as well as poor bone formation. Maintenance of calcium balance is to a large extent dependent upon the intestinal absorption, parathyroid hormone, vitamin D synthesis and calcitonin. Deficiency of either of these coupled with poor dietary intake can not be adequately compensated by renal calcium conservation. Result is negative calcium balance.

Hypocalcaemia. Negative calcium balance can be due to number of factors which include hypoparathyroidism, chronic renal failure, vitamin D deficiency and hypomagnesemia. Hypoparathyroidism may be either idiopathic or following surgical trauma over that region and occurrence of hypocalcemia results due to failure of homeostatic mechanism of parathyroid hormone resulting in loss of calcium from the extracellular compartment at a rate faster than it can be replaced.

Hypomagnesemia of severe degree is associated with severe hypocalcaemia while hyperphosphatemia in chronic renal failure results in reduction in calcium absorption due to formation of insoluble calcium phosphate complexes. Increased demands of calcium during pregnancy and lactation and its poor intake in diet coupled with vitamin D deficiency is another factor responsible for hypocalcaemia.

Clinically cases of hypocalcaemia have a picture of tetany due to increased neuromuscular irritability. Patient is often irritable complaining of tingling or parasthesia in limbs, cramps in calf muscles, muscular twitchings and carpopedal spasm. Spasm of larynx and bronchial musculature may be seen and this often simulates bronchial asthma like picture. There may be sometimes features of impaired memory, anxiety and hallucinations. Hair may be thinned and dental caries is often seen. Latent tetany is demonstrated by certain tests:

1. Chovstek's sign. Here brisk contraction of facial muscles takes place on tapping the facial nerve in front of the external auditory meatus.
2. Trousseau's sign. When pressure is applied on the upper arm by tying a sphygmomanometer cuff and raising the pressure above systolic levels for one to five minutes, corpo pedal spasm occurs in a case of tetany.
3. Erb's sign is an exaggerated, muscular contraction to normal electrical stimuli or increased excitability of motor nerves to galvanic stimulation.

Serum calcium levels are low, generally below 8 mg/dl while phosphorus levels are rather normal or raised. Electrocardiogram shows a prolonged Q-T interval.

Management. In an acute case of tetany 10 or 20 cc of 10 per cent calcium gluconate is to be given intravenously. For subacute or chronic cases of hypocalcaemia due to hypoparathyroidism, chronic renal failure, and vitamin D metabolism defects, supplements of calcium and vitamin D metabolites are given.

Usual dose of Hydroxylated derivative of vitamin D is 0.25-1 µg of 1.25 OHD3 (calcitriol) daily along with oral calcium supplements (2-10 g/day). In addition diet must be rich in calcium and low in phosphate content (more fresh fruits, vegetables, milk, white of egg and less of meat, nuts, cheese and yolk of egg). Oral aluminium hydroxide gel be given 15 ml three times a day to reduce absorption of phosphates in intestinal tract. While patient is on therapy, regular monitoring of calcium levels in blood must be done.

Hypercalcaemia. It is much more common than hypocalcaemia. Hypercalcaemia is commonly associated with hyperparathyroidism. Other causes include presence of malignancy, vitamin D intoxication and diseases associated with high bone turn over.

Clinically hypercalcaemia is characterised by generalized weakness, fatigue, aches and pains, anorexia, nausea, mental confusion, vomiting, abdominal pain, polyuria, nocturia and hypotonia. Excess calcium gets deposited at various sites in the body like lungs, heart, skin and kidneys. Kidney involvement leads to renal insufficiency and calcification. There is progressive deterioration in renal function. Concentrating function suffers, leading to renal failure. Drowsiness and coma supervenes. In electrocardiogram there is shortening of Q-T interval. Cardiac arrhythmias appear and even cardiac arrest may occur. Symptoms due to hypercalcaemia go along with calcium levels in blood. When calcium levels exceed 12.0 mg/dl most of the symptoms appear and levels above 15 mg/dl require emergency medical management.

Causes of hypercalcaemia

1. Hyperparathyroidism (primary, multiple endocrine neoplasia).
2. Malignant diseases (multiple myeloma, lymphoma, leukaemia, carcinoma breast, lung secondary deposits).
3. Vitamin D intoxication.
4. Hypercalcaemia associated with high bone turn over.
   a. Hyperthyroidism,
   b. Prolonged immobilization.
5. Excess calcium intake (milk alkali syndrome)
6. Renal failure.

Treatment. Hypercalcaemia develops because calcium release from bones is excessive along with increase in calcium absorption from intestines as well as excretion of calcium from kidneys is inadequate. So treatment must be aimed at correcting these abnormalities.

First principle is to restore hydration since most of the patients have been having vomiting with drop in glomerular filtration. If the fluid balance is well maintained by intravenous infusion of isotonic saline, there is increased excretion of urinary calcium. This is further helped by giving frusemide twice a day. By this way tubular reabsorption of calcium shall be inhibited.

Causes of hypocalcaemia

1. Hypoparathyroidism
   a. Congenital deficiency
   b. Idiopathic (autoimmune)
   c. Surgical trauma.
2. Poor intake and utilization of calcium
3. Chronic renal failure
4. Severe hypomagnasemia
5. Vitamin D deficiency
6. Drugs like calcitonin, phosphate therapy, resistance to parathyroid hormone.

When patient is on intensive diuretic therapy care must be taken that potassium and magnesium from the body is not excessively depleted. In patients where calcium levels are very high, Plicamycin may be employed. It is a useful therapeutic agent which inhibits bone resorption. Dose is 25 ug/kg body weight in slow intravenous infusion. Major side effects are bleeding, thrombocytopenia, renal failure. Other drugs beneficial in lowering calcium levels include glucocorticoids (prednisolone 40-60 mg/day), Diphosphonates (7.5 mg/kg perday intravenously for 3 days), Biphosphate (15-90 mg in intravenous infusion). For patients with very high levels of calcium and with renal failure, peritoneal dialysis is the treatment of choice.

Hypercalcaemia is a symptom complex of number of diseases. Once calcium levels have been lowered, treatment must be aimed at treating the underlying conditions. Dietary restrictions about calcium intake should also be enforced.

OSTEOPOROSIS

A World Health Organization study has defined osteoporosis as a systemic skeletal disease characterized by low bone mass and microarchitectural deterioration of bone tissue leading to increased bone fragility and a consequent increase in fracture risk. The common fractures are those of neck of femur, vertebral bodies and lower end of radius.

Aetiology. Osteoporosis is common both in men and women and advancing age is an important underlying factor. Post menopausal women and women with menstrual irregularities are most commonly affected. Bone health partially depends on physical stress and on adequate levels of calcium, parathyroid hormone and oestrogens. Excess bone loss most commonly occurs in women who have insufficient levels of oestrogen. Factor of ageing has also role to play and in women beyond 70 years of age along with poor intake of calcium in diet and its deficient absorption as well as less effective production of 1,25-dehydroxy vitamin D_3 are important aetiological factors.

Besides delayed menarche and amenorrhoea other risk factors for the development of osteoporosis in women, include a family history of osteoporosis, low calcium intake in diet. Poor absorption of calcium as in malabsorption syndrome, malnutrition, eating disorders like anorexia nervosa, premature menopause and prolonged use of drugs like corticosteroids, phenytoin.

If females are likely to get osteoporosis then men in advancing years are equally liable to get it. In men osteoporosis again has predisposition in those with a family history especially on father's side, advanced age, lack of physical exercise, and early decline in testosterone levels. History of malignancy and those using corticosteroids, anticonvulsants, frusemide and anabolic steroids is equally significant.

Clinical profile. Patients with osteoporosis present with history of aches and pains and for a long time patient may ignore it. Many times per se there are no symptoms and after the occurrence of fractures it does become clinically evident. Fractures may involve any bone except the skull and the most common sites are vertebrae, wrist and hips. Shortened height, bone pains, low back pain, difficulty in getting up from chair are common complaints in women at menopause with osteoporosis. Women are much more susceptible than men because they start with a lower peak bone mass and have accerlerated bone loss spread over a number of years after menopause.

A number of factors are known to play their role in the causation of osteoporosis ranging from genetic predisposition, poor calcium intake, protein malnutrition, ageing, menopause to prolonged intake of drugs like corticosteroids, and antiepileptic drugs.

Senile osteoporosis

Osteoporosis in elderly patients of both sexes is characterized by uncoupled bone remodeling which is induced by sex hormone deficiencies (Oestrogen or testosterone), by the growth hormone or insulin like growth factor (IGF) deficiency, by Vit D deficiency and importantly by reduced synthesis of D-hormone in kidneys and bone. It is also induced by the lack of receptors in the target organs (gastro intestinal tract, bones and parathyroid). Inadequate 1.25 (OH)2 D3 levels will lead to lower intestinal calcium mobilization from the skeleton and increased bone resorption.

In elderly males and females osteoporosis increased bone resorption is not accompanied by increased formation. As a result of decreased renal production of and reduced intestinal response to 1,25-dihydroxy vitamin D, there is relative hyperparathyroidism which may explain the excessive cortical bone loss and increased hip fracture risk in the elderly.

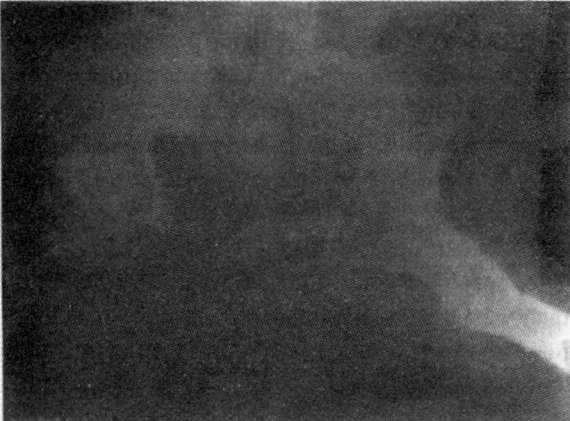

Fig. 9.2. X-ray Pelvis (PA view). There is generalised osteoporosis of bones. There is fracture of head of femur

It is important to diagnose osteoporosis in the elderly. Conventional X-rays are relatively insensitive and bone loss is apparent only when bone mass

has decreased by around 30-50%. Measuring of bone mineral density is the method to detect senile osteoporosis.

Senile osteoporosis is particularly important in post menopausal women and it is estimated that 30% of post menopausal women are oesteoporotic.

Secondary osteoporosis. Certain diseases like hyperparathyrodism, hyperthyroidism or hypothyroidism can also cause osteoporosis. Further bone conditions that mimic some of the features of osteoporosis such as malignancy or osteomalacia must be excluded.

Levels of calcium, phosphate and alkaline phosphatase are abnormal in patients with osteomalacia or bone secondaries. Renal function tests will exclude renal osteo dystrophy, X-rays of thoracic or lumbar spine shall exclude bony secondaries.

Diagnosis. Confirmation of diagnosis shall be by laboratory investigations. Serum levels of calcium, phosphorus, parathyroid hormone and calcitonin which are normal in primary osteoporosis are altered. Serum alkaline phosphatase levels are elevated after a fracture. Routine radiographic studies are not very helpful. Before osteopenia becomes evident, 30 per cent of bone must be lost.

Risk factors for osteoporosis in women

1. Age (older than 50 years).
2. Family history of osteoporosis
3. Poor calcium intake.
4. Malabsorption or poor absorption.
5. Lack of physical activity.
6. Immobilisation due to chronic illness or injury.
7. Excess consumption of alcohol.
8. Cigarette smoking
9. Small body built.
10. Lack of sun exposure
11. Delayed menarche
12. Premature menopause
13. Post-menopause
14. Eating disorders like anorexia nervosa.
15. Prolonged use of corticosteroids, phenytoin
16. Protein malnutrition.

The diagnosis is based on measurement of bone mineral density (BMD). Dual energy X-ray absorptiometry (DEXA) is the most widely used imaging technique. It is a fairly accurate method, can be done rapidly and uses low dose radiation.

Risk factors for osteoporosis in men

1. Family history of osteoporosis
2. Advancing age.
3. Physical inactivity/sedentary habits
4. Prolonged immobility due to injury or debilitating illness.
5. Poor nutrition.
6. History of bone fracture over 45 years age.
7. Early decline in testosterone levels
8. History of malignancy
9. Excessive use of alcohol
10. Smoking
11. Prolonged use of corticosteroids, anabolic hormones, anticonvulsants.
12. Malabsorption.
13. Eating disorders
14. Protein malnutrition.

Dexascanning is the gold standard for identifying osteoporosis and predicting future fracture risk. Any patient with a previous fragility fracture, height loss or kyphosis or radiographic evidence of osteopenia shall require dexascanning. Results from DEXA scans are usually reported as a T score and a Z score. The T score provides a comparison with the young adult mean and relates to absolute fracture risk while the Z score relates to the patients relative risk for his/her age.

T score of above −1.0 is considered normal, a scale between −1.0 and −2.5 is defined as osteopenia and a value more negative than −2.5 indicates osteoporosis. Patient with T score of 2.5 or less who has had one or more fragility fracture has established osteoporosis.

Any patient with a T score of −1 or less should be given advice on improving life style plus calcium and Vit. D.

Computed tomogoraphy (both quantitative CT and peripheral quantitative CT) are other accurate methods but expose the patient to relatively large radiation doses and are not reproducible.

Iliac crest bone biopsy may be done only in doubtful cases.

Pathophysiology. Bones in body are continually being deposited by osteoblasts and resorbed by osteoclasts. This process is called remodelling. Normally this process of bone deposition and resorption is balanced so that the total bone mass in body remains constant. But in osteoporosis bone resorption exceeds that of bone deposition.

For bone remodelling to take place normally it is essential to provide calcium in adequate amounts so that levels are maintained in extracellular space, the repair of old bones takes place and elasticity of skeletal system is maintained. Activity of osteoclasts and osteoblasts govern the bone mass. Low bone mass (osteopenia) leads to osteoporosis which is because of imbalance between bone formation and bone resorption.

There are two types of osteoporosis. Type I results from the predominant loss of trabecular bone associated with menopause while in Type II there is loss of both trabecular and cortical bone associated with the process of ageing. The former (type I) is associated with vertebrae, distal forearm and ankle fractures while in latter (type II) there are commonly hip fractures.

Prevention and treatment. Osteoporosis is a disabling condition. Women who are likely to suffer from it because of risk factors must take preventive measures. The line of prevention and treatment of osteoporosis almost mingle with each other. These are:

1. Weight-bearing activity is essential for developing and maintaining a healthy skeleton. So a person must take part in active physical activity, so that strength, flexibility and coordination of body improves. This shall also lessen chances of falls and subsequent development of fractures. Physical exercise is very important for remodelling and strengthening of bones.

2. Adequate intake of calcium in diet. A daily calcium intake of 1500 mg is recommended in adolescents so that a large bone mass is created. For women in age group 50-65 years who are taking oestrogens, calcium 1000 mg per day and in post-menopausal women older than

65 years and not on oral oestrogens daily intake of calcium 1500 mg is recommended.

Calcium supplements retard bone loss and fracture risk more so when given in combination with oestrogen therapy in menopausal women. Once osteoporosis develops treatment becomes difficult. Addition of 400 to 800 IU of vitamin D supplements are also beneficial. In addition adequate consumption of milk and other calcium rich foods must be ensured.

3. Oestrogens play important role in the maintenance of bone health and proper development. Oestrogen replacement therapy (HRT) is widely accepted for the prevention and treatment of osteoporosis. Oesstrogen not only increase bone mineral density but also reduce the risk of osteoporotic fractures.

HRT is the treatment of choice for preventing osteoporosis in post menopausal women. Patients taking HRT should have yearly PAP smears and Pelvic examination. HRT should begin within 2 to 7 years of menopause and maintained for as long as possible.

Major drawback to the oestrogen use is fear of developing breast and endometrial cancer. But in women who have uterus intact, the risk of cancer is minimized if oestrogen is combined with progestrone.

4. In women where there is contraindication to use of oestrogen replacement therapy, they should be treated with alendronate (second generation Bisphosphonate) dose 10 mg once a day. It is highly effective in increasing BMD and decreasing risk of fractures. Side effects include nausea, abdominal pain, headache, bowel disturbances.

5. Patients where both oestrogens and alendronate are contraindicated (women of child-bearing age because of teratogenic effect) calcitonin (100 IU S/C or IM daily) with calcium and vitamin D supplements be used. Nasal spray of calcitonin (200 IU per activation per day) is equally effective. It has antiresorptive activity and targets osteoclasts directly.

In sum total good nourishing diet, milk, calcium, oestrogens, alendronate/calcitonin with appropriate weight bearing exercises are the basic approach for prevention and treatment of osteoporosis.

DIABETES MELLITUS

Diabetes is widely prevalent all over the world and the number of diabetics in various parts of the world is variable. Probably there are more than 50 million people in this world who suffer from this malady.

Diabetes is not only a disease of civilization but has been in existence since centuries and the early physicians of India, China, Egypt and Africa have all mentioned it in their treatises on medicine.

In India the incidence of disease is increasing and on an average ranges from 2.1 per cent of the urban population and 1.5 per cent of the rural population. Disease is more common in men as compared to women though it is reverse in western countries. Time was when diabetics was considered a dreaded disease as before the discovery of insulin, the life expectancy of diabeties was cut short either by inter current infections or complications. But the credit for bringing hope in the life of diabetics goes to the epoch-making discovery of insulin by Dr. Charles Best and Dr. Banting.

Diabetes is now no longer a dreaded disease since majority of diabetics can lead an absolutely normal life without interference in their normal vocations and activities. The duration of life has been prolonged though in untreated diabetics, a number of complications ensue, cutting short their life.

What is diabetes? Diabetes is a metabolic disorder whose exact cause remains still unknown. There is a disturbance of carbohydrate metabolism and there is deficiency of insulin required for its proper utilization with the result that there is hyperglycaemia. The normal levels of blood sugar are dependent on the adequate amounts of insulin being secreted in the body.

Insulin is produced in the body by the beta cells of the islets of Langerhans of pancreas. Main stimulus for release of insulin is hyperglycaemia caused by ingestion of carbohydrates, hyperamino-acidae-mia due to protein ingestion hormones like gluca-gon, gastrin, secretin pancreozymin and binding of insulin molecules to insulin receptors. Insulin fa-vours the entry of glucose into the liver, into mus-cles as glycogen and builds up adipose tissue by converting glucose into fat.

Insulin secretion decreases with age since by the process of ageing the number of beta cells are lost by degeneration. Normally these cells regenerate but in diabetes there is inherent defect in the regenera-tion of cells. Though mechanisms like lack of syn-thesis and release of insulin are operative in major-ity of diabetics yet other factors like defect in the transport mechanism of insulin, DNA sequence cod-ing insulin receptors and degenration of insulin on the cell surface may be operative.

Aetiology of diabetes. A number of factors are held responsible in the causation of diabetes. It has been considered a related disorder of metabolism rather than a disease entity. The viral aetiology of the disease has been incriminated based on evidence from viral epidemics where inflammation was ob-served in beta cells of recently diagnosed young diabetics. Other factors favouring this hypothesis are the appearance of diabetes abruptly. Seasonal incidence of onset and the frequent failure of hereditarily predisposed subjects especially identi-cal twins to develop the disease. But there are number of other factors which predispose to the development of diabetes and these range from age, sex, socioeconomic status, race, diet, occupation, obesity, autoimmune mechanism to heredity.

Heredity. Diabetes is more common in those who have one or more blood relative suffering from it. Though the exact role of heredity in diabetes is con-troversial yet it is well accepted that the risk of in-heriting diabetes is greater if there are other affected member in the family. It is inherited as mendelian type of recessive trait and is predominant in chil-dren born to parents who are diabetics.

Every person who has a history of diabetes in his or her family is a carrier of disease. The risk per-centage in first degree relatives is generally upto 20 per cent while in second degree relatives it is about

5 per cent and the overall percentage of diabetes among the children of diabetics goes upto 10 per cent. Identical twins of a diabetic have almost 40 per cent chances of developing the disease. Factor of heredity has an important role in insulin depend-ent diabetes as majority of such patients demonstrate HLA antigens (HLA-DR3, HLA-DR4 or both) as well as islet cell antibodies in the blood.

Obesity. Obese people are more prone to suffer from diabetes probably because obesity imposes a strain on the islets of langerhans and there is a rela-tive deficiency of insulin. Obese also show a rela-tive resistance to insulin due to reduction in the number of insulin receptors on target cells.

Obesity results due to uninhibited indulgence in food and lack of physical activity and imposes a constant stress on the pancreas. Thus these people are more prone to get diabetes. The problem of over nutrition is important when one considers the fact that more than 80 per cent of the diabetics of late onset are over weight and the morbidity of the disease is directly proportional to the degree of obesity.

Of the various surveys carried out all over the world it has been shown that more than 80 per cent of the non-insulin dependant diabetics are over-weight. The role of obesity and heredity are prob-ably complementary to each other. Obesity runs in families and so does diabetes. Probably the table manners, dietetic habits and over eating all go hand in hand in producing diabetes. The plethora of calo-ries in obese produces hypertrophy of pancreatic islets with resultant cells dysfunction and an im-paired glucose metabolism. When a person takes more food it acts as a stimulus to further insulin secretion which in turn increases his appetite and thus a vicious cycle sets in. The obese person takes more food, puts a greater demand on his insulin se-cretions with the result that the cells in pancreas at first hypertrophy and later on get exhausted.

When such condition is present, any acute stress or infection aggravates the already existing diabe-tes mellitus.

Race. All races are involved and suffer from diabetes though a number of factors operate in one ethnic group or the other. Jewish race has been known to be more commonly affected than others. Some communities are known to have less incidence of diabetes as compared to others but here the role of diet, physical exercise and environmental factors come into play. There are certain variations in the ethnic distribution of jews belonging to various regions, it being maximum among jews of Eastern, Central and Wester European origin and double that for jews settled in United States.

A certain community in Japan (Ainus) was known to have practically no or little diabetes probably due to undernourishment and poverty but with the rapid industrialization and boom in the economy of the community, the incidence of diabetes among them has gone up.

Interesting are the observations about Japanese Sumo wrestlers who have not only great body size but are also very obese. The incidence of diabetes mellitus is quite high among these active as well as retired sumo wrestlers.

Social and environmental factors. Diabetes has been considered a disease of civilization and its prevalence is closely related to the economic affluence. Diabetes occurs more in richer and affluent classes of society though the poorer class of people are equally liable to suffer from early onset diabetes. Diabetes in richer class of people is closely related to their eating habits, lack of physical effort and obesity.

Exercise. Lack of physical effort and exercise promotes obesity and indirectly predisposes to diabetes. Physical effort and leading an active life goes a long way in keeping one self trim and helps in the proper utilization of body glucose and maintains a homeostatic balance.

Diet. Excessive intake of carbohydrates and refined sugars produces strain on the pancreas and this combined with sedentary occupation goes a long way in predisposing to diabetes.

Parity. Women with repeated pregnancies are more liable to develop diabetes since too many pregnancies are a strain on the carbohydrate metabolism and often there is hormonal imbalance.

Parity is an important predisposing factor in the causation of diabetes in middle aged women having more than seven children.

All these factors go a long way in understanding the primary form of diabetes especially if one keeps in mind the faulty gene, over eating, obesity, lack of physical effort, racial, social and environmental factors in addition to hormonal imbalance.

Pathogenesis. Diabetes is a metabolic disorder of uncertain origin. Normally there is a state of equilibrium between a person's beta cell activity and insulin requirements. But when there are either structural or functional disorder of the pancreas, the beta cells are unable to meet the minimum requirement of insulin in the body.

Deficiency of insulin in the body may be absolute either as a result of genetic defect, pancreatic disorders or it may be relative when insulin secretion balance to the prevailing glucose levels falls as a result of loss or exhaustion of beta cells.

There is either decreased synthesis or storage of insulin in the beta cells. Hyperglycaemia and even ketoacidosis may occur as a result of abnormalities at the insulin receptor level. Further on there is inadequate release of insulin due to a defect in initiation, transmission or amplification of the glucose signal. Autoimmune processes are involved in type I diabetes. The cycle of diabetes starts firstly with genetic predisposition when synthesis of insulin and proinsulin may be defective. Viral infection may trigger an inflammatory response and an autoimmune process with the result that beta cells are destroyed and diabetes new becomes apparent.

Types of diabetes. Diabetes may be classified into:

1. Primary diabetes consisting of growth onset or juvenile diabetes
2. Matuurity onset diabetes.
3. Secondary diabetes which is either as a result of pancreatic disorders (chronic relapsing pancreatitis, haemochromatosis, calcific pancreatitis, carcinoma of the pancreas), endocrine disorders (acromegaly, hyperthyroidism, cushings syndrome) and prolonged use of drugs like corticosteroids, thiazide diuretics and oral contraceptives.

Insulin dependent diabetes mellitus (IDDM type I, young or juvenile diabetes). It occurs in young individuals who are generally lean and thin with classical symptoms of increased thirst, polyurea, polyphagia and rapid loss of weight. These people may present either insidiously or suddenly but majority have a definite onset.

Insulin deficiency is a primary factor which may be either deficient because of decreased production or release (glucose receptor anomaly) or factors which reduce the metabolic efficacy of insulin (insulin antogonism). There is also role of islet cell antibodies, insulin auto antibodies and auto immune mechanism. Most of these diabetics are underweight, undernourished and their symptoms are severe. Presence of ketone bodies in the urine is quite common in such diabetics since their diabetes is brittle. These patients are more liable to develop complications. They are sensitive to insulin but do not respond to oral antidiabetic drugs.

Differences between juvenile and maturity onset diabetes

Feature	Juvenile diabetes	Maturity onset diabetes
Age of onset	Below 40 years	Above 40 years
Constitution	Usually thin & lean	Obese
Onset of disease	Sudden acute	Insidious
Symptoms	All symptoms of diabetes present	Often asymptomatic in the beginning
Tendency to ketosis	Pronounced	Much less marked
Plasma insulin	Low to absent	Normal to high
Response to insulin therapy	Insulin sensitive	Relative insulin insensitivity in the majority
Oral hypoglycamic agent	Poor response	Response good in majority of patients
Complications	Acute more. Ketoacidosis, diabetic coma	More chronic
Direct inheritance	Absent	Present in some cases

Non-insulin dependent diabetes mellitus (NIDDM, type II maturity onset diabetes). It occurs in adults generally above the age of 40 years. Such patients are mostly obese. Many a time such people are detected on a routine medical examination or when they are taking up a life insurance policy.

Onset of symptoms is usually insidious. Many patients come with complications, have little tendency to ketosis and are relatively insensitive to insulin. Plasma insulin levels are either normal or raised. In a majority both growth onset and adult diabetes may be merging into one another.

Genetic factors appear to play a major role in this form of diabetes and transmission is suggested to be due to an autosomal dominant trait. Neither HLA relationship or auto immune mechanisms have been considered. There are two main defects i.e. abnormal insulin secretion and insulin resistance to its action in target organs.

Many obese or overweight diabetics secrete large quantities of insulin but this insulin is ineffective at cellular level. There are insulin receptors on the cell wall and insulin attaches itself to these receptors before exerting its biochemical effect. Lack of adequate number of insulin receptors on the cell surface may be responsible for the induction of diabetes. Weight loss in such persons is known to result in increase in receptors and benefit such diabetics.

In addition to the above two classical types of diabetes there is pancreatic diabetes, J type diabetes and young ketones resistant diabetes.

Pancreatic diabetes. It is mostly seen in Kerala, Tamil nadu, Andhra Pradesh and large parts of south India. These are young patient with history suggestive of chronic relapsing pancreatitis due to protein malnutrition and pancreatic calculi. Patients who are young usually come with recurrent attacks of pain abdomen in the upper abdomen. They are wasted with sunken eyes and cyanotic hue of the lips. Bilateral painless parotid enlargment may be seen. Glucose intolerance is severe. Ketosis is common and insulin is the drug of choice.

J-type diabetes. Type of diabetes seen in Jamaica. Most such patients are grossly underweight, are resistant to ketosis and require insulin for control.

Young ketosis resistant diabetes. This type of diabetes is seen in north India. These are young diabetics who are insulin dependent. Main feature is absence of ketosis. Hyperglycaemia is usually moderate or severe. Disease generally presents acutely.

Prediabetes. It is the state in the life of a diabetic before the diagnosis is made and is called as prediabetes. It is important to recognise such a state which may not be a disease but an aberrant state of normality since control at this stage may help in further arresting the progress of disease.

Potential diabetes. It is suspected in people with a positive family history of diabetes, hereditary predisposition, presence of glycosuria during conditions of acute stress, infections, and in women who have history of repeated still births, spontaneous abortions, toxaemias of pregnancy, glycosuria during pregnancy and have given birth to big babies (weighing more than 10 lbs and above). Potential diabetics have a normal glucose tolerance curve but still have potential risk of developing diabetes.

Latent diabetes. It is form of diabetes present in a person who shows a normal glucose tolerance curve yet shows up abnormal glucose levels at some time during pregnancy, infections or during periods of acute stress.

Chemical diabetes. These are the people who have no symptoms but when subjected to glucose tolerance test, the curve is abnormal. Such cases again manifest with classical diabetes under condition of stress.

Clinical features of diabetes. These are variable and may range from undue fatigue to acute complications like diabetic coma. Diabetes should be suspected if a patient has increased hunger (polyphagia) thirst (polydypsia) and polyuria.

In addition features of generalized weakness, loss of weight, pains and aches in the body and limb, recurrent infections, such as common cold, boils and itching of genitalia are other symptoms. Many patients may come complaining of disturbed vision, requiring frequent changes in the number of glasses. Often the first manifestation of diabetes is in the form of a major complication like diabetic coma, vascular complications like myocardial infarction or cerebrovascular accident or a foot lesion.

Complications of diabetes. Almost all systems in body bear the burnt of diabetes and it is the long term complications chiefly vascular which pose a major challenge. Though to some extent early detection and adequate control of diabetes may minimise the severity of complications yet there are some complications which pursue a relentless course irrespective of the fact whether diabetes is controlled or not.

Complications of diabetes may be acute in the form of diabetic coma which is a medical emergency and requires immediate management or chronic complications which are present in majority of patients.

Vascular complications. Diabetics are six to eight times more liable to heart disease than non-diabetics. Diabetes effects blood vessels both large (macrovascular disease) and small vessels particularly the capillaries (microvascular disease or microangiopathy). Macrovascular disease in the form of premature atherosclerosis accounts for much of morbidity in maturity onset diabetes. There is characteristic thickening of the intimal layer and lipid material gets deposited in the intimal plaques. Aorta, carotids coronary arteries and vessels of the limbs are commonly involved. In microangiopathy there is thickening of basement membrane with hypertrophy and hyperplasia of the lining cells progressing to vascular occlusion.

Diabetic vascular lesions are usually found in patients with diabetes of long standing. In fact coronary heart disease is the major cause of death in diabetics after the age of 40. Ischaemic heart disease in the form of myocardial infarction, angina pectoris is very common in diabetics. Again painless myocardial infarction explained on the basis of autonomic diabetic neuropathy or involvement of coronary vessels is common in diabetics as compared to non-diabetics. Diabetic cardiomyopathy, cerebrovascular accidents and hypertension are other vascular complications.

Peripheral vascular disease. Progressive

involvement of peripheral vessels especially of lower limbs is very common and is characterised by attacks of pain brought on by exertion (intermittent claudication) and relieved by rest. Peripheral vessels are diminished and there may be cyanosis or redness of the limb in dependent position. A number of times there is associated neuropathy.

Gangrene of the foot occurs as a result of neuropathy, microangiopathy and secondary infection. Diabetic gangrene often develops as a result of minor trauma in the form of injury, ill fitting shoe, paring of corns and collosities.

Renal lesions. Diabetics are more prone to get urinary tract infections. Many times the infection may be asymptomatic. Acute pyelonephritis may have a fulminant course in diabetics while chronic pyelonephritis predisposes to chronic renal failure.

Glomeurlosclerosis may develop depending on the duration of diabetes. There is arteriosclerosis of the renal artery, sclerosis of renal arterioles and intercapillary glomerulosclerosis. Glomerulo-sclerosis is diffuse though when it is nodular it is labelled as Kimmelsteil-Wilson lesion. Diabetic nephropathy is characterised by oedema like full blown nephrotic syndrome, Hypertension, proteinuria, pyelonephritis and azotemia leading to chronic renal failure.

Uncommon renal complication in diabetics is renal papillary necrosis where there is ischaemic necrosis of renal papilla. It occurs in middle aged women and is characterised clinically by acute pain in renal area, hematuria, constitutional disturbance and rapidly progressive renal failure. Sometimes there is obstruction in ureter due to necrotic debris leading to pyonephrosis.

Neurological lesions. Involvement of nervous system in diabetics may be in form of either symmetrical sensory neuropathy or isolated peripheral nerve lesions or motor neuropathy in the form of weakness and wasting of muscles especially of the lower limbs (Amyotrophy). In addition diabetics have features of autonomic neuropathy in the form of diarrhoea, difficulty in passing urine leading to atonic bladder. Postural hypotension, disturbances

of sweating and pupillary abnormalities are other manifestations. Trophic ulcers in the foot of diabetics is of common occurrence due to sensory neuropathy.

Gastrointestinal manifestations. Common are gastric atony with stasis of the gastric contents. Gastritis (acute and chronic) diarrhoa with or without steatorrhoea, nocturnal diarrhoea, paralytic ileus, cholecystitis are other commonly seen complications.

Skin. A number of skin diseases are more seen in diabetics as compared to non-diabetics. Diabetics are more likly to suffer from pyogenic and fungal skin infections in the form of furuncles, recurrent boils, acute paronychia, intertrigo and carbuncle. In men chronic balantitis and in females chronic or acute vulvo vaginitis may be seen caused either by candida or monilial infection.

Eye in diabetes. Diabetic retinopathy is the commonest complication of diabetes and may lead to severe visual loss or even complete blindness. Development of retinopathy depends on the age of onset, duration and control of diabetes. Micro aneurysms are the earliest lesions followed by irregular segmental dilatation and tortuosity of retinal vessels, deep dot shaped haemorrhages and hard white, multiple yellowish exudates. As the disease progresses, haemorhages and exudates become numerous and coalesce to form large patches, the large subhyaloid haemorrhages occur along the vein, seriously impairing the vision. Massive vitreous haemorrhages occurring repeatedly and remaining unabsorbed for a long time leading to retinitis proliferans and retinal detachment.

In addition to retinopathy diabetics develop refractive changes and require frequent change of spectacles. Young or juvenile diabetics develop cataract in their eyes at an early age while in middle aged diabetics the development of cataract may be hastened. Patients of diabetes are more prone to suffer from eye infections especially of lids, conjunctiva and cornea. Glaucoma, optic neuritis and paralysis of nerves supplying extraocular muscles and internal muscles of the eye are other complications.

Miscellaneous. The incidence of pulmonary tuberculosis, pneumonia and bronchopneumonia in diabetics is high. In addition infections of the skin (bacterial and fungal) foot (neuropathy, delayed wound healing, trophic ulcers, gangrene) recurrent urinary tract infections, osteoporosis, neuropathic joints, pyorrhoea (poor orodental hygiene), impotence in men. Repeated abortions, miscarriage, still births and big babies are more common in women. Diabetics have dental sepsis, stomatitis, halitosis, loosening of teeth and have poor fitting of dentures.

Acute complications. These include diabetic coma with ketoacidosis and non-ketotic hyperosmolar coma.

Diagnosis. Diagnosis of diabetes in a well developed case with classical features is not difficult. An unexplained loss of weight, asthenia and increased frequency of micturition in a middle age person should make one suspect the disease. Confirmation is to be done by further investigations.

Urine examination. It is a simple screening test but since urinary glucose does not always directly reflect the blood glucose levels so the examination is not the sole criteria for making diagnosis.

Renal glycosuria may be present during pregnancy, and when patient is on drugs like ascorbic acid, salicylates and penicillin. It depends on renal threshold for glucose (normal 180 mg/dl) and is positive when the excretion exceeds the threshold levels. In addition to urine examination for glucose it is important to assess proteins and ketone bodies in urine.

Blood sugar estimation. Both fasting and post-prandial (2 hours after a meal) levels of blood sugar be estimated. Mean values of blod sugar in healthy adults is 70 to 80 mg per cent. When fasting blood sugar levels exceeds 110 mg% the diagnosis is certain. Two hours post prandial blood sugar levels is a further screening test and if value exceeds 120 mg per cent it is strongly suggestive.

Random blood sugar estimations may not be very helpful as a screening test. Value exceeding 160 mg per cent in the presence of glycosuria is suggestive while values above 200 mg per cent is diagnostic.

Glucose tolerance test. In a case where both fasting and postprandial blood sugar levels are diagnostic, glucose tolerance test is not required but where blood glucose levels are borderline orwhere there is glycosuria in the presence of normal blood sugar levels glucose tolerance test is indicated. Procedure involves that the patient to be tested must be on his/her usual diet, exercise and routine for at least three days prior to the test.

Test is carried in the morning when patient has fasted for 8-12 hours. Fasting blod sample is collected, 75 gms of anhydrous glucose in adults and 1.75 gm per Kg of body weight in children dissolved in water is given orally. Blood samples are collected half hourly for next two hours.

Care must be taken while interpreting the test that patient is afebrile, taking proper rest, not smoking and is not on drugs like corticosteroids, thiazides and oral contraceptives.

A fasting value of over 100 mg per cent, one hour value over 160 mg per cent and two hour value of over 120 mg per cent are indicative of diabetes. When the fasting and two hours values are normal but the peak value is high, it is a lag storage curve and requires further investigation.

In patients with equivocal results, patient is to be kept under observation and test repeated after three months. The patient in the mean time is neither on any drugs or dietary control.

Glucose tolerance test may be abnormal in conditions other than diabetes like liver diseases (cirrhosis) chronic renal failure, starvation, myocardial infarction and all other endocrinal conditions (thyrotoxicosis acromegaly) producing secondary diabetes.

Cortisone primed glucose tolerance test. When there is strong suspicion of diabetes and repeat G.T.T. curve is equivocal, cortisone primed test is carrieid out. Here prednisolone in a dose of 0.4 mg/kg body weight in two equal doses is given a day prior and on the day of test. Rest procedure for G.T.T. is followed as such. Cortisone, primed G.T.T. may help in unmasking diabetes in cases with prediabetic or latent state.

Management of diabetes. The main aims to be achieved while treating diabetes are:

1. To relieve the individual from his/her symptoms of disease and to control the blood sugar levels to normality.
2. To make life as normal as possible so that the person's vigour and vitality is restored.
3. To prevent further progress of the disease and to safeguard against various complications.
4. To educate the person suffering from diabetes about various principles of diet, general cleanliness, body care and drug control.

The management of diabetes can be discussed under three main heading:

a. General measures
b. Dietetic
c. Drug therapy

Complications of diabetes mellitus

Acute complications
1. Diabetic coma
2. Non-ketotic hyperosmolar coma
3. Skin infections (boils), urinary tract infections and pulmonary infections.

Chronic complications
1. *Vascular.* Ischaemic heart disease, hypertension, cerebrovascular disorders, peripheral vascular disease, gangrene.
2. *Renal.* Chronic pyelonphritis, recurrent urinary tract infections, K.W. syndrome, papillitis necroticans, renal failure.
3. *Neurological.* Sensory and motor neuropathy, amyotrophy, autonomic neuropathy.
4. *Gastrointestinal system.* Dental sepsis, pyorrhoea, gastric distension, diarrhoea with or without steatorrhoea, cholecystitis.
5. *Skin.* Boils, trophic ulcer of the feet, genital infection, pruritis vulvae.
6. *Eye.* Retinopathy, changes in refraction requring frequent change in glasses, cataract, glaucoma, eye infections (iritis, iridocyclitis).
7. *Respiratory.* Pulmonary tuberculosis, bronchopneumonia, pneumonia.
8. *Bones and joints.* Osteoporosis, neuropathic joint.
9. *Genitourinary system.* Impotence in men, repeated abortions, miscarriage, stillbirths and big babies in women, hydramnios, toxaemia of pregnancy, intrauterine foetal death, prematurity, congenital anomalies and respiratory distress syndrome.

General measures. A diabetic individual must understand that having diabetes is no longer. Much of a disadvantage and with adequate precautions life expectancy is not shortened. Foremost principle for a diabetic is to ensure a regulated life consisting of general hygienic measures, adequate rest, relaxation and proper amount of physical activity.

Regular exercise helps to normalise glycemic control by increasing insulin sensitivity of the tissues to insulin and thus resultant utilization of glucose. Exercise in addition has beneficial effect on lipid metabolism, cardiovascular system, weight control as well as physical and psychological well being of the individual. A regular exercise programme tailor made for every individual depending on age and physical fitness of the person should be undertaken.

It is preferable to have exercises which do not put strain on the cardiovascular system. Walking would appear to be the most appropriate and safe exercise. Strenuous exercises have to be avoided. Excercise during periods of poor metabolic control (blood glucose more than 250 mg and or ketones) should be avoided. There is risk of developing hypoglycaemia and myocardial ischaemia if very vigorous physical activity is indulged in. Regularity in exercise programme is essential for its benefit.

Obesity or overweight must be controlled. Obese diabetics are more likely to suffer from complications. There is increased lipid oxidation in obesity which interferes with glucose oxidation producing insulin resistance and deposits resulting in an increased blood glucose level. There is no obesity without increased nutritional supply and over eating so diabetics have to lose weight. Weight loss shall result in increased insulin sensitivity, increased peripheral utilization of glucose and decrease in blood lipid levels.

A diabetic must avoid infections and even minor colds, cuts or wounds must be got treated properly. Proper cleanliness of the mouth and dental hygiene are very important since infection in the mouth may be constant source of increasing the daily requirements of insulin. This applies to those diabetics who have got pyorrhoea, infected gums and carious teeth.

Diabetics must keep the skin healthy and should always pay attention to any injury or infection. They must avoid exposure to extremes of heat and cold.

Feet must be taken care of since diabetics are more liable to injure their feet because of defective circulation and diminished sensations. Feet must be inspected daily for any break in the skin, any scalds and burn marks, injuries, corns callosities, change in colour of skin and any infection. The feet must be washed daily in lukewarm water and dried. If the feet sweat excessively then daily a mild talcum powder should be sprinkled over the feet after washing and drying.

Nails should not be cut close to the edge. Corns and callosities must be treated with care. Socks must not have a tight elastic top. Patient should be advised not to walk bare foot even at home. Feet should never be warmed over any heating pad or hot water bottle or radiator because there may be decreased sensations and one may unwillingly burn the skin of feet. Shoes must be soft, broad toed and fitting properly. Bad foot wear or too tight shoes must be avoided. Similarly a diabetic be advised not to wear tight clothes like garters etc. so that the circulation does not suffer in any way. Use of too strong or irritant antiseptics must be avoided since diabetic skin being delicate may be injured.

Patient be advised to start taking a broad spectrum antibiotic at the first sign of any foot problem.

Diet. Diet in diabetes must be judiciously planned and adjusted according to needs of the individual. This is governed by age, weight, occupation (sedentary worker or labourer) and eating habits of the individual.

In obese diabetics diet has to be restricted so that reduction in weight is achieved while in young diabetics and growing children the amount of calories must be adequate (40 calories/kg) to provide for growth and physical activity.

The daily requirements of calories must be mapped out on a time table of the patients daily menu with a full description of his/her meals as well as the type of activity the person indulges in.

Ideally a diabetic should eat three main meals with two to three snacks. Meals must be spread all over the day so that energy disribution is evenly placed irrespective of the total caloric intake.

The following caloric distribution is recommended:

1. Breakfast — 20-25%
2. Mid morning snack — 5-10%
3. Lunch — 30-35%
4. Afternoon snack evening tea — 5-10%
5. Dinner — 25-30%
6. Bed time snack — 5-10%

Roughly an obese diabetic with mild diabetes shall require 1000-1400 calories daily while young active, lean and thin diabetic shall require 2000-3000 calories daily.

Carbohydrates form major constituent of the Indian diet and should constitute around 60-70 per cent of the total calories. The carbohydrates should be in the form of complex polysacchrides (starch) and contain adequate amounts of fibre.

Rice, wheat and other cereals which form the main bulk of Indian diet are rich sources of carbohydrates and it is possible to reduce their intake drastically. The optimal amount of carbohydrates for the diabetics is debatable but the daily intake of carbohydrates must be sufficient enough to prevent ketosis. On an average 100-150 gms of carbohydrates per day are sufficient. A simple method of calculating the carbohydrate content of the diet is to allocate one tenth of the total calories to carbohydrates i.e. if a diet of 1800 calories is prescribed it should contain about 180 g of carbohydrates.

There are good and bad carbohydrates. Glycemic Index (G.I.) is a method for classifying carbohydrate foods based on their glycemic index. The index provides an indication of the rate of digestion of carbohydrate. Foods which increase the glycemic index leave the person more hungrier while low glycemic index foods are digested more slowly and so the blood sugar levels rise more slowly. In this way there is less strain on the pancreas.

Common carbohydrate foods with low G.I. are Bran, Porridge, fruit, Rye bread, baked beans. Lentils, apple, apricot, bananas, cherries, apple, juice, orange juice, Milk, Yogurt etc, while foods with moderate G.I. are Basmati rice, whole meal bread, potatoes, Melon, Pine apple squash (Diluted) and foods with high glycemic index include white bread, sweets, French fries, colas, water melon etc. While planning diet, glycemic index should not be used in isolation. Proteins have a role in making you feel full since they take longer to digest than carbohydrates. It may be desirable to take proteins in diet with main principal meals.

The requirements of proteins varies with the age and weight of the individual. On an average 1-2 g/kg body weight must be advised. But the consumption of proteins is largely determined by social and economic considerations and it may not be possible to make much changes in the eating habits of the individual. Meat, fish, milk products, eggs, legumens etc. constitute a rich source of proteins, and proteins of animal origin are always preferable. In our country, since a greater chunk of population is vegetarian on social and religious grounds, one has to make a judicious selection of foods of vegetable origin. Adequate protein intake not only maintains the proper body build but also supplies essential minerals and vitamins.

The intake of fats should be adjusted to bring the total calories to the level desired and to maintain normal body weight. Excess of fats is not desirable and on an average 25-30 g of fat per day are sufficient. Of the fats, unsaturated fats derived from vegetable sources like safflower oil, til oil, groundnut oil etc. are preferred in contrast to fats from animal sources like butter, ghee, margarine etc. One should preferably take proportionate amounts of saturated, unsaturated and polyunsaturated fats. It is misconception to feel that polyunsaturated fats are safe and can be taken freely.

In addition to the three principle constituents of food, the diet must contain adequate amounts of minerals, and vitamins. The diet must be palatable and as near the normal diet as possible. Broadly speaking, after making proper allowance for provision of adequate calories and nutrients in diet a diabetic may follow some of the principles laid down for general guidance.

One must follow strictly the prescribed diet. Nothing should be taken which is not on the diet list. Meals should not be skipped and neither one should cheat by nibbling at sweets etc in between the prescribed meals.

The golden rule for a diabetic on diet therapy should be to eat little and more often. A heavy meal is not desirable since it gives rise to rise in blood lipids.

One must time the meals, Food must have variety and monotony in diet be avoided. Foods should be adjusted in such a way that they form part of the family rations.

1. **A diabetic may be allowed in plenty.**
   a. Vegetables like cabbage, cauliflower, gourd, asparagus, cucumber, lettuce, lemon, ladyfingers, tomatoes, radishes, spinach, watercress, mushrooms, carrots, brinjals, karelas, onions etc.
   b. Tea, coffee (milk from allowance, no sugar).
   c. Tomato juice, lemon juice, soup, spices.
   d. Fruits like grape fruit, mosambi, half-ripe papaya.

2. **A diabetic may take in moderation.**
   a. Vegetables like beets, green peas, pumpkins and turnips.
   b. Fruits like oranges, apples, plums, guavas, pears, cherries etc.

3. **A diabetic must avoid.**
   a. Concentrated foods and sweets like jams, honey, chocolates, marmalade, cakes, biscuits (especially cream), pies, ice cream, fruit squash, tinned fruit in syrup, puddings, thick gravies etc.
   b. Dry fruits like dates, cashew nuts.
   c. Vegetables like potatoes, sweet potatoes.
   d. Fruits like mangoes, grapes, bananas, chekoos.

4. Fresh fruits, vegetables, fish, meat, eggs and skimmed milk should form the major bulk of a diabetic diet. It is important that vegetables are taken liberally since they will tend to

increase the bulk of food and thus try to satisfy the hunger and so reduce the intake of food.

5. Meat, fish and eggs provide rich source of first class proteins for non-vegetarians and be taken in usual quantities but for vegetarians it is essential that they take at least 20 ozs of milk every day and supplement it with curd, cheese etc. Pulses like bengal gram, and groundnuts are rich source of proteins.

6. The quantity of cereals which contain a greater amount of carbohydrates be restricted. Rice, wheat, bread and chapatis be taken in measured quantity but no prathas. Rice contains almost same amount of carbohydrates as wheat but the protein content of rice is of better quality. For people not used to taking wheat, rice be permitted though as per usual quantity and calories.

7. Alcoholic drinks are permitted in diabetics but only in limited amount. Most of the spirits like whisky, gin, rum and brandy produce enough calories in concentrated form. Alcoholic intoxication may produce marked fall in blood sugar and this may sometimes prove dangerous.

8. Sweetening agents like aspartame (equal) and saccharin are allowed in moderation and their high intake is not advisable.

Diet for patients on insulin. The traditional Indian diets with slight modifications are close to what is now considered ideal diabetic diet. When a patient is on a restricted diabetic diet and insulin, it must be ensured that the food is distributed into four principle meals instead of the usual two main meals. Proteins and fats are allowed as per requirements in adequate quantities but the carbohydrate part of the diet should be more or less equally divided throughout the day.

Aim should be to provide a diet which satisfies the patients appetite as well as keeps a control on his/her weight and waist line. In sum total diet in diabetics is so monitored as to meet his/her usual dietary habits with the exception of avoiding refined sugar, adjusting fat intake but at the same time providing adequate nutrition and calories. Diets,

which are not drastic in nature, mean increasing compliance.

Drug therapy. There are two main lines of drug therapy and both have their own indications as well as advantages.

Insulin. Approximately 40 per cent of all diabetes shall require insulin for proper control of the disease and to keep the blood sugar levels within normal limits.

Absolute indications for insulin are:

1. Insulin-dependent diabetes mellitus.
2. Diabetics with significant complications like ischaemic heart disease, CVA, peripheral artery disease, nephropathy, severe infections, injury and acute surgical problems.
3. Diabetic ketoacidosis.
4. Hyperosmolar coma.
5. Pregnant diabetic woman not controlled by diet alone.
6. Diabetics undergoing surgical procedures especially those requiring general anaesthesia.

Relative indications are:

1. Failure of oral hypoglycaemic agents.
2. Contraindications to use of oral hypoglycaemic agents.
3. Underweight diabetes.

Insulin can be either beef (Bovine) or pork (Porcine) or human and they differ in their aminoacid sequence which affects the antigenecity of the molecule. Bovine insulin has three aminoacids while pork insulin has only one which makes it less antigenic. As compared to these two, human insulin is structurally identical to the physiological insulin secreted in the human body and incidence of insulin allergy, resistance and antibody mediated complications is less, making it now more acceptable.

Mixtures of bovine and porcine insulins are also available but their use because of high immunogenicity problems has declined.

Insulin preparations are available in different strength and the commonly available strength, are 40 IU/ml and 100 IU/ml. It is preferable to use syringes corresponding to the strength of insulin.

Purity of insulin is important from the point of view of minimizing immunological problems like allergy, lipotrophy and insulin resistance. Purification of insulin with the help of sophisticated chromatographic techniques has resulted in decline of reactions such as insulin allergy, resistance and lipotrophy, so purified preparations being more effective and less antigenic are preferable.

Conventional insulins. Older conventional insulins are of beef (Bovine) origin and differ from human insulin in that their aminoacids and impurities present in them can lead to formation of antibodies leading to insulin resistance and allergic reactions. But because of economic reasons and easy availability these are widely used. Various types of beef insulin used are:

1. Soluble regular insulin. It is the insulin of choice in emergencies like diabetic coma, infections, surgical procedures and as an initial therapy as well as in those requiring large doses of insulin (more than 150 units daily).

2. Protamine zinc insulin (PZI). It is slow acting insulin with prolonged effect. Action lasts for 24-36 hours. It is mainly used in large majority of patients requiring small to moderate doses of insulin. Advantage is single injection in 24 hours and greater lattitude in timing of meals. Main drawback is chances of developing hypoglycaemia and use not indicated during acute infections.

3. NPH (Isophane) insulin. It is a mixture of regular and PZI and is used as routine in the treatment of moderate to severe diabetes. It is used as a one dose daily injection in mild and moderate diabetes. In severe form of diabetes, supplementary dose of plain insulin is added.

4. Lente insulin or insulin zinc suspension (IZS). It contains 70 per cent amorphous (quick acting) and 30 per cent crystalline (slow acting) insulin. Semilente insulin is insulin zinc suspension amorphous while ultralente insulin is IZS crystalline. Lente insulin is used in the tretment of moderate to severe diabetes and meets the needs of most diabetics. It has rapid onset with prolonged action. Single injection is to be given before breakfast. Local allergic reactions are unlikely.

Newer insulins. These are porcine and human insulins and are indicated when patients on conventional insulins manifest immune problems allergy or resistance. All patients who require large doses of conventional insulin (>80 units/day) may shift to these insulins.

Porcine insulins. These differ from human insulins in only one aminoacid and so are less immunogenic as compared to beef insulins. Moreover impurities are insignificant resulting in decrease in their immunogenicity.

Actrapid (soluble, neutral, rapid acting insulin). It is a highly purified mono component pork neutral insulin, is quick acting and useful in intensified insulin treatment, diabetic coma and in the presence of complications.

Lentard. It is a neutral suspension of porcine chromotographed insulin (30% amorphous and 70% crystalline). It is intermediate acting insulin and is particularly useful when prolonged insulin action is required.

Mixtard. It is a mixture of highly purified biphasic insulin (Porcine) containing a mixture of 30 per cent rapid acting insulin and 70 per cent intermediate acting insulin (NPH). It is indicated in cases with failure of oral hypoglycemic drugs, pregnant diabetics and in diabetics with chronic infections like tuberculosis.

Human insulins. Due to high level of purity (monocomponent purity) and structural identity with physiological insulin, human insulin are the least immunogenic.

1. **Human actrapid (soluble, neutral rapid acting insulin).** It is human monocomponent insulin and is mainly indicated in emergencies like diabetic coma, for control of diabetes during surgery and in juvenile diabetes.

2. **Human monotard lente insulin.** It is intermediate acting insulin. Zinc suspension and

Table showing various types of Insulin

Type of Insulin	Speed of action	Peak action	Duration of action
Bovine insulins:			
1. Regular soluble insulin	Quick acting Rapidly absorbed. To be administered 1/2 hour before food.	2-4 hours	6-8 hours.
2. Protamine zinc insulin (PZI)	Slower action with prolonged effect. Administered 1/2 hr. before breakfast.	8-12 hours	24-36 hours
3. Isophane (NPH)	Intermediate acting. Given 1/2 hour before breakfast	8.12 hours	18-28 hours.
4. Lente insulin	Rapid onset with prolonged action. Single injection before breakfast.	6-12 hours	24-30 hours
Porcine insulin:			
1. Actrapid (soluble, rapid acting insulin)	Quick acting. Onset half hour	1-3 hours	6-8 hours.
2. Lentard intermediate acting insulin zinc suspension.	Intermediate. Onset 2 - 2½ hours	7 - 12 hours	20-24 hours
3. Mixtard (mixture of 30% rapid acting and 70% intermediate acting insulin (NPH).	Onset half hour	2-8 hours	22-24 hours
Human insulins:			
1. Human actrapid (soluble neutral, rapid acting insulin.	Onset half hour	1-3 hours	8 hours.
2. Human monotard insulin (intermediate acting insulin zinc suspension)	Onset 2½ hours	7-15 hours	22-24 hours
3. Human insulatard (intermediate acting Isophane insulin, NPH).	Onset one and half hour	4-12 hours	24 hours
4. Human mixtard (Premixed biphasic insulin) Mixture of 30% rapid acting and intermediate 70% acting insulin, NPH.	Onset half hour Single injection before breakfast	2-8 hours	24 hours

is particularly indicated in cases of oral anti-diabetic drugs failure, chronic infections like tuberculosis complicating diabetes.

3. **Human mixtard.** It is a highly purified biphasic insulin and is a mixture of 30 per cent rapid acting and 70 per cent intermediate act-ing insulin (NPH). Its indications are the same as with human insulatard except that it is more long acting as well as of use in chronic cases as a single injection.

4. **Human insulatard.** It is intermediate acting isophane insulin, (NPH). Onset is after 1.1/2

hours and lasts for 24 hours. Indicated in oral hypoglycaemic drugs failure, pregnant diabetics and in chronic infections complicating diabetes.

Principles of Insulin treatment. Pure insulin is a dried crystalline substance. Regular soluble insulin is clear and available in liquid form to be injected either subcutaneously or intravenously but it can not be given orally since it is destroyed by the gastric secretions.

There is no fixed dosage but to start with after putting the patient on prescribed diet, soluble insulin is given half an hour before lunch and dinner in small doses (10 units). Control of diabetes is monitored by urine sugar estimation two hours after principal meals and frequent blood sugar estimation. Depending on the urine sugar content dosage of insulin is increased.

Some patients may require a third dose before breakfast. If adequate control is maintained, patient may be switched on to a single injection of long acting insulin (mixtard/human mixtard), after finding out the total daily requirements of insulin. If the requirements of insulin per day exceed 200 units then mixture of long acting insulins are not desirable. Dosage of human insulin is to be 10 per cent less than that of porcine or bovine insulins. No fixed rules can be laid regarding dosage of insulin.

It is individualised and has to be followed by trial and error.

Insulin should always be stored in a referigerator. Diabetics especially young diabetics must take it regularly. Proper syringes must be used for injections. Insulin is also available in prefilled syringes. It is a slim, compact all in one unit and little larger than ordinary pen. It is used as a small disposable prefilled insulin cartridge (penfill). Advantage is that it completely eliminates the need for handling syringes and vials and results in increased compliance.

Patient must be taught about proper sterilization of the syringes and needles and also about taking the injection himself/herself. Common sites for injection are anterior abdominal wall or thighs and site of injection should be changed regularly.

Complications of insulin therapy:

1. Insulin lipoatrophy at the site of injections. Sometimes painful reddened lesions may be seen.

2. Allergic reaction to insulin. A change from one form of insulin to the other may solve the problem.

3. Insulin resistance due to formation of antibodies which act against the insulin receptors. Sometimes there are insulin antagonists which make peripheral tissue unresponsive despite the fact that large amounts of insulin are available. Requirements of insulin of such patients exceed 200 units or more per day. Often impurities in insulin cause this condition.

Hypoglycaemia. Many times when either insulin has been given in too large a dose or a meal has been missed or there is unusual exertion, fall of blood sugar occurs. The onset is acute, excessive sweating, hunger, palpitation, trembling and a sense of apprehension. If the condition is not diagnosed early patient may become unconscious going on to stupor or coma. Many patients in hypoglycaemia become confused or show an unusual behaviour. Examination shows a cold sweating skin with tachycardia and a bounding pulse.

Oral hypoglycaemic agents. *Oral antidiabetic compounds are given:*

1. In persons with maturity onset diabetes who are not controlled by diet alone and who are without any major complication.

2. Patients without any history of diabetic coma or severe ketosis.

3. People over the age of 40 whose insulin requirements are not much (40-80 units/day), the use of oral antidiabetic compounds (OHA) may be desireable.

Main groups of OH agents are:

a. Sulfonylureas. These constitute first line of therapy in NIDDM and commonly available include Tolbutamide, chlorpropamide, glibenclamide, glipizide, gliclazide and glimepiride.

b. Biguanides. They are often used in combination with sulfonylureas. Commonly available biguanides are metformin and phenformin.

c. Thiazolidinedione group: These include Pioglitazone, rosiglitazone. They improve insulin resistance in patients with type 2 diabeties.

d. α-glucosidase inhibitors. These cause dose related malabsorption of carbohydrates and include Acarbose.

e. Miscellaneous group consisting of Repaglinide and Nateglinide.

Diagnosis is confirmed by blood sugar estimation where very low blood sugar levels (less than 60 mg/dl) are detected.

A diabetic must be warned about such an eventuality and he/she must always keep with him/her sugar cubes so that at the earliest sign of hypoglycaemia sugar can be taken.

Hypoglycaemia developing after short acting insulins has good prognosis but sometimes when patient is on long acting insulins, hypoglycaemia may develop at night (nocturnal hypoglycaemia) which may prove dangerous. It is better to guard against this type of eventuality either by adjusting the dose of insulin or taking a bed time snack. When hypoglycaemia is severe or the patient goes into hypoglycaemic coma, patient be given 25-50 ml of 50 per cent glucose followed by 5 per cent dextrose saline. Further management shall depend on blood glucose levels which must be constantly monitored.

SULFONYLUREAS

These are the drugs of choice in patients of NIDDM, who are obese with diabetes of recent onset and absent ketosis where there are no overt cardiac, renal or hepatic complications and blood sugar levels are less than 300 mg/dl.

Sulfonylureas primarily stimulate the release of insulin by beta cells of iselts of langerhans and inhibit neoglucogenesis and glycogenolysis by the liver and increase responsiveness of peripheral tissues to insulin.

The beneficial effects of sulfonylureas on the lipids are due to improved control of diabetes and not due to any specific action of these drugs on lipid/lipoprotein metabolism.

Commonly available sulphonylureas are:

1. Tolbutamide. Dose 500 mg either as a single dose before breakfast or twice a day morning and evening before principal meals.

2. Chlopropamide. 125-250 mg once daily after breakfast. Increase or decrease by 50-150 mg daily after 3-5 days. Total dose not to exceed 500 mg.

3. Glibenclamide. In addition to release of insulin by beta cells, it leads to enhanced calcium flux across beta cell membrane leading to degranulation of beta cells. After prolonged administration, the insulinemic action of glibenclamide declines but improvement in glucose tolerance is maintained.

   Dose. 2.5-5 mg daily as a single dose before breakfast increasing gradually. Total dose not to exceed 15 mg.

4. Gliclazide. It is a antidiabetic agent with both metabolic and vascular properties. It restores early peak of insulin secretion and ensures glycaemic control throughout 24 hours without hypoglycaemia. It also combats microthrombosis by decreasing platelet hyperadhesiveness and increasing fiibrinolytic activity.

   Dose is 80 mg daily. Total dose should not increase 320 mg.

5. Glipizide. It is a second generation sulfonylurea having similar properties as that of gliclazide or glibenclamide.

   Dose 5 mg twice a day 1/2 hour before main meals. Dose can be increased at weekly intervals to maximum of 20 mg.

A. Glimerpiride: It is second generation sulfonylurea which lowers blood sugar by stimulating insulin release from beta cells in the pancreatic tissue possibly due to increased intracellular camp.

It interacts with insulin and other oral antidiabetics, ace inhibitors, allopurinol, anabolic steroids and male sex hormones.

Dose. 1mg daily in the morning. Increase in dose is carried out stepwise at intervals of 1 to 2 weeks. Total dose should not exceed 8 mg.

Biguanides. They are completely different from sulfonylureas both in their structure and mode of action. Biguanides act by increasing peripheral utilisation of glucose due to enhancement of aerobic glycolysis. They also delay glucose absorption from the intestines and inhibit hepatic neoglucogenesis.

They do not stimulate insulin release from the pancreas and presence of either exogenous or endogenous insulin is necessary for their action. They are mainly used in combination either with sulfonylureas or insulin in which case they act synergistically. Out of the two biguanides metformin is preferred over phenformin.

Metformin. 500 mg daily. It is comparatively safe. Phenformin 25 mg and 50 mg TD capsule daily.

Biguanides do not inhibit ketogenesis in the liver and diabetics on phenformin may develop ketoacidosis with minimum hyperglycaemia. These drugs produce an unpleasant bitter or metallic taste, anorexia, nausea, and abdominal discomfort. In addition lethargy and muscular weakness may result.

Biguanides are contraindicated in patients with renal failure, severe hepatic insufficiency and diabetic ketoacidosis.

THIAZOLIDINE GROUP

ROSIGLITAZONE

Insulin resistance isa state of reduced insulin, sensitivity, an inability of insulin to lower plasma glucose levels. This drug improves insulin resistance by direct stimulation of a receptor on the nuclear surface causing an increase in the transcriptional processes for the production and translocation of GLUT-4 (glucose transporters). The drug is used in the management of Type 2 diabetes both as monotherapy or combination therapy. It has a unique beta cell sparing effect which may help to prolong the life of these cells. Dosage in adults initially is 4 mg administered either as a single dose or in two divided doses. The dose may be increased to 8 mg once daily or in two divided doses. It should be avoided in patients with liver dysfunction or alcohol abuse. It is not recommended for the treatment of Type-I diabetes or for diabetic ketroacidosis. Long term therapy effectively reduces fasting and prandial glucose levels, Hb AIC and raised insulin levels.

Side effects include weight gain, oedema and rise in total cholesterol levels.

PIOGLITAZONE

This thiazolidenedione antidiabetie agent depends on the presence of insulin for its mechanism of action. It decreases insulin resistance in the peripheray and in the liver resulting in increased insulin dependent glucose disposal and decreased hepatic glucose output.

It also is used as monotherapy and in combination with oral hypoglycemic agent (sulfonylurea, metformin) or insulin.

Patients receiving it in combination with insulin or oral hypoglycemic agents may be at risk for hypoglycemia.

Dosage is 15mg or 30 mg once daily. It can be increased to 45 mg in increments. In combination with other oral hypoglycemic agents initial dose is 15 or 30 mg. The same dose is also initiated with insulin. Side effects include Headache, Myalgia, upper respiratory tract infection, sinusitis, Pharyngitis.

α-glucosidase inhibitor (ACARBOSE). It is a pseudotetrasaccharide of microbial origin which reduces intestinal absorption of starch, dextrin and disaccharide by inhibiting the action of intestinal brush border α-glucosidase. Inhibition of enzyme slows the absorption of carbohydrate and glucose thereby reducing post prandial peaks. It has a direct effect on post prandial peaks without producing hyperinsulinemia.

It is often employed as first line therapy in NIDDM after diet has proved insufficient and also as adjuvant to existing OHA.

Dosage. 50 mg three times and it can be further increased to 100 mg three times a day.

Side effects include abdominal pain, diarrhoea and other G.I. symptoms. It interacts with sucrose and foods containing sucrose causing abdominal discomfort or diarrhoea. There is danger of going into hypoglycaemia when it is taken in combination with sulphonylureas.

Miglitol: It is an alphaglucosidase inhibitor similar in action to acarbose and used in the management of type 2 diabetes either alone or with a sulpfonylurea. Urea 25 mg three times daily with meals. Maximum dose 100 mg three times a day.

Drug is contraindicated in G.I. Motility disorders, colonic ulceration, renal insufficiency. Drug interacts with rantidine, propranolol and digestive enzymes containing carbohydrate splitting enzymes like amylase, pancreatin. Adverse reactions include abdominal pain, diarrhoea, flatulence, etc.

Voglibose. It inhibits the alpha glucosidase enzyme and thus delays the digestion and absorption of carbohydrates resulting in improvement of postprandial hyperglycemia. It is 20–30 times more potent than acarbose.

Dose. 0.2 mg given three times a day just before each meal. It the dose is not enough, the single dose may be increased upto 0.3 mg.

Drug is contraindicated in patients or diabetic coma, precoma or severe ketosis. It interacts with sulfonylureas, biguanides, beta blockers, salicylic acid etc. Side effects include abdominal distension, flatulence, diarrhoea, nause vomiting. Heartburn, jaundice and rise in enzyme levels. Drug is comparatively safe in patients with renal impairment as compared to miglitol.

Miscellaneous OHA

(a) **Repaglinide.** This is a derivative of benzoic acid and its structure is unrelated to sulponylureas. However its mechanism of action resembles sulponylureas. It stimulates insulin release by closing ATP dependant potassium in pancreatic Beta Cells. By its insulin secretagogue action, it acts by lowering post prandial blood glucose as well as fasting blood glucose.

It is rapidly absorbed from the gastro intestinal tract producing peak blood levels within one hour. Its half life is abot one hour.

Dosage: The drug may be administered varying from immediately preceding the meal to as long as 30 minutes before the meal.

Starting dose is 0.5 mg in those not previously treated with OHA. Depending on response the patient may be treated from 0.25 mg upto 4 mg preprandially until satisfactory response is achieved. Atleast one week should elapse to assess the response. The drug may be taken preprandially 2, 3, 4, time a day depending on the meal pattern. It should be used with caution in patients with hepatic insufficiency.

Side effects include mild or moderate hypoglycaemia, nausea, vomiting, arthralgia and headache. Drug may interact with ketoconazole, erythromycin. Its metabolism is inhibited by rifampacin, barbiturates.

NATEGLINIDE

It is a non sulponylurea Insulin secretagogue. It is D-pexylalanine lerivative and belongs to meglitinide class of oral hypoglycaemic agents. It acts by blocking ATP sensitive potassium channels in the pancreatic Beta cells. It produces more rapid but less sustained secretion of insulin than other drugs. Its main effect is in reducing the post prandial increase of blood sugar.

Dosage: Drug should be taken 30 minutes to one hour prior to meal in a dosage of 120 mg three times a day. It is mainly metabolized by liver and should be used cautiously in patients with hepatic insufficiency. Geriatric patients and malnourished individuals are more prone to glucose lowering effect of the drug.

Side effects include nausea, diarrhoea, dizziness, arthropathy flu like symptoms and upper respiratory tract infection. It is contraindicated in those with diabetic ketoacidosis with type I diabetes.

Oral hypoglycaemic agents are contraindicated in:

1. Insulin-dependent diabetes mellitus (IDDM)
2. Pregnancy
3. Cardiovascular complications, hepatic and renal disorders. Some of the commonly used drugs such as salicylates, coumarin group of

Oral hypoglycaemic agents

Type	Generic name	Trade name	Daily dosage	Duration of action
Sufonylurea Compounds	Tolubtamide (0.5-1.0 gm tab)	Rastinon	0.5 to 1 gm in the morning and evening before meals	6-12 hours
	Chlorpropamide (125-250 mg tablet)	Diabinese	Once a day before breakfast	25-30 hours
	(Glibenclamide (5 mg)	Euglucon/ Daonil	Single tablet at breakfast or twice a day before meals.	8-12 hours
	Gliclazide (80mg)	Diamicron	One tablet twice a day	6-12 hours
	Glipizide (5 mg)	Glynase	One tablet twice a day with meals	6-8 hours
	Glimepiride (1 mg)	Amaryl	One tablet before breakfast.	18-24 hours
Biguanides	Metformin (500 mg)	Diaphage Glyciphage	One tablet twice a day with or after meals	4-6 hours
	Phenformin (25 mg)	DBI	Twice a day after meals	4-6 hours
	Phenformin (time Disintegrationcapsule 50 mg).	DBI-TD	Once a day after meals	24 hours
THIAZOLIDINEDIONE				
	ROSIGLITAZONE	REGLIT Rezult Rogilin	4 mg singledose or in 2 divided doses	24 hours
	PIOGLITAZONE	PID-G PIOZIT PIOZONE	15-30 mg once a day	24 hours

drugs, probenecid, chloramphenicol, sulfonamides, NSAIDs and phenylbutazone may potentiate these action while some drugs such as glucocorticoids, thiazide diuretics, oral contraceptives, calcium channel blockers may interfere with their action. Presence of any infection like pulmonary tuberculosis and urinary tract infection may interfere with the action of OH agents.

Out of all oral hypoglycaemic agents, chlorpropamide can lead to prolonged hypoglycaemia for 4-5 days in some people especially the elderly. Similarly an antabuse like effect can also occur with this drug (chlorpropamide alcohol flushing syndrome (CAPF)

Special precuation should be taken about use of alcohol even in moderation in patients on oral hypoglycaemic agents.

Miscellaneous drugs:

1. Guragum granules. It is a high molecular weight hydrocolloidal polysacchride and after ingestion it forms a vicious gel in the gastrointestinal tract which slows carbohydrate absorption and thus reduces post prandial blood glucose levels. It is mainly used as an adjunct to either insulin or oral hypoglycaemic agents. Side effects include nausea, loss of appetite, diarrhoea and feeling of fullness.

   Dose is 5 g in a sachet stirred in water two times a day.

2. Indigenous drugs. A number of indigenous

Difference between diabetic and hypoglycaemic coma

	Diabetic coma	Hypoglycaemic coma
Onset	Slow, insidious	Rapid, quick
Cause	Inadequate insulin, uncontrolled	Excess of insulin, too little food
Complicating factor	diabetes, Infection, stress	None
Symptoms	Generalised weakness, loss of appetite, nausea, vomiting, abdominal pain disturbed vision	Marked hunger and weakness, sweating, palpitation.
Signs	III, skin dry, dehydrated. Pulse thready, low blood pressure, cold extremities, air, hunger, ammonical smell in breath.	Well fed person, skin wet, respiration normal. Pulse full. B.P. elevated or normal No ammonical smell.
Biochemistry Urine	Blood sugar levels high, glycosuria and acetonuria	Blood sugar levels low, Absence of glucose and acetone
Response to treatment	Slow	Quick and rapid intravenous glucose.

drugs have been found useful to some extent. The wood of Indian Kino tree has antidiabetic properties. The chips of this wood are to be soaked in a glass of water over night and the patient drinks the water the next morning. The juice of Karela (bitter gourd) taken as such is also useful in diabetes and is known to lower blood sugar levels.

Indications for oral hypoglycaemic agents

1. NIDDM
2. Persons over the age of 40 years.
3. Obese diabetic
4. Diabetes of recent onset
5. Absence of acute complications
6. No ketosis
7. Absence of serious cardiac, kidney or liver disease.

Monitoring glycaemic control:

1. Urine glucose testing. It is a simple test to monitor diabetic control since appearance of glucose in urine reflects renal threshold and is correlated with hyperglycaemia.
2. Blood sugar levels both fasting and postprandial levels at periodic intervals. It shall give information about the status of patients glycaemic control.

3. Glycosylated haemoglobin (GHb) estimation. It is an excellent test to judge overall glycaemic control over a period of 6-8 weeks prior to the test. Levels of GHb do not fluctuate within short periods though falsely elevated levels may be obtained in patients with renal failure. Hb Alc test is generally described as the gold standard of control of diabetes. During the previous two to three months levels between 6-7 percent reflect excellent control at 8 per cent good control, over 8 per cent not adequate control and over 10 per cent very poor control.

4. Besides monitoring glycaemic control, weight control, blood pressure levels, lipid abnormalities, urine for microalbuminuria should be monitored and long term complications detected at the earliest.

Insulin pumps

There is now more awareness about the use of insulin pumps in the control of glycemia in insulin dependant diabetes. Pumps help stabilize the blood glucose into a more narrow range of control. Insulin requirements can be reduced by as much as 50%.

Insulin pumps ensure better flexibility of insulin dose and even as small a dose as 0.025 units / hour can be delivered with the pump. Moroever by the use of pump fewer injections of insulin are required and more direct control over the disease is achieved.

Surgical problem in diabetes management. Management of any surgical problem with diabetes shall depend on the stage of diabetes and nature of surgery to be undertaken.

For all surgical interventions diabetes has to be kept under control with insulin. General principle is to keep patients blood sugar levels as normal as possible both in preoperative and postoperative stage. On the day of surgery patient shall be given 5 per cent dextrose or dextrose saline neutralised with 12 units of soluble insulin. This method is adopted as long as the patient is not allowed orally.

Management of diabetes during pregnancy. Pregnancy produces a stress in predisposed women resulting in appearance of diabetes. This state generally disappears after delivery but its persistence during and after delivery is called gestational diabetes.

It is essential to maintain good diabetic control throughout pregnancy as it shall result in reduced morbidity in conditions associated with pregnant diabetics in neonatal management such as neonatal hypoglycaemia, hyperbilirubinemia, hypocalcaemia. In uncontrolled diabetes there are increased risk of pre-eclamptic toxaemia, hydramnios, premature labour, spontaneous abortions, congenital anomalies, intrauterine deaths and prematurity in foetus but their incidence is less in women where diabetic control is good.

Optimal control of diabetes during the first 6-8 weeks after conception is essential to reduce the risk of congenital malformations in the foetus.

From about 20th week of pregnancy patient must be controlled by soluble insulin. Oral hypoglycaemic agents preferably are discontinued once pregnancy is detected and patient put on diet and insulin. Target blood glucose values should be 60-90 mg per cent in the fasting state and 100-120 mg% in the postprandial state.

Diabetic coma. It is an acute medical emergency and unless managed promptly may prove fatal. Diabetic coma or ketoacidosis is caused by absolute or relative severe deficiency of insulin leading to hyperglycaemia, glycosuria, presence of ketone bodies in the urine and blood and metabolic acidosis.

Causes of diabetic coma. All cases with insulin dependent diabetes when not cotrolled properly and predisposed to ketoacidosis are liable to go into diabetic coma.

Precipitating causes are:

1. Inadequate insulin dosage or abrupt withdrawal.
2. Uncontrolled diabetes
3. Acute infections
4. Surgical operations
5. Pregnancy
6. Acute medical emergencies like severe dehydration, vomiting, cerebrovascular accident.
7. Use of heavy doses of corticosteroids in uncontrolled diabetes.

Pathogenesis. Insulin deficiency leads to acclerated release of free fatty acids from tri-glycerides stored in adipose tissue. There is incomplete metabolisation of these fatty acids when they reach the liver. Under utilization of free fatty acids in the absence of insulin results in excessive production of ketone bodies. There is ketonuria, Ketonaemia and metabolic acidosis. The metabolic derangements contributing to the severity of ketosis include insulin antagonists like growth hormone and glucocorticoids which are produced in excess. Result is enhanced gluconeogenesis, lipolysis and ketogenesis in the liver. The metabolic consequences of this is fall in bicarbonate levels, abnormal shift of potassium in the extracellular compartment leading to hyperkalemia and decrease in serum magnesium levels.

Clinical features. The earliest symptom is weakness, loss of appetite, nausea and vomiting. Features of uncontrolled diabetes supervene. Slight drowsiness may appear and behaviour changes occur. Pain abdomen is often present. As clinical state worsens coma may supervene.

An established case of diabetic coma is dehydrated, drowsy with rapid thready pulse, low blood pressure, cold extremities with subnormal temperature, rapid deep sighing respiration, characteristically called "Kussmaul's breathing". There is a fruity ammonical smell in breath. Eye ball tension is low. There may be dilation of stomach or paralytic ileus leading to abdominal distension.

WHO criteria of diabetes (venous whole blood glucose mg/100 ml)			
Fasting	<100	<120	>120
2 hours	<120	120-179	>180
levels		Impaired glucose tolerance	Diabetes
	Normal		
		Repeat after putting patient on diet drugs	Treat diabetes with diet and if control required

Diagnosis of diabetic coma is suspected in any cases of diabetes who shows deterioration in general health with fatigue, vomiting and altered senorium. This is confirmed by demonstrating glucose and acetones in urine.

Blood sugar is considerably elevated. Plasma ketones are also detected by dipstick or chemical methods.

Treament. The basis of treatment are:

1. To correct dehydration and collapse.
2. To correct ketosis and hyperglycaemia.
3. To correct electrolyte imbalance and acidosis.
4. To remove or correct any precipitating cause like infection.

Correction of dehydration. Fluids and electrolytes should be given as early as possible. Normal saline is the fluid of choice and depending on the severity of the condition 4-6 litres of fluid may be given in 24 hours. Initially fluids may have to be rushed but a check be maintained on CVP so that there is no cardiac overload.

Correction of electrolyte losses. Monitor serum potassium and bicarbonate levels at two hourly intervals. Intravenous potassium is required for correction of hypokalemia. It is important to maintain potassium levels between four and five mEq/litre.

Since there is acidosis (blood pH below 7.1) sodium bicarbonate is given slowly (200-300 ml of 2.75% solution) and dose adjusted accordingly.

Gastric lavage. It is done to relieve abdominal distension and give relief from vomiting.

Insulin. Insulin is the main stay of treatment of diabetic coma. Give 50 units of soluble insulin intravenously and same dose subcutaneously. Further doses of insulin are to be given after testing urine for sugar and acetones every ½ hour. A rough guide is to give 20 units for orange colour of urine, 15 units for yellow and 10 units for deep green.

At the same time estimate blood glucose levels. Since patient is in shock subcutaneous administration of insulin is not much beneficial.

There are no fixed formulas by which insulin dose is to be calculated but depending on the acuteness of the coma, dose of insulin is adjusted. A rough formula is to calculate initial dose of insulin as one-tenth of the blood sugar level in mg/dl and half of this is to be given intravenously.

The risk of hypokalaemia with large doses of insulin and late hypoglycaemia must be watched carefully. Another method is to gives insulin in an infusion (6 units/hour) till blood glucose levels come down to 180 mg/dl. This low dose insulin infusion is often preferred since fall of blood glucose levels starts immediately. Fall of ketone levels in blood is faster.

Correction of acidosis is smooth and risk of hypokalaemia is minimal so low dose constant infusion method of insulin administration is a logical one.

General measures. The patient should be nursed and care taken of bowel, bladder and general nutrition. Attempt should be made to find out the precipitating cause and treated accordingly. As patient recovers, the necessary dosage of insulin be adjusted and patient be advised about diet, physical activity and drug regimen.

Hyperosomolar non-ketotic diabetic coma. This occurs in elderly maturity onset obese diabetics and is often precipitated by acute infections, surgical stress, diuretic therapy, burns, and administration of drugs like corticosteroids, diphenyl hydantoin and propranolol. Peritoneal dialysis in renal failure may be complicated by it.

Clinically there is dehydration, weakness, sensorium disturbances going to stupor and coma. Pathogenesis of the condition is explained on the presence of endogenous insulin which prevents lipolysis but glucose metabolism is effected since it is unable to utilize it. Result is hyperglycaemia with absent ketoacidosis. Hyperglycaemia leads to osmotic diuresis, intracellular dehydration and electrolyte deficit.

Diagnosis. It is based on:

1. Blood sugar levels exceeding 1000 mg/dl.
2. Plasma bicarbonate levels are within normal limits.
3. There is no ketonuria.
4. Marked elevation in plasma osomolarity. In severe cases the osomolarity may exceed 370 mosmol/litre (normal 280-310 mosmol/litre).
5. Clinical picture of an elderly diabetic on oral hypoglycaemic agents starts showing feature of drowsiness, seizures, ataxia and coma.

Treatment. Principles of management include correction of dehydration and any precipitating cause alongwith administration of insulin. Hypotonic fluids are administered. Half strength normal saline is the fluid of choice and about 4-6 litres may have to be given in 24 hours. Keep a watch on venous pressure.

Patients are generally insulin sensitive and very small doses of insulin are employed (10-20 units soluble insulin every 2 hours till blood sugar level falls to 180 mg/dl).

Potassium supplements be given after carefully monitoring their levels.

Prognosis. Since this complication of hyperosomolar non-ketotic coma occurs in ederly, the prognosis is not good and mortality ranges from 20-30 per cent.

Lactic acidosis. This form of complication occurs in diabetics who are on Biguanides. Patient presents with severe degree of metabolic acidosis without significant hyperglycaemia or ketosis. Treatment is by intravenous infusion of isotonic bicarbonate and withdrawl of the drug.

Diseases of the Nervous System

Nervous system consitutes a major part of the body and its correct functioning is essential for the maintenance of quality of life. A number of disorders affect the mind, cerebral cortex, cerebellum, peripheral nerves and all associated parts of central, peripheral and autonomic nervous system and it is their coordinated efforts which sustain a person. When a patient presents with any neurological disorder it is essential to take a thorough history as to when the patient was alright and how the disease started, whether it is stationary or progressive. Site and nature of neurological deficit must be found out. A detailed physical examination along with that of nervous system must be carried out to arrive at the diagnosis.

Once clinical diagnosis has been arrived at, a number of tests may be done to confirm the diagnosis. Medical science has advanced rapidly during the last few decades and we have now a number of newer techniques to arrive at the diagnosis.

INVESTIGATIONS: NEUROLOGICAL DISORDERS

Various tests in this are:

Lumbar puncture. It is one of the earliest test employed in neurological disorders. Lumbar puncture needle is introduced in the intervertebral space between second and third lumbar vertebrae and cerebrospinal fluid collected. CSF is examined for its colour, biochemical examination and cytology. Before doing lumbar puncture, fundus examination be done to look for evidence of papilloedema which indicates raised intracranial tension. Lumbar puncture is contraindicated in the presence of raised intracranial tension.

By doing lumbar puncture we not only collect CSF for examination but also measure CSF pressure by manometer, use it for diagnostic purposes, introduction of drugs in cases of meningitis and air for encephalography and radio-opaque substance for myelography. CSF is also collected by cisternal and ventricular puncture.

If proper precautions have been taken it is a safe procedure. After lumbar puncure person must rest in bed for few hours. Common side effect is headache which comes after a few hours, is throbbing in character and is often associated with nausea, vomiting and pain in the neck and back.

Normal CSF is colourless, clear. Presence of blood indicates either local trauma or subarachnoid haemorrhage especially fresh. Xanthochromia or yellowish coloration of CSF is found in cerebral haemorrhage and when pus is present in CSF in considerable amount. Turbidity when present indicates excess of polymorphonuclear cells (meningitis). A clot or cob web may form in cases of tuberculous meningitis.

Of the biochemical tests, protein content is 30-40 mg/dl and sugar 80 mg/dl. Normal CSF contains a small number of cells mostly lymphocytes (0-5/cumm).

Excess of cells in the CSF indicate meningeal irritation. In cases of meningitis, CSF is examined for bacteria by gram's staining. A culture examination of CSF is often carried out in suspected infective process for identifying the causal organism.

CSF examination has an important role in diagnosing bacterial and viral diseases but its role in cases of cerebral haemorrhage is now being taken over by CT scan because of hazards involved.

Colloidal reactions in the form of colloidal gold reaction is of value in cases of general paralysis of insane (GPI) and differentiates it from other form of neurosyphilis.

Serological reacions like wasserman reaction (W.R) are also of help in cases of neurosyphilis.

Electroencephalogram. The electrical activity of the brain is recorded by use of electrodes placed at various sites in the skull. These are usually in the order of from 5 to 50 millivolts and have a duration of from one second to 20 milliseconds. Recording is done on a 16 channel recorder for 10-30 minutes.

Various waves are recorded. The area of alpha discharge is usually limited to parieto occipital region. These waves wax and wane spontaneously and usually disappear when the patient opens his/her eyes or fixes his/her attention somewhere. Waves faster than 13 Hz and of lower amplitude are called beta waves and are recorded from frontal region while very slow waves are called delta waves and are absent in normal record. EEG is of use in cases of epilepsy, seizure, coma and space occupying lesions.

Electromyogram (EMG). This involves recording electrical activity of nerve and muscles. It involves inserting a needle in a skeletal muscle and changes produced during relaxation and physical activity are recorded either on a magnetic tape or on paper. EMG is of use in cases of muscle disorders like myopathy, motor neurone disease. In addition to conventional recording with electrodes, specialized techniques are used to record activity of single muscle fibres or of the entire motor unit.

Nerve conduction studies. These are of value in cases of neuropathies and where there is local compression of nerve. The speed of conduction in motor and sensory peripheral nerves is recorded after electrical stimulation of nerve. The whole process involves measurements of latencies for F responses (motor action potential). Sensory action potentials (H. reflexes) and blink reflexes.

Evoked potentials. These are records of electrical activity produced by groups of neurons within the eye, brain stem, spinal cord, thalamus or cerebral hemisphere and are caused by visual, auditory, tactile or other sensory stimuli. The amplitude of these potentials is recorded by EEG electrodes. Evoked potentials provide sensitive objective extension of clinical symptoms and are useful in various neurological disorders. Visual evoked potentials are useful in cases of retrobulbar neuritis, friederich's ataxia while auditory evoked potentials help in diagnosing acoustic neuroma and somato sensory evoked responses help in diagnosing sensory peripheral neuropathy, tabes dorsalis, subacute combined degeneration of cord.

Evoked response document lesions in various pathways and may be used to quantify improvement in patients therapy.

Radiological studies. X-ray skull is often done

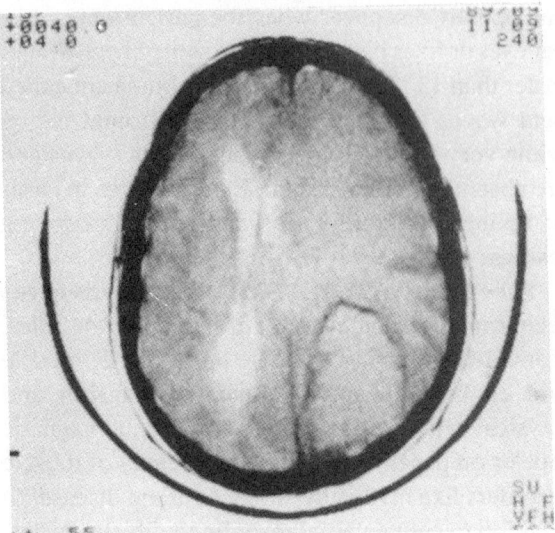

Fig. 10.1. CT Scan Head: An enhancing mass lesion is seen in right temporoparietal region with surrounding oedema. 3rd ventricle is compressed and deviated to left side. Basal cisterns, sylvian fissures and cortical sulci are affected. Right lateral ventricle is compressed. Septum shifted to left side. Space occupying lesion right temporoparietal region (Glioma/Brain abscess).

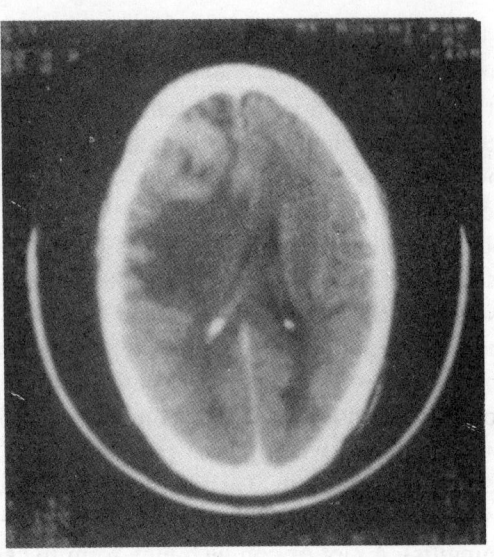

Fig. 10.2. CT Scan Head: A well defined high attenuating mass with central necrosis and significant peritumoral oedema present in the frontal region on left side. Left lateral ventricle is compressed with slight midline shift to the right side. Elsewhere brain parenchyma is normal. Impression: Space occupying lesion probably either a glioma or meningioma.

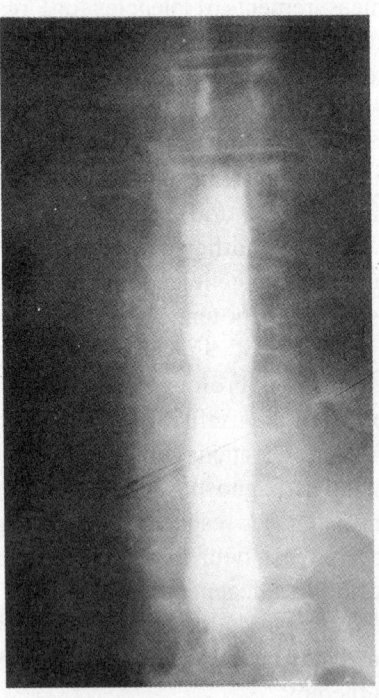

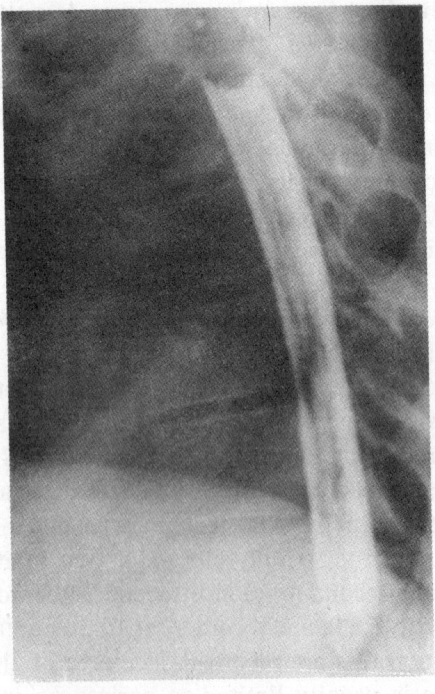

Fig. 10.3 and 10.4. Myelogram in a case of spinal tumour. Note blockage of dye in upper part.

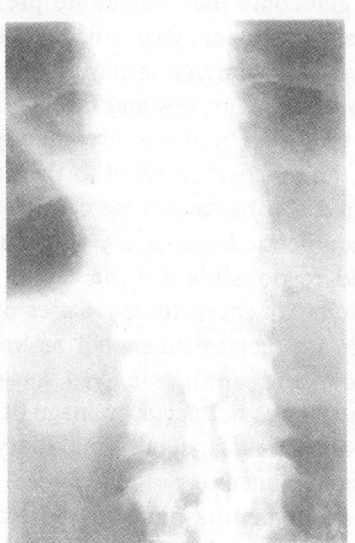

Fig. 10.5. Myelogram in a case of spinal arachnoiditis. Candle on end appearances.

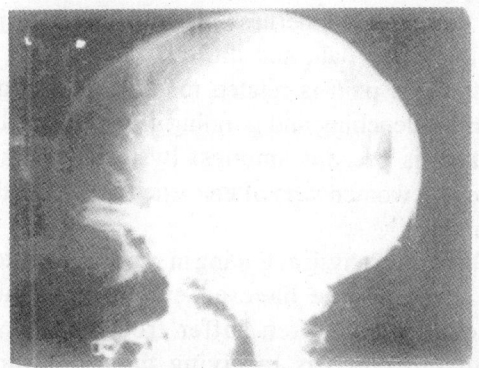

Fig. 10.6. Carotid angiogram to show course of anterior and middle cerebral arteries.

as a routine. Its main use is in detecting enlargement or destruction of sella turcica (tumours, raised intracranial tension) calcification (tubuerculoma, cysticercosis, pineal calcification) and presence of erosions (metastasis, myeloma).

Computed tomography (CT scanning). It is a very important and useful test. It is safe and does not cause much inconvenience. CT is used in the diagnosis of space occupying lesion, cerebral haemorrhage (intracerebral and subarachnoid) cerebral atrophy etc.

The image can also be enhanced by use of intravenous contrast media to delineate areas of increased blood siupply and oedema more clearly.

Main drawback to CT scan is that lesions below one cm in diameter may not be seen in the study.

Magnetic resonance imaging (MRI). MRI is useful technique by making use of the principle that all nuclei when bombarded with radio frequency waves at right angles generate images. It is useful in detecting cases of demyelinating diseases, arteriovenous malformations. Congenital and developmental anomalies, posterior fossa vascular tumours, metastasis, tuberculoma, cysticercosis and lesions which are likely to be missed by CT scanning. Its particular value is in distinguishing between white and grey matter.

Myelography. A myelogram is sometimes required to demonstrate site of spinal tumour. A radio-opaque dye (Myodil) is injected via lumbar puncture needle and conventional X-rays or CT myelogram recorded. It is also useful in cases of cervical spondylosis where an MRI may not be able to demonstrate a lesion.

Cerebral angiography. A contrast is injected either into the carotid or vertebral artery and serial films by a rapid cassette changer are taken and abnormalities in the arterial and venous vessels of the brain like cerebral artery occlusion, arterio venous fistula and aneurysm are visualised. Digital subtraction angiography (DSA) is comparatively safe procedure. Here contrast is injected intravenously while in angiography, procedure is invasive and dye has to be injected intraarterially.

Isotopic brain scanning. Isotopic imaging and flow studies of the brain are usually done in diagnosing vascular tumours, cerebral infarcts, subdural haematoma etc. These studies are more time consuming and incidence of false positive results is high.

Isotopic brain scanning has been largely replaced by CT scan and MRI.

Biopsy. Muscle and nerve biopsies are done in cases of myopathies and polyneuropathy to establish the diagnosis.

FACIAL PAIN

A number of conditions are involved in the pain localised to the face. These may range from pain arising from diseases of teeth, gums, sinuses, tempro mandibular joint to vascular causes.

Common causes of facial pain are:

1. Neuritis of the cutaneous nerves of the face and scalp.
2. Arthralgia of the temporomandibular joint.
3. Trigeminal neuralgia
4. Post-herpetic neuralgia/herpes zoster.
5. Temporal arteritis
6. Miscellaneous causes.

Facial neuritis. It is a form of inflammation of the nerve of the face and scalp. It generally occurs as a complication of a septicaemic state or due to involvement by a neurotropic virus. Onset is usually acute and pain is confined to the face and scalp, occurring in paroxysms lasting for several hours and very often till the end of the day when the patient is exhausted.

The character of pain is dull aching which is intensified by exposure to cold and often occurs in the form of shooting pains in the distribution of the nerve. Sometimes the pain is so severe that the patient is unable to sleep. Physical examination shows presence of hyperalgesia in the distribution of nerves including face and scalp. Nerve trunk is tender on pressure.

Facial neuritis has to be differentiated from number of conditions which have character of facial pain. In infection of the nasal air sinuses (frontal, maxillary and sphenoidal) pain is referred to the disribution of supraorbital and infraorbital nerves. It may be at the root of the nose (ethmoiditis) or forehead or occiput (sphenoidal sinusitis). All cases of sinusitis have a preceding history of a bad cold. Presence of sinusitis can be confirmed by transillumination and X-ray of sinuses.

Teeth are other common source of facial pain. It may be an impacted or unerrupted tooth or a carious tooth. Sometimes an acute inflammation or a growth in the pharynx may cause pain in the ear and face.

Cases of glaucoma may sometime present with referred pain to eyes and face. Uncommonly a case of acute myocardial infarction may present with pain referred to teeth, gums, jaw and face.

Cases of facial neuritis are managed with analgesics and warmth applied to the part of the face effected. At the same time careful search be made for any septic focus or any other cause being considered responsible for the facial pain and appropriate treatment instituted. Cases of sinusitis responsible for facial pain should be treated with antibiotics, and analgesics. In cases where improvement does not occur drainage of pus from the involved sinus especially maxillary sinus is undertaken by puncture.

Cases of glaucoma have to be treated with appropriate drugs while in suspected cases of myocardial infarction electrocardiogram be recorded and if found significant treatment be given on these lines.

Myofascial pain. It is a form of dull constant pain with local tenderness of the muscles of jaw. There is often pain and difficulty in opening the mouth. This pain is related to bad and improper habits of clenching and grinding of teeth. This type of habit is present amongst hysterical persons especially women who often clench and grind their teeth.

There is no physical finding in such people except that these people have an emotionally labile personality and often suffer from depression. Treatment consists in giving them assurance, analgesics and tricyclic antidepressants.

Trigeminal neuralgia. It is a disease of unknown origin seen commonly in middle and elderly individuals and is characterised by attacks of severe pain in the distribution of trigeminal nerve and its branches especially the maxillary and mandibular. Though exact cause is not known but the fact of association of disease with dental and nasal sinuses infection gives credance to the theory of infection at the nerve endings playing a role. Heredity also plays a role since disease may run in same family. Exposure to cold or trauma to the face may bring on an attack.

The paroxysm of pain which is severe and is generally of short duration generally starts with the mandibular and maxillary divisions of the 5th nerve and rarely ophthalmic division is affected. The attack usually is brought on by stimulation of specific area, the trigger zone by exposure to chill, washing, shaving and even while eating and talking. Pain is very severe and intense, putting the patient into great agony. The attacks do not last for more than one to two minute. Pain is present over face in the distribution of nerve involved and there are reflex spasms of the side of face involved (Tic douloureux).

Sometimes trigeminal neuralgia may be part of multiple sclerosis, neuroma of fifth nerve basilar artery aneurysm or cerebellopontine angle tumour. One has to keep these conditions also in mind and look for physical signs.

In cases where no cause for trigeminal neuralgia is operative and there are no physical signs present diagnosis is based mainly on the paroxysmal character of pain coming in attacks with pain free intervals and absence of any signs of organic lesion.

Treatment of trigeminal neuralgia is carbamzepine tablets, initially 100-200 mg twice a day and increasing slowly the dose to 600-800 mg per day. Diphenyl hydantoin (phenytoin) 100 mg two to three times a day is other drug employed but the first drug is better.

In cases which do not respond to medical treatment and the symptoms are severe and intractable, relief of pain can be obtained by alcohol injection of the nerve at various points or ganglion of 5th nerve. In intractable cases resection of the sensory root or its decompression behind the gasserian ganglion is helpful.

Post-herpetic neuralgia. Herpes zoster commonly involves the ophthalmic division of the 5th nerve characterised by vesicular eruption on the face and pain. When herpes heals it leave behind neuralgic pain in the distribution of previous eruptions. It is a form of continuous aching or burning pain at that site on face and patient is often in great agony.

Treatment is by analgesics. Sometimes codeine phosphate may have to be given. In some severe cases the course of post herpetic neuralgia may be prolonged one.

Migrainous neuralgia. It is often called 'Facio plegic migraine' where there are attacks of severe pain especially at night and the pain is confined to face and around one eye. This form of disease is common in men especially middle aged and the attack may be brought on after a bout of alcohol

The pain may last for hour. Because of associated vomiting and paroxysmal nature of disease it is called 'migrainous neuralgia' or 'facioplegic migraine'. There is headache and patient complains of some degree of congestion in the face. Treatment is by analgesics but response is poor.

Arthralgia of temporo mandibular joint. It may be in the form of rheumatoid arthritis or ankylosing spondylitis when there is pain and swelling of the joint. Movements at the joint are limited and patient complains of pain at the site as well as along the jaw confined to face. Involvement of other joints in the body shall favour the diagnosis. Treatment is by heat and antiinflammatory drugs as well as by excercises of the joint involved with adequate periods of rest.

Temporal arteritis. It is a form of collagen disorder of unknown aetiology which involves mainly the arteries. It commonly occurs in elderly age group.

Patient may complain of pain on the face, jaw, mouth and tongue in the distribution of branches of external carotid artery. This pain worsens off on eating and opening of the mouth.

Since temporal arteritis is a collagen disorder there is a form of inflammation of the arteries. Generalized limb pains along with malaise and weight loss is often present. The arteries involved are thickened and palpable. Diagnosis is confirmed by biopsy of the temporal artery. Treatment is by high doses of steroids (prednisolone 60-100 mg per day) which may have to be continued for sometime.

Miscellaneous causes. These include intracranial causes of pain in the face and head. These include lesions of trigeminal nerve in brain stem, syringobulbia and thrombosis of post inferior cerebellar artery. Tabes dorsalis is another cause of pain coming in attacks over the face. This is not of common occurrence and can only be recognised if the condition is kept in mind. Diagnosis of tabes shall depend on establishing involvement of posterior nerve roots, sensory ataxia and diminution and loss of tendon reflexes.

Hysterical pain on face is quite common in women. The pain in such cases is atypical, does not fit into any pattern and there is no relation to any nerve trunk or nerve roots. Very often on sustained equiry an emotional factor underlying the condition may be available. Many patients with this type of malady do not respond to analgesics.

Facial palsy may sometimes present with facial pain especially if the cause is either a trauma or inflammation. Patient here has signs of facial nerve paralysis and it is not difficult to arrive at a diagnosis.

Prognosis. In most cases where the underlying cause is treatable and is responsible for facial pain prognosis is good.

FACIAL PALSY

Facial nerve or seventh cranial nerve is largely a motor nerve supplying muscles of face. It arises from its nucleus located in the pons. The nerve follows a long course within the skull and leaves it through the stylomastoid foramen. While passing through the facial canal, it gives off a nerve to the stapedius muscle and chorda tympani. In its course a small number of sensory fibres going to external auditory meatus carry fibres which excite salivary secretions as well as convey taste impulses from the anterior two thirds of tongue.

Facial palsy may result due to:

1. A supranuclear lesion involving the pyramidal fibres Upper motor neurone (UMN).
2. Infranuclear or nuclear lesion involving lower motor neurone.

Upper motor neurone lesion (UMN). Commonest cause is internal capsule lesion due to cerebral thrombosis or infarction. Characteristically the lower half of face is involved more severely than the upper half. This is because the nuclear centre which controls the movements of the upper half of the face has both ipsilateral and contralateral connections. Thus upper part of face has got bilateral nerve supply.

Patient is able to raise furrows on forehead, close his eyes though lower half of face is involved. Emotional movements such as laughing, smiling are preserved, since these are not dependent on the same supranuclear pathway from the pyramidal tract as voluntary movements.

Lesions in the region of cortical or subcortical produce paralysis of lower part of face on opposite side. This is because of association of facial neurones with pyramidal tracts as they pass through the internal capsule, cerebral peduncle or pons above the level of facial nucleus.

Lower motor neurone (LMN). It may be nuclear or infranuclear type. The facial nerve neurones may be involved within the pons, in the posterior fossa (cerebellopontine angle)within the temporal bone and after leaving the skull. The lesion is lower motor neurone type and the whole half of face on the involved side is paralysed. The clinical features in each group shall vary per the site of lesion.

1. **Pontine lesion.** Massive lesions at this site involve adjacent structure especially 6th nerve resulting in paralysis of external rectus muscle. If there is involvement of spinal tracts, nucleus of trigeminal nerve and of spinothalamic tracts there is sensory loss along with pyramidal lesion of the limbs on opposite side.

    Causes include syringobulbia. Tumours (glioma) vascular lesios, polio, infective polyneuritis and disseminated sclerosis.

2. **Cerebellopontine angle.** Because of proximity of facial nerve at this place to 5th, 6th and 8th cranial nerves, the lesion involves all three. There is facial paralysis, deafness and loss of taste in anterior two thirds of tongue. Causes include cerebellopontine angle tumour, acoustic neuroma and syphilitic meningitis.

3. **Within the temporal bone involvement of facial nerve** is due to fracture of skull,

PLATE XVII

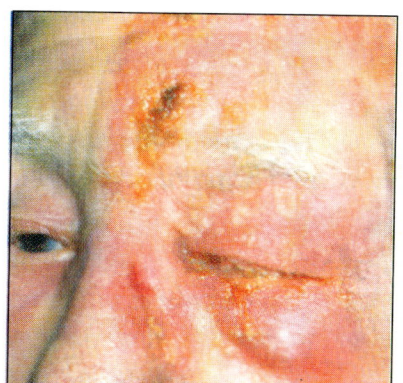

Herpes zoster

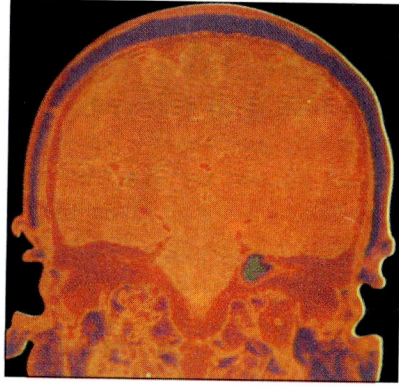

MRI showing acoustic neuroma (green)

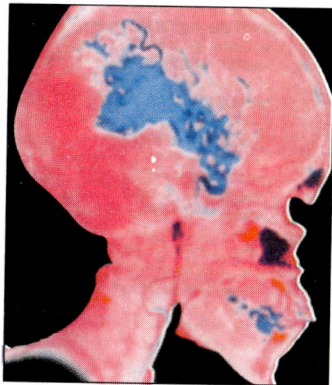

MRI scan showing arteriovenous malformation

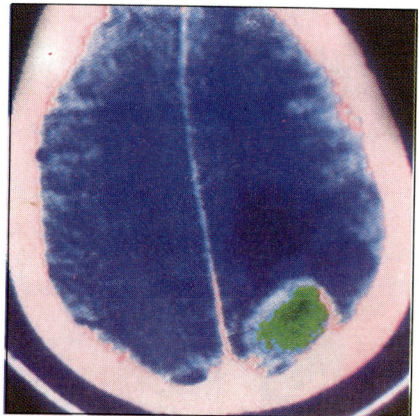

Cerebellar abscess

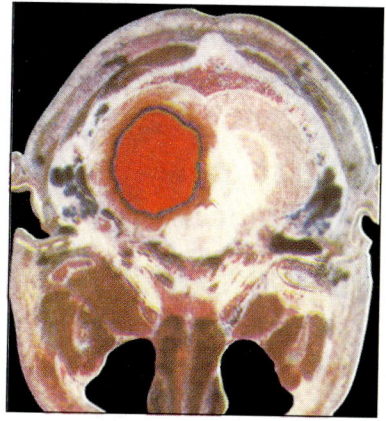

Cerebellar haemorrhage

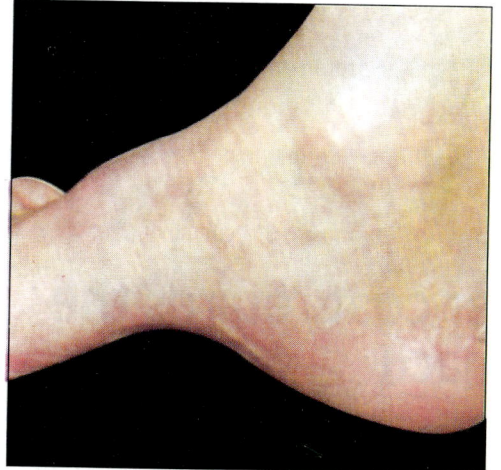

Pes cavus

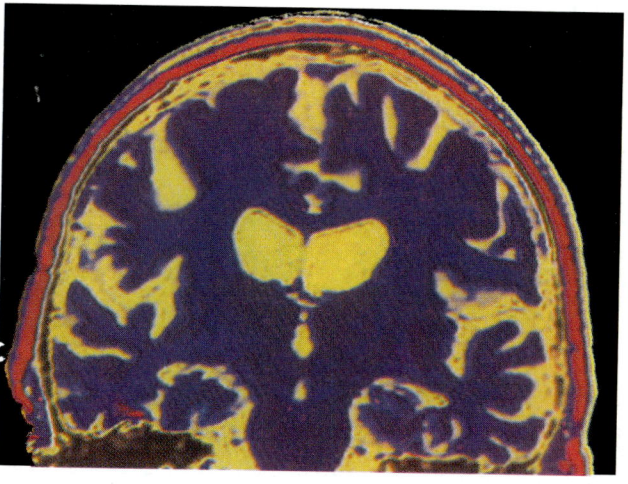

Alzheimer's disease. Brain tissue (blue) shrinks and ventricles dilate

PLATE XVIII

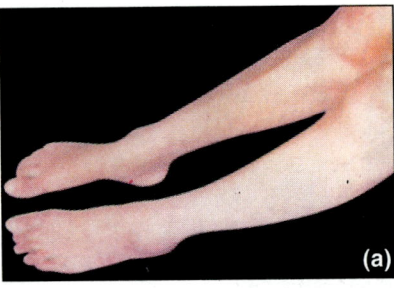 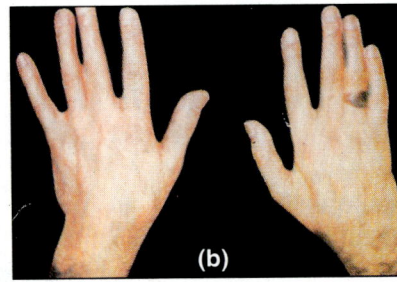 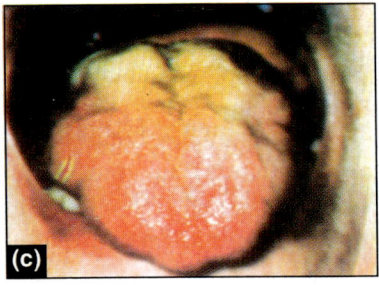

Motor neurone disease: (a) Bilateral foot drop with anterior tibial wasting; (b) Interosseus muscle wasting is an early sign; (c) Bilateral wasting of tongue

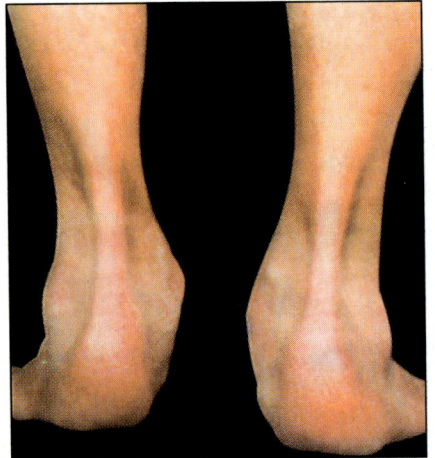 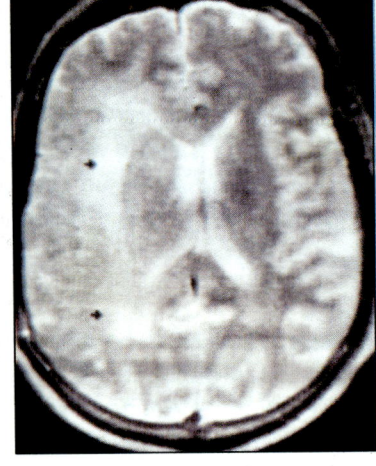 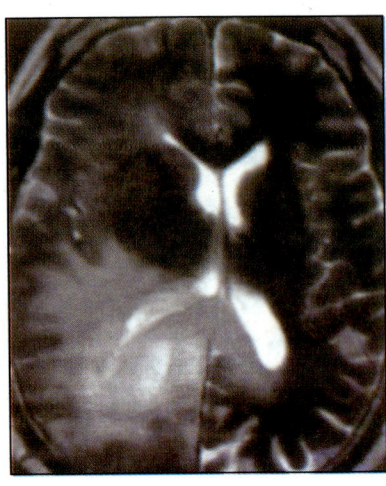

Limb muscle atrophy leading to severe disability

CT scan showing a diffuse glioma

CT scan showing S.O.L.

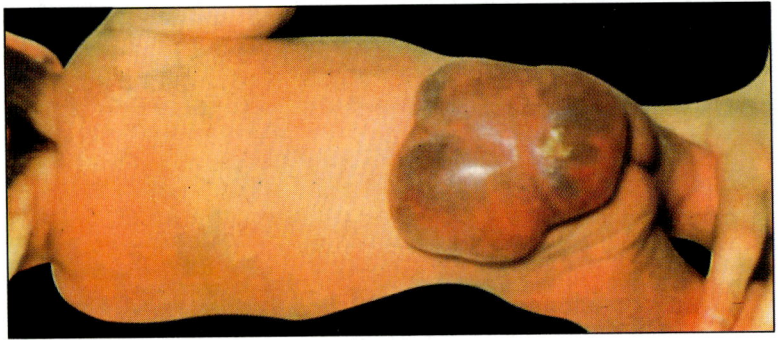 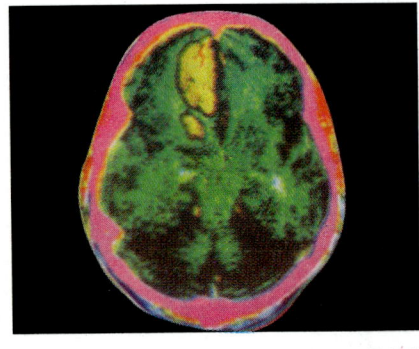

Spina bifida

CT scan: subarachnoid haemorrhage (SAH)

infections of the middle ear and mastoid. Because of proximity of the nerve to temporal bone, middle ear infections, suppuration of temporal bone and mastoiditis involve it as a result of direct spread to nerve.

Facial paralaysis caused by a lesion within the middle ear is associated with loss of taste in the anterior two thirds of tongue and when the nerve is involved in the facial canal between branching of nerve to stapedius and ganglion of facial nerve, in addition to facial paralysis, loss of taste in anterior two thirds of tongue, impairment of salivary secretions and hyperacusis occurs.

Ramsay hunt syndrome is another entity when herpes zoster involves the geniculate ganglion causing facial paralysis through secondary involvement of the motor fibres of the nerve and deafness due to herpetic involvement in the external auditory meatus. Involvement of facial nerve within the stylomastoid foramen occurring generally as a result of exposure to cold or idiopathie produces facial paralysis known as Bell's palsy.

After leaving the skull the nerve may be involved by inflammation from glands behind the angle of jaw, parotid gland tumours, trauma, surgical operations, polyneuritis and sarcoidosis.

Bell's palsy. It is a common manifestation of isolated facial nerve involvement and is quite frequently seen. It may occur at any age. It comes acutely and is considered to be due to acute inflammation of the nerve probably due to viral aetiology. The involvement of nerve occurs in its course within the stylomastoid foramen. Other causes include interstitial neuritis, middle ear disease and periostitis of temporal bone. The nerve is swollen, oedematous resulting in compression of nerve fibres. In a great majority of cases no predisposing cause is seen and often the lesion is ascribed as 'exposure to cold'.

Symptoms. There is unilateral involvement of face on the paralysed side. Often the onset is acute. There may be pain behind the ear, in the mastoid region or around the angle of jaw.

Both upper and lower half of face are equally effected. Patient is unable to raise furrows on forehead, frowning is not possible. Palpebral fissure is widened and patient is unable to close eye on paralysed side. Eversion of lower eye lid, leads to impairment of absorption of tears which overflow. Nasolabial fold is flattened and the mouth is drawn to opposite normal side. Patient is unable to blow his cheeks or whistle. Since mouth is displaced, tongue is deviated to the normal side. There is inability to show teeth. Food may accumulate between teeth and cheeks. When the involvement of nerve is at the point when chorda tympani leaves it there is loss of taste on the anterior two thirds of tongue and when branch to stapedius is involved there is hyperacusis (increased acuity of hearing with undue sensitivity to low tones).

Diagnosis of bell's palsy is made on clinical grounds especially when it is isolated facial nerve involvement and there is no evidence of any other cranial nerve involvement. Onset is acute and generally comes in an apparently healthy individual.

Treatment:

1. Since the eyes are exposed because of eversion of lower eye lid there is danger of developing exposure keratitis. Patient must wear dark glasses to protect the eyes from damage. An antibiotic eye cream may be used two times a day.

2. Steroids (prednisolone 60 mg/day in divided doses) along with course of amoxycillin (250 mg 8 hourly) are started at the earliest. Their use is indicated to reduce oedema round about the nerve.

3. Heavy doses of vitamin B_{12} (1000 ugm per day I/M) have non-specific role but have been found beneficial.

Electrophysiological tests are of help in predicting the outcome. Galvanic current is used to stimulate the facial muscles. As soon as some power returns patient is encouraged to practice closing his eyes as well as retracting the angle of the mouth by gentle finger massage three to four times a day. If no recovoery takes place within 6 to eight weeks, cosmetic surgery including renervation of nerve may be considered. In cases where bell's palsy is due to middle ear disease treatment should be directed towards it but when it has followed an operation in that region or trauma or surgery, recovery is poor.

Course and prognosis. Most cases of bell's palsy recover though complete recovery may not take place and the person is left with residual facial paralysis. Certain sequlae may develop in a number of cases where recovery is not complete. *These include:*

1. Crocodile tears: Because of eversion of lower eye lid patient is shedding tears constantly.
2. Contracture on the side of facial palsy in paralysed muscles, and this is evident when patient smiles.
3. Facial tics
4. Clonic facial spasm.

HEADACHE

One of the commonest problem seen in clinical practice is headache which very often is trivial and benign in nature but there may be some cases where headache is a symptom complex of more serious ailments.

History in a case of headache

1. When did the attack occur?
2. Are there any prodromal symptoms?
3. Is there any aura?
4. What is the site of headache (unilateral, bilateral, frontal, occipital, temporal)?
5. Character of headache (throbbing, dull, band-like pressure).
6. What is the duration of headache?
7. Frequency of attacks of headache.
8. Associated symptoms like nausea, vomiting, photophobia.
9. Relation of headache to posture.

Pain in the head may arise from tissues or structures covering the head or from diseases of the structures inside the skull. It may be classified into primary headache syndrome and headache due to secondary causes such as meningeal irritaiton, vascular causes, intracranial tumours and raised intracranial tension.

Primary headache syndromes:

1. **Neuralgic headache.** Pain in the head may be due to neuralgia of sensory nerves supplying the scalp or the face. The pain in such cases is paroxysmal varying in intensity and is in the distribution of the nerve effected. This group includes cases of trigeminal neuralgia, post herpetic neuralgia and neuritis of nerves supplying the scalp. Quite often ill fitting dentures or infection of carious teeth may cause severe headache. Other causes shall include arthralgia of temporomandibular joint and temporal arteritis.

2. **Migraine.** It is the commonest form of primary headache and generally begins before the age of 40, women being effected more as compared to men.

A classical case of migraine has premonitory symptoms or aura in the form of lethargy, hyperactivity, food craving, constipation and depression lasting for varying period from several hours to a day. The onset may occur during the day and aura is followed by throbbing headache confined to one half of the head (hemicrania) accompanied by photophobia nausea and vomiting. In somce cases aura is not present. In milder forms of migraine vomiting may relieve the symptoms. Very often sleep relieves the symptoms. In severe cases the attack may persist for days.

Above is the classical example of a common form of migraine but there are other forms of migraine. After an attack patient may have urge to go to sleep.

a. *Ophthalmoplegic migraine.* It occurs in younger patients and in addition to attacks of headache there is unilateral third nerve palsy associated with ptosis, dilated pupil and diplopia. The palsy gradually disappears over a period of days and weeks and is replaced by headache.

b. *Facioplegic migraine.* Here migraine pain is restricted to nose, cheek, gums and teeth on one side of face. There is transient facial palsy. As in a typical attack of migraine, nausea, vomiting and photophobia are present.

c. *Retinal migraine.* There is sudden transient monocular blindness followed by retro-orbital headache. It is a rare variant of migraine.

Diagnosis of migraine can be made by classical history of throbbing headache. Photophobia, nausea and vomiting. Patient usually is a female in the age of 20 to 30 years. Family history of migraine is often present. An attack may be precipitated by bright light, fatigue, hypoglycaemia, stress, fatty foods, alcohol, allergy and in females who are on oral contraceptive pills and during menstruation. Attacks come at periodic intervals, usually two to five times per month and patient likes to rest in a dark room undisturbed.

Diagnostic features of migraine

1. Headache preceded by an aura which may last upto 30-60 minutes.
2. Aura may be visual, motor or sensory.
3. Headache varies from moderate to severe. It is unilateral and throbbing.
4. Headache aggravated by normal activity.
5. Headache associated with nausea and vomiting as well as photophobia.

Physical signs are not present. Electroencephalograms recorded in between the attacks are normal.

Treatment of a case of migraine can be:

1. General measures
2. During the acute attack
3. Prevention of attacks

In the first category patient should be assured about the benign nature of the condition and advised to take precautions against factors which may precipitate an attack.

During the acute attack which is not severe Tablet Paracetmol and Prochlorperazine (Stemetil) 5 mg twice daily are efffective. In addition Metoclopramide either by injection or tablet is given if patient is vomiting. Ergotamine preparations are also useful in relieving the attacks. They may be given in form of ergotamine tartrate (1-2 mg daily) or

360 mg by aerosol or 0.25-05 mg by injection. Ergot preparations are contraindicated during pregnancy and in patients with hypertension, ischaemic heart disease and peripheral vascular disorders.

Sumatriptan is another effective drug during the acute attack. It is mainly indicated in severe form of migraine. It is a specific and selective 5HT-1-like receptor agonist. Dose 50 mg tablet twice a day or 6 mg by injection. The drug not only relieves headache but also other symptoms such as nausea and photophobia. The drug is contraindicated in elderly patients, hypertensives and those with ischaemic heart disease.

For prevention of attacks of migraine number of drugs are employed. These drugs definately decrease the frequency of attacks.

Tablet Propranolol 10 mg three times daily to start with. Dose can be increased to 40-60 mg three times a day. Monitor the heart rate for bradycardia.

Flunarizine is a calcium channel antagonist and has anti-migraine effect. Dose 10 mg at night. Side effects include drowsiness, weight gain, depression, dry mouth, gastric pain and extrapyramidal signs. Drug is contraindicated during pregnancy and lactation. Either of the above two drugs is given for a period ranging from 3-6 months.

Cluster headache. It is also called horton headache and histamine cephalalgia. It is severe form of migrainous type of headache and is characterised by intense unilateral non-throbbing periorbital pain, conjunctival injection, lacrimation, nasal congestion, rhinorrhea, miosis, ptosis, flushing sweating and oedema of face. Cluster headache is rare in women and mainly involves men in the age group of 20-40 years. An attack usually lasts for one to two hours and attacks occur in the form of cluster over weeks or months with remissions lasting from months to years. Attacks are often precipitated by stress, over work, emotional disturbances, smoking alcohol and nitroglycerine. Treatment of cluster headaches is like that of migraine. Antihistaminics are also useful in some cases.

Tension headache. It is again a common form of headache and is brought about by any type of stress. It occurs at any age and headache involves the whole head with pain which is either pressing or band like tightness. There are no prodromal symptoms. Often there is anorexia, lack of sleep, depression, anxiety and restlessness. Factor of tension or stress is operative. Headache may last for days. Duration of pain is variable. Treatment is by analgesics and antianxiety drugs (Alprazolam 0.25 mg twice a day).

Diagnostic features of tension headache

1. Bilateral headache often frontal, occipital and across neck and soulders.
2. Pain is like a pressure or band like.
3. Headache is mild to moderate.
4. Patient is able to do normal functions.
5. No associated symptoms as in migraine.
6. Headache may be worsened by some physical activities.
7. Headache may last for days.

Secondary headache. As compared to primary forms of headache, there is always some organic disease responsible for causing headache. Among the important causes of secondary headache are head trauma, disorders of cranio facial structures, cerebrovascular defects. Intracranial tumours, meningeal irritation (meningitis) raised intracranial tension, encephalitis, metabolic disorders (hypoxia, hypoglycaemia) substance exposure or abuse, and withdrawl of certain drugs (alcohol, nitrates, ergotomine).

Disoders of craniofacial structures. These include disease of cranial bones in the form of osteits. Patient has got a boring or burning type of headache along with local tenderness. Sinus headache causes a sense of congested feeling in the sinuses and heaviness in the head which resembles tension type headache. Sinus headache is worsened by bending forward. Often there is history of allergy and nasal discharge available.

Temporomandibular joint dysfunction is also associated with tension type headache. There is limitation of movements of jaw and jaw clicking or locking may be present.

Trigeminal neuralgia also produces a stabbing type of pain and headache evoked by trivial stimuli on the face. Nausea and vomiting are absent but the attack may occur several times during the day and the duration of attack is only for seconds to minutes.

Abnormalities in CSF pressure. A dull throbbing headache follows lumbar puncture. It is worsened on standing up but is relieved by lying down. This headache may last for few days.

Benign intracranial hypertension (Pseudotumor cerebri) is associated with headache which is mild to start with. It is generally bitemporal or occipital and is intensified by coughing and straining. It generally occurs in young women and subsides gradually. Nausea and vomiting accompanies headache. Because of raised CSF pressure there may be papilloedema.

Head trauma. Headache is always present following head trauma. A post concussion headache is accompanied by dizziness, blurred vision and anxiety. This type of syndrome may develop even following minor trauma. Patients with head injury have persistent headache which may last for months and these headaches are worsened by neck movement and change of posture.

Referred headache. Disorders of the structures of the face, and neck like glaucoma, iritis middle ear disease, tongue spondylosis and injury to neck produce sometimes a severe headache often unbearable in nature.

Vascular headache. Throbbing or bursting headache may be present in cases of hypertension. Cases of intracranial aneurysm produce severe headache often unbearable before rupture. An abrupt rise in blood pressure as in hypertensive encephalopathy, phaeochromocytoma produces a pounding headache accompanied by nausea, tachycardia, pallor and profuse sweating.

Subarachnoid haemorrhage produces sudden severe generalized pain of thunder clap headache. Cases of cerebral thrombosis may have headache before developing hemiplegia. Temporal arteritis is characterized by a throbbing or burning sensation accompanied with headache involving one or both temporal region along with anorexia, malaise fatigue and night sweats.

Meningeal irritation. It is an important cause of severe headache. The pain is severe, throbbing and is usually associated with neck rigidity. Causes include bacterial meningitis, viral encephalitis and fungal infections of the brain and spinal meningitis. Headache is accompanied by photophobia nausea and vomiting. Fever is invariably present along with features of toxaemia.

Miscellaneous causes. This group includes cases of intracranial tumours, brain abscess, hydrocephalus, metabolic disorders, uraemia, hypoxia, alcohol over indulgence, following general anaesthesia and abuse of various drugs.

Diagnosing headache. Once a patients present with persistent headache of some duration or headache coming in attacks, a detailed history about its duration, character of headache (location, severity and frequency) and any factor which may trigger the attack. Family history, psychological background are other important point.

In primary form enquire about accompanying symptoms like nausea and vomiting and as to what worsens the headache. First try to distinguish whether one is dealing with a primary or secondary form of headache. History in the group shall be different like trauma, infection and worsening of symptoms. Cases of space occupying lesions or meningitis have a down hill course. Sudden onset of headache severe throbbing and unbearable in character is more suggestive of a leaking aneurysm.

Check list suggestive of secondary headache

1. Severe headache in a person over age of 50.
2. Intense headache.
3. Neck rigidity.
4. Papilloedema/diplopia
5. Hypertension
6. Worsening of headache by exertion
7. History of head injury, trauma.
8. Worsening and progression of headache.

In physical examination look for neck rigidity (meningitis) presence of tenderness over scalp, sinuses and cranial nerve involvement. Fundus examination must be done in every case to look for papilloedemna, suggestive of raised intracranial

tension. Diagnostic tests mainly include CT scan to evaluate intracranial haemorrhage or space occupying lesion.

In cases of meningitis or encephalitis a lumbar puncture is done to arrive at diagnosis and CSF examined CSF culture is carried out to isolate the oroganism. MRI can also be done since it offers better soft tissue contrast as well as better detection of small lesions and old bleed. In suspected intracranial aneurysm MRI with angiogram is done to visualize it.

Characteristics of migraine

1. Family history
2. Throbbing headache confined to one half
3. Nausea and vomiting
4. Photophobia
5. Altered mood, irritability
6. Often precipitating factor present
7. Polyuria.
8. Patient does not want to be disturbed.
9. Prodromal symptoms present
10. Attack lasts for variable period (4 to 24 hours).

EPILEPSY

Epilepsy may be defined as abnormal transient disturbances of the cerebral function, paroxysmal in nature due to abnormalities in the electrical activity of brain cells. An attack of epilepsy is characterized by tonic and clonic convulsions with loss of consciousness coming on suddenly preceded by an aura, the attack ceasing spontaneously. This is typical form of epileptic attack though a number of variations are there depending on the site of origin in the brain and its spread.

Epilepsy may be primary where no cause responsible for it can be demonstrated. Patients suffering from primary or idiopathic form generally have hereditary predisposition while in secondary form of epilepsy a number of causes both local and general are responsible for causing it. In fact epilepsy in such cases is a symptom complex.

Pathophysiology. In epilepsy there are abnormal

changes in the electrical potentials of the brain and a large number of neurones are activated repeatedly. The abnormal physiochemical state of the neurones is inhibited by certain changes at the cell levels and failure of this activity leads to repeated uncontrolled neural discharge. Initially it is confined to one area in the brain but in some it may spread throughout the brain. Post epileptic symptoms characterised by loss of consciousness, transient motor or sensory disturbances result due to exhaustion of neurones which have been discharging impulses actively.

Classification. *Epilepsy is classified according to type of seizures:*

Primary epilepsy

1. *Generalized seizures:*
   a. Grand mal epilepsy (tonic clonic seizures)
   b. Petit mal (absence seizure)
   c. Myoclonic seizures
   d. Tonic seizures
   e. Atonic seizures
   f. Infantile spasm.
2. *Partial seizures*
   a. Simple partial seizures
   b. Complex partial seizures (temporal lobe or psychomotor seizures)
   c. Secondary generalization of partial seizures.

Secondary epilepsy. Here a cause either local or generalized responsible for causing epilepsy is operative. Causes of secondary form of epilepsy are varied and include.

1. *Local causes*
   a. Increased intracranial pressure (space-occupying lesion, cerebral haemorrhage).
   b. Inflammatory conditions (meningitis, encephalitis)
   c. Trauma (head injury)
   d. Congenital abnormalities (cerebral diplegia)
   e. Degenerative (diffuse sclerosis, Alzheimer's disease)
   f. Vascular (cerebral atherosclerosis, hypertensive encephalopathy).

g. Parasitic (neurocysticercosis)
2. *General causes.* Poisons, cerebral hypoxia, disturbances of metabolism (hypoglycaemia), uraemia, alkalosis, hypopituitarism.

Clinical features:

Grand mal epilepsy. It comes suddnely without warning in some patients while in others it is preceded by prodromal symptoms which are present for hours or even for a day and consist of irritability, depression, abnormal feelings, giddiness and abdominal cramps. Often the patient is able to recognize these symptoms and know that a fit is coming.

Characteristics of hysterical fits

1. Gradual onset
2. Fits only in presence of people
3. Consciousness not completely lost
4. No aura
5. Fits are bizarre and do not fit any pattern
6. Person does not hurt himself/herself
7. No incontinence of urine
8. No biting of tongue or injury
9. Generally a young female
10. EEG is normal

These symptoms are followed by aura which may be reflected in abnormal sensations like flashing of light, hallucinations of hearing words or sounds, sensation of tingling or numbness, pain in the epigastrium and unnatural sensations in some part of the body. Aura is warning of the attack and is produced by activation of epileptic discharge in the brain. In some before patient looses consciousness there is turning of the head from side to side and flexion of the upper limb. The onset of fit is characterized by sudden loss of consciousness, patient falling to ground, tonic contraction of the muscles and an epileptic cry produced by forcible expiration though the partly closed vocal cords. While falling the patient may injure himself. Tonic convulsions of the two sides of body occur with head and eyes rotated to one side. Tonic phase is followed by clonic phase which lasts for variable period of time. There are alternate to and fro movements of the limbs, frothing of the mouth and increased salivation. During this phase patient may bite his/her tongue and pass urine and stools.

Factors precipitating an epileptic fit

1. Physical fatigue
2. Mental stress
3. Hypoglycaemia
4. Flashes of bright light
5. Violent exercise
6. Alcohol
7. Infection

Clonic phase is followed by phase of unconsciousness lasting for a few minutes to half an hour. After recovery patient is confused, irritable and may go to sleep. When patient wakes he complains of severe headache. In post epileptic phase, an automatism may develop. Often there is amnesia. Sometimes patient may perform harmful or dangerous acts without being aware of them.

EEG shows a low voltage fast activity during the tonic phase while during clonic phase there are bursts of sharp waves associated with rhythmic muscular contractions. In attack free period EEG may show spike waves and occasionally sharp and low wave discharge.

Petit mal (Absence seizures). This type of epilepsy is generally seen in children. Transient loss of consciousness without any convulsions is the main symptom. These attacks usually last for a few seconds to few minutes when all motor activity including speech stops. During the attack the child looks dazed and eyes have a staring look. Recovery takes place soon. In severe forms of attack, the patient looses consciousness and falls to the ground. There may be slight motor activity like fluttering of eyelids, chewing movements and rigidity.

EEG is abnormal and shows classic, "three per second". Spike and wave discharges. Absence seizure may occur, many times during the day but in one third of these chiddren the attacks disappear once they reach adolescence while one third may develop tonic-clonic form of seizures in addition to them.

Myoclonic seizures. These are sudden brisk brief single or repetitive muscular contractions involving a single limb or whole body. These are often violent and uncontrollable. They may occur alone or coexist with other forms of epilepsy. EEG shows polyspike and wave discharges or sharp and slow waves.

Atonic seizures. These usually occur in children and are characterized by sudden loss of consciousness and postural tone. There are no tonic muscular contractions and the child falls to the ground without any cause. These atonic seizures may be accompanied by other forms of seizures. EEG is abnormal and shows polypikes and slow wave.

Tonic seizures. This is a form of grand mal epilepsy where person adopts a sudden rigid posture of the limbs or body. There is deviation of the head and eyes. Tonic seizures are of short dration and are not followed by clonic seizures.

Infantile spasms (Hyposarrhythmia). These fits occur in infants below one year of age. There are brief synchronous jerky movements of the neck, body and limbs. These spasms often occur in children with a preexisting neurological disorder. Prognosis in these cases is not good because of neurological disorder. EEG is grossly abnormal and is characterized by a very disorganized background.

Partial or focal seizures. These seizures start with the discharge from an epileptiform focus in one area of the cortex. The seizure has a focal onset usually from either thumb, index finger or part of face. When a muscular contraction starts it involves the whole limb followed by generalized clonic movements and loss of consciousness.

Jacksonian epilepsy is the term applied to the partial seizures when contractions start from one part, involves that side and soon spreads, to the same side of the body. This has been called Jacksonian march (right thumb to right hand to right arm to right side of face) and may not be followed by loss of consciousness or involvement of opposite side. EEG consists of regularly occurring spike discharges in the area of cortex involved. Partial seizures may have behavioral disturbances (Sensory, autonomic and psychic symptoms). The seizure discharges occur in other areas of cortex like temporal, and frontal lobes.

Complex partial seizures (Temporal lobe or psychomotor epilepsy). This is the form of epilepsy where the aura is either auditory, visual, olfactory or gustatory. There may be feeling of an unusual smell, an emotional feeling or hallucinations. These may constitute the only form of seizure. There is temporary cessation of activity followed by lip smacking, chewing movements or the patient may walk about aimlessly or do some complicated movements. When the seizure ends there is amnesia. Recovery may take place ranging from minutes to hours. Most of these seizures originate from temporal lobe but may also arise from other parts of limbic system or orbital frontal regions. EEG may be normal or show spike discharge or focal slow activity during the seizure.

Reflex epilepsy. This is the form of epilepsy which is precipitated by some form of external stimuli like sudden loud noise (acoustico motor epilepsy) music (musciogenic epilepsy) or visual (photogenic epilepsy) or by certain stimuli of the skin.

Diagnosis. Epilepsy is diagnosed by clinical history about the type of fit, its onset and acompanying symptoms like biting of tongue, passing of urine in clothes injury to the patient, loss of consciousness and post epileptic features. Primary epilepsy has to be differentiated from numerous organic causes responsible for causing secondary form of epilepsy.

Main differential diagnosis of primary seizures is from hysteria where generally convulsions are bizarre type, occur in the presence of people to draw attention and patient never injures himself or herself. The seizure does not follow any specific pattern and patient usually is a young female. Electroencephalogram may be helpful in diagnosing epilepsy when it is abnormal but a normal EEG does not exclude the diagnosis. CSF is normal in cases of epilepsy. CT scan is important in excluding any organic pathology in the brain.

Management of epilepsy. Patients of epilepsy must be warned about working at hazardous occupations like working at heights, near fire or machinery.

General hygiene must be maintained. Any factor which may precipitate an attack must be avoided.

Prescription of antiepileptic drugs. Antiepileptic drugs should be started only when one is convinced about the diagnosis. They are not curative but help in controlling seizures and give symptomatic relief. Most patients will be controlled by a single drug but if response is not adequate, another drug may be added. Aim should be to have seizure free period and once treatment has begun it has to be continued for sometime after seizure free period. Sudden withdrawl of the drugs is also not advisable. When another drug is to be substituted the first drug should be slowly withdrawn and the new drug introduced.

Drugs for tonic clonic seizures. Commonly used drugs are phenytoin, phenobarbitone, carbamezapine and valporate.

Phenytoin. It is an effective drug and useful in abolition of tonic clonic seizure. It is not a CNS depressant but some sedation occurs at therapeutic doses. It limits spread of seizure activity but has little effect on intellectual impariment. Dosage 100 mg two or three times a day. Maximum dose 600 mg per day. Side effects include gum hypertrophy rashes, hirsuitism, cerebellar and vestibular disturbances, ataxia,and diplopia.

Phenobarbitone. It is also effective like phenytoin in abolishing generalized tonic clonic seizures. It causes sedation and a dulling of intellect. Drug is started with a dose of 60 mg perday in adults and 4 mg/kg in children. Main draw back of the drug is sedation which is dose dependent. In patients where control is achieved without producing excessive sedation, it is an ideal anticonvulsant. Side effects include mental confusion, Rashes, impaired performance, dizziness and ataxia.

Sodium valproate. It is a broad-spectrum anticonvulsant and has little sedative effect or other central effects. Drug action is by potentiating the inhibitory transmitter GABA. It is the drug of choice in myoclonic epilepsy and primary generalized epilepsy. Starting dose is 600 mg once or in two

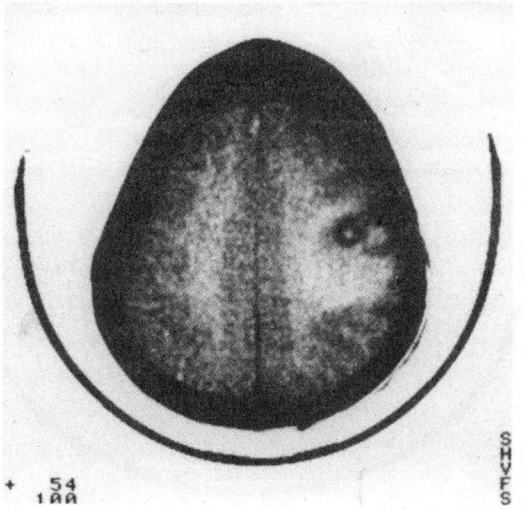

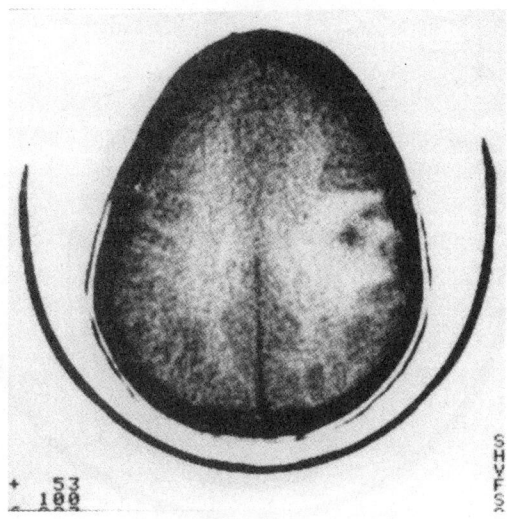

Fig. 10.7. CT Scan head: There is an enhancing ring lesion with perifocal oedema present in right posterior frontal region. Regional cortical sulci effaced. Right ventricle mildly compressed. Left lateral ventricle is normal in size. This type of lesion is non-specific and is usually seen after focal seizures.

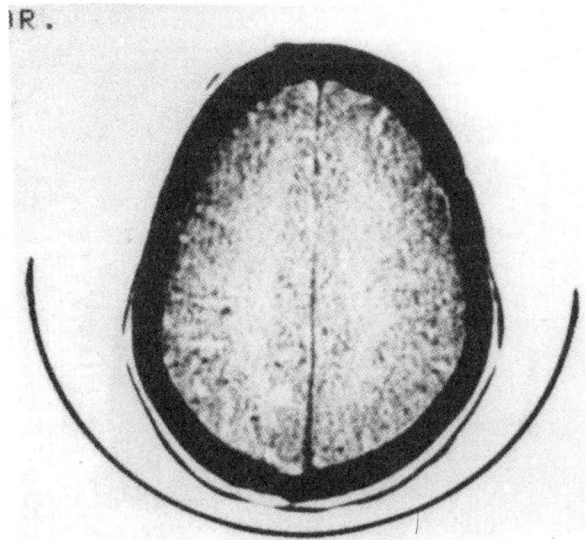

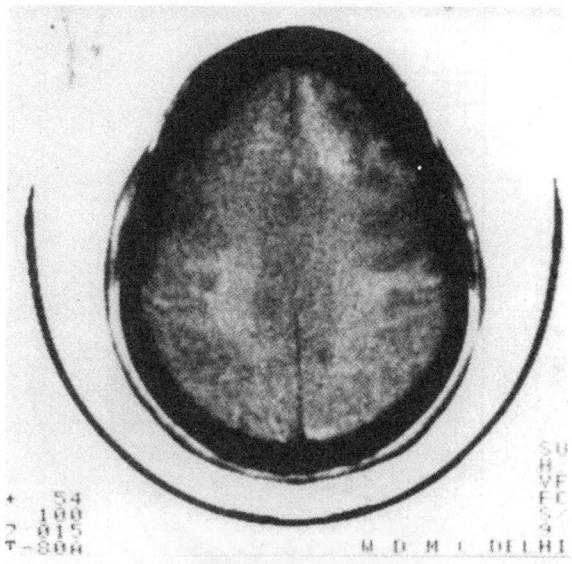

Fig. 10.8. CT Scan Head: Multiple hyperdense shadows are seen scattered all over the brain parenchyma. These findings are suggestive of cerebral cysticercosis with diffuse cerebral oedema. Neutocysticercosis is an important cause of epilepsy.

Fig. 10.9. CT Scan head. Multiple small high density enhancing disc cum ring lesions present, scattered diffusely in the supratentorial compartment. Most of the lesions are surrounded by perifocal oedema in both frontal and parietal regions. Multiplicity of small lesions suggest neuro-cysticercosis. This scan is from a 45 years old male presenting with epileptic fits.

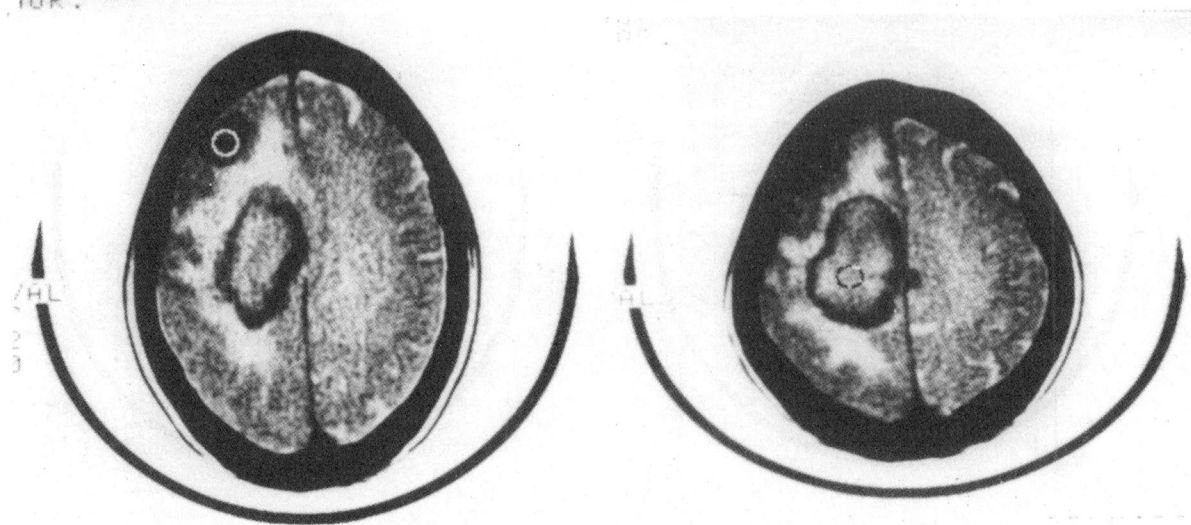

Fig. 10.10. CT Scan head. Multiple ring enhancing lesions of varying sizes are seen scattered all over the brain parenchyma some having surrounding oedema. A solitary enhancing focus is seen in left cerebral hemisphere. *Impression.* Nueorcysticercosis is an important cause of epilepsy.

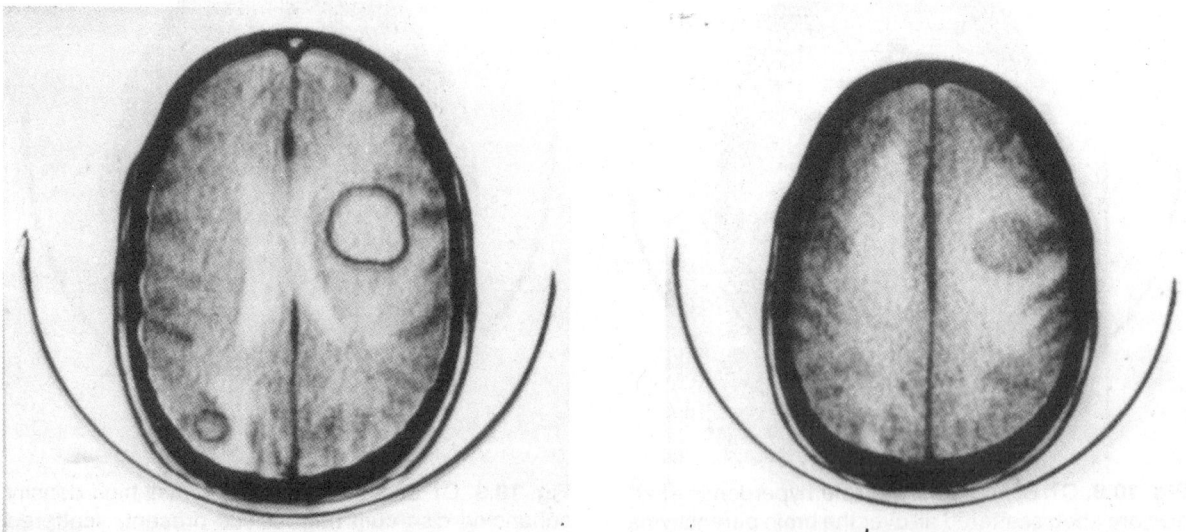

Fig. 10.11. CT Scan head. A 20 years old female presented with focal epileptic fits. Scan shows calcified lesions in the right frontal and parietal region. These lesions are not associated with any oedema. Rest of the brain parenchyma shows normal attenuation values. Impression is of old calcified lesions in right cerebral hemisphere. Probably tubercular in aetiology.

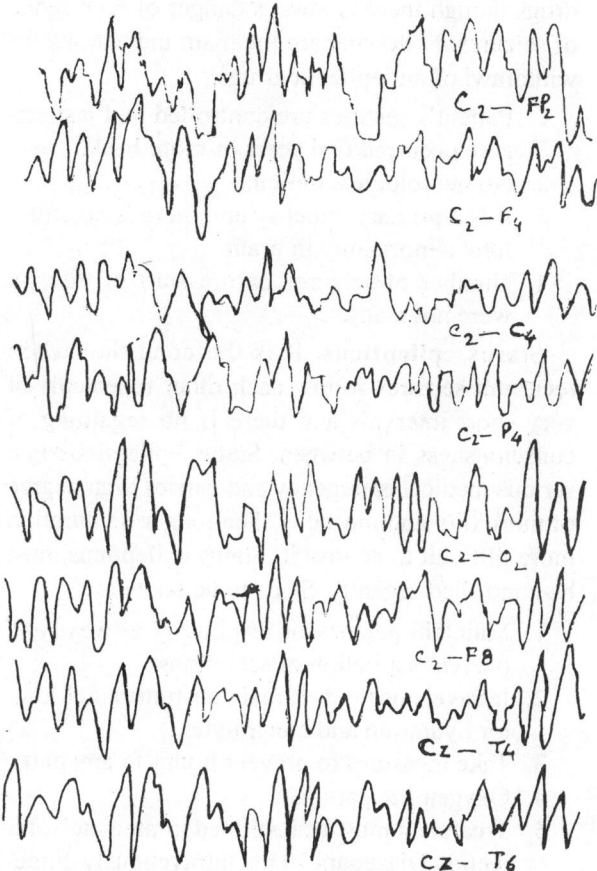

Fig. 10.12. Electroencephalogram (EEG) in a case of epilepsy. Alpha background activity seen sporadically. Graph consists of slow high voltage waves and spikes. This is grossly abnormal graph record seen in grand mal epilepsy.

divided doses daily and subsequent increase by 200 mg daily at three days interval till seizures are controlled. Side effects include anorexia, vomiting, drowsiness and tremors. Weight gain, rashes, fulminant hepatitis, thrombocytopenia and oedema are other side effects.

Carbamazepine. It has both antiepileptic and psychotropic activity. It is used either as monotherapy or in combination with other antiepileptic drugs. It is indicated in the treatment of partial and generalized tonic clonic seizures.

Dosage initially 200 mg once or twice a day to be raised slowly to 400 mg two to three times daily. Side effects include loss of appetite, dryness of mouth, headache, dizziness, ataxia, disorders of visual accommodation. It may produce liver impairment so blood counts and liver functions should be monitored before and at 2 weeks intervals after starting the therapy.

Partial and complex partial seizures. Drugs which are effective for tonic clonic seizures are also effective in partial seizures and these are phenytoin and carbamazepine. Complex partial seizures may be difficult to control and require more than one drug. In addition to a primary drug, methsuximide is employed.

Trimethadione is the drug of choice for petit mal epilepsy while ethosuximide and valproic acid are used for simple and atypical absence attacks.

Trimethadione (Tridione). This drug is effective in the treatment of petit mal epilepsy or absence attacks. Initial dose is 0.3 gm three times a day. Maximum dose is 2.1 gm a day. Side effects include visual glare, sedation and dyspepsia. Blood changes include leucopenia, neutropenia, bone marrow depression and aplastic anaemia.

Ethosuximide. Its action is mainly on thalamocortical system which raises seizure threshold. It is used for patients with uncomplicated absence seizures or in other cases where petit mal co-exists with other forms of epilepsy. Dose 500 mg daily, slowly increasing thedose to 1.5 g/day. Side effects include gastrointestinal intolerance, mood changes, headache, drowsiness, rashes and blood dyscrasias.

Clonazepam. It is effective in treatment of typical and atypical absence infantile spasms, myoclonic jerks, temporal lobe epilepsy and tonic clonic seizures. It reduces excitability of neurones and also suppresses the spread of epileptiform discharges. Dose in adults initially 1.5 mg/day increased by 0.5 mg/day. Maximum dose 20 mg per day. Side effects include drowsiness, fatigue, ataxia, muscular incoordination, vertigo, nausea and vomiting.

In addition to the above drugs there are other drugs which are effective in those patients who are refractory to main drug therapy.

Clobazam. Its antiepileptic activity is related to

its binding to one or more specific GABA receptors. It is most beneficial to patients with partial seizures and refractory epilepsy. Dosage single bed time dose starting 10-20 mg increasing upto 60 mg. Side effects include sedation, dizziness, depression and aggression.

Gabapentin. It is of use in adult patients who have not obtained adequate control of partial seizures with the drugs already employed. So its main use is as an adjuvctive therapy in the treatment of partial seizures with secondary generalization. Dose 900-1800 mg per day in three divided doses to a maximum of 2400 mg perday. Side effects include fatigue, headache, nausea, dizziness, diplopia and ataxia.

Lamotrigine. It is effective in all types of epileptic seizures and is mainly used as an adjuvctive therapy in patient of simple partial seizures, complex partial seizures and secondary generalized tonic colonic seizures. Initial dose is 50 mg daily for two weeks followed by 100 mg/day given in two divided doses for two weeks. Thereafter dose should be increased by 100 mg every one to two weeks till the optimal response is obtained. Side effects include skin rashes, diplopia, dizziness, drowsiness, G.I. disturbances, irritability, agitation and confusion.

Use of antiepileptic drugs. While using antiepileptic drug, select the drug which is most effective in that type of seizure. Start with a small dose and depending on the patients response dose should be increased at 1-2 weeks interval till seizure control is achieved. Dose of the drug should be minimised to the lelvel when major side effects do not occur.

Since half-life of phenytoin and phenobarbitone is such that the total daily requirement can be given in a single dose at bed time. Sometimes even when maximal dose of an antiepileptic drug has been achieved and still seizure have not been controlled it is advisable to add another antiepileptic drug like phenobarbitone with phenytoin in grand mal epilepsy.

Withdrawal of antiepileptic drugs. When patient is free of seizures for two years or more it is desirable to gradually withdraw the antiepileptic drugs though there is always danger of recurrence of seizures. Following are the main indications for withdrawl of antiepileptic drugs:

1. Patient's seizures are controlled and last seizure occurred two years or more back.
2. No neurological deficit.
3. It is a primary epilepsy and there is no structural abnormality in brain.
4. Number of seizures before start of therapy were not many.

Status epilepticus. It is the condition when recurrent seizures follow each other repeatedly at very short intervals and there is no regaining of consciousness in between. Status epilepticus is a serious medical emergency and carries high degree of morbidity and mortality. The longer its duration more difficult to control it. Status epilepticus must be controlled urgently. Steps to be taken are:

1. Maintain patency of respiratory airways and prevent aspiration of secretions.
2. Intravenous fluids to maintain nutrition. Monitor hydration and electrolytes.
3. Take measures to prevent injury to any part.
4. Oxygen inhalation.
5. Treatment must be instituted immediately. Injection Diazepam 10 mg intravenously immediately followed by intravenous infusion of 100 mg in one liter fluid during the next 24 hours. Other drugs employed are Injection Dilantin 0.5-1 g intravenously stat. This achieves optimal effect. Further control is maintained by Dilantin 200 mg alternating with phenobarbitone 60 mg given parenterally every 6 hourly.

Choice of drugs in the various types of epilepsy.

Type of epilepsy	*Drug of choice*
Grand mal epilepsy	Phenytoin sodium, phenobarbitone, sodium valproate, carbamazepine.
Petit mal seizures	Tridione, sodium valproate.
Partial complex seizures	Carbamazepine, sodium valproate.
Absence attacks	Sodium valproate, ethosuximide.
Myoclonic epilepsy	Sodium valproate, clonazepam.
Infantile spasms	ACTH/Pednisolone, clonazepam.

6. A broad-spectrum antibiotic (Injection Ampicillin 500 mg I/V 6 hourly) to prevent infection. Failure to control status epilepticus is due to inadequate dosage of antiepileptic drugs as well as delay in starting treatment.

Surgical management of epilepsy. In some cases of epilepsy not responding to medical treatment, surgical removal of the epileptogenic focus has been carried out. This has been done in temporal lobe epilepsy after identifying the area. Procedures include cortical excision and hemispherectomy (amputation of anterior temporal lobe). Results are statisfactory only in small percentage of cases.

SYNCOPE

It may be defined as transient loss of consciousness which comes suddenly, lasts for a short time and is due to diminished blood supply to the brain. The symptoms (fainting, vasovagal attacks) are produced as a result of disorder of circulation in which cardiac output is not sufficient to maintain normal cerebral blood flow. The causes of syncope are many and range from disorders of the heart to emotional factors.

Aetiology:

1. *Simple faint.* It is of common occurrence and occurs commonly when a person has been standing for long periods (in parades and drills), exhaustion, starvation and excessive heat. Pain especially when severe and unbearable results in syncope.

2. *Carotid sinus syncope.* Changes in carotid sinus pressure are important. Pressure on carotid sinus either as a result of digital pressure, tight collar and any disease in its neighbourhood shall produce syncopal attacks due to cerebral anoxaemia.

3. *Diseases of the heart.* Disorders of cardiac rhythm (varying degrees of heart block, auricular flutter, supraventicular, and ventricular tachycardias, ventricular fibrillation, adams stokes attacks) are important causes. In cases of tachycardias and heart block, syncopal attacks occur during periods of cardiac asystole. Other cardiac conditions responsible are congential cyanotic heart disease, aortic stenosis and cardiac temponade.

4. *Orthostatic hypotension.* This may occur in some people while suddenly getting up as in cases of addisons disease and in people on antihypertensive drugs (ganglion blocking drugs). Levodopa and phenothiazines. In eld-

Clinical efficacy of commonly used antiepileptic drugs

Drug	Dosage/day	Indications	Side effects
Phenytoin	200-400 mg	Grand mal, focal	Gum hypertrophy, hirsutism, depression
Carbamazepine	400-600 mg	Tonic clonic, focal complex, partial	Diplopia, rashes, dizziness, aplastic anaemia
Phenobarbitone	60-120 mg	Tonic clonic, focal	Ataxia, sedation, rash, depression
Sodium valproate	500-1500 mg	Absence, atypical, grand mal, myoclonic	Weight gain, dyspepsia, oedema, hepatic insufficiency
Ethosuximide	500-1000 mg	Petit mal	Agitation, headache, rash.
Clonazepam	2-8 mg	Atypical, myoclonic, absence seizures	Fatigues, dizziness, ataxia, sedation
Trimethadione (tridione)	900-1200 mg	Absence, atypical seizures, petit mal	Skin rash, bone marrow, depression, visual glare.

erly people due to impaired autonomic functions, postural hypotension results on standing up and while micturiting.

5. *Psychological causes.* Fear and sudden anxiety in cases of heightened tension may produce syncopal attack. An unpleasant sight or experience may sometimes be responsible for it. Sudden psychological shock on hearing an unpleasant news produces syncope due to fall in blood pressure as well as slowing of the heart rate.

6. *Physical injury.* It may be as a result of trauma to deep lying tissues or a form of minor surgical procedure like venepuncture, lumbar puncture, pleural and ascitic tap where reflex action results in syncope.

7. *Blood loss.* Sudden loss of blood which may be excessive produces syncope due to cerebral anoxaemia. Sometimes site of blood in a patient may provoke it.

8. *Hypoglycaemia.* Low blood sugar levels may result due to starvation, following over dosage of insulin, antidiabetic drugs when food intake has been poor. Tumour of islets cells of pancreas (insulinoma) is an important cause of hypoglycaemia lasting for months to years.

9. Miscellaneous causes include sudden rise in intrathoracic pressure due to bouts of coughing resulting in diminution of venous return to the heart. Other causes include vertebro basilar, artery insufficiency when blood supply to the brain is effected, sudden movements of neck and allergic reactions.

Clinical picture. Onset of a syncopal attack is sudden. There may be prodromal symptoms in the form of tingling or numbness in limbs, sudden darkness before eyes and patient may have a feeling of blacking out. He is cold and sweating and may fall to the ground suddenly becoming unconscious. Unconsciousness lasts hardly for more than two minutes. Patients respiration is sighing, pulse is slow and limbs cold and clammy. Pupils may react to light sluggishly and deep reflexes are diminished. Sometimes patient may show convulsive movements

though it is not a typical epileptic attack. Patient regains consciousness shortly and may complain of exhaustion and weakness.

Physical examination may not be contributory except in cases of cardiovascular disorders. Postural hypotension when present is helpful. Presence of cardiac murmurs (aortic stenosis), cyanosis (congenital cyanatic heart disease) and cardiac irregularities are helpful in making an aetiological diagnosis. Carotid pulsations are diminished in cases of vertebro basilar artery insufficiency.

Diagnosis. It is based on number of factors. Hysterical syncope occurs in young females while carotid sinus syncope and cardiac rhythm irregularities occur in elderly individuals. Diagnosis of syncope due to history of prolonged standing, heat exhaustion, starvation, sudden rotation of neck, fall of blood sugar levels in diabetes is made on thorough detailed history. History of drug intake especially antihypertensives. Insulin, antidiabetics is also helpful. A detailed physical examination shall confirm any aetiological factor which might be operative. Young females who exhibit emotional lability apprehension and sweating excessively shall favour a diagnosis of hysterical cause of syncope.

Investigations. No specific investigation is required except to diagnose any organic ailment if so present. A blood sugar estimation may be done when hypoglycaemia is suspected. Cardiac monitoring may be required in cases with cardiac rhythm disturbance.

Treatment. No treatment except reassurance is required for an ordinary syncopal attack since it is a self limiting disease. Smelling salts are often used in hysterical cases. A case of syncope must be laid on bed, in an airy room. Foot end of the bed be elevated. If blood pressure is on the lower side, vasopressor drugs may have to be administered. For hypoglycaemia intravenous glucose be administered immediately. Monitor pulse and blood pressure. Where a cause is operative it should be treated with proper medication especially cases of cardiac arrhythmias.

MENINGITIS

Inflammation of the meninges is called meningitis and may be caused by bacteria, viruses, fungi and other organisms in immunocompromised patients.

Infection may reach meninges as a result of direct spread from without as in case of fracture of skull or penetrating wounds or spread from within in cases of intracranial abscess. Infection through the blood stream may result from focal infection, somewhere in the body such as empyema, pneumonia or osteomyelitis. Disseminated miliary tuberculosis is an important cause of tubercular meningitis. Similarly focus of infection in the cranium like mastoiditis, nasal air sinuses shall spread the infection to meninges.

Aetiology. Meningitis may be classified according to the organisms responsible for it.

1. Acute pyogenic meningitis due to Streptococcus pneumoniae, Staphylococcus aureus, Haemophilus influenzae, Staph. epidermidis, Listeria monocytogenes and organisms like E. coli, Proteus, Pseudomonas. Uncommon organisms include Salmonella, Shigella.
2. Meningococcal meningitis
3. Tuberculous meningitis
4. Acute lymphocytic choriomeningitis

Acute pyogenic meningitis. Commonest organism for acute pyogenic meningitis is streptococcus pneumoniae responsible in 30 to 50 per cent of cases in adults followed by haemophilus influenzae type B which mainly effects children. Other organisms include staphylococcus aureus which generally occurs postoperatively in neurosurgical patients Staph. epidermidis producing meningitis associated with shunting procedures and group B streptococci and gram negative bacilli which are associated either with brain abscess, head injury or neurosurgical procedures. Listeria monocytogenes is also a major pathogen responsible for causing meningitis in infants, elderly debilitated patients or those who are immunosuppressed.

Pathology. Irrespective of the organisms causing meningitis pathology in all cases is the same. Infection once it breaches the protective wall of the meninges, rapidly spreads over the surface of the brain, spinal cord and ependymal lining of the ventricles. The brain and spinal cord are swollen and congested. The cortical veins become congested and convolutions on the surface of brain become flattened because of internal hydrocephalus which is due to inflammatory adhesions obstructing outflow of CSF from fourth ventricle. Whole of CSF becomes turbid and purulent. Depending on the type of organism, inflammatory exudate may be located at various sites. In pneumococcal infection it is located more often on cerebral convexity while in H. influenzae, it is mainly basal. When the process is fulminant it may spread and involve the cranial nerves as well as ependymal surface of the ventricles.

Clinical features. All cases of acute pyogenic meningitis have the same clinical picture. Most of the time onset is acute characterised by fever coming with rigors, and headache which is very severe almost bursting in character. Increasing severity of headache may be main symptom confined to frontal region and radiating down to the back. Vomiting is often present. Convulsions are seen more often in children especially with H. influenzae meningitis.

Because of meningeal irritation patient may be curled up in bed. There is neck rigidity, head retraction and Kernig's sign is positive. Delirium is common and as the disease progresses patient passes into drowsiness and coma. There is severe degree of photophobia. Pupils are unequal and reaction is sluggish. Later on these become dilated and fixed. Ptosis may be seen because of raised intracranial tension and there is paralysis of occular muscles. Papilloedema is usually present.

Onset of meningts may be insidious in children and elderly people. Rapid progress of the disease takes place in adults, it following a fulminant course. Limbs become flaccid. Reflexes are diminished. Incontinence of urine may take place and within 24-48 hours, course becomes downhill.

Diagnosis of pyogenic meningitis shall depend on history (head injury, infection on skull air sinuses, respiratory infection like pneumonia, lung abscess, neurosurgical operations etc) and clinical picture (fever, headache, neck rigidity, toxaemia). Any patient coming with fever, neck rigidity and confusion the diagnosis of meningitis should be considered.

Investigations:

1. *Blood count.* There is leucocytosis with rise in polymorph count.
2. *CSF examination.* It is the most important test. CSF pressure is raised. It is turbid and purulent pus like. Formation of a coagulum is often seen. Protein content is markedly increased while chloride content is reduced to 650 mg and glucose content is markedly diminished. Cells on microscopic examination are polymorphs and are present in thousands per cmm.

   Lange's colloidal gold curve is meningitic type. Grams stain of sedimented CSF is done to identify the causative agent. Pneumococci and H. influenzae are identified more readily. In cases where bacteria are not seen by Gram's stain, staining with acridine orange and examination under a fluorescence microscope may be helpful in demonstrating bacteria not stained by Gram's stain. CSF cultures are positive in 70 to 80 per cent of cases.

   The measurement of bacterial antigens in the CSF by Latex Agglutination, radioimmunoassay and ELISA may be done to determine the presence of specific capsular polysacchride especially in cases of H. influenzae B and S. pneumoniae. Blood cultures are equally important since they shall provide clue to the causative agent.
3. All patients must have X-rays of chest, skull and sinuses to exclude the presence of infection (pneumonia, lung abscess, sinusitis, skull fracture etc).

Complications. A small percentage of cases of bacterial meningitis may be left with cranial nerve palsies and some with sensory hearing loss. Deafness is equally common. If focal neurological damage takes place there may be local signs of cerebral damage. Some children may be left with mental retardation. Epilepsy may develop. Persistent changes in level of consciousness should raise suspicion of internal hydrocephalus. Some children may be left with learning defects. Cases of pneumococcal meningiis in adults may pass into coma.

Meningococcal meningitis. It occurs both in epidemics and sporadic forms. The causal organism is meningococcus (Nissseria meningitidis) a kidney shaped gram negative organism which can be classified into eight groups and out of which group A,B and C are the ones responsible for most of the infections. The organisms are commonly found in the nasopharynx of people who act as carriers and often the disease spreads by droplet infection. Carriers often outnumber overt cases, infect other people without themselves developing the disease. Principal causes of spread of the disease are over crowding and catarrhal disorder of the nose and throat. Children and young infants are more susceptible to suffer from it. It is uncommon after the age of 40.

Pathology. It is like in other cases of bacterial meningitis except for that in meningococcal meningitis brain is diffusely involved with resultant congestion, oedema, perivascular haemorrhages and suppurative lesions. There may be focal areas of involvement. In fulminant form of meningitis, haemorrhages are found in the adrenals leading to adrenal failure and shock (Water House friederichsen syndrome).

Clinical features. Onset of meningococcal meningitis generally is acute with headache, fever, chills, neck rigidity and signs of meningeal irritation. Commonest age group is young children and adults. Incubation period is 3-5 days and there is history of preceding upper respiratory tract infection.

Onset may be gradual in some cases and fulminant in others. Pulse is slow. Headache and vomiting are rather of severe nature. Delirium may be severe and patient may pass into stupor and coma. Signs of meningeal irritation (photophobia: neck rigidity, kernig's and brudzinski's signs) are invariably present. Meningococcal meningitis is characterised by purpuric eruption and maculopapular rash in areas subjected to pressure. While purpuric eruption takes the form of petechiae appearing during the first 24 hours of illness, maculopapular rash appears before the fourth day first on the trunk and then on thighs and forearms.

As the disease progresses rise in intracranial pressure occurs. Pupils are dilated and react sluggishly. Diplopia, slight ptosis and divergent squint are common. Papilloedema may be present. Limbs are flaccid. Reflexes are diminished. There is loss of sphincter control. Development of stupor and coma are bad prognostic signs. Cases with fulminating type develop water house friederichsen syndrome characterised by cyanosis collapse and shock.

Diagnosis. Meningococcal meningitis is to be differentiated from other forms of bacterial meningitis by its rash (purpuric and maculopapular). Other diseases to be differentiated include encephalitis, cerebral haemorrhage, meningism and general infections (pneumonia, influenza, typhoid) simulating meningitis.

Investigations:

1. Blood count shows leucocytosis with rise in polymorphs.
2. Blood culture for meningococci may be positive in early stages.
3. CSF examination is the most important diagnostic aid. CSF pressure is raised. It is turbid and purulent in appearance. Protein content is raised. There is often a cob web formation. Sometimes CSF may coagulate due to high albuminous content. Glucose content is markedly reduced as well as chlorides (650-680 mg/100 ml). Cell count is increased, the cells being mainly polymorphonuclear. About 1000-2000 cells per cmm are present.
4. Gram's stain of sedimented CSF does not readily identify meningococci. Meningococcal antigen may be demonstrated by immune electrophoresis (CIE) and ELISA test.

Complications and sequelae. A number of complications may occur in cases of meningococcal meningitis. These may be in the form of internal hydrocephalus, focal neurological damage (hemiplegia), paraplegia, aphasia, deafness and loss of vision. Uncommon complications include fibropurulent pericarditis, endocarditis, arthritis and nephritis. In the fulminant type, patient rapidly goes into stupor and coma. Death may occur in a short time. Cases of water house friederichsen syndrome carry poor prognosis.

Cases where treatment has been delayed or inadequate these may be left with a chronic form of basal meningitis characterised by cranial nerve palsies, Hydrocephalus, neck retraction and paralysis.

Treatment of bacterial meningitis:

1. Bacterial meningitis is an acute medical emergency and treatment must be instituted immediately. For adult patients with pneumococcal, meningococcal or Listeria meningitis drug of choice is Penicillin G 5-10 million units intravenously every 6 hourly. Ampicillin in a dose of 300-400 mg/kg body weight daily intravenously is also an effective drug.

   The third generation cephalosporins, cefotaxime (2 g I/V 4 hourly) or Ceftriaxone (2 g I/V once a day) are effectivie in pneumococcal, H. influenzae and meningococcal meningitis but not in listeria meningitis where trimethoprim, sulpha methoxazole (160 mg TMP+ 800 mg SMX) intravenously in drip twice a day is used.
2. Patients who are allergic to penicillin they can be treated with chloramphenicol (dosage 1 g I/v 6 hourly) or third generation cephalosporins.
3. Since these drugs (penicillin and ampicillin) enter the blood-brain barrier, intrathecal administration is not recommended.
4. Treatment must be continued for at least 7-10 days. Progress of the case is observed by CSF. Examination which becomes clear and its biochemistry returns to normal.
5. Look for any focus of infection in para nasal sinuses, mastoid or intracranial region. It should be adequately treated.
6. For raised intracranial tension intravenous

Mannitol be given. It can be accompanied by high doses of steroids (Injection Dexamethasone 4 mg I/V 6 hourly). Supportive treatment consists of maintaining nutrition, fluid and electrolyte balance. Cases of Waterhouse friederichsen syndrome shall require intravenous fluids saline and high doses of steroids.

Prevention. A 23-valent pneumococcal vaccine is advocated in children with sickle cell disease, nephrotic syndrome, asplenia for prevention against pneumococcus meningitis. This vaccine is effective in older children and not of use in children below two years of age.

Similarly vaccine against serogroup A, C, Y and W-125 is effectively used for immunoprophylaxis against meningococcal meningitis. It is also not effective in children below two years of age. It takes one to two weeks for antibodies to develop after immunization. Since the period of risk is first two weeks after exposure, vaccination is not of much use in sporadic cases. However when there is an on going epidemic it may be used as part of an immunization programme.

For contacts chemoprophylaxis with rifampicin (600 mg daily for five day) is effective for eliminating colonization with the meningococcus and to prevent development of meningococcal infection.

Tubercular meningitis. Tubercular meningitis constitutes a major form of meningitis and is widely prevalent in our country. It generally occurs in children and young adults though it may occur in other age groups as well.

Pathogenesis. Disease generally spreads via blood stream from a focus in lungs as in miliary tuberculosis or from any tubercular focus situated in the glands (mediastinal, abdominal) bones or genitourinary tract. Another source of infection is from a caseous focus in the brain which spreads to the meninges. Meninges are generally filled with a yellowish gelatinous exudate which mainly is involving the base of the brain and extending into the lateral sulcus. Miliary tubercles are seen spread over the leptomeninges and are crowding round the vessels. Microscopically the exudate consists of

chronic inflammatory cells including lymphocytes and plasma cells. There is little inflammatory

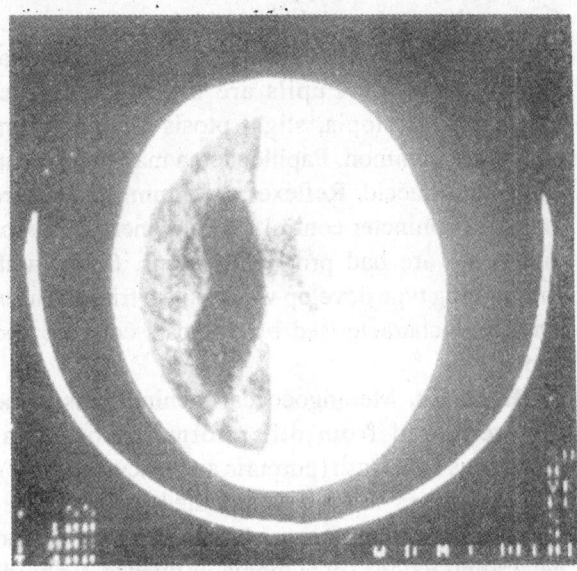

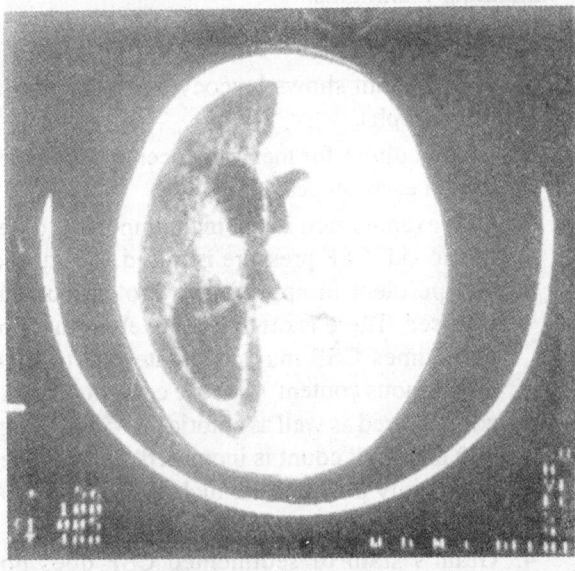

Fig. 10.13. CT Scan in a child with meningitis. Left cerebrum is small in size. Left ventricle shows significant dilatation. Ipsilateral subarachnoid spaces dilated. Generalised decrease in attenuation values of left cerebrum. Right cerebrum shows normal attenuation values. CT Findings suggestive of cerebral hemiatrophy. Post meningitic sequaelae.

CSF picture in various forms of meningitis

Type	Tension	Colour	Proteins	Sugar	Chloride	Cells
Normal	Normal	Clear	30-40 mg/dl	60-80 mg/dl	720-750 mg/dl	0.5 lymph/cmm
Bacterial meningitis	Raised	Turbid	Markedly increased	Reduced	650-680 mg/dl	Increase in cell count mainly polymorph. (1000-2000 per cmm).
Tubercular meningitis	Raised	Clear or Cloudy, Cob web formation on standing	Moderately increased 200-300 mg/dl	Very low 30 mg/dl	500-510 mg/dl	100-350 cells (mainly lymphocytes)
Acute lymphocytic Chorio-meningitis	Raised	Clear	Increased 50-100 mg/dl	Normal 60 mg/dl	Normal 700-720 mg/dl	Cell count ranges from 50-1500 per cmm, mainly mono-nuclear.

reaction of substance of nervous system but marked toxic degeneration of nervous tissue.

Tubercles and adhesions involve almost the whole of the brain spreading to the course of cerebral vessels and inner surface of the ventricles. There may be endarteritis and thrombosis of vessels leading to cerebral infarction.

Clinical picture. The onset is insidious and patient has a history of ill health. There may be history of evening rise of temperature, lassitude, loss of weight and anorexia. In adults there is often confusion and odd behaviour. These prodromal symptoms may last for two to three weeks and are followed by features of meningeal irritation in the form of neck rigidity, vomiting and convulsions. These signs are of lower intensity as compared to cases of pyogenic meningitis. Headache varying from moderate to severe in intensity may be the presenting feature in some.

Phyical examination generally shows an ill nourished person with fever ranging upto 102°F, a slow pulse and neck rigidity. In eyes there is diplopia. Pupils to start with are contracted but later on become dilated and fixed. Oculomotor palsies may develop. Papilloedema is present in some. Deep reflexes are diminished to start with but later on become exaggerated. Organic reflexes get involved

in late stages. As disease progresses patient may show delirium, stupor and even coma. There is presence of tubercular lesion in the lungs. Enlarged glands may be present in mediastinum abdomen or axilla. Presence of a tubercular sinus will be another diagnostic help.

Diagnosis. Any case of tubercular lesion somewhere in the body or a person with history of contact with a tubercular patient presenting with low grade fever, ill health, weight loss, odd behaviour, head-ache should make one suspect tubercular meningitis. Diagnosis shall be confirmed by lumbar puncture.

CSF in tubercular meningitis is under pressure. It is clear on naked eye examination but a cob web forms on standing. Protein content is increased while chloride content is much reduced. CSF sugar content is markedly reduced (less than 50 mg per cent). Cells in the CSF are increased and are mainly lymphocytes (500-1000 cells per mm) Sometimes a mixture of mononuclear and polymorphs is present.

Lange's colloidal gold curve is of meningitic type. Acid fast bacilli may be demonstrated by staining CSF sediment or cobweb. Culture of CSF and animal inoculation may grow mycobacteria tuberculosis in some.

Complications and sequelae. These are varied

depending on the stage at which the patient presents. Earlier the diagnosis is made and treatment instituted, better the prognosis and less chance of complications. Most serious complication is spread of infection into the parenchyma of brain producing meningoencephalitis. Involvement of cerebral vessels produces obliterative endarteritis and thrombosis of cerebral vessels leading to cerebral infarction. Delayed complications include development of hydrocephalus optic atrophy, spinal cord compression and cranial nerve palsies. Some patients may be left with a chronmic tuberculoma in the brain.

Treatment. *It shall be general and specific:*

General measures include maintenance of nutrition, hydration and electrolyte balance along with good nursing, care of bowel and bladder. If there are convulsions anticonvulsants (Phenytoin) be given regularly.

Complications of tubercular meningitis

1. Meningoencephalitis
2. Obliterative endarteritis of cerebral vessels
3. Hydrocephalus
4. Optic atrophy
5. Spinal cord compression
6. Cranial nerve palsies
7. Tuberculoma

Specific treatment consists of institution of antitubercular therapy. Injection Streptomycin (1 g I/M daily). Tablet Isonex (600-900 mg per day), Tablet ethambutol 800 mg per day and rifampicin 600 mg per day. In addition prednisolone 40-60 mg per day is added. Isonex is given in higher dosage because of its ability to cross blood brain barrier.

Treatment is to be given for at least 9 months. Progress of the case is monitored by repeated CSF examinations. Earlier on intratheccal administration of streptomycin was advised but now it is discarded since it does not have any advantage when four drugs are being used. Moreover intrathecal administration of the drug may introduce infection and cause adhesions formation.

Prognosis. It is good if treatment is instituted

early and diagnosis made at appropriate time. Further monitoring of the treatment and response of the patient to it shall tell the prognosis. In patients developing serious complications, prognosis becomes poor.

Acute lymphocytic choriomeningitis. Acute lymphocytic choriomeningitis occurs spordically and has almost the same clinical picture as of bacterial meningitis though the course generally is less fulminant.

Aetiology. The disease is caused by a filterable virus which has been recovered from the CSF of patients. It is an Arena virus which is an RNA virus seen in mice and monkeys. A large number of other viruses like Echoviruses, Coxsackie, Epstein bar, Herpes simplex type-I and Mumps virus havealso been isolated in these cases though it is difficult to document them in all cases.

Pathology. There is intense lymphocytic infiltration of the lepatomeninges along with degeneration of the ganglion cells. Cytoplasmic inclusion bodies may be seen.

Clinical picture. Onset is abrupt with high fever, toxaemia, irritability, photophobia and features of meningeal irritation, Neck rigidity is only slight. Fever comes down by lysis in about a weeks time.

Diagnosis. Lymphocytic choriomeningitis has to be differentiated from tubercular and pyogenic meningitis. CSF in this case is under pressure, clear and rarely turbid. Protein content is raised but sugar and chloride content of CSF is normal. There is excess of cells mainly mononuclear, count ranging from 100 to 1000 cells per cmm.

Treatment. Acute lymphocytic choriomeningitis is a self-limiting disease. Treatment mainly is supportive in the form of maintaining nutrition, hydration and electrolyte balance. No specific drug is indicated but if secondary infection is suspected a cover of broad spectrum antibiotics (Injection Ampicillin 500 mg I/V 6 hourly) may be given.

Prognosis. Since recovery from the condition is good and there are none of the life threatening complications associated with pyogenic meningitis, prognosis is most of the cases is good though recovery may be slow.

ENCEPHALITIS

Central nervous system is involved by a number of neurotropic viruses and these produce number of conditions ranging from meningitis, encephalitis to myelitis etc. Some of the viruses may remain latent in the nervous system and get reactivated later. Most viruses have a phase of extraneural viral replication before involving the nervous system.

Viruses vary in size ranging from 10-25 mμ and are destroyed by heat at low temperatures but are resistant to cold. The common characteristics of virus include a genome which is either RNA or DNA surrounded by a protective protein shell. Acute viral infections come on suddenly and have a short course ranging from days to weeks. Common viruses involving the central nervous system include entero viruses (Poliovirus, coxsackie, ECHO, EV-70). Arena virus (Lymphocytic choriomeningitis) Herpes virus (HSV (1 & 2) varicella zostier virus (VZV). Epstein Barr virus (EBV). Retroviruses HIV and influenza, Adenoviruses and arboviruses. Viruses enter the body through haemotagenous route in most of the cases though herpes virus remains latent in cells and enteroviruses replicate in the gastro intestinal tract.

Acute viral encephalitis

It is an acute inflammation of the nervous system where brain, brain stem or cerebellum is involved due to a virus. It may be primary or post infectious. Primary form occurs when there is direct invasion or replication of virus in the nervous system while post infectious follows either other viral infections or after administration of certain vaccines. The involvement of meninges and other parts of nervous system when inflammation spreads to spinal cord is termed encephalomyelitis.

Aetiology. A number of viruses can cause clinical picture of encephalitis and these viruses range from Arboviruses (Japanese, ST Louis, Westren Equine, Kyasanur forest disease (KFD). Rhabdovirus (Rabies) Entero viruses (Cox'sackie, ECHO), Herpes virus (VZV, EB virus, CMV). Influenza para influenza, viruses to other like measles, rubella, mumps etc.

Clinical picture. In most of the cases of encephalitis there is prodromal period lasting for a few days and symptoms range from headache, myalgia, bodyaches, malaise and features of upper respiratory tract infection. Mild fever is often present. The above symptoms lasting for a few days are followed by neurologic symptoms which come acutely and abruptly. There is headache, photophobia, vomiting and alterations in state of consciousness. Signs of meningeal irritation appear followed by convulsions, confusion, disorientation, stupor and even coma. Focal neurological deficits are found depending on the site of involvement. These defects range from hemiparesis, sensory defects, aphasia, ocular palsies and ataxia.

Brain stem involvement can effect the respiratory center and other vital centers.

Investigations. Blood counts are within normal limits. CSF is usually under normal or slightly elevated pressure. It may be clear or slightly turbid. Protein content is slightly elevated with normal glucose content. There is rise in cell count ranging from 50 to 500 per micro liter.

Viral isolation from blood and CSF is generally not possible. Serological tests may help in identifying the causative organism if there is four fold increase in antibody titres. EEG shows a slow wave activity with disruption of normal rhythm with high amplitude bursts and spike and wave complexes.

CT and MRI may show changes in the form of generalized or localized foci of infection.

Diagnosis. It is based on clinical picture of acute onset of illness which generally comes in epidemics and involves large number of people.

Course of the disease is variable. It may have a short lived benign course or a severe fulminating course leaving behind a number of sequlae.

Treatment. It is mainly supportive. Steroids are employed empirically though their benefit is doubtfull. If a patient is having convulsion then anticonvulsants (Phenytoin 100mg three times a day) are given. Cerebral oedema is relieved by mannitol (20% solution in 20 minutes every 6 hly), Furesmide and steroids.

Cases where Herps simplex virus encephalitis is suspected, antiviral therapy (acyclovir) may be employed with good results.

JAPANESE ENCEPHALITIS

It is a non contagious, mosquito transmitted disease caused by a flavavirus and is the most common cause of epidemic encephalitis in India. It mainly affects young adults and children.

Japanese encephalitis (JE) is a zoonotic illness with man as a dead end. The natural host is the pig and the reservoirs of virus are migratory birds of Ardridae family (Cattle egrets, Pond Herons). The virus which is 45-50 nm RNA virus having 3 structural proteins and five non-structural proteins, is transmitted from birds to pigs by mosquitoes of culex family (Culex vishnui and culex tritaeniohyclinus). It is a rural mosquito which breeds in stagnant water in rice fields. Man is an accidental host in the transmission cycle. When viral load in mosquito gets heavy, man gets infected by its bite. But man to man transmission does not occur.

Epidemiology. It is endemic in Japan, China, Thailand, Siberia, Taiwan, Korea, Nepal etc. In India first epidemic was noted in 1955 in Tamil Nadu and it is now endemic in Karnataka, Andhra Pradesh, West Bengal, Pondicherry, Goa, Maharashtra, UP, Bihar and North Eastern States.

JE involves primarily children in endemic areas while in non-endemic areas, all age groups are affected. Incidence of JE is generally higher in males as compared to females (2 : 1).

Clinical features

The incubation of the disease varies from 5-15 days. A large number of cases may be subclinical and it is only an occasional cases (1 in 300-1000) who presents with clinical picture of the disease.

Onset may be abrupt (1-6 hours) Acute (6-24 hours) and subacute (2-4 days) but in majority of cases it is subacute onset.

Course of the disease is divided into three phases.

1. Prodromal stage which is characterized by malaise, fever, headache, vomiting and diarrhoea. This stage lasts for 2-5 days.
2. Acute encephalitic stage. It is characterized by severe rigors, headache, convulsions and deterioration of mental status. Neurological defects (Cranial nerve palsies, involuntary movements like chorea, myoclonus tics, Hemiparesis, Monoplegia etc.) may appear. Extrapyramidal features like dystonia and sometimes frank parkinsonism may appear late in the course of disease lasting from several days to several weeks.
3. Convalescent stage. This varies from a week to months and generally recovery takes place. Mortality varies from 20-35%. Many patients on recovery are left with sequelae such as presistant paralysis, ataxia, mental retardation and seizures.

Pathogenesis. After the mosquito bite, CNS is affected by haematogenous route and the neurons are the main target of viral attack. There is intense vascular congestion and cerebral oedema. Main pathological changes are in the form of severe inflammation in the basal ganglia, brain stem and the white matter of the brain. The brain shows ganglion cell degeneration, gliomesen chymal nodules and focal necrolytic lesions.

Investigations. A peripheral rise in leucocyte count is present. CSF pressure is usually raised with rise in CSF proteins (50-150 mg/dl) and normal sugar content. There is lymphocytic pleocytosis (10-1000 cells/mm^3) usually in the range of 150-200 cells/mm^3.

Confirmation of the diagnosis is made by demonstrating rising titers of JE specific IgM antibodies in the CSF by IgM capture ELISA. A four fold rise in antibody titres is diagnostic. Viral culture generally is not successful.

EEG shows diffuse slowing and sometimes burst suppression pattern. CT/MRI studies show evidence of diffuse cerebral oedema.

Treatment. No specific antiviral drugs for

treating JE are available. It is mainly supportive and includes:

1. Maintenance of vital functions
2. Nutritional support
3. Monitoring of fluid and electrolyte balance
4. Control of seizures (use of phenytoin and barbiturates)
5. Reduction of cerebral oedema by use of mannitol, frusemide and cortico steroids.
6. Management of Hyperthermia by use of paracetamol / lytic cocktail.

Prognosis. Mortality in JE is variable ranging from 20-35%. Certain indicators herald a poor outcome.

1. Adults fare worse as compared to children.
2. Acute onset; severity of encephalitic stage.
3. Profound slowing in EEG.
4. Presence of immune complexes in CSF.
5. Presence of adverse sequelae.

Commonest cause of death in most cases is extensive and widespread neuronal damage and cerebral oedema as well as respiratory complications.

A significant number of cases develop (50%) sequelae ranging from mental deficiency, Behaviour changes, Motor weakness, speech disorders to convulsions. Uncommonly there is ataxia, parkinsonism, cerebellar deficit and autonomic disturbance.

Prevention. Main thrust should be on mosquito control measures (Fogging of fields with malathion and pyrethrim).

Inactivated suckling mouse brain vaccine given in two subcutaneous doses (7-14 days apart) with a booster 1 year later and then every three years gives good protection. Main drawback is that this vaccine has to be given at least 4-6 weeks prior to the onset of the epidemic and to be effective, at least 80-90% of the population has to be vaccinated.

CEREBROVASCULAR DISEASES

Cerebrovascular disorders constitute one of the commonest form of disorders of central nervous system involving cerebral vessels. These disorders come suddenly and interfere with the blood supply of the brain leading to neurological damage. The incidence of these disorders is on the rise and persons with uncontrolled diabetes, hypertension and heavy smokers are more liable to fall victim to them. Since most of them are due to atherosclerotic and degenrative changes in the vessels their incidence is mainly in the age group of 50 years and above.

The common forms of cerebrovascular diseases conist of:

1. Transient ischaemic attacks (TIAs)
2. Cerebral thrombosis
3. Cerebral embolism/infarction
4. Cerebral/subarachnoid haemorrhage.

Predisposing factors. A number of causes may act as risk factors, like uncontrolled diabetes, hypertension, obesity, hyperlipidaemia heavy cigarette smoking, polycythaemia, arteritis and use of oral contaceptives in women. Embolic strokes are as a result of valvular heart disease, ischaemic heart disease and congenital heart disease where embolism in the cerebral vessels occurs either due to arrhythmias like atrial fibrillation or infective endocarditis. Sometimes atheromatous plaques may get dislodged and produce a picture of cerebral emlolism. Further fall in blood pressure leading to hypotension, the process of autoregulation of blood supply in the cerebral blood vessels fails and depending on the degree of involvement it may be in the form of ischaemic stroke or thrombosis.

Transient ischaemic attacks (TIAs). These are transient attacks of loss of function of one part of the brain coming suddenly and lasting for variable period of time ranging from minutes to hours. Since arteries supplying the brain are end arteries so any pathology which produces obstruction to the flow of that vessel shall produce symptoms in the distribution of that blood vessel.

Internal carotid artery is one of the commonest cerebral vessel which is involved by atherosclerosis and patient complains of transient disturbances due to localized cortical ischaemia in the form of confusion contralteral hemiparesis and sensory loss.

There may be aphasia (if lesion on left side) and hemianopic visual loss. Most commonly occlusion is in the common carotid artery and one may be able to appreciate diminished pulsation in the vessel in the neck. When obstruction is severe a bruite may be auscultated at the site.

Obsturction of other arteries like anterior cerebral artery, middle cerebral artery and posterior cerebral artery produce picture almost like above except for little variations depending on the occlusion site. On the other hand involvement of posterior circulation (basilar artery, vertebral artery, post inferior cerebellar artery) produces a picture of crossed hemiplegia, hemisensory loss and hemianopic visual loss. In addition patient has impairement of consciousness, small fixed pupils, pseudobulbar palsy and quadriplegia seen mainly in basilar artery lesions while cases with posterior inferior cerebellar artery involvement are associated with severe vertigo, vomiting, dysphasia and diplopia. In addition there is some degree of cerebellar deficiency with hypotonia and incoordination on the side of lesion, analgesia and thermo anaesthesia on the face on the side of lesion and on the trunk and limbs on opposite side. Again neurological deficits shall be depending on which branch of the vessel is involved.

Diagnosis. It is based upon the previous hitory of such transient episodes of neurological deficit coming suddenly and lasting for a short time. In some these attacks are very transient and may have to be differentiated from other causes of transient loss of function like focal epilepsy. In cases of TIA there is presence of diseases like diabetes, hypertension etc. Person generally is in the age group where atherosclerosis is common.

Confirmation of the diagnosis is made by carotid angiography when transient ischaemia or narrowing of vessel is seen. Doppler echo flow studies are also important for assessing the blood flow and presence of any narrowing in the vessels.

Management of ischaemic stroke. A case of ischaemic stroke requires careful management since patient is in the twilight zone of cerebral ischaemia and stroke. When the attack has lasted for sometime it is better to use decongestant therapy in the form of Mannitol, infusion and Injection Dexamethasone 4 mg I/M 6 hourly. After the acute stage is over orally Glycerol 15 ml three times a day is given.

When a patient is having repeated attacks of ischaemic stroke or stroke in evolution, use of anticoagulants is consideried though it is risky and there is danger of cerebral leak or haemorrhage. Usually Injection Heparin 5000 units I/M six hourly is given for first few days. Dosage is monitored by keeping control of PTTK levels which should not exceed one and half to two times the pre-treatment values.

Once results have been obtained, patient is switched on oral anticoagulants (Table Dindevan 50 mg). Dosage has to be adjusted individually keeping a watch on bleding tendency.

Antiplatelet drugs are of use in prevention of thrombotic or ischaemic stroke. A daily dose of Aspirin (Dispirin) 75 mg is effective in inhibiting platelet aggregation. All coexisting disease like hypertension and diabetes must be treated and controlled properly. Hypertension is no contraindication to the use of anticoagulants though in such case caution has to be employed.

Cerebral thrombosis. It means occlusion of one of the branches of the carotid artery and is often preceded by one or two transient, ischaemic attacks. Common sites may be carotid artery in the head, basilar or vertebral artery in the neck. Cerebral thrombosis commonly results due to atherosclerosis when there is narrowing of the lumen of the vessel, thickning of the intima of the vessel wall and a thrombus results because of increased coagulability of blood and slowness of circulation.

Though cerebral atherosclerosis remains the commonest cause yet other diseases like syphilitic, thromboangitis obliterans and acute infections also are causative factors in some cases. Obstruction of the artery leads to an area of infarction in the brain and softening may take place at the site.

Symptoms. Onset is often preceded by prodromal symptoms in the form of transient attacks of paresis, and confusion. Sometimes this may take few days to evolve. Headache and giddiness are usually present. Deterioration in neurological symptoms starts within 48 hours when the thrombus extends and cerebral oedema develops. Commonly lesion is in internal capsule and patient has got an acute upper motor neurone lesion of body of one side. Face is also involved. At first the limbs are flaccid because of a state of shock. Aphasia is present if lesion is on the dominant side. Gradually there is recovery, tone in the limbs is increased, deep reflexes become exaggerated and plantar reflex is extensor (Babinski reflex).

In addition to a full fledged picture of hemiplegia, some patients have lacunar infarcts which are smaller in size (less than 2 cm) and occur in the subcortical area in the distribution of perforating arteries. Common sites are internal capsule, basal ganglia and pons. Generally the patient is dazed and unconsciousness does not occur. Multiple lacunar or large infarcts may produce a picture of generalized intellectual impairment. Depending on various localising signs, site of lesion can be clinically judged.

In lesion at the cortex, there is generally monoplegia. There is aphasia and sensory loss of cortical type. Convulsions may occur.

Subcortical. No convulsions, Weakness as well as sensory loss in contralateral limb may develop. Homonymous hemianopia if optic radiations involved.

Internal capsule. Complete hemiplegia, face may be involved.

Mid brain. Ipsilateral 3rd nerve palsy with crossed hemiplegia.

Brain stem lesion. Diplopia, nystagmus, vertigo, ipsilateral ataxia with contralateral sensory loss and hemiparesis.

Pons. Nuclear type of facial paralysis with crossed hemiplegia.

Progress of the case. It shall depend on the size and site of vessel involved. Thrombosis of the basilar artery carries poor prognosis. Depending on underlying conditions like hypertension, diabetes and atherosclerosis the progress of further attacks shall be assessed. Many patients fall prey to intercurrent infections. But once recovery starts

taking place the limbs tend to regain their power though it may take months to recover.

Investigations:

1. CSF is generally normal.
2. CT scan skull is essential to make a diagnosis. It will show low frequency infarcted areas or a low dense lesion.
3. Doppler echo flow studies will demonstrate narrowing of carotid vessels in its extracranial course.

Management. It consists of supportive and specific measures.

In general measure care of the patients nutrition, and feeding. Hydration and electrolyte balance be maintained. Prevention of bed sores, passive movements of hemiplegic side daily and active exercises as power returns, Massage of the limb is equally beneficial.

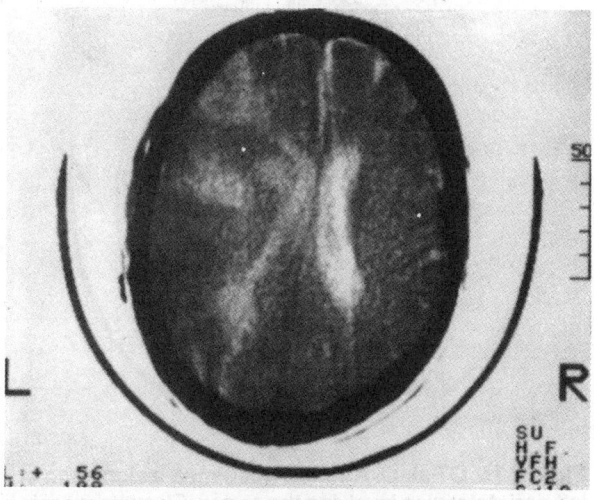

Fig. 10.14. CT Scan head. Multiple low density areas seen in left cerebral hemisphere. Third ventricle is normal and in midline. Left lateral ventricle compressed. Left sylvian fissures and cortical nuclei are effaced. Findings are suggestive of infarcts in the territory of left middle cerebral territory.

Specific treatment consists of decongestant therapy. Injection Mannitol 1 vial I/V twice a day. Inj. dexamethasone 4 mg I/V 6 hourly along with prophylactic cover of antibiotics (Injection Ampicillin 500 mg I/V 6 hourly) and antiplatelet drug dispirin 75 mg daily orally. If a patient comes within three hours after formation of clot. Tissue type plasminogen. Activator is administered 100 mg I/V slowly. This is called clot buster regimen and helps in improving supply of blood to dead part of brain.

Attempt should be made from the very beginning to do physiotherapy and massage of the paralysed limb. Role of anticoagulants in cerebral thrombosis is controversial and should not be employed because of the danger of start of haemorrhage in the brain. As the patient improves, mannitol is replaced by glycerol 15 ml twice a day along with dispirin (75 mg) orally once a day. Other antiplatelet drug Dipyradimole 75 mg once a day has also been employed. While giving antiplatelet drugs look for any bleeding tendencies.

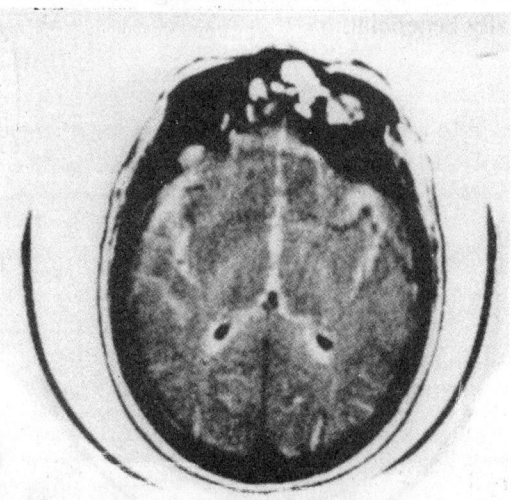

Fig. 10.15. CT skull. A small hypodense lesion seen in left parietal region involving the cortex. Elsewhere brain parenchyma shows normal attenuation pattern. Impression: Cortical infarct

In patients with aphasia language training must be started at the earliest. Recovery in a case of thrombosis depends on the extent of lesion, presence of accompanying diseases like diabetes, hypertension, age of the patient (very old and debililated patients have poor prognosis) and response of the patient to drug therapy as well as physiotherapy. Patients who become ambulatory early their prognosis is definately better since they are saved from development of bed sores, contractures and intercurrent infections.

Cerebral embolism. Sudden occlusion of a cerebral vessel due to a thrombus arising from the carotid, artery or its branches or from a diseased heart constitutes the picture of cerebral embolism which develops suddenly with production of neurological signs. Common causes of cerebral embolism are:

1. Thrombosis arising from the right subclavian artery.
2. Clot arising from aortic aneurysm or atheromatous ulcer in the innominate artery.
3. Embolus arising from a dilated left ventricle following myocardial infarction.
4. Vegetations detached from mitral or aortic valve in cases of infective endocarditis.
5. Pulmonary vein thrombosis and an infected emboli passes from the lung to the brain.
6. Chronic atrial fibrillation in cases of rheumatic, heart disease or atherosclerotic heart disease where a clot may get detached and lodges in the brain.

Pathology. The most common arteries involved are that of the left side of the brain as compared to that of the right. Left middle cerebral artery is the one which is most commonly effected. Following an embolus which lodges in one of the branches of the vessel, it may fragment and get inpacted in the smaller vessels. Thrombosis takes place at that site and produces cerebral infarction. Result is that blood supply to that part of the brain suffers. Infarct produced is generally haemorrhagic and if the embolus is infected, meningitis may develop later on.

Symptoms. Onset of the disease is sudden. A convulsion may occur at the beginning. Headache is variable and slight loss of consciousness may develop though it is never deep. Focal neurological disorder like monoplegia or aphasia may develop. Complete hemiplegia is not very common. Symptoms may be transient and become less in severity owing to the dislodgement of embolus.

Diagnosis. Based on clinical history and sudden onset of neurological features which may be transient, diagnosis is made. Confirmation is by CSF examination which shall exclude haemorrhage. CT scan helps in confirming the diagnosis.

Treatment. Treatment of cerebral embolism is mainly preventive. Patients of infective endocarditis must be adequately treated with antibiotics.

In those with atrial fibrillation complicating myocardial infarction, cardiac valve prosthesis and rheumatic heart disease, attempt should be made to restore sinus rhythm and maintain the patient on long term anticoagulation. If cerebral embolism has developed and there is neurological deficit treatment is on the same lines as in cases of cerebral thrombosis. Prognosis in a case of cerebral embolism is good since in majority of cases neurological deficit is not extensive and is transient.

Cerebral haemorrhage. Haemorrhage in the brain may be intracerebral, subarachnoid or intraventricular. The commonest cause of an intracerebral haemorrhage is rupture of an atheromatous artery in a person suffering from hypertension which in most of the cases is uncontrolled. Factor of degeneration of the cerebral blood vessels along with fluctuations of blood pressure levels account for most of the cases.

Most of the cases suffering from cerebral haemorrhage are either in elderly age group or late middle age. Young persons do not commonly suffer from it.

Cerebral haemorrhage may occur at any site though internal capsule is the commnest site. Other sites are lateral ventricle and subarachnoid space. Once haemorrhage takes place that part of the brain gets swollen and oedematous. The gyri are flattened. Midbrain is displaced to the side opposite the haemorrhage. Cerebral ventricles get distorted. As the site of haemorrhage is occupied by a clot it may get absorbed later on and is replaced by a scar tissue.

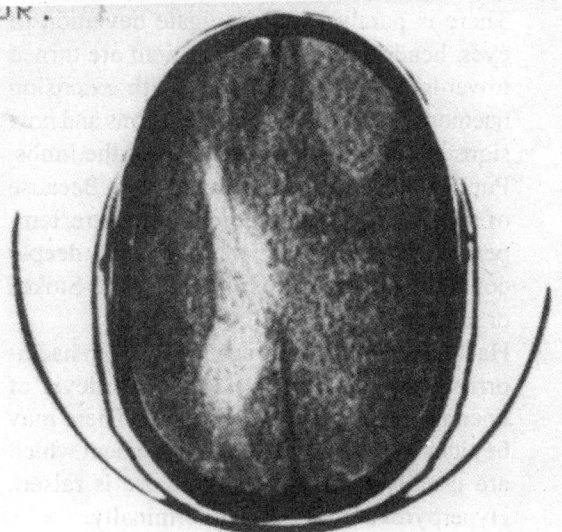

Fig. 10.17. CT Scan Head: A large chronic subdural haematoma is present in the right fronto parietal region. Midline structures show a contralateral shift. The right lateral ventricle and third ventricle show effacement. *Impression.* Chronic subdural haematoma in right frontoparietal region. It could be due to cerebral haemorrahage or following injury.

Symptoms. A known case of hypertension complains of severe headache accompnied by nausea, vomiting There may be premonitory symptoms in the form of transient speech disturbances or weakness of limbs. Once haemorrhage occurs patient become unconscious over a very short period.

In addition to general picture of an unconscious patient signs in a patient of cerebral haemorrhage shall depend on the site of the lesion.

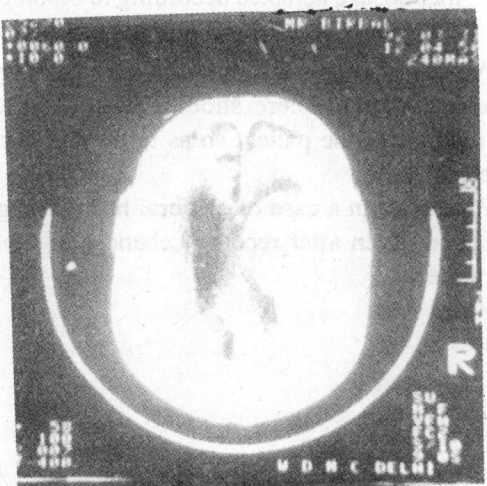

Fig. 10.16. CT Scan Head: This scan is from a 50 years old male, hypertensive who presented with sudden unconsciousness. There is evidence of intracerebral haemorrhage on right side.

1. In the region of internal capsule. Patient is unconscious and its depth depends on the degree of haemorrhage. Pulse is slow, and breathing is Cheyne-Stokes type. Neck rigidity is present. Head is rotated and eyes are deviated towards the side of lesion. Pupils are often unequal though they react to light. Papilloedema is present. There is flattening of nasolabial folds of face and absence of movements on the paralysed limb. Retention or incontinenece of urine may be present.

2. Pontine haemorrhage. In early stages there is facial paralysis on the side of the lesion with flaccid paralysis of limbs on the opposite side. There is paralysis of conjugate deviation of eyes, head and eyes of the patient are turned towards the paralysed side. With extension haemorrhage involves the whole pons and now signs include paralysis of face and the limbs. Pupils are contracted and pin pointed. Because of involvement of heat regulating centre, temperature levels rise. Patient is generally deeply comatose, respiration is either Cheyne-Stokes or laboured.

3. Haemorrhage into the ventricles. When haemorrhage extends into the ventricles, level of unconsciousness further deepens. There may be signs of pyramidal tract involvement which are usually bilateral. Temperature is raised. Hyperpyrexia may be seen terminally.

Diagnosis. Clinical picture of sudden unconsciousness preceded by severe headache, nausea and vomiting in a hypertensive patient should make one suspect it. CSF shows raised pressure. It is haemorrhagic, protein content is markedly raised. CSF sugar and chloride levels are normal. Cell count of CSF shows innumerable RBCs. CT scan skull is the most important diagnostic aid to locate the site of cerebral haemorrhage.

Treatment:

1. Patient should be put to complete bed rest and nursed with as little disturbance as possible. Maintain nutrition, hydration and electrolyte balance. Care of the bowel and bladder, keep respiratory passage clear.

2. For raised intracranial pressure Injection Dexamethasone 4 mg I/V 6 hourly in the acute stage.

3. *Epsilon amino caproic acid (EACA).* It is an analogue of amino acid lysine and is effective in cases of intravascular bleeding. Drug is to be given slowly intravenously in drip (5 g/20 ml). Rapid injection may result in hypotension, bradycardia and arrhythmias.

4. Use of antibiotics (Injection Ampicillin 500 mg I/V 6 hourly) to prevent any secondary infection).

5. Hypertension must be controlled since high levels of blood pressure shall further aggravate the condition. But rapid lowering of blood pressure is also not desirable. Usually injection Serpasil 1 mg i/m stat is given and further dosage adjusted according to blood pressure levels.

A case of cerebral haemorrhage requires great care in nursing. There should be no untoward disturbance of the patient so as to prevent further bleeding.

Prognosis in a case of cerebral haemorrhage is not good. Even after recovery chances of rebleed are there.

CHAPTER 11

Tropical and Infectious Diseases

1. Measles
2. Chickenpox
3. Smallpox
4. Mumps
5. Diphtheria
6. Whooping cough
7. Typhoid fever
8. Malaria
9. Syphilis
10. Gonorrhea
11. Acquired immunodefeciency syndrome (AIDS)

MEASLES (RUBEOLA)

It is a highly infective disease and spreads from person to person by droplet infection or by close contact. Humans are the natural host and disease may occur in epidemic form. Infants, young children, pregnant women and immuno compromised persons run the risk of getting the disease. Children below five years of age are more prone to suffer from measles and the disease generally is common below the age of ten years. Infants below six months rarely suffer from the disease because of transmitted maternal immunity.

Incubation period. It is usually between 9-12 days. Period of infectivity is from the onset of symptoms i.e. 4-5 days after exposure to virus to the appearanceof rash lasting 4-5 days afterwards. It is most infective during the catarrhal stage of the disease. The infectivety declines with the appearance of the rash.

Etiologic agent. Measles is caused by a Paramyxovirus which is an RNA enveloped virus possessing six major proteins. The virus is present in nasopharyngeal secretions and enters the body either through respiratory passages or conjunctive. Virus multiplies in the epithelium of respiratory passages and can be isolated from respiratory secretions, blood and conjunctive a few days before and one or two days after the appearance of rash.

Pathology. The primary change is hyperplasia of the lymphoid tissue which is generalized and shows multinucleated giant cells, histiocytes and cytoplasmic inclusion bodies. Secondary infection may occur in the respiratory tract and bronchial glands get inflamed. Lungs may show interstitial pneumonia and there is aggregation of lymphoid tissue in the small intestines.

Clinical picture. The initial features are malaise, fever, cough i.e. three C's Coryza, Conjunctivitis and Cough. It is the catarrhal stage when in addition to fever patient has got running nose, excessive lacrimation or watering from the eyes, photophobia, swelling of the eyelids and a cough which is dry hacking type as well as hoarseness of voice. The catarrhal stage lasts for 3-4 days and before the appearance of rash, small greyish irregular lesions surrounded by erythema appear on the buccal mucosa opposite the second molar tooth. These are called Koplik's spots and are diagnostic of the disease especially in early stages.

Measles	
1. Incubation period	9-12 days
2. Etiologic agent	Paramyxovirus
3. Clinical picture	Coryza, conjunctivitis, cough
	Catarrhal stage
	Stage of rash
	Convalescence
4. Complications	
Respiratory	Laryngitis, bronchitis, broncho or lobar pneumonia
Ear Nose Throat	Otitis media, mastoiditis
GI tract	Stomatitis, gastro-enteritis, hepatitis
Cardiac	Myocarditis, pericarditis endocarditis
Nervous system	Encephalitis, ence-phalomyelitus

The rash appears one to two days afterwards. The viraemia which was earlier present now gets exaggerated. Temperature rises sharply and nasal and conjunctival discharges become purulent.

The rash appears first at the back of the ear, forehead and spreads rapidly to the face, neck, extremities and trunk. The rash is dark red macular, maculo papular giving a brownish red appearance. At some places it may fuse. Face is the most densely effected area. Itching may be present. Skin is moist and may give a peculiar musty smell.

The rash disappears in 5-6 days in the same order in which it appeared leaving behind brownish discoloration and desquamation. During the period of rash there are signs of generalized toxaemia and malaise. Headache, irritability a sore congested throat with a feeling of wretchdness are common symptoms. Pulse is rapid, tongue is coated and

furred. With disappearance of rash, fever comes down with crisis and malaise and toxaemia subsides.

Varieties of measles. One may come across severe forms of measles and these are toxic, pulmonary and haemorrhagic.

Toxic form is characterised by malignant form of the disease and is manifested by high fever, delirium, circulatory failure and often proves fatal.

Pulmonary form has predominantly fulminating respiratory infection with high temperature and a rapid respiration.

Haemorrhagic type of measles is rare. Here there are haemorrhages into the mucous membranes, skin and subcutaneous tissues.

Complications. Measles generally runs a mild course but malnourished children, persons in immunocompromised conditions, and pregnant women run the risk of getting complications involving respiratory passages G.I. Tract and nervous system.

Various systemic complications include respiratory, (bronchitis, laryngitis, broncho or lobar pneumonia) and in ears (otitis media) mastoid inflammation, G.I. system (gastroenteritis, stomatitis, hepatitis) cardiac (myocarditis, endocarditis and pericarditis) and neurological (encephalomyelitus).

Diagnosis. It is generally based on clinical picture. Serological tests include identification of immunoglobulin M (IgM) and measles antibody by ELISA test.

Acute and convalescent sera are sometimes tested for rise in specific antibodies by hemagglutination-inhibition (HI) complement fixation (CF) and neutralizing antibody techniques.

Treatment. Measles is a self limiting disease and the treatment is usually supportive. The patient should preferably be nursed in a slightly dark room if there is photophobia. Semi solid nutritious food should be given. Where there is secondary bacterial infections antibiotics should be used.

Anti viral drug Ribavirin has been found to be effective against measles virus in vitro but its use is not recomended.

Prevention. An attack of measles results in high degree of immunity and so second attacks are not common.

In people who have been exposed to infection, human immunoglobin 0.25 ml/kg within five days of exposure effectively protects from the disease or the attack is of minimal nature. Children below three years, pregnant women and those suffering from debilitating illnesses should be given this form of passive immunization.

For active immunization live attenuated measles vaccine 0.5 ml is given subcutaneously. It provides immunity lasting for about 10 years. This vaccine is not to be given to infants below 15 months of age since these children fail to respond due to presence in the circulation of residual measles antibody of maternal origin. A combined vaccine consisting of measles, rubella and mumps is also employed.

CHICKENPOX (VARICELLA)

It is an acute infectious disease, universally prevalent and mainly effects children below 10 years of age though elder children and young adults are also effected.

An acute attack of the disease is characterised by fever and a rash which appears in crops. It is highly contagious and in most cases it is self limiting. One attack of chickenpox usually affords complete protection from future attacks.

Etiologic agent. Chickenpox is caused by varicella virus which is closely related to herpes simplex virus, cytomegalovirus and epstein bar virus (EBV). It is a DNA virus and multiplies in the nuclei of infected cells.

The major source of virus are discharges from the respiratory tract and skin lesion. Virus enters the respiratory passages by droplet infection and when patient scratches the skin lesions it becomes aerosolized. Although respiratory tract remains an important source of conveying the virus yet it is difficult to culture the virus from respiratory secretions.

Incubation period. It is between 10 to 21 days.

The spread of disease is air borne and person to person contact. The infectious period is one to two days before the appearance of the rash and lasts till all the skin lesions have crusted which is usually 5-7 days.

Clinical picture. It consists of a stage of invasion or prodromal stage and stage of eruption.

Stage of invasion. The prodromal symptoms are mild and consist of fever, headache backache, malaise and sore throat. This stage usually lasts for 2-3 days. Child is irritable and restless. This is followed by the appearance of eruption which is generally taken to be the first day of the disease.

Chickenpox	
1. Incubation period	10-21 days
2. Etiologic agent	Varicella virus
3. Clinical picture	(i) Stage of invasion or prodromal stage
	(ii) Stage of eruption
	(iii) Convalescence
4. Complications	
Respiratory	Laryngitis, bronchitis, Bronchopneumonia
Skin	Erysipelas, cellulitis, impetigo
Renal	Nephritis
Systemic	Arthritis, encephalo myelitis, myocarditis, purpura

In majority of patients this is a mild stage but in debilitated children, adults and immuno-compromised person it is a fulminating course.

Before the appearance of skin rash, enanthem develops over the palatal, buccal and pharyngeal mucosa.

Stage of eruption. The eruption of chickenpox first appears on the back and then spreads to the other parts of body like face, scalp, chest, abdomen and lastly the proximal part of limbs. The rash appears in the form of crops, at first macular then papular, vesicular and becomes pustular in 24 hours. Distribution of rash is centripetal maximally affecting face, trunk and limbs from above and sparing the distal part of extremities. Appearance of crops of rash after a lapse of a day or two may produce skin lesions in various stages of development at the same time. Pruritis is intense and often leads to rupture of the vesicles. Vesicles present on the mucous membranes may rupture leaving behind shallow grey ulcers.

Rashes generally last for 3-4 days and after that are followed by the formation of scabs which fall off in a few days leaving behind superficial scars. Complete clearance of skin may take few days.

Varieties of chickenpox. Generally chickenpox is a mild disease but sometimes variable form of the disease may be seen. There are three varieties:

1. Varicella bullosa characterised by formation of bullous eruptions.
2. Varicella gangrenosa: It is seen in ill nourished children and there are dark crusts formed in the eruptions which on separation leave behind ulcers.
3. Varicella haemorrhagica: It is uncommon but a very virulent form of varicella. Haemorrhages occur into the vesicles and bleeding may take place from mucous membranes.

Complications. Generally the extent of rash is a good indication of mildness or severity of the disease. In patients with serious illness the number and extent of skin lesions is massive. Various forms of complications include respiratory (laryngitis bronchitis, bronchopneumonia) skin (secondary infection with staphylococci or haemolytic streptococci may produce erysipelas, cellulitis or impetigo) kidney (nephritis) and arthritis.

Neurological involvement is not common but may be in the form of encephalomyelitis, ataxia, transverse myelitis and optic neuritis. Myocarditis, purpura and keratitis are some of the other complications.

Since herpes zoster is closely related to varicella, a scattered rash simulating chickenpox may precede or accompany an attack of herpes zoster though the reverse in cases of chickenpox is not common.

Diagnosis. Clinical picture of a case of chickenpox is very typical. A child presenting with a rash with its typical distribution and coming in crops and presenting with macule, papules, vesicles pustules and scabs at the same time is quite diagnostic.

In cases of doubt diagnosis is confirmed by staining of skin scrapings with fluorescein labelled monoclonal antibody and the diagnosis is made within a few hours. Skin lesions can also be cultured for the presence of virus.

Treatment. Since it is a contagious disease the patient should be isolated till every scale has separated. In the majority of cases only symptomatic treatment is required. Child should be confined to bed especially in the stage when rash is developing.

Analgesics like Paracetamol syrup 1 teasponful thrice a day is given to relieve pain and fever. Many times the child is irritable. In such case phenergan syrup 1 teasponful twice a day is advised. It shall also relieve pruritis.

In immunocompromised patients and those either with serious complications or virulent form of the disease antiviral drug Acyclovir (20 mg/kg body weight) in four divided doses is given for five days. Secondary infection should be treated with broad spectrum antibiotics.

Prophylaxis. It is always advisable to isolate children with chickenpox and care should be taken to protect the contacts.

Passive immunization is produced by use of varicella zoster immune globulin (VZIG) in a dose of 0.5-1 ml/kg body weight within 72 hours of exposure.

Live attenuated varicella vaccine (varivax) in a dose of 0.5 ml is administered in all children above the age of 12 months for immunization. It induces cell mediated immunity and protects against or significantly reduces the morbidity associated with primary VZV infections. A booster dose after six years of vaccination is also given in some children.

Prognosis. A case of chickenpox has a self limiting course and in an uncomplicated case prognosis is good.

PLATE XIX

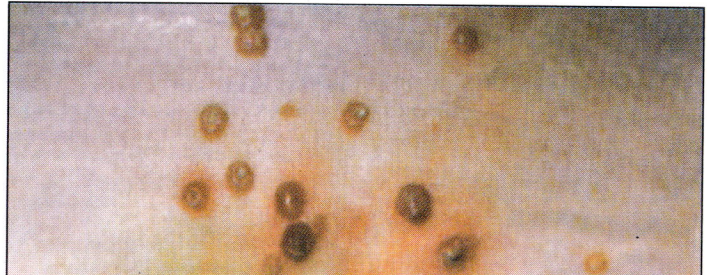

Molluscum contagiosum

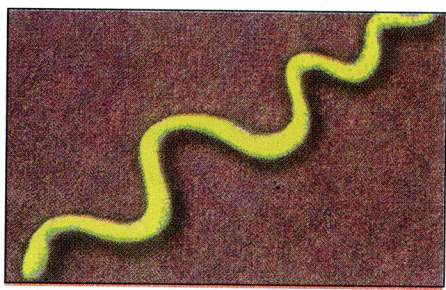

T. pallidum organism

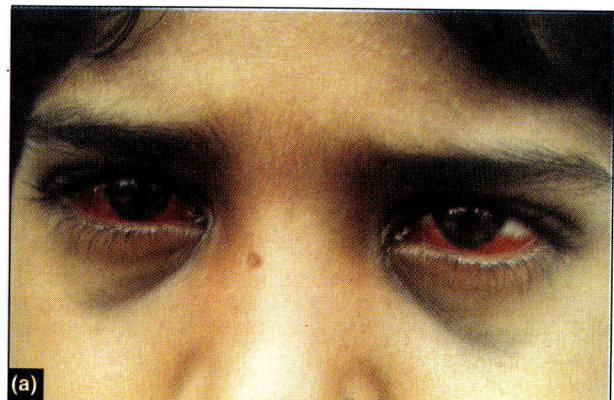

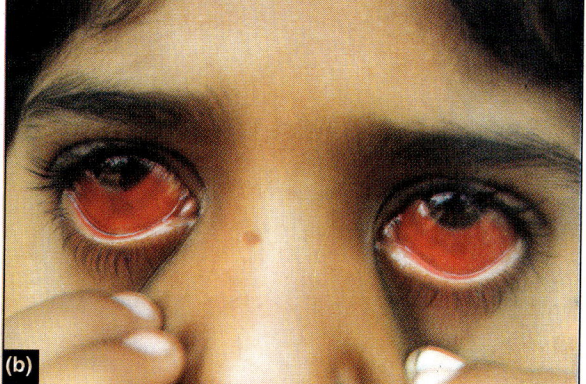

Figs. (a) & (b) showing subconjunctival haemorrhages in a child suffering from whooping cough

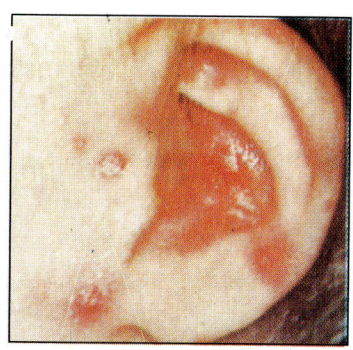

Chickenpox: Lesions around the ear

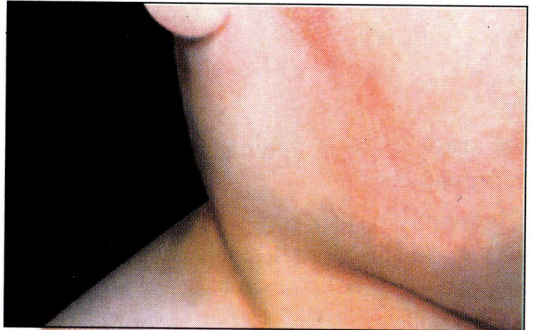

Mumps: Note parotid swelling

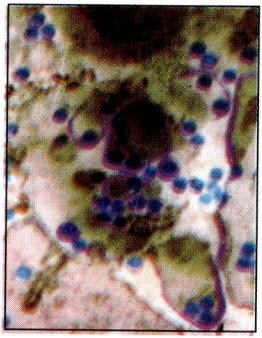

Dengue fever virus

PLATE XX

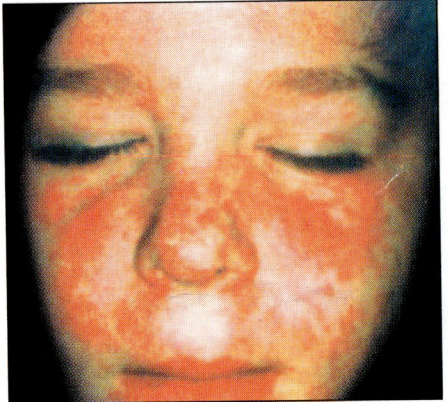

Maculopapular rash in measles

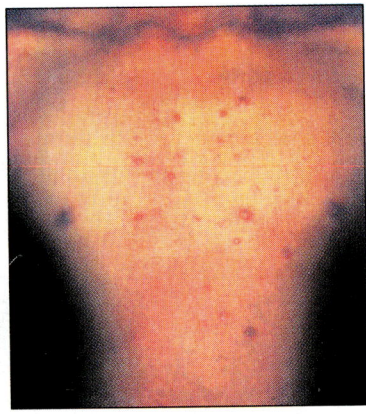

Chickenpox rash

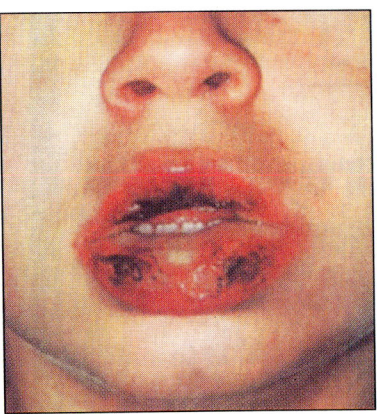

Herpes simplex stomatitis

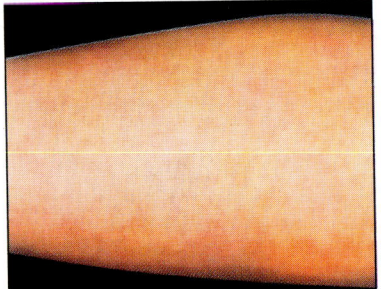

Rubella

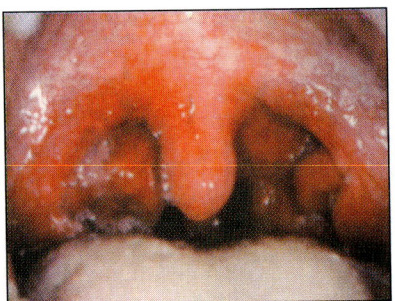

Glandular fever

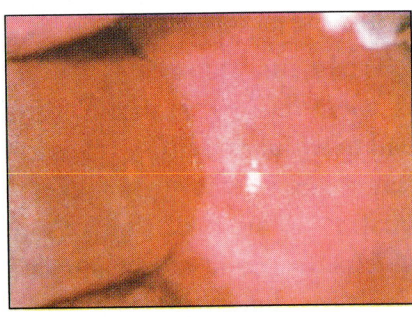

Koplik's spots in measles

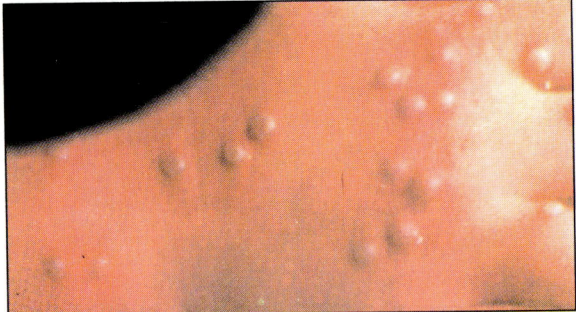

Smallpox rash

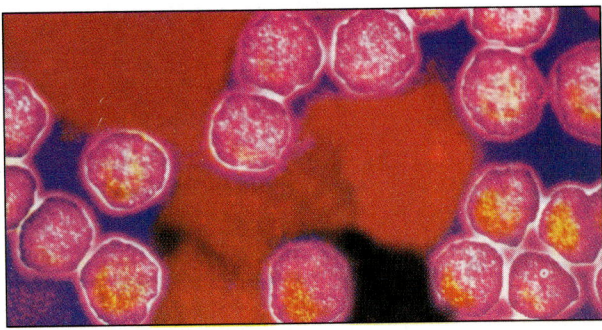

Rubella virus

SMALLPOX (VARIOLA)

It is a highly infectious disease caused by variola virus which belongs to group of pox viruses which are DNA viruses. For centuries disease has been endemic in various parts of the world often occurring in epidemics especially during winter and spring months but with the introduction of mass vaccination the disease has been almost eradicated though one does come across an occasional case of smallpox.

Infection spreads via the respiratory tract and may be by direct contact with the patient or through fomites or the objects contamined by the sick person. Infection may also be conveyed by aerial route.

The *incubation period* ranges from 10-14 days. Infectivity of the disease is slight at the onset of symptoms but increases with the appearance of eruption till the shedding of last scale. Virus is present in nasal secretions, vesicles and dried scabs. It is very resistant to dry heat and may persist in scabs for even one year. Characteristically after virus enters the body it reaches circulation via lymphatics and lymph nodes after multiplying there. There is wide spread involvement of skin and mucous membrane. Epithelial cells of pocks of smallpox contain intracellular bodies known as Guarnieri bodies which are in fact aggregation of virus particles.

Clinical picture. It consisits of a prodromal stage where there is abrupt onset of high fever, frontal headache, backache, sore throat, delirium, insomnia and vomiting accompanied by abdominal pain. These symptoms vary in intensity and may precede the eruption for one or two days. Stage of toxaemia generally lasts two to three days.

Stage of eruption. On the third day of infection the rash starts appearing. First part to be involved are buccal, faucial and pharyngeal mucosa, followed by appearance of rash which appears on the face and distal parts of the limbs. Fever which was high on the first day of illness now comes down to reappear again when pustules form. Rash typically is centrifugal in distribution appearing first on the forehead, face, arm, trunk and legs. Spread of the rash is rapid and often symmetrical. Initial lesions are small pin head macules which become papules in few hours progressing to vesicles in two days followed by pustules lasting for four days. Pustules tend to dry up on the 9th and 10th day. Brown or thick black crusts may be formed by the collapse of these pustules and by the end of thirteenth or fourteenth day when the scabs are separated, deep pitted scars may be left behind. Temperature falls and scabbing continues in the third week. Depending on the severity of the lesion, depressed scars with pitting are distributed at various sites in the body but mainly on face.

Smallpox	
1. Incubation period	10-14 days
2. Etiologic agent	Variola virus
3. Clinical picture	(i) Prodromal stage
	(ii) Stage of eruption
	(iii) Convalescence
4. Complications	
Respiratory	Bronchitis, broncho-pneumonia
Systemic	Parotitis, arthritis, conjunctivitis, panophthalmitis
Cardiac	Myocarditis, pericarditis, endocarditis
Nervous system	Encephalomyelitis

Varieties of smallpox:

1. *Confluent smallpox.* Here rash is profuse and more on face. There is fusion of rash. Toxaemia is severe and patient lies in moribund state. Pus may ooze from the lesions and an offensive odour comes out. Some patients may pass into circulatory collapse.

2. *Haemorrhagic smallpox.* It is the most malignant form. Pupuric spots and haemorrhages appear on the skin, conjunctiva and mucous surfaces. It carries high degree of morbidity and mortality.

3. *Modified smallpox.* It is a mild form of modified type of smallpox where the initial symptoms may be severe, the rash appearing early

and tends to resolve early. It generally occurs in vaccinated individuals.

4. *Variola minor.* It is a mild form of disease with mild course. It has less infectivity and there are no residual pitting or scars. It occurs more in adults than in children.

Complications. These include secondary infection the rash becoming septic. Deep seated abscesses or cellulitis with sloughing of skin may develop. There may be development of parotitis, otitis media, bronchitis, broncho pneumonia, septic arthritis. Mucous membranes of the eyes, nasal cavities may be involved. Involvement of eye is the most dangerous complication Pustules may form in the conjunctive and cornea leading to Panophthalmitis and blindness. In nervous system encephalomyelitis and neuropathy may occur while myocardial failure and pericarditis may be other serious complications.

Diagnosis. It is based on clinical picture of the case. Main difference is from chickenpox. Here the rash is centrifugal, more on face and distal parts of limbs, palms and soles of feet and less on covered parts of body. While in chickenpox it is centripetal i.e. more on the body and tends to avoid the extremities. The eruption comes in crops. The lesions are superficial and do not umbilicate.

Laboratory diagnosis:

1. Demonstration of variola virus in material derived from vesicles.
2. Paul's test which depends on the production of guarnieri bodies by scarification of the cornea of rabbit with fluid derived from vesicle.
3. Demonstration of viral antigen by complement fixation test or precipitation test in the fluid derived from eruptions.

Prognosis. It is guarded in a case of smallpox and shall be guided by age of the patient, nature of the attack and previous vaccination.

It is poor in malnourished children, very small children and infants as well as those who are immunocompromised. Serious complications and haemorrhagic form of the disease carry poor prognosis.

Treatment. It is mainly symptomatic. Patient should be nursed in isolation with strict barrier nursing. Care of nutrition, hydration and electrolyte balance be taken. For contacts vaccinia immunoglobulins offer some protection.

In cases where secondary infection is suspected prophylactie use of antibiotics is advisable.

For prevention of smallpox vaccination is the ideal method. It consists of killed or freeze dried vaccinia virus. Children between the ages of six to 12 months and again after five to seven years are vaccinated. Complications include pyogenic infection at the site, post vaccinal rashes, generalised vaccinia and post vaccinal encelphalitis.

MUMPS

Mumps is a widely prevalent infectious disease and is endemic in most parts of the world. The disease commonly involves children and young adults. It is usually seen during winter months or spring.

It is caused by mumps virus belonging to group of Paramyxoviruses and contains single stranded RNA in a helical nucleocapsid.

Humans are the only natural host and infection spreads by droplet infection as well as by direct contact with respiratory secretions of the patient. *Incubation period* usually ranges from 12 to 22 days average being 16-18 days.

Clinical picture. The onset of the disease is by moderate fever, sore throat and stiffness in the region of masseter muscles, pain or tenderness on pressure beneath the angle of the jaw. Sometimes fever comes with rigors and chills.

A day or two after the prodromal symptoms the swelling of the parotid gland is seen and may be first indication of the disease. Parotid swelling at first is unilateral, often on the left side the gland enlarges in size reaching maximum in about two to three days time. The swelling is ill defined and often obliterates sulcus between mandible and mastoid process. Sometimes i.e. 24-36 hours after the start of illness swelling may appear in the other gland. Skin over the gland may be red and shiny. There is often trismus and pain on opening the jaw. Fever may rise to 103°F or 104°F. Other salivary glands are also now involved and become enlarged and tender. Cervical glands are also enlarged.

In addition patient has features of toxaemia. Tongue is furred and there is diminished salivation. Breath is foul smelling. Parotid duct is also involved generally bilaterally. After a week the fever subsides and glandular enlargement starts regressing.

Blood picture in acute stage is that of moderate leucocytosis with relative lymphocytosis.

Complications. Generally a case of mumps runs a mild self limiting course but in young adults a number of complications may arise.

Orchitis occurs in 15-25 per cent of persons generally on the seventh or eighth day of illness. Sometimes it occurs on the second or third day. Onset is characterised by pain in the testes which are swollen, tender and tense. Fever ranges upto 103°F. Delirium and collapse may accompany orchitis. Not only testes are swollen but there is involvement of scrotum, epididymis, spermatic cord etc. Orchitis to start with is unilateral but in small percentage both testes get involved. Recovery takes place in a week to ten days time but it may result in sterility.

In females, oophoritis, inflammation of the breast (mastitis) and swelling of the vulva may occur.

In the second week pancreatitis characterised by acute pain in the epigastric region, and vomiting may develop. Glycosuria and raised blood sugar levels are seen.

Nervous system also gets involved though not very commonly. Neurological complications include meningismus and meningoencephalitis developing towards the end of first week or beginning of second week.

Other complications include otitis media producing deafness, papilloedema, retrobulbar neuritis, optic atrophy, bronchopneumonia, myocarditis, pericarditis and arthritis which comes after two to three weeks of acute illness.

Suppuration of the parotid gland with involvement of the floor of the mouth, cervical glands and gangrene may develop in some cases especially those who are debilitated and immunocompromised.

Diagnosis. Clinical diagnosis of mumps can be made in any young child coming with fever, malaise and a parotid gland enlargement.

Confirmation can be made by isolating and culturing the virus obtained from throat, saliva, urine and CSF fluid.

Complement fixation, haemagglutination inhibition or ELISA tests will show significant rise in titre between acute and convalescent serum specimen.

Treatment. It is mainly supportive and symptomatic. Child is put to bed rest. Mouth hygiene must be maintained meticulosly. Analgesics and antipyretics are the main stay of treatment (Paracetamol/Nimulid syrup 1-2 teasponful two to three times a day).

Diet should be soft, bland and preferably in liquid form.

In cases where complications like orchitis or neurological complications develop, prednisolone 40-60 mg per day in divided doses for about seven days is given along with antibiotics (Ampicillin/Amoxycillin/Cefazolin/Ceftizoxime).

Prevention. A patient of mumps is contagious upto seven days before the onset of parotid swelling

Mumps		
1. Incubation period	12-22 days	
2. Etiologic agent	Mumps virus (Paramyxovirus)	
3. Clinical picture	(i) Prodromal stage	
	(ii) Stage of Parotid swelling	
	(iii) Convalescence	
4. Complications		
Systemic	Orchitis, Epididmo-orchitis (in men)	
	Oophoritis mastitis (in women), Arthritis	
G.I.Tract	Pancreatitis	
Nervous system	Meningismus, Meningo-encephalitis, optic atrophy, retrobulbar neuritis	
Cardiac	Myocarditis, pericarditis	

and may remain so for about nine days after onset. During this period attempt should be made to isolate the child so that the disease does not spead.

As such mumps runs a benign course but it is the development of complications which pose a serious challenge. For persons exposed to infection gamma globulins derived from convalescent serum are administered and have protective role.

A live attenuated mumps virus vaccine should be given to all children between the age of 12-15 months. It generally is given as combined measles-mumps-rubella vaccine (MMR). A single dose confers almost long lasting immunity. A second dose may be given between four to 12 years of age.

Prognosis. Recovery from mumps is generally uneventful. Prognosis as a rule is good. Mortality occurs in small percentage of cases who have got seious complications, are ill nourished and immuno compromised.

DIPHTHERIA

Diphtheria is of world wide distribution being commonest in temperate climates. It is highly contagious disease and infection spreads mainly through droplet infection, by speaking coughing or sneezing. The organisms reside in secretions from the nose and throat, in membrane formed in throat, infected wounds and spread occasionally through close contact.

The causative organism is corynebacterium diphtheriae, a gram positive, non sporing organism which is slender rod like, straight or slightly curved with a tendency to branch. Based on biochemical reactions and haemolytic properties C diphtheriae has been divided into three main types, gravis, mitis and intermedius type. All these three strains produce a potent toxin responsible for its virulent effects.

The incubation period of disease is usually two to six days and spread of infection is through close contact. Children are the most prone to suffer from it though occasionally it may involve adults. Untreated patients are usually infective upto a period of two weeks.

Diphtheria	
1. Incubation period	2-6 days
2. Etiologic agent	Corynebacterium diphtheriae
3. Varieties of diphtheria	Pharyngeal, laryngeal, nasal, cutaneous, conjunctival
4. Complications	
Cardiovascular	Toxic myocarditis, acute circulatory failure
Respiratory	Bronchitis, bronchopneumonia, otitis media
Nervous system	Paralysis of palate, bulbar, facial paralysis, cerebral thrombosis
Renal	Toxic nephritis

Pathology. The main constitutional symptoms are as a result of toxins being absorbed from the primary lesion whose severity guides the degree of toxaemia.

There is epithelial necrosis with formation of a sero fibrinous exudate resulting in a bluish white membrane. This membrane contains fibrin, epithelial cells, blood and leucocytes. It is adherant to the underlying tissue and when removed leaves behind a raw bleeding surface.

Formation of membrane at tonsils, soft palate faucial pillars, pharynx and larynx is common. It may extend downwards to the trachea Toxins may be absorbed from the primary site and involve various organs including heart, kidney, liver and nervous system. There may be extensive degeneration and inflammation in these organs.

Clinical picture. Diphtheria may have a mild, moderate or severe course. The clinical picture of any case shall depend on the site which is involved.

All cases have prodromal symptoms in the form of headache, sore throat, malaise, nasal discharge, vague aches and pains in the body and loss of appetite. Fever is moderate in intensity but may come on with chills.

Varieties of diphtheria. *The various form are:*

1. Pharyngeal diphtheria
2. Laryngeal diphtheria

3. Nasal diphtheria
4. Cutaneous diphtheria
5. Conjunctival diphtheria.

Pharyngeal diphtheria. It is the commonest form of diphtheria and is characterised by toxaemia, congestion and oedema of palate with formation of a membrane in pharynx which is generally thin glistening pearly white in early stages and becomes thick, greyish and opaque later on. It is adherent to underlying structure and has well defined borders. It bleeds on forcible removal. It may extend to palate, uvula.

There are feature of lymphadenopathy in neck (bull neck appearances), breath is foul smelling. Fever does not correspond to the gravity of the disease.

In second week patient may pass into circulatory collapse. There is lethargy and restlessness. Pulse may become irregular. Respiration is rapid and shallow. Repeated vomiting takes place. Some patients may pass into cardiac failure. Neurological complications occur in the third week. It may be in the form of paralysis of palate and pharynx.

Laryngeal diphtheria. It is common in young children and is characterised by hoarseness, brassy cough followed by attacks of inspiratory stridor, and laryngeal spasm. Membrane is generally limited to larynx and may spread to air passages. These children suffer from respiratory obstruction and may run a fatal course.

Nasal diphtheria. It is in the form of a serous discharge followed by a mucopurulent one often blood stained. Here the membrane is confined to the anterior part of nasal septum. The disease is often unilateral. There is foul smell coming. It may be the only way of presentation. It may extend to other parts of pharynx. Nasal diphtheria is not very common and is present in only two to three per cent of cases.

Cutaneous diphtheria. C diphtheria organism when it gains entry through abrasions and wounds produces punched out ulcers often covered by greyish membrane.

Conjunctival diphtheria. It is due to direct involvement of the eyes by the organism or may spread from nose. It generally occurs in very small children and is chracterised by severe congestion in eyes and a discharge.

Complications. Various complications can be:

1. Acute circulatory failure. It may develop in the first few days.
   Toxic myocarditis in a case of diphtheria is a serious complication. It is characterised by tachycardia, feeble heart sounds, cardiac enlargement, tic tac rhythm and arrhythmias. Sudden death may occur.
   Congestive heart failure is not very common. Electrocardiographic changes are generally non-specific.
2. Respiratory complications like bronchitis, bronchopneumonia, respiratory obstruction and respiratory paralysis.
3. Toxic neurological damage generally occurs in 3rd to 6th week. It may be paralysis of palate, paralysis of accommodation, facial paralysis, bulbar paralysis and muscles of respiration. Peripheral neuropathy also develops though at a late stage.
4. Renal complications like toxic nephritis. It is generally seen on 10th day.
5. Vascular involvement especially of middle cerebral artery leading to a picture of thrombosis or monoplegia.
6. Other complications include otitis media and arthritis.

Diagnosis. In addition to clinical picture of a sore throat toxaemia and a greyish membrane adherent to the pharynx diagnosis is confirmed by direct smear and culture of secretions either by a nasopharyngeal or laryngeal swab and demonstrating the organism.

Schick test is done to determine whether an individual is susceptible to diphtheria or not. Intracutaneous injection of 1/50 MLD of toxin contained in 0.1 cc of diluent is injected. Susceptible person shall show a reddish reaction in 24-36 hours. Late positive reaction may be observed after one week.

Treatment. General supportive measures like soft semisolid food analgesics and antipyretics.

Specific therapy consists in the administration of anti-diphthertic serum (ADS) in thedose ranging from 20,000 units to 120,000 units depending on the extent of involvement and severity of disease process. Drug is to be given by intramuscular route. Before giving ADS sensitivity test be done.

Since C. diphtheriae is sensitive to erythromycin and penicillin these drugs are given as adjuvant to antitoxin. Injection Penicillin 5 lacs unit I/M or Erythromycin 40 mg/kg body weight in four divided doses for seven days. These drugs are sufficient to take care of the disease as well as secondary infection.

Management of complications. Cardiovascular complications are the major risk. In addition to antitoxin, antibiotics, vasopressor drugs in circulatory collapse. Injection Betamethasone 8 mg four times a day is beneficial. Cases who develop arrhythmias shall require appropriate drugs. Digitalis is indicated if congestive failure develop.

In cases where there is palatal paralysis in acute stage nasogastric tube feeding may be required. Respiratory paralysis is managed by oxygen and ventilator.

Prevention. For passive immunization 1000-2000 units of diphtheria antitoxin for temporary protection to all close contacts be given. Immunity lasts for two weeks. In addition all close contacts be given erythromycin (40 mg/kg/day for seven days) as anti-microbial prophylaxis.

Active immunisation of all children with triple vaccine containing diphtheria. Tetanus and pertussis (DPT) is done at third month followd by further two doses at monthly interval.

Prognosis. It depends on the severity of disease process as well as on the type of diphtheria. It is poor in severe and malignant form. Very small children carry poor prognosis.

Haemorrhagic symptoms, cardiovascular collapse and respiratory paralysis carry poor prognosis.

WHOOPING COUGH (PERTUSSIS)

Whooping cough or pertussis is a disease of young children and is highly contagious. The disease is of world wide distribution and carries a high degree of morbidity.

It is caused by Pertussis borderella, a gram-negative coccobacillus responsible for 90-95 per cent of cases and by B. parapertussis in about 5 per cent of the cases. Small outbreaks of whooping cough like illness may also occur due to B. bronchiseptica. The clinical picture by these three organisms is almost similar though the disease with the last two is of mild form.

The only natural reservoir of these organisms is human being and spread occurs through droplet infection and from aerosals generated by intense cough and sneezing of the infected patients. Since in early stages the disease resembles an upper respiratory tract infection the diagnosis is not suspected and the patient goes on infecting other people. The incubation period is usually seven to ten days but may be prolonged to 15-20 days.

Disease generally involves children below five years of age and children in most intimate contact are likely to get infected. The incidence of disease declines after the age of ten.

Whooping cough	
1. Incubation period	7-10 days
2. Etiologic agent	Borderella pertussis
3. Clinical picture	(i) Catarrhal stage
	(ii) Paroxysmal stage
	(iii) Convalescence
4. Complications	
Respiratory	Bronchitis, broncho-pneumonia, bronchiectasis, pneumothorax
Systemic	Conjunctival haemmorrhages, intracranial haemorrhage, encephalitis, ulceration of tongue.

Clinical picture. *The disease can be divided into three stages:*

1. Catarrhal stage
2. Paroxysmal stage
3. Convalescence

Catarrhal stage. Disease has an insidious onset and starts with fever, running nose, sore throat and cough which is troublesome. Cough to start with is simple but soon assumes a paroxysmal character with intense severity at night. Picture at this stage is like that of an upper respiratory catarrah. This is the most infective period. The catarrhal stage lasts for seven days to a fortnight.

Paroxysmal stage. It starts at the end of second week. Cough now is severe and occurs in the form of repeated paroxysms. Each paroxysm of cough is followed by a long drawn inspiratory effort through a narrowed glottis resulting in 'Whoop'. There may be single or repeated paroxysms of cough punctuated by whoops and terminated by vomiting or expectorating thick mucus. During the paroxysm the face becomes congested. Superficial veins are engorged, eyes are filled with tears and sometimes subconjunctival haemorrhages may develop. Child is irritable and sweating.

Physical examination of chest shows diffuse crepts and rhonchi. This stage may last from few days to three to four weeks.

Incubation period of various infectious diseases	
Disease	Days
1. Measles	09-12 days
2. Chickenpox	10-12 days
3. Smallpox	10-14 days
4. Mumps	10-22 days
5. Diphtheria	02-06 days
6. Whooping cough	07-10 days
7. Typhoid fever	10-14 days

Convalescent stage. This begins in the fourth week. There is now decrease in the intensity and frequency of paroxysms. Whoops disappear. Vomiting declines and cough also disappears. Since the childs immunity is at low level and he is exhausted because of prolonged illness, chances of super infection by other pathogens is there and may lead to development of various complications.

On an average this stage generally lasts for one to two weeks and by this time the child is fully recovered.

Complications. These may be mechanical or inflammatory: Mechanical is in the form of rupture of emphysematous bullae leading to pneumothorax, or ulceration of the tongue due to biting of tongue or prolapse of rectum or subconjuctival haemorrhages due to bouts of coughing.

Respiratory complications include bronchitis, bronchopneumonia, bronchiectasis. Nervous system, complications include convulsions due to anoxia, rarely encephalopathy. Haemorrhage may occur in mucous surfaces. Haemoptysis is commonly seen. Retinal haemorrhage may occur. Rarely intracranial haemorrhage may occur.

Diagnosis. It is based on clinical profile of the disease when child has cough and a typical whoop.

Confirmation is by culture of the organism obtained from nasopharyngeal secretions. Organisms are most likely to be obtained during catarrhal stage. It can also be done by placing border-gengou agar medium plate directly before mouth and growing organisms.

Early diagnosis can be made by fluorescent antibody staining of conjugated B. pertussis and B. parapertussis antiserum. Serological tests are not much helpful in early stage.

Laboratory investigations. Total leucocyte count is raised (20,000 to 50,000 cells/cmm) with absolute increase in lymphocyte count. X-ray chest may show mediastinal enlargement of glands and inflammatory shadows in lungs.

Treatment. Supportive care is very essential. Give small feeds at frequent intervals to maintain nutrition and prevent vomiting as over filled stomach is more liable to vomit.

Maintain hydration by giving adequate amount of fluids. In cases where vomiting is severe intravenous fluids are administered.

Antimicrobial agents are mainly employed to prevent secondary infection though their role to shorten or abort the paroxysmal stage is limited.

Erythromycin in the dose of 40-50 mg/kg/day in four divided doses is given for 10-14 days. If given in catarrhal stage it will decrease severity of the disease. Other drug is Clarithromycin (250 mg twice a day)which is superior to erythromycin and is to be given for shorter period (5-7 days). In addition to antimicrobial agents, antipyretics and bronchodilators have beneficial effect. Albuteral in the dose of 0.3 to 0.5 mg/kg/day in three divided doses is effective. Use of corticosteroids in dosage of 1-2 mg two to three times a day is helpful in reducing the severity of cough paroxysmas.

Prevention. For susceptible individuals who come in close contact with the child and have not previously been immunised. Gamma globulins may be given for passive immunisation.

Active immunisation is achieved by use of a combined vaccine (DPT) containing killed B pertussis alongwith diphtheria and tetanus toxoid. It is given at three month and next two doses repeated at one month interval each. Booster doses may be given at second and 5th year. Adverse reactions include fever and local irritation at the site of injection. Rarely encephalitis following vaccination has been reported.

TYPHOID FEVER

Typhoid is widely prevalent all over the world and millions of people fall victim to the disease every year. Though the incidence has considerably declined in developed countries due to improvement in sanitation, socioeconomic factors and quality of public health measures yet in developing countries in tropics and south East Asia, typhoid is a major health problem taking with it great toll of human lives.

Typhoid involves all age group though less in infants and the incidence of disease declines as the age advances with the result that one hardly observes people in the age group of seventy and above to be suffering from typhoid.

Aetiology. Typhoid is a potentially lethal infection and is caused by Salmonella typhi which is flagellated, gram-negative, non acid fast, non-capsulated, non-sporing and actively motile organism. Salmonellae belong to enteric group of organisms which include both S. typhi and S. paratyphi. The organisms are quickly killed by boiling water and within 15 minutes by exposure to temperatures above 60°F. It survives for considerable time in ice and also for some days in fresh water and for weeks in sewage. The Salmonellae also resist drying so that they may be propagated by dust or soiled articles. Propagation of typhoid is from such as human source, a patient having active disease or a convalescent patient or a carrier. Contamination of drinking water either by sewage or excretions of a patient or of a carrier are a common source of spreading infection. Infection is mainly through the fecal oral route. Articles of food like milk, ice cream etc. which have been contaminated may act to spread the disease. Flies play important role in carrying infection from place to place.

Pathogenesis. Incubation period of the disease is 10-14 days. Ingestion of more than 105 bacteria is required to cause the disease. Development of lesions shall depend on the dose of organisms ingested, their virulence gastric acidity and hosts defence mechanism. The organisms after ingestion reach the small intestines, penetrate the mucosa and enter the lymph nodes and lymphatics where they rapidly multiply to enter the blood stream. Bacteremia of short duration may result. From here they go to liver, spleen and from liver the bacilli pass into the bile, multiply rapidly to re-enter the intestines and get lodged in the Peyer's patches and lymphoid follicles.

The characteristics lesions are in the Peyer's patches which are swollen and inflamed. Other lymphoid follicles in the intestines are also effected and a diffuse inflammation of the intestinal tract may be seen. There may be necrosis and ulceration in the Peyer's patches and lymphoid tissue sloughing takes place and lesions heal with minimal fibrosis. Ulcers in the intestines are not very deep and are present along the long axis of the intestines on the terminal portion of ileum. Blood vessels lying in these ulcers may erode and cause haemorrhage while their extension to the deeper layers causes perforation. Other organs in the body are equally effected. Spleen is enlarged, soft with marked proliferation of cells of sinusoids and red pulp. Liver shows cloudy swelling with collection of phagocytic mononuclear cells and lymphocytes with formation of typhoid nodule.

Salmonella also involves other sites like heart, kidney, gall bladder, joints. Diffuse inflammatory reaction develops. Muscles especially of abdomen show Zenker's degeneration. Nervous system may show meningitis like picture.

Clinical features. The onset of the disease is insidious with malaise, headache, anorexia and fever which is continuous in majority of patients rising in a step ladder pattern during the first week. Sometimes it is intermittent or remittent coming with rigors and chills. Pulse is slow and there is bradycardia. Headache is a common symptom and mainly frontal. The tongue is furred. Abdominal symptoms in the form of dull pain, constipation and even diarrhoea with meteorism are present.

On the seventh day, rose spots appear on crops over the abdomen and chest. These are flattened papules 2-3 mm in diameter, slightly raised lasting for a few days and then fadeaway. Rose spots are seen in fair coloured skins. In paratyphoid infection the spots are more numerous and large. Sometimes neuropsychiatric features like delirium encephalopathy, convulsions and psychosis may dominate the picture.

Clinical profile of typhoid

1. Staircase or stepladder type of temperature
2. Headache, cough, dry coated tongue
3. Abdominal symptoms
4. *Pulse rate slow.* Disproportionate in relation to temperature
5. Rose spots
6. Splenomegaly
7. Confusion or delirium (at height of temperature)
8. Pneumotyphoid, nephrotyphoid, meningotyphoid.

In the second week, patient becomes more toxic and delirious. Fever rises and there are signs of dehydration. Prostration increases, Spleen is enlarged. Pulse rate rises. There is delirium in the form of tremors, convulsions and picking movements of the hands. Abdomen becomes tumid and a gurgling sound is felt in right iliac fossa (gurgling caecum). Complications usually develop by the end of second week. Stools are loose. Pea soup diarrhoea is characteristic.

By third week patient is now in a more moribund state typically called 'Typhoid state' where patient lies listless with sunken eyes and a staring look (coma vigil). Pulse now is feeble and thready. Temperature now falls by lysis i.e. coming slowly and even pass into subnormal temperature. Major complications of typhoid occur during the third week. By fourth week the temperature comes down to normal. The patient now is generally very weak. There may be loss of hair on head. Convalescence may take another seven to ten days.

Above is the description of a typical case of typhoid but now the clinical profile of the disease is changing and classical picture like step ladder temperature, bradycardia. Dry coated tongue, cough, malaise, and abdominal symptoms may not be observed in more than 50 per cent of cases. Some patients of typhoid may present with fever coming with rigors and chills and often mistaken for malaria or in some patients with upper respiratory tract infection or in some nerulological complications may dominate the clinical picture.

Clinical varieties of typhoid fever. Depending on which system in body is predominantly involved due to typhoid the cases which have mainly respiratory system involvement are called 'pneumotyphoid' while those with neurological symptoms are labelled meningotyphoid and where renal involvement predominates it is labelled as 'nephrotyphoid'.

Complications. Typhoid is a multi system disease and hardly any organ in the body escapes its involvement. *Main complication in a case of typhoid are:*

1. *Intestinal haemorrhage.* It occurs in the second week of illness and is characterised by bleeding from intestinal ulcer.
2. *Paralytic ileus.* There is abdominal distension and intestinal movements are diminished. It is due to extensive intestinal involvement and endotoxaemia.

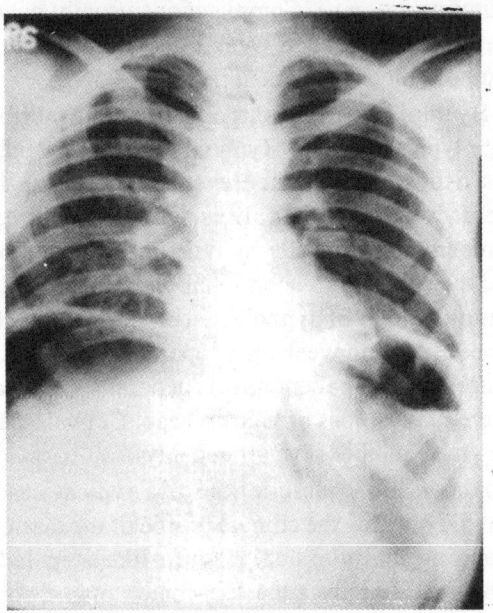

Fig. 11.1. Typhoid Perforation: Note air under right dome of diaphgram.

3. *Intestinal perforation.* It is a serious complication and carries high degree of mortality. It occurs in second week and also during relapse. Poor nutrition, inadequate treatment, and late onset of disease predisposes to this. If patient reports within 24 hours of perforation surgery is of help. Perforation is diagnosed by presence of air under the right diaphragm.
4. *Neuropsychiatric complications.* These include delirium convulsions, confusion, encephalopathy, psychosis meningismus, transient parkinsonism, focal neurological defects, hemiplegia, peripheral neuropathy, mania, hypomania and catatonic schizophrenia. Typhoid meningitis may be seen in an occasional case especially in children.

Neuropsychiatric complications in cases of typhoid are on the increase and often dominate the clinical picture. Anaemia and poor social background along with endotoxaemia are factors known to predispose to the development of these complication.

5. *Respiratory complications.* Bronchitis is the commonest complication. Typhoid pneumonia may be seen in second or third week. It is generally unilateral. Typical signs of consolidation are present in lungs.
6. *Cardiovascular complications.* It may be in the form of myocarditis or cardiogenic shock. Pulse is rapid, heart sounds are feeble and there is gallop. Cardiac arrhythmias (conduction defects and heart blocks) may be seen. Electrocardiogram may show non-specific ST segment and T wave changes.

Enzyme levels are raised and persistence of electrocardiographic changes carry poor prognosis.

7. Acute circulatory failure or collapse is a very serious complication and is as a result of severe toxaemia. It carries high degree of mortality.
8. *Hepatobiliary complications.* Hepatomegaly in seen in 20-40 per cent of cases. Jaundice is seen in few cases. Typhoid hepatitis is a well defined complication characterised by elevations of SGOT/SGPT levels. Chronic cholecystitis may occur in later months and these patients act as carriers.
9. *Haematological complications.* There is depression of bone marrow. Blood count shows leucopenia with relative lymphocytosis. Haemolytic anaemia in patients of typhoid with G6PD deficiency may occur, DIC is uncommon complication.
10. *Genitourinary complications.* Renal involvement (nephrotyphoid) is in the form of toxic nephritis. Sometimes renal failure may occur secondary to septicaemia and shock.
11. *Musculoskeletal complications.* Typhoid may involve ankle or hip joints. Involvement of spine (typhoid spine) is a late complication. Degeneration of abdominal muscles may occur (Zenker's degeneration).

12. *Miscellaneous*. These include parotitis, cancrum oris, venous thrombosis in deep leg veins and abscess formation.

Relapse in typhoid. A relapse may be defined as return of fever within the next fortnight and fever which reaches its maximum in two to three days time accompanied with symptoms attributable to typhoid though in much milder fever. Relapse occurs in 5-15 per cent of all cases of typhoid. Blood culture may become positive again. Relapse is more likely to occur in patients who remained vaguely ill and never really settled after treatment or those who were treated inadequately with antibiotics. Relapse has to be differentiated from recurdescence which is a spurious form of relapse in the way that fever occurs only for very short duration.

Most cases of relapse occur in those treated with chloramphenicol cotrimoxazole, ampicillin and amoxycillin while in those treated with quinolones relapse rate is almost nil.

Diagnosis. A classical case of typhoid presents with continous fever, headache, malaise, dry furred tongue, bradycardia. Presence of physical sign like gurgling caecum is helpful in making diagnosis. Difficulty arises when a case presents with fever coming with rigors and chills when it has to be differentiated from a case of malaria or when neuropsychiatric features dominate the clinical picture. Here differentiation has to be made from meningits, encephalitis and various forms of psychiatric ailments.

Laboratory investigations:

1. Blood count shows leucopenia with relative lymphocytosis. There is eosinopenia.
2. Blood culture for S. typhi is positive in 70-90 per cent of the cases during the first week and falls to 40 per cent in the third week of illness.
3. *Clot culture*. It is said to give positive result in 65-80 per cent of the cases when blood culture is negative.
4. *Bone marrow*. Bone marrow culture is important in establishing the diagnosis especially when a case of typhoid has already received antibiotics. This is because the organisms lurk in the bone marrow for long time after leaving the blood stream. Rate of positivity is upto 95 per cent.
5. *Stool culture*. It is positive in 40-50 per cent of cases in first week and this positivity increases upto 75 per cent in third to fourth week. After eight weeks it is only 10 per cent and three per cent of these patients continue to excrete organisms even after one year.

Diagnosis of typhoid

1. Clinical profile
2. TLC & DLC. Leukopenia with relative lymphocytosis.
3. Blood cululture. Most dependable
   +ve in 70-90 % cases first week
   +ve in 30-40 % cases third week
4. Bone marrow culture. Important when blood culture –ve after anti-microbial therapy. +ve in 95% of cases.
5. Stool culture.
   +ve 40-50 % 1st week
   +ve 75% 3rd - 4th week
   After eight weeks only 10% and 3% continue to excrete organisms even after one year.
6. Urine culture. Runs parallel with stools culture.
7. Widal test. Somatic antigen O, flagellar antigen H
   Four fold or more increase in agglutinins in the absence of recent immunization (by TAB) is diagnostic but by no means specific.
   'H' agglutinins subject to non-specific variations. No value in diagnosis.
8. Clot culture. Higher rate of isolation than blood culture.
9. Counter immunoelectrophoresis (CIE). Highly specifid, rapid diagnostic test, useful for detecting S.Typhi antigen and antibody in sera.
10. Slide haemagglutination test (SHA) useful for detecting antibodies to flagellar antigens of S. Typhi in unvaccinated subjects.
11. Indirect haemagglutination test. Superior in typhoid serology but elaborate.
12. Duodenal string capsule culture. Valuable aid in diagnosing carrier state.
13. Limulus test for detection of endotoxins.
14. Elisa test
15. L. adenosine deaminase (LADA). Increased activity. May serve as prognostic indicator in serious cases of typhoid.

6. *Urine culture.* Its positivity runs parallel with stool culture. It is positive in one third to one fourth of cases. Salmonella are shed irregularly and infrequently in urine and for establishing diagnosis of typhoid in early weeks they may not be of much use. Kidney acts as purely excretor of organisms. Culture of urine when excretion of organisms is persisting helps in identifying carriers.

7. *Bile culture.* Duodenal intubation is done by a string capsule and bile collected. Bile culture is helpful in establishing diagnosis of carrier state.

8. *Culture of rose spots.* It is useful in patients who have taken antibiotics.

Serological tests:

1. **Widal test.** It is a helpful in making a presumptive diagnosis. It has low sensitivity because a significant number of culture positive patients do not develop antibodies as detected by the test. Of the two antigens Somatic antigen 'O' is more important than Flagellar antigen. In an uninoculated patient living in an non-endemic area if the titres are 1:80 and above the diagnosis should be suspected. A four fold or more increase in O antigen titres in excess of 1:160 shall provide presumptive diagnosis. 'H' antigens are not so specific since they remain elevated after a recent infection or immunization.

2. **Other tests include.** Latex agglutination test for quick diagnosis of typhoid fever especially in those who have previously taken antibiotics.

   a. *Staphylococcal slide coagulation test (SSCOAg).* It is positive in 80-86 per cent of cases where widal is negative and is always positive in culture positive cases.

   b. Adenosine enzyme activity (ADA) is elevated in patients of typhoid.

   c. Elisa test mainly used to detect Vi antibodies which rise after three to four weeks of illness.

3. CSF culture for Salmonella organisms in cases of meningitis.

Management of a case of typhoid. An uncomplicated case of typhoid is not difficult to manage. General supportive measures include bed rest, maintenance of satisfactory fluid and electrolyte balance, adequate nutrition and general as well as personal nursing care. In acute stage of illness hyperpyrexia shall require hydrotherapy and if patient is unable to take sufficient fluids orally intravenous hydration is employed. Presence of shock shall necessitate use of vaso pressor drugs and steroids.

Antimicrobial agents:

1. *Choramphenicol.* It has been the first line of therapy in cases of typhoid. It has been effective in cutting febrile toxic course of the disease in great proportion of cases in shortest time and in reducing the fatality rates. But its major drawback is the production of toxic reaction in the form of bone marrow depression which may be either dose related or hyper sensitivity reaction which is genetically controlled. Because of the toxicity and emergence of drug resisitant strains of salmonella the use of chloramphenicol in the treatment of typhoid has almost been reduced to nil.

   Dose is 50 mg per kg body weight in four divided dose (3 to 4 G per day). When patient becomes afebrile, after 48 hours the dose is reduced (30 mg/kg body weight). Total dose of chloramphenicol should not exceed 10-14 gm. Resistance to chloramphenicol is because of its indiscriminate use and acquisition of transferable extrachromosal factor (R-factor).

2. *Trimethoprim (80 mg) + Sulfamethoxazole (400 mg) combination.* It is an effective bactericidal combination but the average time until defervescence is prolonged. It has also got bone marrow depression effect especially in cases of typhoid with anaemia.

   Dose is 2 tablets orally twice a day for 10-14 doays.

3. *Ampicillin/Amoxycillin.* The dose of ampicillin in typhoid is 4-6 g/day in adults or 200 mg/kg/day in chidren given in four divided doses. Dose of amoxycillin is 4 g/day given

in three divided doses in adults and in children 100 mg/kg/day in three divided doses.

Both these drugs are good alternative to chloramphenicol though inferior. Major benefit is that these drugs can be safely given in typhoid complicating pregnancy. G.I. disturbances, nausea and vomiting are main side effects. Total course of the drugs is 10-14 days. Drug resistant strains to these drugs have also developed.

4. *Aminoglycoside.* Gentamycin is effective against salmonella especially when given in combination with amoxycillin. Dose is 1-2 mg/kg eight hourly intramuscularly. Main side effect is neuro and ototoxicity.

5. *Quinolones.* These have emerged as potent drugs against salmonella both orally and parenterally and are able to attain appropriate levels in gut, liver and gall bladder. These are bactericidal and very effective against intracellular organisms.

They achieve rapid clinical and bacteriological cure and most of the patients become afebrile in three to four days. Dosage of Quinolones is:

   a. Oxfloxacin 400 mg/d for 7-14 days.
   b. Pefloxacin 400 mg/BD for 7-14 days.
   c. Ciprofloxacin 750 mg twice a day for seven to 14 days. After the patient has been afebrile for two days dose of Ciprofloxacin is reduced (500 mg twice a day).

But due to its indiscriminate use, resistance to Quinolones is on the rise. It is also due to an altered DNA gyrase.

All the three quinolones are effective against typhoid and paratyphoid organisms but out of them Ciprofloxacin is the drug of choice because of its therapeutic response.

6. *Third generation Cephalosporins.* In cases resistant to Quinolones, third generation cephalosporins are the drug of choice. Ceftriaxone is used. Dose is 4 G per day for two days and then 2 G/day for two days. It is used both in children and adults and total course of the drug is for four days.

Role of steroids. Use of steroids in cases of typhoid often raises controversy. An uncomplicated case of typhoid does not require any additional use of steroids and it is only in seriously ill patients where these are indicated.

Oral prednisolone in the dose of 40-60 mg per day is effective and in those who are very ill toxic or in shock, dose recommended is 2 mg/kg body weight of Dexamethasone administered intravenously and repeated six hourly.

Use of steroids is based on the assumption that adrenocortical functions are impaired in the acute stage of illness. It is a transient phenomenon and patients of typhoid who do not have severe toxaemia do not require supplementation with steroids.

Management of typhoid with complications. Cases of typhoid with predominant neuropsychiatric features will require in addition to general supportive measures, institution of appropriate antimicrobial agent (Ampicillin/Amoxycillin/Genticyin/ Ciprofloxacin) along with steroids. Convulsions, psychiatric features shall require drugs like Dilantin, diazepam, prochlorperazine etc.

In patients with intestinal perforation coming within the first 24 hours and preferably within six hours. Operative management of perforation is indicated. But where the patient is moribund and very ill, conservative medical treatment has to be instituted. There is often confusion in a suspected patient of perforation whether surgery has to be undertaken or not. No generalization can be made and the treatment will vary from patient to patient. Mortality shall depend on number of factors like nutrition of the patient and the stage at which the patient comes.

Intestinal haemorrhage in most cases is to be managed by general supportive measures including replacement of blood loss. Cases of myocarditis, hepatitis have to be managed on conservative lines with the use of appropriate antimicrobial agents and steroids. Cases of typhoid myocarditis with persistent arrhythmias shall require in addition antiarrhythmic drugs.

Treatment of carriers. Ideal drug for the use in cases of carrier stage is Ciprofloxacin 500 mg twice a day for four to six weeks. It is effective because of its tissue penetration properties and is also effective in patients who have got infection in their gall bladder.

Prophylaxis. Prevention of typhoid is a major health problem in any developing country. It means provision of clean water supply, food and milk. Adequate sewage control along with excellent sanitary and public health measures are must in any society as safeguard against typhoid.

Immunization against typhoid may not give 100 per cent protection but it does lower the incidence and morbidity of the disease.

TAB vaccine. It has been in use since long but has a short lived effect on individuals resistance. It does not protect an individual from typhoid completely and severe forms of typhoid can occur in vaccinated individual.

Prophylaxis against typhoid

TAB vaccine. Contains S.typhi (1000 million) S.paratyphi A (500-700 million) and S.paratyphi B (500-700 million) organisms per ml.

    Primary immunisation consists of two doses. Each (0.5 ml) given S/C at four to six weeks interval. Booster dose every three years.

    Immunity develops 10-21 days after inoculation and maintained for three years.

Reactions. Local (pain, tenderness, swelling) general (fever,malaise). Protection. Only partial

Liver attenuated oral vaccine (Ty 21a). Three doses of enteric coated capsule at 1,3 and 5th day one hour before meals with cold or luke warm milk.

Protection rate of 70-95 % for three years.

Vi capsular polysaccharide vaccine (Typhim Vi). Single 25 µg given I/M, effective and free from major side effects. Protective efficacy 65-75%.

TAB vaccine is generally either acetone killed or heat killed phenolysed preparation containing S. typhi (1000 million), S. paratyphi A (500-750 million) and S. paratyphi B (500-750 million) organisms per ml. Immunization consists of two doses of 0.5 ml given subcutaneously at an interval of four to six weeks.

Side effects include fever, malaise and local pain at the site of injection. TAB vaccine is not preferred these days because of its weak protective effect and failure to stimulate cell mediated immunity.

Vi capsular polysaccharide typhoid vaccine (Typhim Vi). It is a single parenteral vaccine containing 25 µg of purified Vi capsular polysaccharide of S. typhi in each immunizing dose. It provides protection against the disease for three years and this ranges between 65-75 per cent. Reactions include pain, fever, nausea and swelling or erythema at the site of injection.

Complications of typhoid:

1. **General.** Hyperpyrexia: Acute peripheral circulatory failure. Deep vein thrombosis: Toxaemia, typhoid state.
2. **Gastrointestinal.** Parotitis, meteorism, diarrhoea (pea soup diarrhoea), intestinal perforation, intestinal haemorrhage, paralytic ileus.
3. **Neurological.** Encephalopathy, delirium, meningismus, convulsions, catatonic schizophrenia, melancholia, mania, hypomania, transient parkinsonism, cranial and peripheral neuropathies, focal neurologic defects, transverse myelitis, meningitis.
4. **Cardiovascular.** Cardiogenic shock, myocarditis, ST-T changes and T wave inversion in electrocardiogram, cardiac arrhythmias.
5. **Respiratory.** Bronchitis, pneumonia, ARDS (acute respiratory distress syndrome).
6. **Hepatobiliary.** Hepatomegaly, typhoid hepatitis, chronic cholecystitis.
7. **Haematological.** Bone marrow depression, leucopenia, haemolytic anaemia, DIC.
8. **Genitourinary.** Toxic nephritis, glomerulonephritis, pyelonephritis, renal failure.
9. **Musculoskeletal.** Arthritis, typhoid spine, osteomyelitus, Zenker's degeneration of abdominal muscles, post-typhoid anhidrosis.

Live attenuated oral vaccine (Ty21a). It is a plasmid containing enzyme deficient and genetically crippled strain and its capacity to survive in the intestinal tract gives a protection rate of 70-95 per cent. Three doses of the vaccine (one capsule on day 1,3, and 5) irrespective of age one hour before meal with a cold or lukewarm drink e.g. milk is advocated. Protection commences two weeks after taking the last capsule and lasts for at least three years. Liver oral typhoid vaccine is indicated for immunization of adults and childrlen above five years of age. Booster dose of the vaccine which consists of same three doses is recommended once every three years. Side effects include mild gastro-intestinal disturbances and a transitory exanthema. Results with oral vaccine are good though it may not protect all people.

Paratyphoid fevers. These are caused by salmonella paratyphi A and B. The clinical picture resembles typhoid but the course and morbidity of the disease is mild, complications are also comparatively less. Management is on the same lines as of S. typhi.

Prognosis in typhoid fevers. In any case of typhoid it shall depend on severity of the disease process. Toxaemia, state of nutrition of the patient, presence of complications, cell mediated immunity and presence of drug resistant strains of salmonella. A correct and early diagnosis coupled with institution of treatment shall go long way in reducing morbidity and mortality in a case of typhoid.

MALARIA

It is one of the commonest tropical diseases which affects millions of people in many parts of the world. Easy travel and migration of population has intro-duced the disease in almost all the countries. It is caused by various species of plasmodium, the ma-larial parasite. Though more than three hundred species of this parasite have been identified but in humans only four species i.e. P. vivax, P. falciparum, P. malariae and P. ovale cause infection. Of these four species P. vivax is the most common and along with P. falciparum accounts for 90-95 per cent of all cases of malaria. Benign tertian is caused by P. vivax, maligant tertian by P. falciparum, Tertian malaria due to P. ovale and Quartan malaria by plas-modium malaria. The disease is conveyed by the bite of infected female mosquito of genus anoph-eles which bites from sunset to dawn.

Life cycle of malarial parasite. There are two stages in the life cycle of the malarial parasite.

1. Asexual cycle in man (Endogenous cycle. Schizogony).
2. Sexual cycle in mosquito (Exogenous cycle. Sporogony).

Sexual cycle in mosquito. When female anopheles mosquito bites an infected person gametocytes from its blood are ingested. These are either round or oval bodies in benign tertian infection and crescent like in malignant tertian malaria. In the mosquitos stomach, the corpuscles rupture and they form into circular shape, the gametes which develop further. By a process of flagellation and exflagellation the male gamete fertilizes into a female gamete known as Zygote. This develops into ookinete which penetrates the stomach wall and becomes circular in shape and forms oocyst. About 10,000 sporozoites develop within each oocyst. These oocysts subsequently rupture and sporozoites make their way to the salivary gland. Depending on the temperature and humidity the whole cycle takes from eight to 20 days. Now when the mosquito bites, the sporozoites from the salivary secretions are passed into the victim.

An infected mosquito can carry the infection for the duration of its life span which generally is one month.

Asexual cycle in man (Schizogony). It consists of pre-erythrocytic, erythrocytic and exoerythrocytic cycles.

Pre erythrocytic schizogony. This is the stage when sporozoites after inoculation by the mosquito completely loose their infectivity and enter the parenchyma cells of the liver and multiply within them. Here they undergo changes and metrozoites come out of the liver cell and invade the blood stream after a variable number of days. During this period only local inflammatory chnges occur. Man is not infective and there are no clinical symptoms.

Erythrocytic cycle. This is the stage which is harmful to the host. The merozoites invade the red blood cells, grow into a ring and form trophozoites.

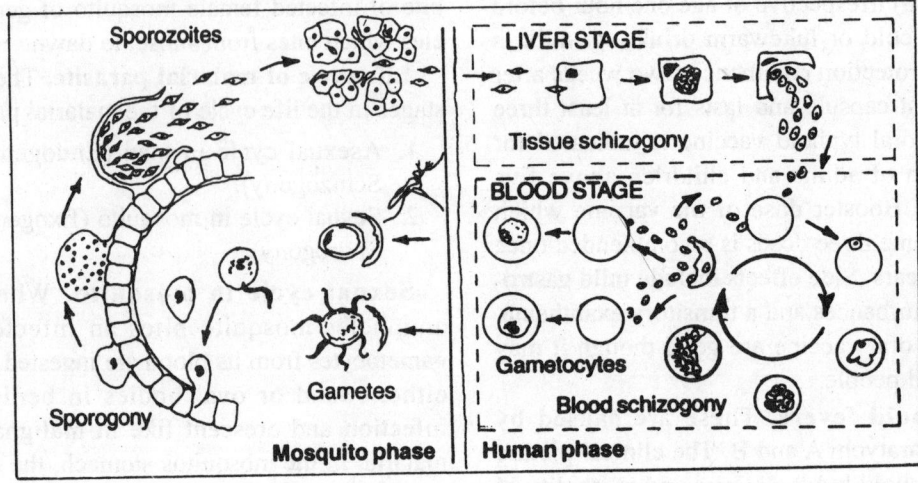

Fig. 11.2. Life cycle of Malarial parasite.

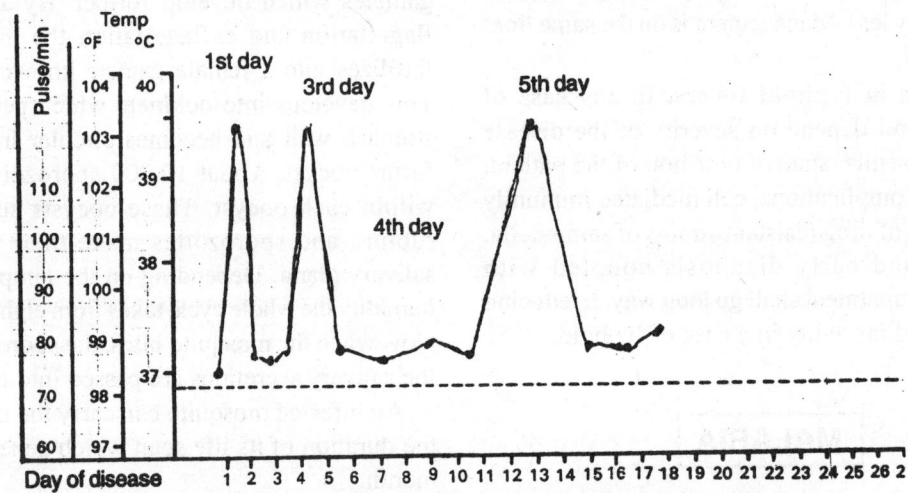

Fig. 11.3. Temperature chart in a case of benign tertian malaria.

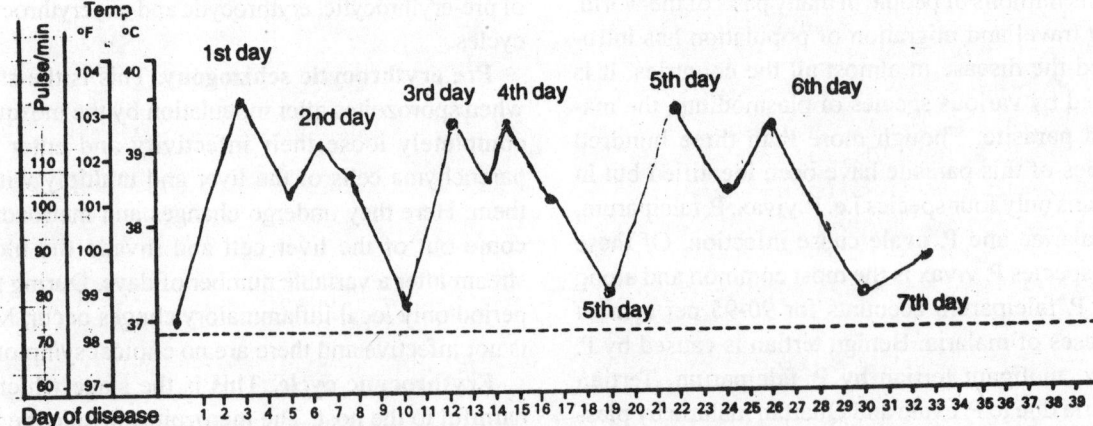

Fig. 11.4. Temperature chart in a case of malignant tertian malaria.

PLATE XXI

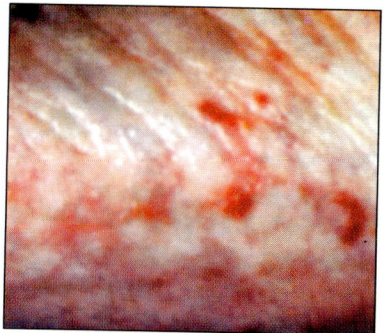

Discoid eczema

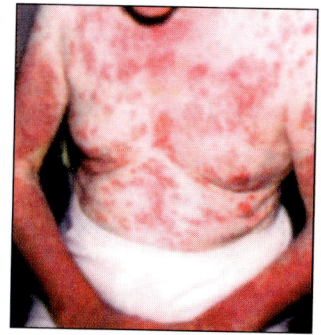

Bullous pemphigoid

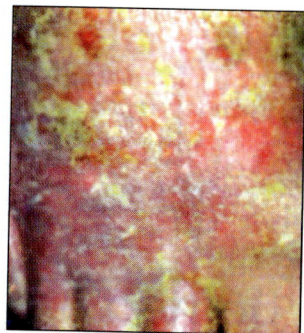

Infected eczema

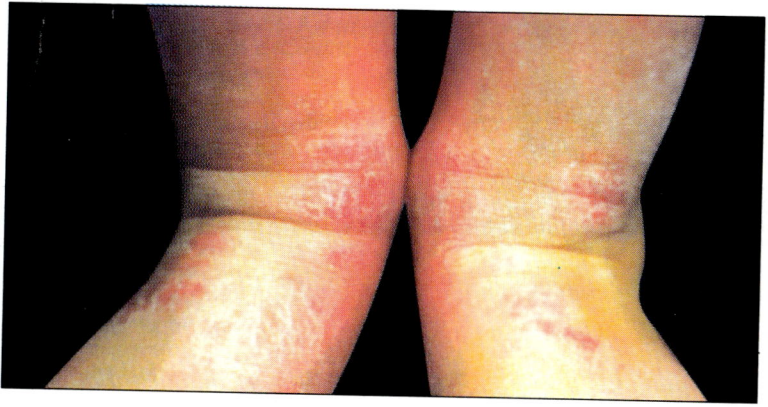

Atopic eczema

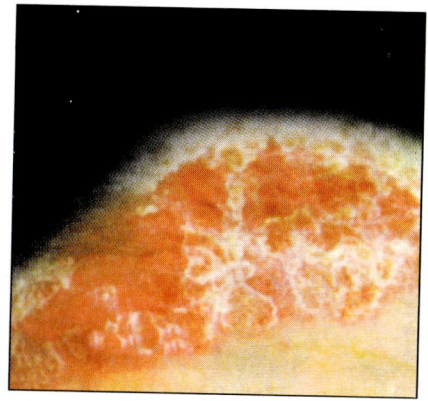

Chronic psoriasis

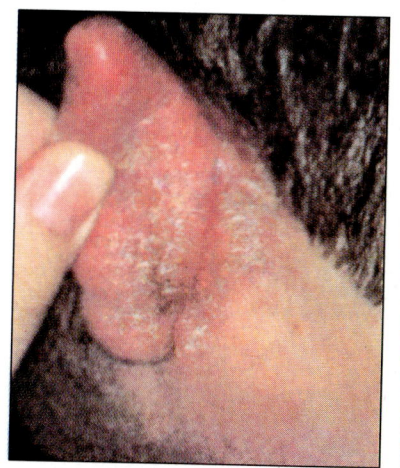

Flexural eczema

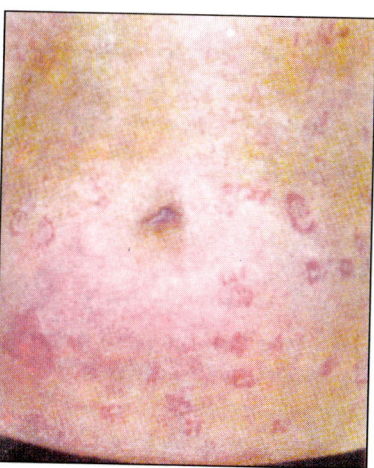

Pityriasis rosea

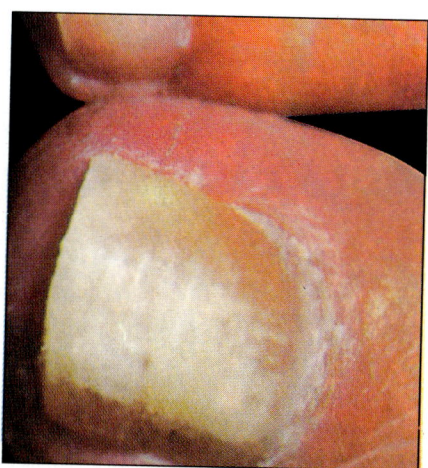

Psoriasis of the nail

PLATE XXII

ADDISON'S DISEASE

THYROID

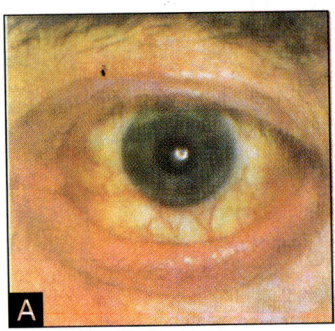
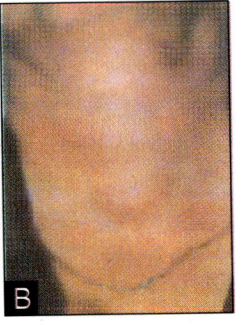

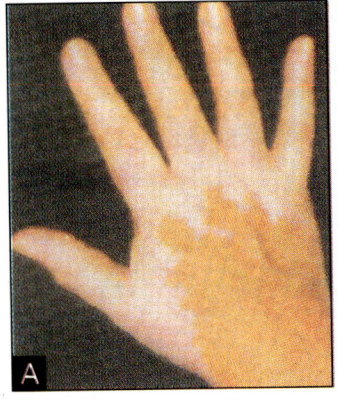
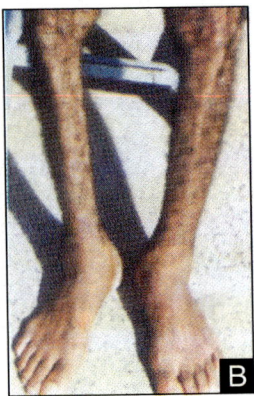

(A) Exophthalmos with proptosis, periorbital oedema, inflammation and dilated conjunctival vessels. This is a case of thyrotoxicosis. (B) Nodular goitre.

(A) Vitiligo in a case of Addison's disease. (B) A case of tubercular abdomen with Addison's disease. There is marked wasting with pigmentation.

VITAMIN DEFICIENCY

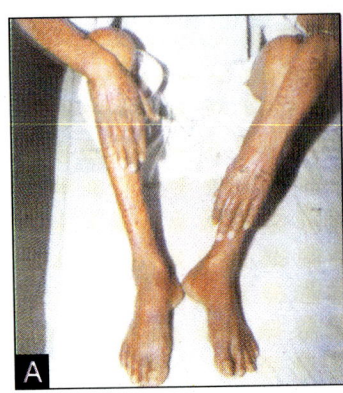
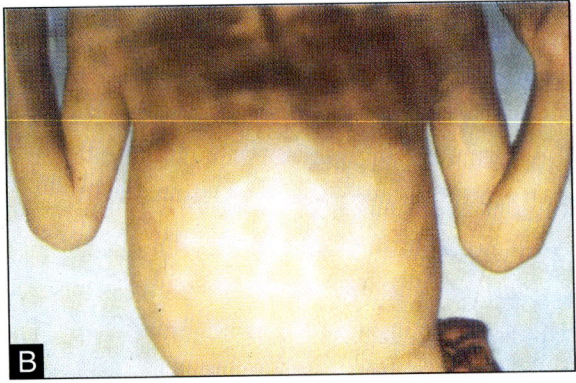

(A) Pellagra. There is pigmentation and desquamation of exposed surfaces. Observe pavement type skin. (B) Rickets. Observe rickety, rosary and Harrison's sulcus.

DIABETES

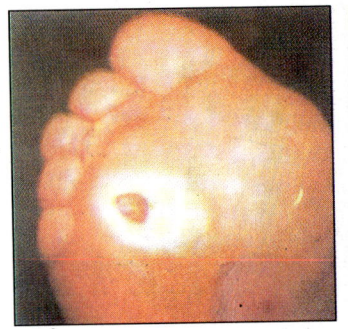
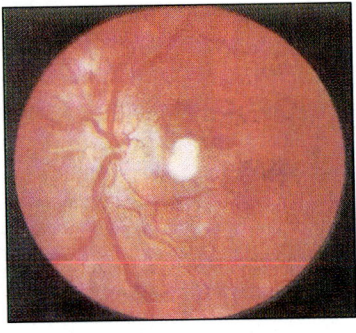
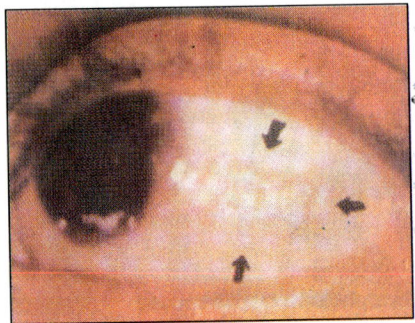

Neuropathic foot ulcer in diabetes.   Proliferative diabetic retinopathy.

Bitot's spots.

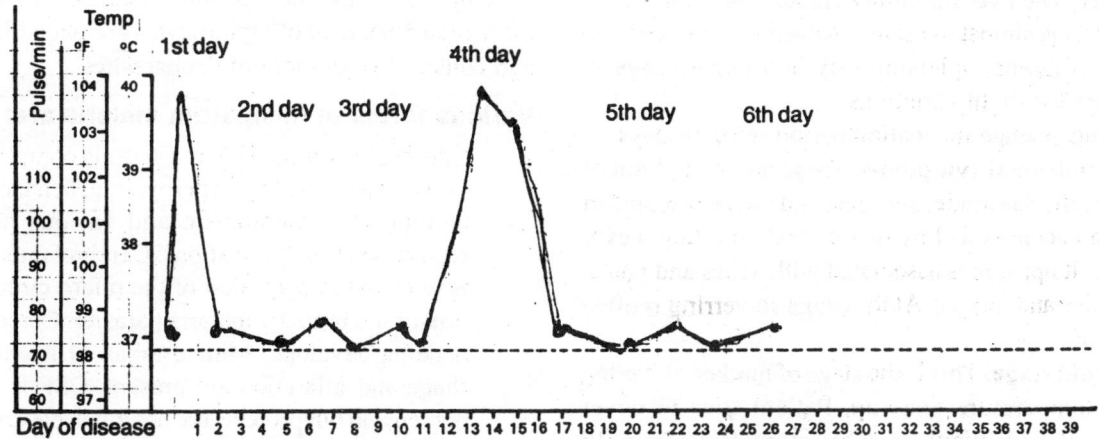

Fig. 11.5. Temperature chart in a case of quartan malaria.

These further divide by binary fission to form a schizont which contains number of merozoites. These asexual forms of parasites are found in blood stream at variable intervals depending on the species involved. These when released into the blood stream, some are destroyed while others attach to fresh erythrocytes and repeat the cycle of multiplication.

The erythrocytic phase may continue for sometime before the stage of gametogony occurs when some of the merozoites develop into the male and female gametocytes. They continue further only if ingested by the vector other wise they die within variable time lasting from two to eight weeks. This is the stage of infectivity of patient.

Exoerythrocytic stage. This stage is only seen with P. vivax, P. ovale and P. malariae infections and does not occur with P. falciparum infection. This phase mainly occurs in the liver when some of merozoites liberated in the pre erythrocytic phase re enter the liver cells and continue the cycle. This stage is reponsible for persistence of infection and relapses. The parasites in this phase are called hypnozoites.

Pathology. The malarial parasites engulf and destroy large number of red cells and this coincides with a paroxysm of febrile illness. The result is haemolysis. A brown malarial pigment (hemozoin) is released from ruptured red cells along with merozoites and this is taken up by spleen and other

organs of the reticuloendothelial system like liver, lymph nodes and bone marrow. Malarial pigment is deposited in these organs giving them a brownish appearance. The pathological changes mainly include parenchymal degeneration of the organs and fibrosis with marked reticuloendothelial hyperplasia throughout thebody. Degenerative changes due to toxic action or anoxia or both are seen in liver, kidney and supra renals. Multiple haemorrhages may be seen, parasitised cells block the capillaries and because of vascular spasm there are small areas of haemorrhage and necrosis. Spleen is massively enlarged, congested with dark red pulp. As the disease progresses fibrosis sets in and now spleen which contains malarial pigment, parasitized cells becomes fibrosed and firm. Liver may also get enlarged and it is mainly due to congestion and hyperplasia of the cells.

The clinical picture of a patient depends on his immune status. Spleen plays an important role in natural immunity. An attack of malaria is known to produce partial immunity due to stimulation of macrophages by T. cells. Presence of abnormal haemoglobins (Thalassaemia haemoglobin-S, glucose-6-Phosphate-dehydrogenase deficiency) or altered metabolism of red cells is also unfavourable for the development of P. falciparum infection.

Clinical picture. It consists of premonitory symptoms followed by cold, hot and sweating stages. The over all clinical picture in all forms of malaria is almost the same (Anaemia, fever coming in paroxysms, splenomegaly and hepatomegaly) except for slight variations.

The average incubation period is 10-14 days.

Prodromal symptoms. These are in the form of headache, lassitude, anorexia and vague discomfort often accompanied by nausea and vomiting. Fever when it appears is associated with aches and pains, malaise and fatigue. At this stage shiverring is often absent.

Cold stage. This is the stage of marked shivering and temperature goes up. Patient tries to cover himself with blankets. This stage lasts from 30 minutes to one hour.

Hot stage. This follows cold stage which stops abruptly. There is a feeling of intense heat and uncomfortable sensation. Patient now throws away the blankets. The face is flushed. Headache, burning skin and vomiting may be present. This stage lasts for two to four hours.

The sweating stage. It follows hot stage and there is profuse perspiration. The bed clothes now are drenched with sweat. Temperature comes down but the patient is exhausted and dehydrated. Often the patient feels refreshed after a paroxysm of fever which is repeated generally after 24 to 48 hours depending on the parasite involved.

P. vivax and P. ovale produce a picture of benign tertian fever occurring every other day. The infection is mild.

P. malariae. The paroxysms of fever occur after an interval of 48 hours. These are mild of short duration and generally run a chronic course. Involvement of kidney in the form of nephritis can complicate this illness. Liver and spleen are enlarged. Patient has a sallow complexion and anaemia.

Falciparum malaria. This is the malignant form of malaria and has a more serious profile. It may start acutely with body aches, headache and vomiting. Fever may follow no specific pattern. It may come daily (quotidian) or after 36 hours (subtertian). In between the paroxysms of fever patient is not well. Various pernicious complications

develop with it and these should be expected when more than 5 per cent of erythrocytes are parasitized and contain two or more of the parasites.

Various forms of falciparum malaria are:

1. *Cerebral malaria.* This is a serious complication characterised by hyperpyrexia, headache, convulsions, meningism and various neuropsychiatric complications. Cerebral malaria results due to occlusion of the micro circulation of the brain by malaria parasite. Cerebral oedema develops. Minute areas of haemorrhage and infarction are present. CSF is under tension but proteins are not much elevated. A case of cerebral malaria carries poor prognosis and it may prove fatal.

2. *Algid malaria.* There is picture of severe shock, vomiting and peripheral circulatory failure. Pulse is rapid thready and weak. Blood pressure levels are low. Respiration is shallow. Temperature is subnormal. Algid malaria is characterised by presence of plenty of parasites in the peripheral film.

3. *Septicaemic malaria.* There are signs of marked toxaemia, fever, vomiting with pulmonary and cardiac involvement.

4. *Cardiac.* Breathlessness, cyanosis, respiratory distress, congestive failure may be present. This is not very common.

5. *Gastrointestinal malaria.* There is severe degree of nausea, vomiting, epigastric discomfort, diarrhoea and even haematemesis. Some patients may develop severe jaundice and picture resembling hepatic failure.

6. *Purpuric as haemorrhagic malaria.* There is epistaxis, haematemesis petechial eruptions, haemolysis and DIC.

7. *Nephritic.* There is albuminuria with granular and blood casts in the urine.

8. *Pulmonary.* It is in the form of congestion bronchopneumonia or acute resparatory distress syndrome.

Black water fever. It occurs in cases of falciparum malaria who have been inadequately treated and have heavy infection. Poor immunity in the patient sensitises the erythrocytes. Sometimes small quantities of Quinine in sensitive persons brings out the condition. Both parasitized and non-parasitized cells are destroyed. There is severe degree of intravascular haemolysis, jaundice, shock. Fever comes with rigors and chills. There is pain in the loins and high coloured urine is passed. A series of haemolytic crisis occur. Nausea, vomiting and hiccough are present. Signs of collapse quickly appear. There is haemoglobinuria and hyper-bilirubinemia. Urine shows granular, epithelial and haemoglobin casts. Generally black water fever has a severe fulminating course and may prove fatal. Death is generally due to shock, renal or cardiac failure.

Diagnosis of malaria. It is made by demons-tration of malarial parasites in thick and thin blood smears after staining with one of Romanowsky dyes (Leishman: Giemsa or Wright). Repeat blod smears should be taken daily for two to three days before finalising the diagnosis.

The use of flurochrome dyes like acridine orange and quinacrine hydrochloride and direct fluorescent antibody method is useful for rapid detection of malarial parasites in patients with low levels of parasitaemia.

Serological tests like complement fixation, indirect haemagglutination, gel diffusion, counter current immunoelectrophoresis, indirect fluorescent antibody ELISA and radio immuno assay are the other tests employed. These tests have variable degree of sensitivity. Indirect haemagglutination has better sensitivity and sepecificity. Detection of malarial antigen is useful in diagnosis of active infection. Demonstration of malarial parasites in bone marrow smear and after splenic puncture are other ways of looking for parasite.

Treatment. It can be prophylactic, suppressive, curative and treatment of complications.

Prophylactic. It includes destruction of adult mosquitoes by use of DDT and pyrethrin. In endemic areas mosquito nets and proper clothing to protect against mosquito bites. Use of mats and coils in the room while sleeping is also beneficial.

Suppressive drug treatment. Quinine is the drug of choice for suppression of benign tertian or malignant tertian infections though it may fail to suppress heavy infection with P. falciparum. Dose 300 mg - 600 mg per day. Other drug is chloroquine diphosphate given in a single dose of two tablets (0.5 g) once a week.

Treatment of an acute attack. An acute attack of malaria which generally is due to P. vivax infection, treatment is by chloroquine (4 tablets stat 600 mg base) followed by two such tablets (300 mg) after six hours andthen 150 mg twice daily for three days. After the acute attack is over, the patient should be continued on two tablets (300 mg) every week for 10 weeks. Alternative would be 8-amodiaquine hydrochloride 600 mg followed by 400-600 mg daily for two days. Total dose should not exceed 2400 mg.

If the causative organism is P. falciparum and infection is not very severe Quinine sulfate 650 mg twice a day for seven days. For chloroquine resistant malaria treatment of choice is Quinine 650 mg three times daily for five days. This may be combined with pyrimethamine 50 mg daily for three days and sulphadiazine 500 mg twice daily for five days.

Alternative to above regimen, Quinine may be followed by a single dose of three tablets each containing sulfadoxine 500 mg combined with pyrimethamine 25 mg. Mefloquine is another drug effective against multiresisitant P. falciparum infection. Dose 15 mg/kg (maximum 1 g) taken with plenty of water and preferably after meals.

Another regimen is to combine Quinine with a course of Tetracycline for seven to ten days (quinine 650 mg thrice day for seven day + Capsule Tetracycline 250 mg four times daily for seven to ten days).

Eradication of infection. For eradication of infection and relapses in cases with P. vivax, P. malariae and P. ovale infection, treatment is by chloroquine combined with primaquine 15 mg twice daily for 14 days. Primaquine not only effects the exooerythrocytic stage but also destroys the gametocytes in the blood. But this drug is contraindicated in patients with G-6-PD deficiency because of risk of producing haemolysis and methaemoglobinaemia.

In P. falciparum infection chloroquine alone or in combination with either pyrimethamine 25 mg or primaquine 45 mg given as a single dose produces radical cure. This course is effective since there is no exoerythrocytic cycle in falciparum infection.

Treatment of acute infection. Cases of malaria presenting in pernicious form require treatment on emergency lines. *It should consist of:*

1. Intravenous fluids, maintain hydration and electrolyte balance.
2. Patient's urinary output must be adequate.
3. Quinine is to be given intravenously in slow drip form in a dose of 10 mg/kg body weight over a period of 20-30 minutes (600 mg I/V stat followed by eight hourly infusion). Once the acute stage is over, oral drug be substituted. Chloroquine is also given in a dose of 5 mg/kg body weight in a slow intravenous drip thrice a day.

Treatment of cerebral malaria. *Broad principles are:*

1. Intravenous fluids to maintain hydration, monitor electrolyte balance.
2. Intravenous quinine infusion eight hourly (600 mg slow intravenously over a period of half an hour eight hourly).
3. Injection Dexamethasone 8 mg intravenously six hourly.
4. Injection Tetracycline 500 mg I/M six hourly.
5. Low molecular weight dextran, to reduce sludging by parasites.

Treatment of black water fever:

1. Intravenous fluids (Dextrose + Dextrose saline). Monitor electrolyte balance, urinary output. Sodium bicarbonate (100 ml 20% solution intravenously twice a day to combat acidosis. If a patient has renal failure, then dialysis has to be done.
2. Injection Tetracycline 500 mg six hourly.
3. Injection Dexamethasone 8 mg intravenously six hourly.
4. Injection chloroquine (500 mg intravenously 8 hourly). It is preferred to quinine since quinine is known to precipitate an attack of black water fever. Blood transfusion if there

is circulatory failure or severe degree of anaemia.

1. Mefloquine is the drug of choice for both P. vivax and Falciparum infections (250 mg tablet once a week). Other drugs are doxycycline 100 mg daily.
2. Chloroquine 300 mg (2 tablets each containing 150 mg base) once weekly. Proguanil 200 mg daily. Quinine as chemoprophylaxis is not preferred. Prophylaxis should be continued for four weeks after the person leaves the endemic area.

Newer antimalarials:

Artemisinin. It is the active principle of a plant used in traditional medicine as Quinghaosu. This drug is effective against resistant forms of P. falciparum infection.

Recommended doses of Artesunate is 100 mg twice a day (4 mg/kg) on first day followed by 100 mg per day in one or two doses for five days. For serious cases parenteral use is recommended (120 mg I/M or I/V on first day followed by 60 mg daily for four days)

The drug use should be restricted to acute attacks of multiresistant falciparum malaria. Side effects include nausea, vomiting, abnormal, bleeding and ST segment changes in electrocardiogram.

Complications of malaria. These include chronic anaemia ill health, herpes simplex, hepatitis and nephritis. Women if suffer from malaria during pregnancy they are likely to abort or have premature delivery.

Splenic complications include perisplenitis and rupture of an enlarged spleen. There may be subcapsular haematoma and torsion of the pedicle, Rupture and torsion of the spleen are grave emergencies and require operative interference.

Chemoprophylaxis. It should start seven days before a person visits an endemic area.

Prognosis. Depending on the acuteness of the attack and body's defence mechanisms as well as immune status prognosis in a case of malaria is variable. Presence of relapses at frequent intervals is not good. People living in endemic areas must

Commonly used anti malarial drugs

Drug	Route	Use	Side effects
1. Chloroquine (4-amino quinoline group) diphosphate and sulphate	Oral 150 mg base	Rapidly acting erythrocytic schizontocide. No effect on pre and exoerythrocytic phase. Effective in all forms of malaria. Does not prevent relapse in P.vivax and P. malariae	Nausea,vomiting, headache, rashes, photophobia, confusion psychosis. Contra-indicated in G-6-PD deficiency.
Chloroquine hydrochloride	500 mg 1/M, or I/V	In pernicious form of malaria.	
2. Amodiaquine (camoquin)	200 mg oral	Same as chloroquine	Hepato toxic, visual disturbances, nausea, vomiting, skin pigmentation,neuropathy.
3. Quinine sulphate	300/325 mg tablet	Erythrocytic schizontocide. Most chloroquine and multidrug resisitant strains respond, effective in perniciousforms.	Headache, tinnitus, blurred vision, acute haemolytic, anaemia, vomiting, diarrhoea
Quinine Dihydrochloride	500-650 mg intravenous	For pernicious and malignant forms of malaria.	Use with caution in pregnancy and those with cardiac ailments.
4. Primaquine	7.5 mg orally	Active against exoerythrocytic forms of P. vivax and P.falciparum. Kills gametocytes. Radicalcure of vivax and other relapsing malaria.	Abdominal cramps, Anaemia, epigastric distress.
5. Sulfadoxine 500 mg+ pyrimethamine 25 mg (Croydoxin - FM)	Oral single dose (3 tabs.)	Schizontocide chloroquine Resistant P. falciparum malaria	G.I. disorders, pruritis, erythema multiforme.
6. Mefloquine	Oral 05 g	Schizontocide. Used as second line treatment in chloroquine resistant malaria and severe malaria. due to P. falciparum and vivax	Confusion, anxiety, hallucinations, dizziness, nausea, vomiting
7. Artesunate	Oral 100 mg BD first day followed by 100 mg daily 4 days. Parenteral 120 mg on first day followed by 60 mg daily for next 4 days.	Rapidly acting schizontocide. No effect on hypnozoites or gametoeytes. Effective in chloroquin resistant falciparum malaria.	Drug fever, drug rash, bradycardia, First degree hurt block, nausea, vomiting, dark unine
8. Tetracycline Doxycycline	250 mg Q/D 100 mg B.D.	Slow acting'schizontacide Used as prophylaxis and curative, use along with other antimalarials	G.I. Disturbances Tooth discoloration
9. Cotrimoxazole Trimethoprim 80 mg + sulfam-ethoxazole 400 mg	2 tabs. B.D. for 3 days	Schizontocide resistant P. falciparum.	Drug eruptions. Bone marrow depression

guard against repeat attacks. Once malaria becomes chronic there is anaemia, nutritional deficiencies and liability to suffer from intercurrent infections. The prevalence of malaria in a community is asessed by spleen rate (percentage of children between two and 10 years with splenomegaly), parasite rate (percentage of positive cases of malaria) and infant parasite rate (percentage of children below one year of age with positive malaria parasites) and this factor of high prevalence governs the prognosis of people living in that community.

SYPHILIS

This is a systemic disease prevalent all over the world and is due to treponema pallidum, a spirochacte which is usually transmitted by sexual contact. Syphilis may be congenital or acquired which is further divided into three stages. Primary, secondary and tertiary. Primary form is characterised by a primary lesion which generally appears after an incubation period of three weeks. In the secondary stage there are generally mucocutaneous lesions widely distributed and abundant with generalized lymphadenopathy. This stage may remain latent for a number of years when it manifests with neurovascular and distinctive lesions in many tissues.

Aetiology. This disease is caused by a thin delicate aerobic organism called Treponema pallidum which survives only for a few hours under natural conditions but survives in stored blood for 72 hours. It is destroyed by heat, antiseptics and the process of drying.

Humans are the only natural host. Though many mammals can be infected by this organism yet only humans and apes show syphilitic lesions.

Infection spreads generally by sexual contact. It may also be conveyed by contamination of skin abrasions with secretions from infected lesion, the most dangerous being primary sore and moist secondary lesions.

It is not necessary for a person transmitting the infection to be suffering from external genital lesions. The period during which a person suffering from syphilis may convey infection varies. After second year infectivity declines and is reduced to minimum after five years. In case of congenital syphilis infection occurs in the second half of pregnancy.

Pathology. After gaining entry into the body, treponema rapidly develops and within a few hours reaches the lymphatics and blood stream to produce infection. It nearly effects all organs or tissues in the body making a pattern of tissue injury. The syphilitic lesions at every stage are in the form of granuloma consisting of epitheloid cells, plasma cells, numerous small lymphocytes and some giant cells. There is vasculitis leading to obliterative arteritis. This results in necrosis and ulceration of the tissues leading to scar formation. The immune responses and immunologically mediated protection do have a role to play in initial response. Late stage of tissue injury is seen many years after the primary infection and is in the form of gumma seen any where in the body and consists of a centre of coagulative necrosis surrounded by macrophages, inflammatory reaction and obliterative endarteritis. Erosion of gumma leaves behind a shaggy ulcer.

Clinical picture. Acquired syphilis consists of three distinctive stages, primary, secondary and tertiary. Of these the first two stages are most infective.

Primary syphilis. This stage is characterized by the appearance of a small papule, which is painless and single called chancre. It appears at the site of inoculation usually on the penis, vulva or cervix after an incubation period ranging from ten days to three months after sexual contact. In homosexuals the lesion may be found in the anal canal or rectum. The papule quickly enlarges, surface becomes eroded and ulcereates forming a punched out ulcer with a dull red areola and induration round about. The sore does not bleed easily and oozes out serum which is teaming with spirochaetes.

The course of primary sore varies. In some it is just a fleeting lesion and may not be noticed. Ordinarily a sore which remains untreated lasts for eight to ten weeks leaving behind a button of indurated tissue and a thin scar.

Soon after the appearance of primary lesion the nearest lymph glands become enlarged. The glands are firm, rubbery and discrete. Shortly generalized lymphadenopathy particularly in cervical axillary and epitrochlear areas appears. Even after healing of the lesion the lymph node enlargement persists.

Secondary stage. One to three months after the appearance of the chancre, secondary stage of syphilis develops. It is characterised by wide spread diffuse or patchy mucocutaneous rash accompanied by symptoms of malaise, sore throat, weight loss, headache, anorexia, arthralgia, low grade fever and generalized lymphadenopathy.

The rash is wide spread, distributed symmetrically and abundantly. Earliest lesion is macule which is rose coloured round or oval with ill defined margins. It is present on chest, flanks, back, abdomen, palms and soles. Papules which are round, brownish red or coppery firm to feel also appear at this time.

The character of rash is polymorphic (macules papules or pustules) with little variation in size. Mostly rash is maculopapular, non-itching but in some cases pustular, follicular, annular or scaly lesions are seen.

A more severe form is ecthymatous type in which papule breaks down quickly and the underlying tissue becomes ulcerated. In addition to skin lesions, papules may become large flashy looking masses due to constant moisture and rubbing. These are called moist papules or condylomata. They are rounded in outline with broad base and flat top. These are the most infective lesions of syphilis, and exude serum packed with treponema. Condylomata are seen at the mucocutaneous junctions e.g. round the anus, on the labia, between the buttocks, on the lateral aspects of scrotum and other warm moist areas of the body. Mucous surfaces of the oral cavity especially lips and pillars of fauces show snail track ulcers. On the tongue the mucous lesions appear as pink, bald spots after the papillae have been shed in the necrotic process. Mucous patches are also found in the nose, septum, floor of the mouth and extend downwards to larynx causing hoarseness of voice.

In addition to eruptions patients in secondary stage shows involvement of other organs in the body. There is generalized lymphadenopathy with glands being non-tender, discrete rubbery; joints and bursae involvement with limitation of movements. Aching pains in the long bones are due to mild periostitis. These pains are very severe and are worse at night time. Eyes shows acute iridocyclitis, pupillary abnormalities, optic neuritis and retinitis pigmentosa picture. Syphilitic hepatitis is characterised by jaundice and high levels of alkaline phosphatase. Renal inovement may take place in the form of nephrotic syndrome or immune complex glomerulonephritis.

Latent syphilis. After a variable period ranging from three to twelve months after the primary and secondary stages the patient enters into a latent period. It may be early or late latent phases. Early latent stage is the first year after infection while in the late latent stage patient may have latent fom of the disease persisting for years. In both these phases the organisms are present in the tissues and may intermititently be shed in the blood stream. This stage is diagnosed by treponemal antibody tests.

Tertiary syphilis. The pathogenesis of this stage began in early stage of the disease. Sometimes secondary and tertiary stage may merge into each other. The classical lesion is a typical distinctive lesion called 'gummata' which tends to be localised and asymmetrical in distribution. The gummata may be in the form of small pea shaped nodules joining together to form a continuous ridge present on areas exposed to friction or injury. But the commonest lesion is a painless rounded swelling, rubbery in consistency which to start with is a small nodule and progressively increases in size and involves deeper tissues such as muscle or bone. The central portion of gummata undergoes necrosis forming a gummatous ulcer. On healing a tissue paper scar is formed.

The mucous membranes of mouth and throat are often involved and the process may commence either in the hard palate or musculature of the tongue. In the tongue gummata may reach the surface and cause diffuse gummatous infiltration and even punched out ulcers. Chronic superficial glossitis and leukoplakic patches appear on the margins of tongue, mucous surfaces of cheek and at angle of the mouth. Patient generally complains of pain in the tongue and is unable to tolerate spicy and acidic foods.

Tertiary stage also involves bones and often the diagnosis is difficult. Bones most commonly involved are tibia, skull, clavicle, sternum and femur but any bone in the body can be involved. Patient complains of a gnawing boring pain which is very severe at night. It may be in the form of periostitis. Radiologically some bones show sclerotic lesions while in some bones especially of skull there are osteoporotic areas surrounded by sclerosis (moth eaten appearance). Gummata may produce destruction and there may be perforation of palate, or bridge of nose destroyed.

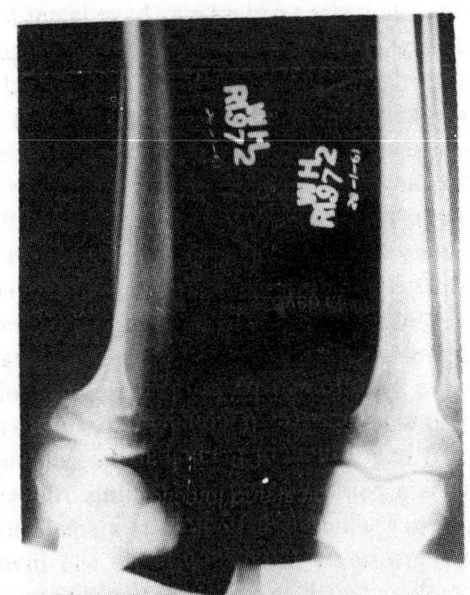

Fig. 11.6. Xray lower legs showing periosteal reaction (Syphilitic periostitis).

Central nervous system involvement in tertiary stage probably began in the early phase of disease though it may not be clinically apparent for number of years. The major involvement is in the parenchymatous or meningovascular forms.

Meningovascular syphilis is associated with diffuse involvement of meninges along with local or wide spread involvement of small medium or large vessels. It may produce acute syphilitic meningitis, basal meningitis, retrobulbar neuritis and hemiplegia. In parenchymatous form the lesions generally are tabes dorsalis, general paralysis of insane (GPI) and optic atrophy. In the spinal form of meningovascular syphilis there is meningo-myelitis, acute transverse myelitis, syphilitic pachymeningitis, erb's paraplegia and amyotrophy.

Cardiac involvement is mainly limited to large vessels. Common lesions are syphilitic aortitis, aortic regurgitation, saccular aneruysm of the ascending and arch of aorta and coronary ostial stenosis. Cardiac symptoms generally occur at periods varying from ten to thirty years after the primary infection. Asymptomatic aortitis may be suspected if there are linear calcification in the ascending aorta on X-ray abdomen.

Congenital syphilis. Treponema pallidrum are passed from an infected mother to the foetus, transmission occurring at any time during gestation. But the lesions of congenital syphilis develop only in foetus affected after the fourth month. This suggests that the pathogenesis of congenital syphilis depends on the immune response of the host. Depending upon the degree of the infection the foetus may die in utero or soon after birth or it may survive. Adequate treatment of mother before the sixteenth week of pregnancy can prevent foetal damage.

Surviving infants usually show a wide spread, fulminant picture of disease. The manifestations may be early appearing within the first two years of life and late which appear after two years and leave late stigmata.

The early manifestation are in the form of running or blocked nose (snuffles) fever, wasting. The infant is undersized marasmic with a hoarse cry, and maculopapular erruptions which are wide spread and involve almost the whole body. Sometimes bullae appear and contain serum or pus which is highly infective. Condylamata appear on the muco-cutaneous junctions. Baby has a wrinkled skin and a wizened look. Alopecia is there. Occasionally growth of black hair on head occurs (syphilitic wig).

Radiating fissures form along the angle of the mouth. Liver usually is enlarged. Kidneys may show albuminuria. Bony lesions in the form of osteochondritis develop within six months of birth. These occur at the end of long bones and are very painful. The infant may not move the limbs because of pain (pseudoparalysis). Knee joints may show painless effusions.

In the late stage which develops after two years, lesions may appear at any time. There is generally interstitial keratitis in the eyes with choroiditis and retinitis. Neurological symptoms resemble juvenile general paralysis of insane. Meningovascular syphilis or optic atrophy is rare. Eighth nerve deafness is common. Gummatous lesions of palate and periostitis resemble that of adult syphilis.

Stigmata of congenital syphilis include Hutchinson's teeth (upper central incisors are notched, widely spaced, broader at the base than at the cutting edge with central notches—peg-shaped) and mulberry molars, the sixth year molars which have poorly multiple developed cusps numbering more than usual four.

Skull shows frontal bossing. There is saddle shaped nose and maxilla which is poorly developed. Palate is high arched. Other stigmata include nerve deafness, optic atrophy, chorioretinitis and intrstitial keratitis.

Sero diagnosis of syphilis. It may be made by:

1. Non-specific tests like Wasserman's test, Kahn's test and venereal disease research laboratory (VDRL) test. These tests use cardiolipin antigen and are useful for screening purposes. They become positive within three to four weeks after primary infection and the titre progressively increase in secondary stage. These generally become negative by six months after treatment. False positive results may occur in patients of infectious mononucleosis, malaria, leprosy, hepatitis, tuberculosis, mycoplasma infection and connective tissue disorders.

2. Specific tests include treponema pallidum immobilization test (TPI) and T pallidum haemagglutination assay (TPHA) and fluorescent treponema antibodies absorbed test (FTA-ABS). These are highly specific tests. FTA-ABS becomes positive in early part of infection while TPI is positive in late stages. Also FTA-ABS is positive in patients with latent and late syphilis and remains positive for life even after treatment.

    TPI test is the most specific treponemal test but is more laborious. Out of all the tests both specific and non-specific all the tests are positive almost 100 per cent in secondary stage while FTA-ABS gives almost hundred per cent (96-100%) positivity in primary secondary and tertiary stages of syphilis.

3. Treponemas in chancres, condylomata, mucous patches and infected secretions may be visualised by dark-field microscopy. In cases of neurosyphilis, CSF is examined for increased protein concentration and pleocytosis. VDRL test may be specific if it is not contaminated with blood. Higher sensitivity is seen in meningovascular syphilis and low in asymptomatic neurosyphilis and tabes dorsalis, Lange's colloidal gold curve may show a paretic or luetic curve. FTA-ABS test is more specific.

Treatment of syphilis. The aim should be to achieve cure as well as make the patient noninfective at the earliest. In all patients with primary or secondary forms of syphilis a daily injection of 600,000 units of procaine penicillin intramuscularly for ten days is the treatment of choice. For patients sensitive to penicillin, Cap. Tetracycline 500 mg four times a day or Erythromycin 500 mg four times a day for two weeks is the alternative treatment.

Classification of syphilis

1. Acquired
   a. Primary
   b. Secondary
   c. Latent—Early latent (within 2 years of infection)
      —Late latent (after two years of infection)
   d. Tertiary syphilis.
2. Congenital
   a. Early manifestations (within 2 years of life)
   b. Late manifestations (after 2 years of birth)
   c. Residual stigmata of syphilis.

For latent and tertiary syphilis treatment is as above but for longer periods (2-3 weeks).

For cardiovascular and neurosyphilis procaine penicillin 600,000 units I/M a day for 14-21 days. The course may have to be repeated after an interval of 2 to 3 months. In cases of neurosyphilis dose of procaine penicillin is 2-4 mega units given intramuscularly daily with probenecid 500 mg four times a day for 10-14 days.

Patients of syphilis who are receiving penicillin may develop Jarisch-Herxheimer reaction due to destruction of large number of organisms. It may develop in 50 per cent of patients with primary disease and follows a few hours after first injection. It is charactrised by general malaise, headache, rigors and fever lasting for few hours. Cases of secondary syphilis are liable to get in 90 per cent of the cases while in neurosyphilis the disease may be exaceberated. In a number of cases the reaction is transient and subsides within a few hours. This reaction can be prevented by giving prednisolone 20 mg 24 hours before giving penicillin and continued for two days. Penicillin should not be witheld for fear of this reaction.

In infants with congenital syphilis Injection procaine penicillin 25,000 units/kg/dose intra-muscularly twice daily for 10 days or crystalline penicillin G. 25,000 units/kg/dose intravenously twice daily for ten days.

TESTS FOR SYPHILIS

1. Dark field examination of treponema
2. Serological tests:
a. Non-specific Kahn's test, W.R. and VDRL tests.
b. Specific
    i. Treponema pallidum immobilization test (TPI)
    ii. T. pallidum haemagglutination assay (TPHA)
    iii. Fluorescent treponema antibodies ab-sorbed test (FTA-ABS).

Follow up. All patients should be followed up for two years. CSF be examined after one year. After successful treatment VDRL progressively declines and becomes negative in 12 months time. If a patient is negative in all counts (clinically and serologically) at the end of two years he is declared cured.

GONORRHOEA

Gonorrhoea is one of the commonest sexually trans-mitted disease prevalent all over the world. It is caused by a gram negative diplococcus called Neis-seria gonorrhoea which is found in pairs with adja-cent surfaces flattened. A number of strains of neisseria are present and it is differentiated from them by its ability to utilize glucose and immuno-logic reactions. Gonococcal strains can be typed on the basis of nutritional requirements or surface antigenic variation of protein 1. It is an intracellular organism and depends for its spread upon direct transfer from host to host. The only natural hosts for the organism are humans.

The organism is rapidly killed by antiseptics, heat and by drying. It does not survive for more than a few hours outside the body.

Pathology. Sexual intercourse is the commonest mode of infection. Sometimes newly born children may be infected by infection from the mothers genitalia.

The organism after gaining entry gets attached to the columnar or transitional epithelial cells pene-trating deeply to reach the subepithelial connective tissue. Attachment of gonococci to mucosal cells is mediated in part by pili genes and protein II. In subepithelial tissue, gonococci interact with serum antibody to initiate inflammatory reaction. Exten-sion from the site of infection leads to complications such as urethritis, epididy-moorchitis and prostatitis in men while in females urethritis, endometritis, bartholinitis and salpingitis may develop.

Clinical features. The clinical picture in a case of gonococcal infection depends on the virulence of the organism, duration of infection local or systemic spread and body defence mechanism as well as immunity. The disease presents variations in its presentation and course both in males and females.

Gonorrhoea in male. Usual incubation period is from two to seven days following sexual contact. Longer intervals are also known. Some men may not develop symptoms. Earliest symptoms is burning or tingling sensation in the urethra followed by a discharge which soon becomes mucopurulent. There is dysuria and increased frequency of micturition. Pus which is greenish yellow is teeming with gonococci and is highly infective. Patient may have slight malaise. Infection soon spreads to epididymis, testes, spermatic cord and prostrate. The margins of external meatus are often inflamed and reddened.

If patient is not treated the infection may reach posterior urethra and patient now has more severe dysuria. Sometimes in severe cases a few drops of blood may be passed after micturition.

Local complications include involvement of cowper's glands and ducts, prostate gland and extension of suppuration into periuretheral tissues and scrotum often resulting in fistulous openings.

Rectum is important site of involvement in homosexual men. There is anorectal pain, tenesmus and a bloody mucopurulent discharge from rectum. Ulceration develops in the rectum and anal canal. Gonococcal organisms from homosexual men tend to be more resistant to antimicrobials as compared to those from hetrosexual contact.

Gonorrhoea in females. An uncomplicated case of gonorrhoea generally has urethritis, cervicitis and sometimes infection of vaginal orifices. Symptoms are as that in men like burning micturition, dysuria but they are less marked. There is often leucorrhoea, and features of pelvic infection. Extension of infection leads to salpingitis, bartholinitis and abdominal pain. Coexisting trichomonas infection may further increase inflammatory reaction. Chronic salpingo oophritis and tubo ovarian masses may develop. Exacerberation of disease may occur during mensturation. Pelvic infection may lead to abscess formation with resultant toxaemia.

Complicatios of gonococcal infection. These occur both in males and females and include gonococcal arthritis conjunctivitis, iridocyclitis, cutaneous lesions and septicaemia. Endocarditis and pericarditis are rare complications. Men who suffer from gonococcal infection are left behind with stricture urethra which may take some time to develop.

Laboratory diagnosis:

1. Diagnosis of gonorrhoea may be made by demonstration of intracellular gram negative diplococci in smears obtained from urethral discharge and staining with gram's stain.
2. Organisms can be identified by culture, sugar utilisation test, rapid enzyme test or agglutination reaction using antibodies that are specific for N. gonorrhoae.
3. Immunofluorescent antibody technique test is important for quick diagnosis.
4. ELISA test is done for detecting gonococcal antigens in urethral or cervical secretions.

Treatment. Various regimens are followed: Penicillin has long been used in dose of 2.4 to 4.8 mega units (Procaine penicillin intramuscular once only along with probenecid 1 G.) Alternative therapy consists of Ampicillin or Amoxycillin in a dose of 3 G orally as a single dose along with Probenecid 1 G or Co-trimoxazole 4 G in single dose.

Present trend is to give Ceftriaxone 250 mg I/M single dose and Doxycycline 100 mg twice daily for seven days. For patients who are sensitive to penicillin or in pregnant women with gonococcal infection Erythromycin 500 mg four times a day for seven days is the line of treatment.

Treatment of complicated gonorrhoea. These are the patients who have pelvic inflammatory pathology or disseminated gonococcal infection. These patients may require hospitalization. Treatment is by Ceftriaxone 1 G I/M or I/V once in twenty four hours or Cefotaxime 1 G I/V eight hourly. This has to been given for period ranging from seven to ten days.

ACQUIRED IMMUNE DEFICIENCY SYNDROME (AIDS)

Acquired immune deficiency syndrome may be defined as an opportunistic disease as a result of infection with human immunodeficiency virus type-1 (HIV-1) which produces progressive deterioration of the immune system of the body and results in develoment of persistent constitutinal symptoms ultimately leading to secondary infections, malignancies, neurologic disorders and other diseases related to acquired immunodeficiency syndrome (AIDS).

Epidemiology. AIDS is widely prevalent all over the world and primarily occurs in young adults. Humans are the only known reservoires of HIV.

The earliest case of the disease was reported in 1981 in USA and by mid 1990, approximately 120,000 cases among adults and 2000 cases among children had been seen. It is estimated that between one and 1.5 million people are infected with this virus.

The spread of HIV and AIDS in sub-Saharan Africa is probably the worst. In 13 countries of the region prevalence of HIV infection is more than 10 per cent and in some as high as 30 per cent. At the end of 1998, 22.5 million people out of the regions population of 600 million were living with HIV or AIDS and this number includes one million children. The epidemic of AIDS in sub-Saharan Africa accounts for two thirds of the world wide total of 34 million people with HIV/AIDS. On a rough estimate about 7500 people are being infected daily.

Situation in India is equally grim. Close to 3.5 million people which is about one per cent of the adult population are living with the AIDS virus in India. Abolut seven lakh of those infected could be living in rural areas and a large number of women are among those infected. HIV spreads from urban areas to rural areas, the highest prevalence in Maharashtra, Karnataka, Tamil Nadu, Andhra Pradesh and Manipur. For every infected woman there are 12 infected men in these areas.

Mode of spread. Sexual contact is the major mode of transmission. Adults at highest risk of acquiring infection include men who have sex with men (Homosexual or bisexual males) and people both men and women who have multiple sex partners. People who share infected needles or syringe, with an infected person inject drugs, and use crack cocaine are other probable victims.

A great percentage of patients are those who have received blood transfusions or blood products which are HIV infected. Haemophilics without any previous history of risk factors fall easy victim because of repeated transfusions of factor VIII and other plasma concentrates that are received intravenously. They are at further risk because of HIV contamination of blood products.

Direct inoculation of infected blood or tissue through use of contaminated needles, or a penetrating injury with a contaminated object are other modes of infection. Patient receiving transplants also run higher risk.

Children of HIV infected mothers run the risk of getting infected through perinatal transmission from the mother to the foetus or at delivery or post natally during breast feeding. This mode of transmission accounts for more than 90 per cent of HIV infection in children while the risk of an infant acquiring HIV from an infected mother before or during delivery ranges from 15 to 25 per cent.

But transmission of HIV/AIDS does not occur through touching, hugging or shaking hands with an infected person. Insect or mosquito bites, sharing food, clothes, utensils or even toilets with HIV person or through food water or casual contact in household or work place.

Etiological agent. AIDS is caused by HIV (Human Immune deficiency virus) which is a RNA cytopathic retrovirus not known to infect other animals. Humans are the only reservoirs of the virus. Two major types of HIV have been identified and these are HIV-1 and HIV-2. HIV-1 is the one responsible for most cases of AIDS all over the world while HIV-2 is less common and is said to be less pathogenic. While HIV-1 infection is more common in western countries HIV-2 is more prevalent in western African countries.

Incubation period. It is variable and depends on the mode of transmission. In adults an acute illness may occur within a few weeks after sexual contact. But onset of chronic infection varies from one to ten years. In infants and children, clinical illness is apparent within first or second year of life. When infection follows blood transfusion, clinical illness may not be detected for number of years.

Pathogenesis. Following infection with HIV, the virus attaches to the cell through interaction between the viral envelope and its receptor the CD4 molecule present on the surface of the cells. The cells worst infected are CD4+ lymphocytes and cells of monocyte-macrophage series. Following binding, virus integrates with the host cell DNA and thus establishes a persistent chronic infection.

There is generally an abrupt, slight to moderate decrease in circulating T4 lymphocytes reflecting containment of HIV infection by immune responses. Once the T4 lymphocytic count falls (200 cells per microliter or less) the chances of developing opportunistic infections are high. The relationship between depletion of T4 lymphocytes and immuno suppression is significant as subsets of these cells is responsible for regulation of immune system. Any defect in this results in global impairment of immunity.

In addition to opportunistic infection, cases of AIDS have increased incidenceof neoplasms such as Kaposi's sarcoma, Hodgkins disease, B-cell lymphomas and some malignancies. Increased levels of cytokines (cachetin) produce hypercatabolic wasting syndrome.

Clinical features. Following infection with HIV most of the patients have no signs or symptoms initially but after three to six weeks acute illness may present with non-specific features like fever, rigors, myalgia, joint pains, rash, urticaria, abdominal cramps and diarrhoea. Some of the people have features of aseptic meningitis in the form of headache and vomiting. This phase lasts for two to three weeks and resolves of its own.

This stage is followed by asymptomatic period which generally lasts from three to 10 years. Some patients develop deterioration of immune system within three years though there are no symptoms. Some develop persistent generalized lympha-denopathy which persist for more than three months, and may go on to disease progression. This is followed by AIDS related symptoms after symptom free period lasting for several months to years. Patients now have fever, fatigue, weight loss, chronic diarrhoea, skin rash, oral hairy leukoplakia, herpes and oral thrush.

Oral Lesions in HIV Disease

1. Candidiasis
   - Pseudomembranous
   - Erythematous
   - Hyperplastic
2. Hairy Leukoplakia
3. Kaposi's Sarcoma
4. Non-Hodgkins Lymphoma
5. Periodontal Disease (Gingivitis, Periodon-titis)
   - (i) Necrotising Ulcerative Periodontis
   - (ii) Linear Marginal Gingival Erythema
6. Ulcerative Stomatitis
7. Human Papilloma Virus Infection
8. Fungal Infections Other Than Candidiasis
9. Hyper Pigmentation of Oral Mucosa
10. Angular Chelitis
11. Herpes Simplex infection

Since there is progressive deterioration of immune system, ultimately development of opportunistic infections, malignancies, wide spread Kaposi's sarcoma and encephalopathy takes place. A full blown picture of AIDS develops depending on the degree of infection. It may take even 10 years for the disease to become symptomatic.

Of the various clinical manifestations of AIDS various opportunistic infections occur and produce manifestations varying on the type of infection.

Pneumocystis carinii produces pneumonia, usually interstitial and rarely disseminated. There is fever, dysponea, anaemia andsigns of toxaemia.

Cytomegalovirus infection causes retinitis, pneumonitis, intractable diarrhoea, interstitial pneumonitis and adrenalitis. Candida albicans produces oral thrush or oesophagitis. Cases of AIDS are more susceptible to suffer from tuberculosis. Cryptococcus neoformans causes meningitis while toxoplasma gondii which is responsible for one of the most common CNS infection in AIDS patients produces encephalitis. Herpes simplex infection manifests with severe mucocutaneous disease. In addition to these persistent diarrhoea, wasting and bacterial infections are common.

Thrombocytopenia may occur as the initial presenting sign of HIV infection. Kaposi's sarcoma clinically may present with multifocal vascular nodules in the skin and viscera. Neurological disorders include encelphalopathy dementia, peripheral neuropathy, myelopathy and aseptic meningitis.

Laboratory Diagnosis of HIV Infection

1. Elisa Test
   Easy to Perform
   Highly Sensitive & Specific
   Disadvantage - False Positive may occur
2. Western Blot Test (WB Test)
   Confirmatory
   Highly Specific
3. Immunofluoresence Assay (IFA)
4. Radio immuno precpitation assay
5. CD_4 Counts
6. Plasma Viral Load (PVL)

Classification system for HIV infection.
(Based on center for disease control classification).

Group I	Acute infection with transient symptoms.
Group II	Asymptomatic infection
Group III	Persistent generalized lymphadenopathy.
Group IV	Other manifestations.
Subgroup A	Chronic constitutional disease (fever, lassitude, diarrhoea).
Subgroup B	Neurologic disease (dementia, encephalopathy, aseptic meningitis, peripheral neuropathy).
Subgroup C	Secondary infections
Subgroup D	Secondary neoplasms (Kaposi's sarcoma, lymphomas, squamous carcinoma).
Subgroup E	Other conditions (diarrhoea, thrombocytopenia).

Diagnosis. The most commonly employed test is ELISA (Enzyme linked immuno sorbent assay) where presence of antibody to HIV is tested. The test may give false positive results but is a useful screening test.

Confirmation is by Western Blot Test. Other confirmatory tests are immunofluorescence assay (IFA) and radio immuno precipitation assay (RIPA).

Detectable antibodies to HIV do not appear for weeks or months following infection though in majority (95%) antibodies appear within five months of infection. Virus can be detected by assays for circulating viral protein particularly the P24 core antigen. This test is of value in children below 24 months of age.

Guidelines for Therapy

Antiretroviral therapy is indicated for all patients of HIV infection who is symptomatic. This regardless of CD_4 counts and Plasma Viral Load levels (PVL). In asymptomatic patients, ART is indicated if CD_4 count is < 350 mm^3, while patients with CD_4 count more than this, no treatment is required (ART) Except in these persons who have coexisting HIV/HBV/HCV infection.

Anti retroviral therapy has significantly reduced mortality and morbidity rates in HIV Disease. Its main goal is to ensure minimal and durable suppression of the virus as will as to reconstitute and maintain immunologic quantity and quality. Further the therapy can be used to reduce situations like prevention of transmission of infection from infected mother to child.

Treatment is divided into two major catagories.

(1) Drugs active against HIV virus

(2) Drugs to treat the opportunistic infections and malignancies.

Anti-retro viral drugs: These include five classes of drugs which are mainly used for the treatment of infected patients and includs Nucleoside and Nucleated reverse transcriptase inhibes (NRTI) (NERTI), non-nucleoside reverse transcriptase inhibitors (NNRTIS) Protease inhibitors (Pis) Entry inhibitors (Fusion and Chemokine inhibitors) and integrase inhibitors.

NRTIS (Nucleoside and Necleotide Reverse Transcriptase inhibitors)

Mechanism of action of these group of drugs is inhibition of viral reverse, Transcriptase and termination of growing DNA chain, Drugs in this group are Zidovudine (ZDV) Stavudine (d4T) Lamivudine (3TC) Didanosine (dd1) Zalcitabine (ddC) Abacavir (ABC) Tenofovir (TDF)

NNRTI'S (Non-nucleo side reverse transcriptase inhibitors)

These inhibit reverse transcriptase but are not incorporated into the viral DNA. Examples are Nevirapine (NVP) Delavairidine (DLV) Efavirenz (EFV) and Etravirine.

PI's: (Protease Inhibitors) Protease enzyme is critical for the motivation of newly formed virus. Protease inhibitors are anti viral drugs and inhibit this enzyme thereby preventing the maturation of viruses capable of infecting other cells. Drugs in this group are Saquinavir (SQV) Indinavir (IDV) Ritonavir (RTV) Naive (NFV) Lopinavir (LPV/r) Atazanavir (ATV) Tripranavir (TPV) Darunavir (DRV) and Amprenavir.

Entry Inhibitor: These are Enfurirtide (T-20) and Maraviroe. These block the entry of HIV into cells.

Integrase Inhibitor: Only drug in this group is Raltegravir and is not available in India. Its use is limited. It targets a different enzyme of HIV virus and might help prevent resistance with other medications.

Initiation of Therapy: Mono-threapy is not recommended because this does not have potent and sustained anti viral acivity. The combination of reverse transcriptase inihibitors with protease inhibitors are effective line of approach in suppressing HIV infection, reducing viral overload and prolonging life. The initial regimen shall consist of NRTI and NNRTI (two different entities in one group of drugs) and combined with a protease inhibitor later on. Commonly used combinations are
(a) Two Drugs

   (1) Stavudine + Lamivudine

   (2) Zidovudine + Lamivudine

(b) Three Drugs

   (a) Stavudine + Lamivudine + Nevirapine

   (b) Zidovudine + Lamivudine + Nevirapine

   (c) Zidovudine + Lamivudine + Elavirenz

NNRTI: Based regimens are potent and have shown comparable efficacy to retonavir boosted Pl based reginens. Use of NNRTI based regimens as initial therapy have the advantage of preserving PI's for later use.

Once the treatment has been instituted patient should be monitored for Declining viral load and improvement in CD_4 counts. Once the goal of threapy has been achieved it should be continued indefinately while monitoring all parameter. Anti retrovial therapy restores immune defects in HIV patients partially and this results in sharp decline in the opportunistic infections. Suppression of HIV is accompanied by atypical manifestations of other inflammatory diseases in some. This condition is often labelled as IRIS (Immune Reconstitution inflammatory syndrome) which is a new occurrence of worsening of existing clinical condition despite a favorable result of CD_4 counts and viral load.

Treatment of opportunistic Infections

This is important since these often kill the pateint by their over whelming complications. These range from Pneumocystis Carini, Cytomegalovirus infection, Candidiasis, Cryptococcal meningitis, Lymphoma, Kaposis Sarcoma etc. Patients with Pneumocystis infection are treated with Trimethoprim-Sulfamethoxazole/Pentamidine/Primaquine while patients with Cytomegalovirus infection shall be put on acyclovir/valaciclovir and for candida infection Ketoconazole/Fluconazole are the drugs commonly employed.

Kaposi's Sarcoma shall be present in the form of limited oral lessions on hard palate and gingiva (reddish brown or purple flat zones of discoloration which do not blanch with pressure). Treatment is either by radiation or inter lesional Vinblistine.

Course and Prognosis

It shall depend on how early the diagnosis of AIDS was arrived and when was the ART initiated. At the same time patient must be given palliative treatment with due attention to pain control and adherance of therapy. Further CD_4 Counts, viral load, presence or absence of opportunistic infections shall further guide the prognosis.

Guidance on Oral Hygiene to HIV Patients

1. A soft/super soft tooth brush be used for cleaning of teeth.
2. Interdental plaque be regularly removed. Patient be advised to use Dental Flossing for removal of plaque.
3. Regular mouth wash with Chlorhexidine (0.12%) twice a day. It shall reduce the incidence of gingivitis.

WHO Clinical Staging System of AIDS in Adults

1. Clinical Stage 1

Asymptomatic

Persistent generalized Lymphadenopathy

2. Clinical Stage 2

1. Moderate unexplained Weight Loss (under 10% of body weight)
2. Recurrent Respiratory tract infections
3. Angular Chelitis
4. Recurrent oral ulcerations
5. Fungal infections of Nails

3. Clinical Stage 3

1. Unexplained severe weight loss; Chronic Diarrhoea Persistent Fever
2. Persistent oral Candidiasis
3. Acute necrotizing ulcerative Stomatitis, gingivitis or periodontis
4. Oral Hairy Leukoplakia
5. Pulmonary tuberculosis
6. Severe bacterial infection

4. Clinical stage 4

1. HIV Wasting Syndrome
2. Kaposis Sarcoma
3. HIV Encephalopathy
4. Oesophageal Candidiasis
5. Recurrent Severe Bacterial infections/septicaemia
6. Disseminated Mycosis
7. Extra Pulmonary Cryptococcosis
8. Lymphoma (Cerebeal or B Cell Non-Hodgkins)
9. Symptomatic associated nephropathy or Cardiomyopathy

Commonly Used Anti Retroviral Drugs

NRTI	Dose	Side effects
1. Zidovudine	600 mg in two divided dose	Anorexia Nausea, malaise, Anaemia, Abdominal pain, Fever, Neutropenia, Leucopenia
2. Zalcitabine	0.37 - 0.75 mg three times daily	Hepatitis Stomatitis Peripheral Neuropathy
3. Stavudine	40 mg twice daily	Peripheral Neuropathy, Headache, Chills Rise in liver enzymes, Abdominal Pain. Pancreatitis
4. Lamivudine	150 mg orally twice daily	Skin Rashes Neuropathy, Headache, Nausea Insomnia, Dizziness
5. Abacavir	300 mg orally twice daily	Fever; Hyper sensitivity Reaction Fatigue, nausea, skin rash, vomiting Diarrhoea
NNRI's		
6. Nevirapine	200 mg daily for 2 weeks then 200 mg twice daily	Drug Rash, Malaise, Hyper Sensitivity Cutaneous eruptions
7. Efavirenz	600 mg orally once daily	Rash Dizziness, Nausea, Headache Insomnia
Proteose inhibitors		
8. Saquinavir	1200 mg three times daily	Dry Mouth, Night sweats, Dizziness, Ataxia, confusion
9. Ritonavir	600 mg orally twice daily	Nausea, Palpitation, Bloody Diarrhoea, Vomiting, Cachexia

Miscellaneous

ALLERGY

Allergy is defined as 'altered reactivity' which is immunologically mediated reaction. An individual becomes sensitilized to any agent and reacts to it or to an extract of it by process of allergic reaction (swelling, inflammation and oedema). The change responsible is in tissue cells and not dependent on presence of an antibody in the blood. Thus anaphylactic sensitivity is transferable from one individual to another by serum, but allergy is not.

Hypersensitivity reaction. This is dependent on the introduction of an antigen which may be in the form of dust, pollens, fungi and food particles. This leads to the production of IgE antibodies in sensitive persons which get attached to mast cells producing excessive damaging reaction termed hypersensitivity reaction. Six types of hypersensitivity reactions have been described and most of them occur in combination with one another.

Type I reaction (anaphylactic immediate hypersensitivity reaction). This is an allergic reaction which occurs within 15-30 minutes of exposure to an allergen. This reaction is mediated by IgE antibodies which get attached to surface of mast cells. This type of reaction occurs in cases of asthma, allergic rhinitis and anaphylaxis in people who are genetically predisposed atopic individuals.

Type I reaction can be transferred to another person by injection of IgE containing serum and this reaction is abolished by use of drugs like adrenaline and antihistamines which compete with the released histamine. Type I reactions are diagnosed by skin-prick tests, when an allergen is injected into the skin and observed for the development of weal and induration within 15 minutes. There is a good correlation between diameter of weal and levels of specific IgE antibodies in the serum.

Type II reactions (cytotoxic/membrane reactions). Here antibodies are produced against the patients own cells and antibodies of the IgG or IgM class are directed against cell surface or tissue antigen. They also block the receptor site, thus preventing its normal functioning. This reaction results in production of auto immune haemolytic anaemia, pernicious anaemia, myasthenia gravis and transfusion reactions.

Type II reaction is diagnosed by Coombs' test, red cell agglutination and indirect immuno-fluorescence methods.

Type III reactions (immune complex mediated hyper sensitivity reactions). The presence of antigen continuously results in persistent antibody production. Antibodies (IgG, IgM and IgA) react with antigen to form immune complexes which circulate in the body.

The antigens in this type of reaction are generally exogenous (bacteria, fungi, parasites) or may be auto-antigens. It takes between 4-12 hours for the reaction to develop.

The immune complexes are usually removed by the cells of reticuloendothelial system but in the presence of an hypersensitivity reaction, inflammatory reaction leading to tissue damage occurs. If the antibody is in excess, it tends to precipitate the complexes which are localised at the site of entry of antigen. Conversely if antigen is in excess, soluble complexes are formed which get precipitated in all tissues.

This type of reaction is diagnosed by skin tests which show Arthus type reaction.

Common diseases in this group are glomerulonephritis, S.L.E., rheumatoid arthritis, farmer's lung.

Type IV reactions (Cell mediated/delayed hypersensitivity reaction). This type of reaction is mediated by T cells and generally takes between 12-48 hours to develop. This type of reaction can not be transferred by serum and is mediated by delayed hypersensitivity cells which have become sensitized to a particular antigen previously. Further T cells from sensitised individuals may directly damage injected target cells like virus infected cells.

Type IV reactions are diagnosed by skin tests (tuberculin test) and are seen in viral infections, tuberculosis brucellosis, autoimmune diseases such as Hashimoto's thyroiditis and homograft rejection.

Type V reactions (Stimulating antibody reaction). Here antibodies of IgG act against some component of the receptor producing continuous stimulating activity rather than destroying them. This type of reaction is important in the production of neonatal hyperthyroidism where long acting stimulator (LATS) produces TSH like activity.

Type VI reaction (antibody-dependent cell-mediated cytotoxicity). Here the effects cells are K cells which lyse target cells coated with antibody. Only very small amounts of antibody is required to produce this reaction. The K cells react with cell bound antibody and destroy target cells by means of an enzyme.

This type of reaction is important in autoimmune diseases and defence against helminthic infections.

Diseases related to allergy. A number of diseases ranging from respiratory, eyes, skin and gastrointestinal tract are known to result due to an allergen provoking an allergic response. In some persons pseudoallergic reaction takes place where the allergic response is there but without immunologic response. In this category are substances which release histamine and other mediators directly from mast cells without involving an antigen antibody reaction. e.g. aspirin may produce flushing, urticaria, rhinitis, bronchial asthma, conjunctivitis and angioneurotic oedema without an antigen antibody reaction.

Common diseases are:

1. *Respiratory.* Allergic rhinitis, hay fever, bronchial asthma, bronchopulmonary allergic aspergillosis.
2. *Eyes.* Phlyctenular conjunctivitis, allergic iritis.
3. *Skin.* Urticaria, angioneurotic oedema, drug rashes, contact dermatitis, eczematoid dermatitis.
4. *GI tract.* Food allergy.

Allergic rhinitis. It is one of the commnest and obvious form of allergy. Here the patient is susceptible to very small doses of some substances to which he has become sensitized but to these substances normal people are completely immune.

Allergic rhinitis occurs in atopic individuals i.e. in persons with a family history of allergy or a personal history of some form of allergy.

The substances which may cause the disease are diverse and numerous.

A person may inhale pollens of certain plants, weeds or grasses, moulds or fungi. This type of rhinitis is generally seasonal and depends on the pollination of these flowers and plants. Other sources include animal products like hair feathers and even small particles present in their desqumating skin. House dust which contains numerous such substances is notorious for causing allergic rhinitis.

Ingestion of some common food items such as eggs, fish may produce allergic sensitization. Often a focus of infection in the nasal sinuses may induce allergic response.

In some people allergic rhinitis is seasonal while in others it is perennial where person is sensitive to an allergen like house dust.

Clinical features. Disease shows itself in early adolescence and improves with age though in some patients symptoms start in the third or fourth decade. The symptoms come and go rapidly. There is rhinorrhoea, sneezing, lacrimation and itching of the conjunctiva along with obstruction of the nasal passages due to swelling of nasal mucosa.

The nasal mucosa is pale and swollen. Swelling of the nasal passages may induce secondary infection by obstructing eustachian tubes. The mucosal fluid contains eosinophils, IgA and IgE antibodies. The mast cells present in the nasal mucosa and submucosa generate and release mediators through IgE associated reactions resuling in not only tissue oedema but also eosinophilic infiltration.

Diagnosis of allergic rhinitis depends mainly on seasonal occurrence and clinical profile of sneezing, running and blocked nose, excessive lacrimation are important in making diagnosis. Often an offending allergen can be located. Blood count shows eosinophilia. Nasal smear also shows eosinophils. Total serum IgE is frequently elevated. Further skin tests shall also confirm the offending allergen.

Treatment is by avoidance of exposure to the allergen which may be offending agent.

Temporary relief is obtained by antihistamines. Immunotherapy which consists of repeated injections of gradually increasing concentrations of preparation obtained from the allergen responsible for the disease produce hyposensitization and is helpful in some.

Topical use of steroids ameliorates symptoms especially in seasonal type of allergic rhinitis.

Food allergy. Food allergy or intolerance is one entity which is very common but often missed. In some people, allergic reactions to some foods occur in the form of vomiting, diarrhoea, pain abdomen, indigestion and general symptoms like headache, palpitation etc. Allergy to food starts immediately after taking the food and there may be sometimes urticaria, swelling of lips and anaphylactic shock. These symptoms are in addition to G.I. symptoms.

Allergic reaction may be due to a constituent of food or reaction to chemical mediators released by food or to toxic chemicals present in preserved foods. Though the exact mechanism of cause of food allergy is not clear but this term is often restricted to patients who demonstrate immunologically hypersensitive reaction which is being mediated by IgE.

Clinical features. These are immediate which start within a short time of ingestion of that particular food while the delayed symptoms are rather vague and generally consist of indigestion, dyspepsia etc..

Foods which may cause allergy are diverse and generally consist of eggs, fish, sea food, cheese, milk, bananas.

Diagnosis of food allergy can be made by a good history. Skin prick tests may be helpful. Dietary challenge is other form of arriving at diagnosis when the patient is given small quantity of that food and response studied.

Treatment is by exclusion of the food responsible for allergic reaction. Here the cooperation of the patient should be sought as by constant experimentation, the food responsible can be isolated.

DRUG REACTIONS

Drugs form essential part of treatment of any disease. They may be employed as effective agents against disease or as replacement in certain diseases where there is deficiency of a substance like in cases of myxoedema, addison's disease. But the main aim is to achieve therapeutic cure.

While achieving therapeutic levels, a drug may produce unwanted side effects or toxicity. This reaction of drug is called adverse drug reaction and has been defined as drug reaction which is unintended and harmful and which occurs when a drug is given in usual therapeutic doses for therapeutic, diagnostic or prophylactic purpose. Drug reactions may be in the form of side effects, over dosage, intolerance, idiosyncrasy and hypersensitivity reaction.

Broadly there are predictable reactions (side effects, toxicity, overdosage) while unpredictdable reactions include idiosyncrasy and hypersensitivity reaction.

These may vary from mild to severe forms of reaction and may be dose dependent in some while in others factors of sensitivity reaction may play major role and even exposure to a very small dose of drug may induce severe reaction. Let us look at some of these adverse reactions.

Side effects. These are those undesireable effects which accompany therapeutic effects of the drug and so does not necessitate stoppage of the drug. In this group are examples of anticholinergics for treatment of peptic ulcer where dryness of mouth results. Another example is use of sorbitrate in cases of angina pectors and an undesirable side effect is headache.

Toxic effects. These effects develop when a drug is used for long periods in therapeutic doses. The period for which the drug is used may vary from person to person.

Tubercular patients on isoniazid may develp peripheral neuropathy and those on ethambutol develop optic neuritis/atrophy. Toxic effects of any drug may be potentiated if the patient is suffering from hepatic or renal insufficiency. Cardiotoxic effect of dehydroemetine and vestibular damage due to streptomycin toxicity and ototoxicity due to aminoglycosides are other examples of toxic effects. Similarly use of antimalarial drugs in patients of G-6-PD deficiency shall result in haemolytic anaemia or black water fever.

Poisoning. It results when large doses of the drug has been consumed over prolonged periods or by accidental consumption or for suicidal and homicidal purposes.

Drug intolerance. Some people are intolerant to a drug even in very small therapeutic doses. This is because of low threshold of the person to the drug, e.g. chloroquine in usual dosage produces nausea and vomiting but an intolerant person may develop vomiting even with a single tablet. Ataxia results after prolonged use of carbamazepine but in some it develops after a few doses.

Idiosyncrasy. It is abnormal reaction to any drug which occurs in individuals who are genetically predisposed to it.

Example is people with G-6-PD deficiency who remain alright but when exposed to antimalarials, quinidine, nalidixic acid develop haemolytic anaemia. Quinine may cause cramps, diarrhoea and vascular collapse in some.

Drug allergy. Allergy to any drug is independent of the dose of the drug. Even very small doses of the drug may initiate sensitivity reaction. These reactions generally occur in patients who have previously been exposed and sensitized to the drug or to another drug of the same chemical class. These reactions are based either on humoral factor or cell mediated. IgE mediated drug reactions usually manifest in the skin, G.I. tract, respiratory and cardiovascular system.

Photosensitivity. Exposure of skin to ultraviolet rays of the sun results in cutaneous reactions from drug induced sensitization. It may result in metabolic disorders in which photosensitizing chemical is produced. Drugs or their metabolic products which accumulate in the skin undergo a photochemical reaction on first exposure and the phototoxicity results due to concentration of sensitizer and amount of light resulting in erythema, oedema and skin eurptions. Drugs in this group include tetracyclines, fluoroquinolones, and phenothiazine.

Teratogenicity. This is the type of drug reaction which should always be kept in mind when prescribing any drug to a pregnant women. A drug is teratogenic if it harms the foetus. The harm can be anatomic where child is liable to be born with anatomical congenital anomalies or the growth being retarded.

A foetus can be effected depending on the time the drug is given.

First trimester of pregnancy is the most vulnerable period in the growth of foetus. In the earlier part, a drug is likely to produce deformities while in the latter part functional and developmental abnormalities occur. The type of malformation depends on the drug as well as on stage of exposure of the foetus to the drug. A whole lot of drugs are known to be teratogenic and it is a wise policy to avoid any drug during pregnancy until and unless it can not be avoided.

Cytotoxicity. Certain substances like radio isotopes, are known to act as cytotoxic and may produce cancer later on. An example is use of radio active iodine in the treatment of hyperthyroidism. Such patients may suffer from carcinoma of thyroid after a period of 10-15 years. Chemical carcinogenesis is also recognised and may take number of years to develop e.g. parenteral iron may lead to development of sarcoma at the site of injections after number of years.

Drug induced diseases. A number of drugs have side effects which sometimes if persistent produce major illnesses.

1. Use of salicylates, NSAIDs for long periods produces hyperacidity and peptic ulcer.
2. Corticosteroids use produces Cushing's syndrome-like picture, peptic ulcer, diabetes, hypertension and cataract.
3. Hepatitis may be induced by isoniazid, rifampicin/pyrazinamide.
4. Parkinsonism-like picture by phenothiazines.
5. Aplastic anaemia is one of the commonest haematological abnormalities which is secondary to drugs either dose dependent or idiosyncrasy to the drug or as a result of immunologic mechanism. Drugs in this group include chloramphenicol, phenylbutazone and gold salts.
6. Leukopenia results due to cytotoxic drugs and corticosteroids. Drugs like stibophen, quinine cause haemolysis by immune complex mechanism.

Cytotoxic drugs such as cyclophosphamide, cytosine arabinoside, 6-mercaptopurine and 5-fluorouracil block DNA synthesis and produce megaloblastic change in dose dependent manner. while thrombocytopenia may be caused by drugs like phenylbutazone, isoniazid, nitrofurantoin, sulfonamides and acetaminophen. Acute attacks of intermittent porphyria are precipitated by barbiturates, oral contraceptives, alpha methyl dopa, sulfona-mides, griseofulvin and phenytoin.

7. Cardiac disorders may be caused by drugs used for cardiac illnesses like cardiac arrhythmias induced by sympathomimetic agents and anti arrhythmic drugs. Hypotension may result due to use of diuretics. Most of antiarrhythmic drugs (Digoxin, quinidine, lignocaine, verapamil) and other drugs like carbamazepine, phenothiazines, imipramine, levodopa and theophylline produce a number of cardiac rhythm irregularities either by exaggerating the existing arrhythmia or new arrhythmia (proarrhythmias) while drugs in the latter group produce these irregularities either as a result of central action or effect on autonomic nervous system.

Myocardial depression results due to digitalis, verapamil, anti parkinsonian drug (amantadine), chloroquine, tricyclic antidepressants while toxic myocarditis may be produced by drugs like emetine, adriamycin, fluorouracil, cyclophosphamide, lithium and phenothiazines. Hypersensitivity myocarditis has been observed after use of methyl dopa, hydralazine, chlorthalidone, spironolactone, sulfonamides, indomethacin, acetazolamide, amitryptiline, sylfonylureas, carbamazepine and diphenylhydantoin etc.

8. Drug-induced respiratory disorders are equally common and a number of drugs produce not only parenchymal but also interstitial lung disease.

Drugs that may cause parenchymal lung injury include mitomycin, busulfan, melphalan, cyclophosphamide, methotrexate, vinblastine, nitrofurantoin, sulfasalazine, carbamazepine, lidocaine, amiodarone propranolol, and gold salts while drugs causing pneumonitis or fibrosiitis include methotrexate, busulfan, mitomycin, chlorambucil gold salts, penicillamine and nitrofurantoin.

Cutaneous drug eruptions. Cutaneous eruptions are the most common adverse effect of drugs and these are of varied forms ranging from fixed drug eruptions to bullous and toxic epidermal necrolysis. Various common forms of eruptions are:

1. *Urticaria.* Here there is itching, red wheals and lesions vary from a small point to large areas. Itching is the most distressing part. This generally results from either IgE dependent mechanism circulating immune conmplexes or as a result of non-immunologic activation of effective pathways.

   Common drugs producing urticarial eruptions include aspirin, penicillin, NSAIDs, radiographic dyes. In fact any drug can cause immediate acute urticarial eruption.

2. *Photosensitivity or phototoxic eruptions.* These are in the form of increased pigmentation on the exposed surfaces and often simulate sun burn. Drugs commonly known to cause these reactions include chlorpromazine, tetracycline, thiazides, nalidixic acid and piroxicam.

3. *Pigmentary changes* in the skin may be caused by antimalarials, phenothiazines and heavy metals like gold, bismuth and mercury. Clofazimine, a drug used in the treatment of leprosy causes red colour of skin while oral contraceptives may produce chloasma.

4. *Maculopapular eruptions* are very common form of drug induced reaction which generally start from the trunk or areas of pressure or trauma. These eruptions tend to become confluent and are often associated with itching and malaise. These eruptions generally appear after a week or so of taking the offending drug. Drugs commonly responsible are ampicillin, amoxycillin, trimethoprim-sulfamethoxazole,.

5. *Erythema multiforme* is a form of inflammatory lesion of skin and mucous membranes.

Drugs like phenyl butazone sulfonamides, penicillin and phenytoin produce this type of lesion. A more severe form of this type of eruption associated with fever, arthralgia, ulceration in the mucous surfaces is known as Stevens-Johnson syndrome and is often produced after intake of long acting sulfonamides and trimetoprim-sulfamethoxazole.

6. *Fixed drug eruptions.* These are erythematous lesions ococurring on the face, genitalia and oral mucosa. These are associated with sulfonamides, tetracyclines, barbiturates and phenyl butazone.

7. *Bullous eruptions.* These are severe pemphigoid like eruptions and occur after nalidixic acid, frusemide, penicillamine and clonidine use.

8. *Toxic epidermal necrolysis.* It is a very serious form of drug eruption and may even prove fatal. This type of reaction has been seen with sulfonamides, phenytoin, NSAID's and after measles vaccination.

Factors influencing adverse drug reactions:

1. **Age.** Small infants especially premature because of their hepatic drug metabolizing enzymes being not efficient and renal functions unsatisfactory have more chances of developing drug reactions. Example is production of grey baby syndrome in premature infants on chloramphenicol. Premature infants have a relatively low glomerular filtration rate and renal plasma flow as compared to adults with the result that because of decreased excretion of drugs chances of developing reactions increase. Similarly people in elderly age group there is reduced kidney efficiency and hepatic drug metabolism is effected and this contributes to the development of adverse drug reactions. As glomerular filtration falls with age so the result is accumulation of drugs which are principally excreted by the kidney. Moreover elderly have reduced body mass. Chances of adverse drug reactions increase in geriatric patients if the dosage of drugs administered is not adequately reduced.

2. **Sex.** Women are more prone to suffer from adverse drug reactions. No explanation is available for this except that this may be sex linked.
3. **Pregnancy.** A large number of drugs have teratogenic properties and produce anatomical defects and retard growth of the foetus when given in early months of pregnancy.
4. **Race.** People of certain races are more prone to suffer from adverse drug reaction. In Egyptians who are poor acetylators, chances of isoniazid and hydralazine toxicity increase. Similarly incidence of G-6-PD deficiency is more in American blacks, so use of antimalarials can cause haemolysis in them.
5. **Hepatic and renal disorders.** Persons who suffer from chronic hepatic or renal insufficiency are more likely to get adverse drug reaction because of poor metabolism and excretion of drugs.
6. **Enzyme activity.** Differences in enzyme activity which may either be inherited (genetic linked) or acquired shall interfere with the metabolic pathway of the drug administered increasing its adverse effects. Examples are administration of barbiturates in a case of acute porphyria. Similarly when there is interference with hepatic drug metabolizing pathway or in the excretion of drugs by the kidney, adverse effects of the drug result. Changes in urinary pH also control the excretion of the drug.

Physiological changes in the body tissues also govern the adverse effects of the drug. In cases of congestive heart failure when there is hypokalaemia, this leads to increased concentration of digitalis in the cardiac muscle thus enhancing its toxic effects.

Thus when administering drug to any patient one must consider the age, sex, weight and built of the individual. Dose of the drug must be as per the body's weight. People at extremes of age group (infants and elderly age group) shall require lesser amount of drugs. Similarly in patients with chronic hepatic or renal insufficiency since drug metabolism or excretion is going to be effected, dosage of the drug has to be given in reduced quantity.

While prescribing more than one or two drugs one must be aware that there is no interaction between these drugs. It is equally important to elicit history of any drug allergy in the past. People who suffer from allergic diathesis are more prone to get allergic drug reactions. So if the drugs are prescribed in judicious manner, adverse drug reactions can be minimized.

Drugs which have adverse effects on the foetus if given to mother during pregnancy.

Drug	Abnormality
Tetracyclines	Deformed and discoloured teeth.
Aminoglycosides	Eighth nerve deafness
Antithyroid drugs	Foetal hypothyroidism, goitre
Anti-epileptic drugs	Various congenital malformations, spina bifida.
Corticosteroids	Foetal and neonatal adrenal suppression, congenital anomalies.
Androgens	Virilization, cardiac anomalies.
Oral antidiabetics	Foetal and neonatal hypoglycemia
NSAIDs	Premature closure of ductus arteriosus, delayed labour.
Anti-cancer drugs	Foetal death
Lithium	Foetal goitre, cardiac and other anomalies.
Beta agonists	Foetal tachycardia
Beta antagonists	Foetal and neonatal bradycardia

Haematological manifestations:

Agranulocytosis. Chloramphenicol, Co-trimoxazole, gold salts, antithyroid drugs, tricyclic antidepressants, phenylbutazone.

Haemolytic anaemia. Chlorpromazine, dapsone, phenacetin, quinidine, isoniazid, levodopa, rifampicin.

Haemolytic anaemia (in G-6-PD deficiency). Antimalarials, cotrimoxazole, nalidixic acid, phenacetin. **Quinidine.** Sulfonamides, dapsone, nitrofurantoin.

Thrombocytopenia. Co-trimoxazole, gold salts, indomethacin, methyldopa, quinine, quinidine, thiazides, chlorpropamide.

PLATE XXIII

ALLERGY

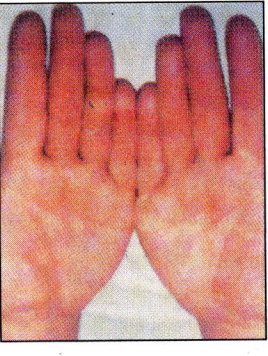

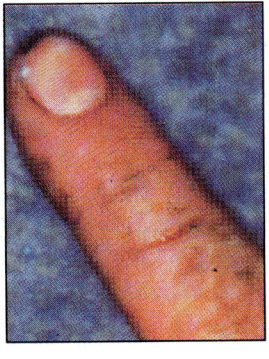

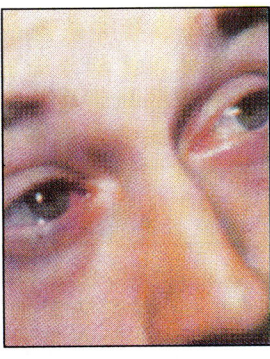

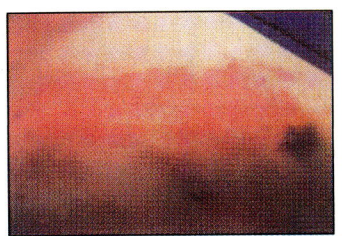

Allergic contact dermatitis.

Allergic dermatitis.

Primary irritant dermatitis due to contact with detergents.

Arc welders' eyes.

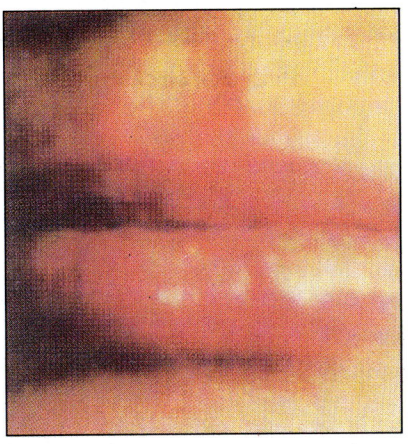

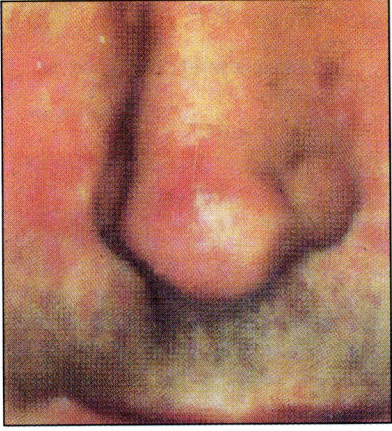

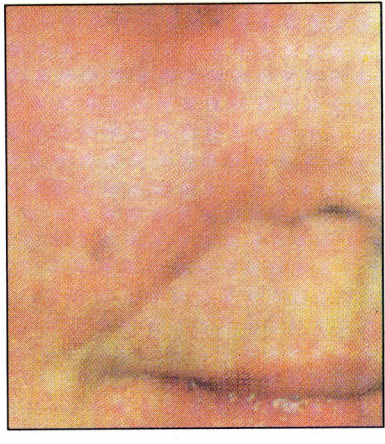

Herpes simplex triggered by ultraviolet light to produce actinic cheilits.

Photoallergy. Drugs like tetracyclines, thiazides & phenothiazines can react with ultraviolet light to produce photoallergy.

Butterfly eruption in a patient of systemic lupus erythematosis. This followed exposure to sunlight.

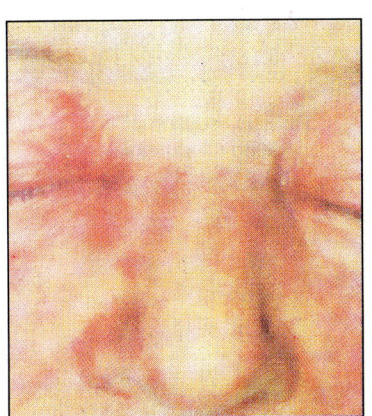

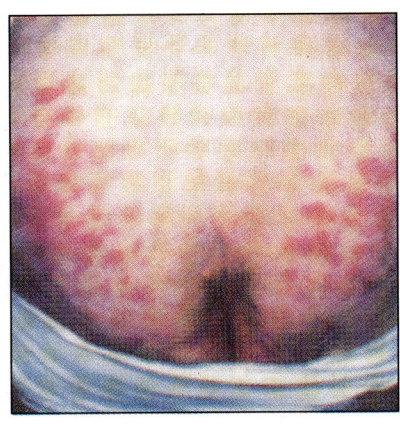

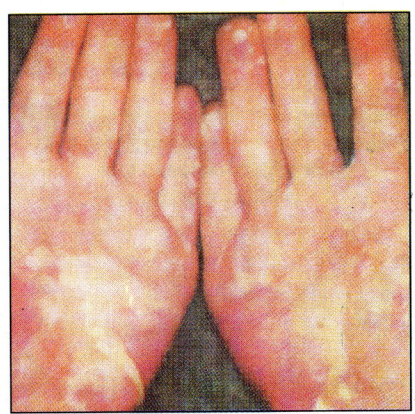

Phytophotodermatitis as a result of reaction of sunlight with the plant primrose.

Erythema multiforme following nitrate therapy.

Stevens-Johnson syndrome. This followed after ingestion of cotrimoxazole.

PLATE XXIV

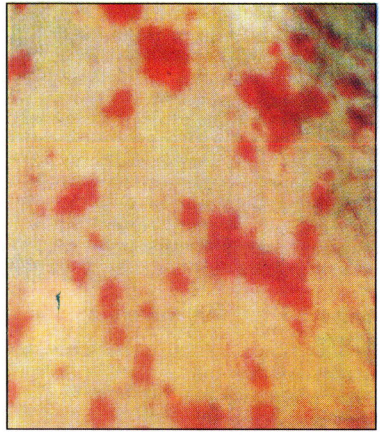

Purpuric eruptions due to phenytoin

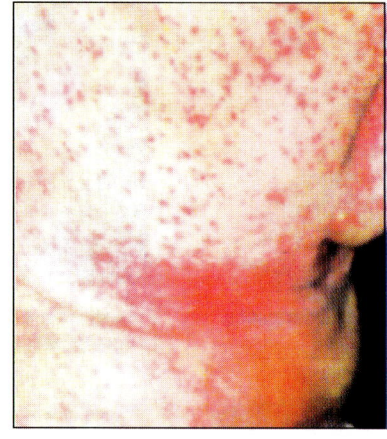

Rash following cotrimoxazole

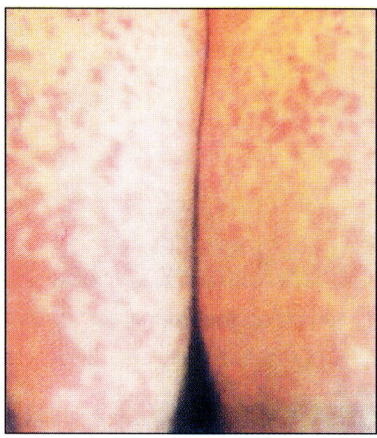

Rash after ampicillin

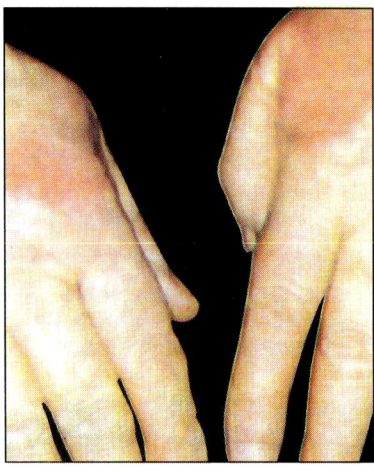

Fixed drug rash following tetracycline (reaction that recurs at the same time a person is exposed to a particular drug)

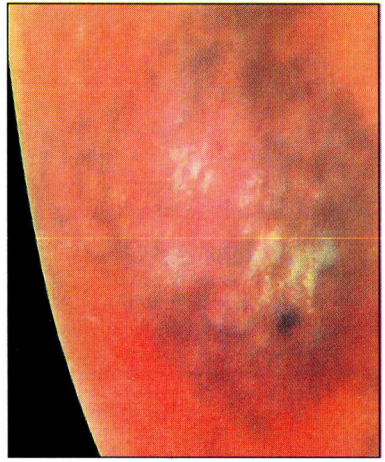

Lichenoid reaction after chloroquine

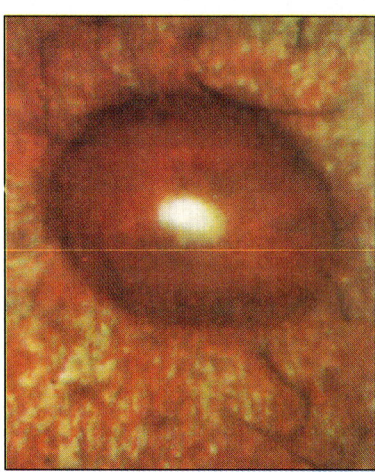

Bullous eruption after taking allopurinol

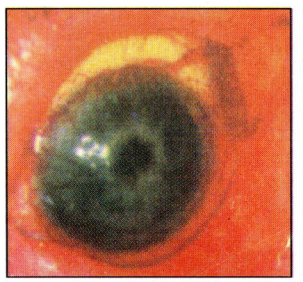

Phytophotodermatitis caused by combination of reaction between a plant chemical and ultraviolet light

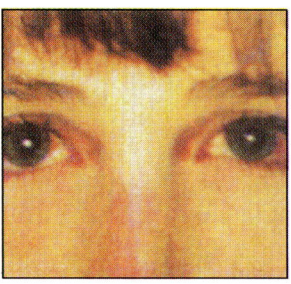

Reaction to soft contact lenses. Increase in vascularity of area and marked redness

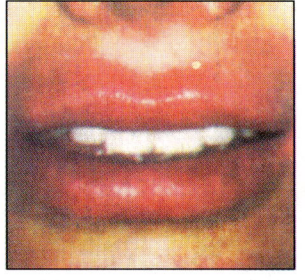

Contact cheilitis after using a balm containing lanolin

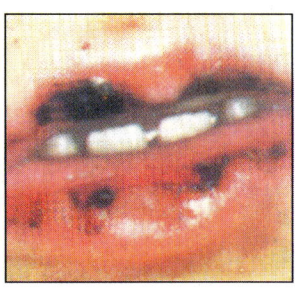

Stevens-Johnson syndrome

Clinical manifestations of adverse reaction to drugs:

Anaphylaxis	Fever
Penicillin	Antipsychotics
Streptomycin	Antihistaminics
Ampicillin	Amphotericin-B
Amoxycillin	
Lidocaine	
Cephalosporins	
Iodine	
Radioactive dyes	
Contrast substances	

Drug-induced lupus erythematosus:

1. Barbiturates
2. Hydralazine
3. Iodides
4. Isoniazid
5. Methyldopa
6. Phenytoin
7. Quinidine
8. Procainamide

Metabolic manifestations:

1. *Hyperglycaemia.* Frusemide, oral contraceptives, glucocorticoids, thiazides, beta-blockers.
2. *Hyperuricaemia.* Aspirin, diuretics
3. *Hyperkalaemia.* Digitalis, spironolactone, triamterene
4. *Hypokalaemia.* Diuretics, laxatives, corticosteroids.

Cardiac manifestations:

1. *Arrhythmias.* Digoxin, quinidine, atropine, emetine, lithium, phenothiazines, thyroxine, tricyclic antidepressants, verapamil, lignocaine, sympathomimetic drugs, diuretics, theophylline.
2. *Cardiomyopathy.* Emetine, lithium, phenothiazines, adriamycin, sulfonamides, sympathomimetics, daunomycin.
3. *Congestive failure.* Minoxidil, propranolol, steroids, estrogens.
4. *Hypotension.* Nifedipine, diuretics, nitrates, phenothiazines, quinidine, procainamide.

5. *Hypertension.* Oral contraceptives, corticosteroids, sympathomimetics.
6. Pericarditis. Hydralazine, emetine, procainamide, quinidine.

Pulmonary manifestations:

1. Asthma. Beta blockers, aspirin, indomethacin, penicillin, cholinergic drugs.
2. Pneumonitis/fibrosis. Mitromycin, busulfan, melphalan, methotrexate, nitrofurantoin, gold salts, sulfasalazine, amiodarone.
3. Pulmonary parenchymal injury. Mitomycin, busulfan, cyclophosphamide, nitrofurantoin, diphenyl hydantoin, haloperidol, lidocaine, procainamide, propranolol, gold salts, isoniazid, colchicine, penicillamine.

DRUG INTERACTIONS

Drug interaction is an important problem in clinical practice since a number of drugs being taken simultaneously either for one ailment or in a patient where there are more than two or three diseases (Diabetes, hypertension, coronary heart disease) at the same time, result is that number of drugs being prescribed are essentially going to be numerous. In this way the examples can be multiplied ad lib. When confronted with such situation, it is important for the prescribing doctor to be aware that there is no interaction between the drugs being prescribed. While drug interaction is being considered it is equally important to know the relationship between drugs and diet.

Drug interaction has been defined as the action of an administered drug upon the effectiveness or toxicity of another drug administered earlier, siumltaneously or later.

When two or more drugs are prescribed either simultaneously or in quick succession they may exhibit either a synergic or antagonistic action. When two drugs are combined and given in single dose they potentiate the action of each other. Examples are ephedrine + theophylline (Bronchodilator) amlodipine + atenolol (antihypertensive) sulfonamide + trimethoprim (anti microbial). Antagonistic action of drug is demonstrated when one drug inhibits the action of another. Thus while frusemide leads to potassium depletion from the body, spironolactone retains potassium leading to hyperkalaemia. When these two drugs are combined though some of their action is antagonistic to each other yet results are beneficial.

Mechanism of drug interactions. These are varied since the drugs have the potential of acting in an almost infinite number of ways at several sites in the body, starting from their ingestion, absorption to their excretion.

Many drugs may influence gastrointestinal function like reduction in the rate of their absorption or in the total amount of drug absorbed so that the effects of the drug are reduced. One drug may alter the absorption of other drug by changes in the pH of GI tract, formation of complex substances, alterations in gastric emptying and GI motility. Thus absorption of tetracyclines is inhibited when given along with antacids or iron preparations. Similarly colchicine by its action on intestinal mucosa shall interfere with the absorption of vitamin B_{12} and may cause megaloblastic anaemia.

Interaction between drugs may occur at levels which involve the body's metabolic enzyme system. Drugs may enhance or inhibit the production of liver microsomal enzyme system. One of the administered drug causes a change in the amount of metabolizing enzyme or its activity in relation to the other drug. This may change the rate of biotransformation in the body and the action of one or both of the drugs may be either enhanced or decreased. Examples of this shall be barbiturates which stimulate the metabolism and reduce activity of drugs like coumarin anticoagulants, cortisol, doxycycline, oestrogen, digitoxin, chloramphenicol Similarly Rifampicin shall decrease the effect of oral contraceptives, propranolol, quinidine, and oral anticoagulants.

One drug may inhibit the metabolism of another drug by inhibiting the activity of hepatic microsomal enzymes or by competing for the same enzyme or coenzyme. Isoniazid inhibits the metabolism of diphenylhydantoin thereby increasing its toxicity manifold especially in patients who are slow acetylatorsof isoniazid. MAO inhibitors interfere with the metabolism and enhance the effect of drugs like oral antidiabetics, tricyclic antidepressants and narcotic analgesics.

Warfarin by competitive inhibition reduces the metabolism of phenytoin and thus a patient on usual doses of phenytoin may exhibit signs of its toxicity.

Food drug interactions. Food has an important role to play in the body metabolism, and equally so when drugs are to be administered. Drugs when taken orally are absorbed in the G.I. tract and then through blood stream travel to various sites. A food item may sometimes interfere with the absorption, distribution or excretion of a drug. Thus if tetracycline is taken with milk, its absorption is delayed and so its potency is effected.

The effect of chlorpromazine is weakened if taken with tea or coffee, while erythromycin effect is reduced if taken with fruit juices or aerated drinks. Diazepam absorption is enhanced if taken with food. Absorption of iron salts is faster if taken with fruit juices while cereals, eggs and milk inhibit their absorption due to formation of insoluble chelates.

Food has a definite role to play. Many drugs if taken on empty stomach cause gastric irritation. Rifampicin, erythromycin are absrobed faster when taken on empty stomach while ethambutol is absorbed rapidly if taken after meals.

Alcohol drug interactions. Alcohol acts on a large number of drugs as it acts on the microsomal enzyme system in the liver which also handles the metabolism of a number of drugs. Aspirin taken before or after alcoholic drinks may give rise to severe gastrointestinal bleed. Isoniazid is rendered ineffective if taken with alcohol. Alcohol enhances the effect of sedatives, hypnotics, antidepressants, tranquilizers, analgesics like opioids leading to central nervous system depression. When a patient is on antiamoebic drugs like metrogyl, tinidazole, if alcohol is consumed patient develops disulfiram like reaction while in those who are on oral hypoglycaemics, this effect is enhanced and sometimes even fatal hypoglycaemia has resulted.

Interaction of drugs with other drugs.

As already described interaction of a drug with other drug is controlled by a number of factors ranging from its absorption, distribution, biotransformation excretion andenzyme system in the liver. Let us look at some of the common drugs and their action with other drugs and resultant side effects.

Drug	Administered in conjunction with	Effects
Morphine and other opiods	Antidepressants, alcohol, barbiturates phenothiazines,chlorpromazine	Increased sedation and respiratory depression. Sedative effect of barbiturates enhanced.
	Isoniazid	Adverse effects enhanced.
Barbiturates	Corticosteroids, Oral Anticoagulants, digitoxin, doxycycline, oral contraceptives, phenytoin	Decrease effect of these drugs.
Phenytoin	Chloramphenicol, isoniazid, sulfonamides, oral anticoagulants	Increased plasma concentration of phenytoin.
Tricyclic antidepressants	Phenyl butazone, aspirin, phenothiazines, phenytoin, oral contraceptives	Action of tricyclic anti-depressants increased.
	Barbiturates	Action of tricyclic antidepressants decreased.
	Alcohol	Action potentiated.
	Anticholinergics, oral anticoagulants	Enhanced anticoagulant and anticholinergic effects.
Anticoagulants (Warfarin, Dicoumarol, phenindione)	Anabolic agents, salicylates, phenylbutazone, chloramphenicol, metrogyl, tricylic antidepressants.	Increased risk of haemorrhage due to their enhanced effect.
	Phenytoin	Increase in toxicity of phenytoin.
	Sulfonamides	Increase in toxicity of sulfonamides.
Antipsychotic drugs like chlorpromazine	Sedatives, hypnotics, antihistamines, alcohol	Chlorpromazine potentiate their action.
Salicylates	Tricyclic antidepressants,	Action potentiated
	Warfarin, oral hypoglycaemics	Action of these increased
	methotrexate Spironolactone	Diuretic action is decreased.
Oral hypoglycaemic agents	Sulfonamides, propranolol, salicylates, phenylbutazone, chloramphenicol, monamine oxidase inhibitors, alcohol.	Increased risk of hypoglycaemia.
Adrenocorticosteroids	Barbiturates, phenytoin, rifampicin	Action of corticosteroids decreased.
	Thiazide diuretics	Increased hyperglycaemic effect.
Propranolol	Antidiabetic agents	Enhanced hypoglycaemic effect.
	Aminophylline	Antagonistic effect.
Quinidine	Oral anticoagulants	Enhanced hypoprothrombinemic effect.
	Phenothiazines	Cardioactivity of quinidine is potentiated.
Neomycin	Quinidine	Ototoxicity enhanced.
Aminoglycosides like streptomycin Gentamicin, kanamycin	Amphotericin, Frusemide	Nephrotoxicity potentiated
	Mannitol	Ototoxicity increased.
Tetracycline	Antacids, sodium bicarbonate	Antacids inhibit action of tetracycline.
	Oral anticoagulants	Anticoagulation is enhanced
	Heparin	Anticoagulation action decreased.
Amoxicillin	Aspirin	Serum levels of drug are increased.

(Contd.)

Drug	Administered in conjunction with	Effects
	Antacids	Effect of amoxicillin decreased
	Erythromycin	Action of amoxicillin may be enhanced.
Ampicillin	Probenecid	Ampicillin action enhanced.
	Antacids	Antacids decrease the action of ampicillin
	Chloramphenicol	Decreased action of ampicillin.
Cephalosporins	Frusemide	Enhanced nephrotoxicity.
	Gentamicin	Possible enhanced nephrotoxicity.
Chloramphenicol	Anticoagulants	Anticoagulant activity enhanced.
	Oral antidiabetics	Enhanced antidiabetic effect.
	Diphenylhydantoin	Enhanced antiepileptic activity, Metabolism of drug blocked.
Doxycycline	Antacids	Activity of doxycycline is decreased
	Anticoagulant	Anticoagulant activity enhanced.
Griseofulvin	Anticoagulants	Anticoagulant activity inhibited.
	Barbiturates	Griseofulvin efficacy is decreased.
Nalidixic acid	Oral anticoagulants	Enhancement of anticoagulant effect.
	Nitrofurantoin	Effect of nalidixic acid gets antagonized.
Rifampicin	Oral contraceptives	Reliability of oral contraceptives decreases.
	Paraaminosalicylic acid (PAS)	Absorption of rifampicin delayed.
Sulfonamides	Oral anticoagulants	Anticoagulant effect enhanced.
	Methotrexate	Methotrexate toxicity enhanced.
	Oral antidiabetics	Effect increased, may lead to hypoglycaemia.
	Antacids	Effect of sulfonamides is inhibited.
Metronidazole	Alcohol	Disulfiram like effect
	Oral anticoagulants	Increased effect of oral anticoagulants.
Antihistamines	Alcohol, hypnotics sedatives	Increased depressing effect on central nervous system.
	Anticholinergic drugs	Increased anticholinergic effect.
Frusemide	Allopurinol	Uricosuric action of allopurinol may be decreased.
	Aminoglycosides antibiotics	Ototoxicity is enhanced.
	Antidiabetic agents	Blood sugar levels increased
	Antihypertensives	Hypotensive action potentiated
	Lithium carbonate	Lithium toxicity may be enhanced.
Spironolactone	Digoxin	Digoxin activity may be decreased.
	Antihypertensive agents	Hypotensive action potentiated
	Salicylates	Diuretic action decreased
Thiazide diuretics	Antidiabetic agents	Inhibition of antidiabetic effect
	Corticosteroids	Enhanced potassium loss
	Lithium carbonate	Increased possibility of lithium toxicity.
Dapsone	Probenecid	Antileprosy effect of dapsoneenhanced.
Haloperidol	Antihypertensive drugs	Antihypertensive effect potentiated.
	CNS depressants	Sedative effect enhanced
	Diazepam	Helps controlling restlessness
Ibuprofen	Oral anticoagulants	Anticoagulant effect potentiated.
	Corticosteroids	Ulcerogenic effect increased.
Indomethacin	Aspirin	Aspirin tends to block analgesic, anti inflammatory effect of indomethacin.
	Salicylates, steroids, phenylbutazone	Effect of indomethacin enhanced.

(Contd.)

Drug	Administered in conjunction with	Effects
Levodopa (anti Parkinsonism drug)	Phenothiazines, pyridoxine, reserpine	Inhibition of levodopa effect.
Tinidazole	Alcohol	Flushing nausea, abdominal cramps
	Oral anticoagulants	Anticoagulant effect potentiated.
Pentazocine (Fortwin)	Alcohol, antidepressants	Depressive action of alcohol enhanced Antidepressant effect enhanced.
	Sedatives, tranquilizers,hypnotics	Effect enhanced.
Theophylline	Ephedrine, pseudoephedrine, aminophylline	Effect of theophylline potentiated.
	Antigout drugs	Decreased effect of antigout drugs.
Methotrexate	Salicylates, sulfonamides	Increased risk of toxic effects of methotrexate.
Cimetidine	Antacids	Absorption of cimetidine reduced.
	Beta blockers, phenytoin, procainamide	Action potentiated.
Ranitidine Famotidine	Antacids	Interfere with. absorption of ranitidine
Omeprazole	Diazepam, warfarin, phenytoin, aminophylline	Excretion prolonged.
Lansoprazole	Diazepam, phenytoin	Inhibits their metabolism.
Sucralfate	Tetracyclines, phenytoin, cimetidine, warfarin	Reduces their absorption.
Cisapride	Diazepam	Rate of absorption increased
	Anticoagulants	Effect enhanced
	Anticholinergic drugs	Effect antagonised.
Simvastatin	Anticoagulants	Bleeding may increase
	Digoxin	Effect enhanced
	Cyclosporine, erythromycin, immuno suppressive drugs, nicotinic acid	Increased risk of rhabodmyolysis and acute renal failure.
Norfloxacin	Nitrofurantoin	Antagonises the effect of norfoxacin
	Probenecid	Reduces urinary excretion
	Theophylline	Theophylline levels are increased.
	Oral anticoagulants	Anticoagulant effect enhanced.
Flunarizine	Phenytoin, carbamazepine, valproic acid	Effect reduced.
Sumatriptin	Ergotamine, lithium, MAO inhibitors	Effect enhanced, risk of side effects increased.
Sodium valproate	Aspirin	Effect enhanced
	Carbamazepine, phenobarbitone, phenytoin, primidone	Effect reduced.
Amantadine	Levodopa	Enhances the effect
	Diuretics	Increased plasma levels may cause toxicity
Primidone	Anticoagulants, corticosteroids, oral contraceptives	Effect reduced
Carbamazepine	Oral contraceptives	Effect of oral contraceptives reduced.
	Phenytoin, phenobarbitone, primidone	Serum level reduced
	Lithium	Neurotoxic reactions.
Artesunate	Chloroquine	Effect potentiated
	Pyrimethamine, sulfonamide	Antagonistic effect.
Fluconazole	Phenytoin oral anticoagulants, oral antidiabetics	Effect enhanced.
Isosorbide dinitrate	Calcium channel, blockers, antihyper-tensives, phenothiazines, tricyclic antidepressants.	Orthostatic hypotension may occur
	Alcohol	Severe hypotension and collapse.
Amiodarone	Oral anticoagulants, beta blockers, calcium channel antagonists	Effect enhanced.

MEDICAL EMERGENCIES IN DENTAL PRACTICE

Medical emergencies in dental practice are of common occurrence and a dental surgeon must' be well prepared to meet them since correct and early management can not only prevent morbidity but also mortality in such patients.

To a large extent most of these problem can he prevented. This is best done by taking a careful history about allergy to any drug or substance, of any ailment the patient is suffering from and the drugs he/she is taking.

The important questions in the history should be especially directed towards following aspects:

1. Has the patient suffered from any fainting fits or spells (vaso vagal attacks) convulsions (epilepsy)?
2. Does he suffer from hypertension. If so is it under control and which drugs the patient is taking?
3. History of pain chest suggestive of coronary heart disease, angina pectoris. History of valvular/congenital heart disease and surgical procedures on heart (heart valves replacement, by-pass surgery, Pace makers).
4. Does the patient has chronic cough or is suffering from bronchial asthma and as to what treatment be is on. Is he a smoker?
5. Any history of postural hypotension?
6. Any major cadiac, renal or endocrinal ailment from which the patient is suffering?
7. *History of diabetes.* Is the patient on oral anti-diabetic drugs or insulin. In case of diabetics it must be ensured that surgery of patient or treatment must be done at that time when chances of hypoglycemia developing are less.

   Prolonged starvation in a diabetic is not desirable. If dental procedure is likely to take long time then morning dose of insulin he omitted and in that case, I/V glucose drip neutralised with insulin must be started.
8. Does the patient suffer from any bleeding disorder?

Physical examination should include examination for anaemia, blood pressure levels, presence of any murmurs in the heart, signs of congestive heart failure, any organomegaly, chest for any evidence of infection (chronic bronchitis, bronciectasis, lung abscess, pulmonary tuberculosis) respiratory insufficiency. Patients above the age of fifty must have an electrocardiogram, X-ray heart and blood sugar levels (fasting and post prandial) estimated.

Prophylaxis against infection in cardiovascular disorders. All patients who suffer from valvular heart disease or congenital heart disease or those with prosthetic heart valve or a pace maker, prevention against infective endocarditis is required when dental procedures are to he carried out. The risk to the patient following these procedures is very high. In all such patients oral antibiotic prophylaxis is advised.

Usual procedure is to give prophylactic antibiotics for two days prior to dental procedure and follow it up afterwards for five to seven days. Capsule Doxycycline 200 mg first day and 100 mg next day followed by 100 mg for seven days daily or Capsule amoxicillin 500 mg 8 hourly for two days before and for seven days after wards . Or Tablet Erythromycin 500 mg six hourly initially for two days followed by 250 mg six hourly for seven days.

Emergency management. For management of any medical emergency every dental clinic must be fully equipped to manage the problems which are likely to rise.

Of the various emergency equipment, O_2 cylinder, endotracheal tube and set, laryngoscope, suction apparatus and catheter. I/V fluids and administration sets, disposable syringes and needles, stethoscope, blood pressure apparatus, sterilized pads and tourniquet must be available. A fair amount of emergency drugs like the following must be readily available.

1. Injection Adrenaline (1 in 1000 dilution 1 ml ampoules).
2. Injection Atropine (0.4mg/ml)
3. Injection Avil/Pheniramine malcate (22.75 mg/ml)
4. Injection Aminophylline.(0.024 g/l0 ml)

5. Injection Deriphylline (Etophylline 162.4 mg + Theophylline 50.6 mg) per 2 ml injection.
6. Injection Mephentine (30 mg/ml).
7. Injection Dopamine (200 mg/5 ml).
8. Injection Lidocaine (Xylocard) 20 mg/ml.
9. Injection Mexiletine (250 mg/10 ml).
10. Injection Digoxin (0.25 mg/ml).
11. Injection Propranolol.(1 mg/5 mg/ml)
12. Injection Lasix (20 mg/2m1)
13. Injection Diazepam.(10 mg/ml)
14. Injection Dilantin(50 mg/ml)
15. Injection Stemetil (12.5 mg/ml)
16. Injection Isoproterenol.
17. Injection Fortwin (Pentazocine).(30 mg/ml)
18. Injection Pethidine (50 mg/ml).
19. Injection Morphine (15 mg).
20. Injection Analgin (500 mg/2m1)
21. Injection Diclofenac sodium (250 mg/ml).
22. Injection Dexamethasone (4 mg)ml)
23. Injection Betamehasone. (4 mg/ml)
24. Oxygen
25. Tablet Isosorbide dinitrate (10 mg)
26. Capsule Nifedipine (5 mg).
27. Injection Serpasil (lmg/ml).
28. Injection Calcium carbonate/chloride
29. Injection Glucose (10%) or 5% dextrose saline
30. Dextrose 50% 50 ml
31. Aromatic salts

Vasovagal attack (Syncope). It is one of the commonest medical emergency in dental practice and is characterised by transient loss of consciousness. It can occur during any phase of dental procedure and often causes lot of anxiety all round.

Most commonly the person who faints is an anxious patient who is afraid of pain and of the procedure. Factors like sight of blood, unfavourable environment, apprehension, lack of sleep, fasting predispose to the condition.

Vaso vagal attack is generally harmless condition but if it lasts for prolonged period it may harm leading to reduction in cardiac output and cerebral blood flow.

A syncope is often preceded by prodromal symptoms lasting from few seconds to minutes. The patient during this period has a feeling of weakness, discomfort and quisiness. It is followed by sweating, pallor, dizziness and darkness before the eyes. The patient often falls to the side becoming unconscious. Now he is pale, ashen coloured with shallow respiration. Pulse may become weak and thready. Often blood pressure levels fall. Extremities are cold and sweaty. This phase generally lasts for a few minutes and then patient recovers. The patient may not remember about the whole episode but there is feeling of generalized weakness.

Prevention. To a large extent vagovasal fit can he prevented. If a patient who comes for dental consultation is found to be anxious and apprehensive, it is better to explain to him the whole procedure which is likely to be carried out. It is better if patient is put on an antianxiety drug (alprazolam 0.25 mg twice a day) at least 24 hours before the procedure. Patient can take a light breakfast before coming for the procedure.

Management. *Once syncope develops immediate measures be taken:*

a. Make the patient lie supine with legs elevated to improve blood supply to the heart and brain.
b. Loosen the collar round about the neck.
c. Maintain the patency of airways. Head tilt chin manouver may be required to maintain it. Suck out secretions from the throat and oral cavity.
d. Check respiration, pulse and blood pressure.
e. If patient appears to be cyanotic, O_2 be administered.
f. Inhalation of aromatic spirits of ammonia generally helps. Application of cold towel on the forehead is useful.
g. If patient feels cold, blanket may be given.
h. As patient recovers, reassure him.
i. Prevent recurrence of syncope by going into the factors which precipitated it.
j. If patient remains unconscious for more than 10-15 minutes other causes of syncope (cardiac arrhythmias, C.V. accident, hypoglycaemia) must be looked into.
k. Once patient has come out of syncopal attack it is better to postpone the dental procedure for 24 hours. Patient be sent home along with a relation or a friend.

Electric shock. It is not of common occurrence but sometimes due to faulty connections in the dental chair, patient may get an electric shock. Its intensity shall be dependent on the wetness of the skin, degree and duration of exposure to the current.

A severe electric shock will cause immediate loss of consciousness. If it does not occur there is severe degree of pain alongwith sensory disturbances in the distribution of nerve. Temporary paralysis of limb may occur. There may be burn at the site of passage of current. Most serious side effect is development of ventricular fibrillation or apnoea. Patient often becomes unconscious which lasts for varying periods of time.

Treatment consists of switching off the electric connection. Cardiopulmonary resuscitation must be carried out immediately. Artificial respiration may be required. In some cases when shock is present it must be treated by intravenous fluids and vasopressor drugs. A case developing ventricular fibrillation may require defibrillation.

Allergic reactions, anaphylaxis. Allergic reaction to a drug may be either immediate (humoral) or delayed (cellular). These occur when a patient is exposed to a particular allergen and hypersensitivity occurs, the response being produced due to exaggerated reaction of immune system of the body. It may manifest in the form of skin reactions like urticaria, drug fever, pruritis and angioedema or more severe anaphylactic response like respiratory symptoms (bronchospasm) circulatory collapse and shock.

Generally previous exposure to the drug is needed for an allergic response to take place. The fact that patient has taken that drug several times before without developing an allergic response does not mean that allergy to that drug can not develop. While allergy to any drug can develop at any time. Persons who suffer from allergic disorders like urticaria. Bronchial asthma, Hay fever have increased tendency to develop allergic reaction. As compared to allergic reaction to the drugs, there is idiosyncratic reaction which can neither be explained on any pharmacologic or biochemical basis.

The severity of idiosyncratic reaction is unpredictable since it is not dose related. Of the drugs, commonly employed in dentistry. Local anasthetics are the ones which are likely to produce an allergic response. Very often the patient may be sensitive to the preservative employed in the anaesthetic agent. Inadvertent intravascular injection of anaesthetic agent may sometimes produce an allergic response which develops within seconds and is of more severe intensity. An allergic reaction must be identified. The most frequent being skin eruptions (Urticaria. Bullous eruption) along with severe itching and angioneurotic oedema. There is often excessive lacrimation in eyes. Lips and tongus are swollen. For skin reactions it is best to adminster an antihistaminic (Inj Pheniramine Maleate (Avil) 50 mg I/m) immediately. If no response then 1 mg Adrenaline (1 in 1000 dil/ml) followed by inj Dexamethasone 8 mg. intravenously.

This is followed by oral tablet of an antihistamine twice a day for next two days. Respiratory symptoms are in the form of a bronchospasm and asthma like picture. The line of action here shall be:

1. O_2 inhalation.
2. Injection epinephrine 0.5 to 1 ml given subcutaneously or intramuscularly.
3. Injection Dexamethasone 8 mg intravenously. Circulatory collapse in the form of shock often develops. It is more of an anaphylactic reaction. *The following regimen is advised:*

   a. Put the patient in a supine position.
   b. O_2 inhalation.
   c. Intravenous fluids rapidly to be administered.
   d. Injection Adrenaline (1 in 1000 dilution) 1 ml subcutaneously or intramuscularly.
   e. Injection Dexamethasone 8 mg intravenously stat, to be repeated every six hourly.
   f. Injection Avil (Pheniramine maleate)50 mg intramuscularly.
   g. Monitor pulse, blood pressure and respiration. Keep respiratory passages clear.

h. In patients with low blood pressure levels, Dopamine infusion be started. Alternatively Injection Mephentermine 15-30 mg) be given intramuscularly.

As a rule patient should recover within half an hour. If no recovery takes place or it is not satisfactory patient should be hospitalized.

As drug reaction or anaphylaxis develops, dental procedure shall have to be terminated. Sometimes in some patients laryngeal oedema may develop which may produce severe degree of respiratory difficulty and is a grave emergency.

Treatment in such emergency situation is again by antihistaminics, steroids and O_2. If respiratory obstruction is severe and causing respiratory distress, tracheostomy as an emergency procedure may have to be undertaken.

Airway obstruction by foreign body. Airways obstruction is an important emergency in dental practice.

It may occur due to swallowing of food particles, vomitus, secretions being swallowed during operations in oral cavity or passage lower down of partial dentures.

During operative procedures it is known to follow sometimes with swallowing of very small surgical instruments, blood, loosened teeth and secretions which pass on to the respiratory passages. Foreign body passage into the airway generally occurs when patient is either under sedation or even when some dental procedures are being carried out and some nerve block has been done.

When a foreign material passes into the respiratory passages there is generally a bout of cough, and choking sensation. Depending upon the nature of foreign body the symptoms may be mild in case of a very small matter but if it is in the form of a denture, surgical instrument or copious secretions symptoms are very severe. Patient is acutely breathless with wheezing sounds in the chest. In a mild case confimation can be made by radiological examination of chest which may show a solid foreign body or patch of segmental or lobar pneumonia.

Treatment consists in aspiration of secretions from the respiratory passage. Simple procedures like turning the patient to side, thumping of the back and if foreign body is lying in the upper respiratory passages, manual removal be attempted.

Most of the times the attempt is not successful. In such cases bronchoscopic aspiration of secretions and removal of foreign body should be done. In case the foreign body (denture) gets lodged peripherally, it may require thoracotomy.

Bronchial asthma. In a patient who is suffering from bronchial asthma, an acute attack of bronchial asthma may be triggered off when patient is waiting for the dental procedure or even when any procedure is being carried out. As we have already discussed every patient must be thoroughly screened for such ailments.

An enquiry should be made regarding history of asthma or allergy and whether the patient is on some drugs for that purpose and the frequency of such attacks. Any precipitating factors should be specially looked into. If patient is not under control for his/her condition dental procedures should be postponed till the patient is symptom free.

In patients who are symptom free but on maintenance therapy it is essential to ensure that the patient is on drug therapy. It is a good practice if an asthmatic takes inhalations of salbutamol and corticosteroids daily for three days prior to the dental procedures. Drugs like aspirin, penicillin and sulfonamides which are likely to induce allergic reactions be avoided and substituted by cephalosporins and acetaminophen.

But despite all the precautions when a bronchial asthma attack develops, clinically it can he recognised by acute breathlessness, wheezing sounds in the chest both during inspiration as well as expiration. There is cough, laboured breathing with use of accessory muscles and intercostal retraction. Patient sits up fighting for air. He is very anxious, apprehensive with cold sweats.

Recognition of an asthmatic attack is not very difficult since most of the times the clinical picture is very characteristic.

Treatment should always be prompt and taken as an emergency measure. Firstly terminate the dental procedure. Administer a bronchodilator immediately. In young persons administer Injection Epinephrine (1 in 1000 dilution) 1 ml by subcutaneous Hurst method. Generally relief is obtained. If no relief then Injection Aminophylline (0.24 G in 10 cc glucose) intravenously slowly. It may be combined with Injection Decadrone 8 mg I/V for more quick response. In elderly patients or those with hypertension or coronary heart disease, epinephrine is contraindicated. In such patients aminophylline/deriphylline is the first drug to be given with or without corticosteroids.

O_2 inhalations be given. Use of narcotics be avoided because of their constricting effect on smooth muscles of bronchi and respiratory depression as well as drying of secretions.

Once the patient has come out of the acute attack, dental treatment is postponed and patient asked to take rest so that he recovers from the acute episode. Within 24 to 48 hours repeat dental procedure be carried out after ensuring that the disease is under control and giving prophylactic therapy (salbutamol + corticosteroids inhalations).

Acute left heart failure. Patients of chronic heart disease like coronary, hypertension, valvular heart disease may be slowly progressing towards heart failure over a period of time and generally have features of weakness, undue fatigue and progressive dysponea. In some there may be history suggestive of orthoponea and attacks of nocturnal dysponea.

In any patient suffering from myocardial disease, a detailed history about attacks of breathlessness, the drugs patient is on and whether the patient is in a compensated stage or not should always be taken.

Cases with heart disease who have got decompensation or those sitting on the border line picture of early left heart failure, dental procedures are likely to trigger the attack of acute left heart failure or pulmonary oedema.

This complication can be recognized with the presence of acute breathlessness, patient finding it difficult to lie in bed and is often panting for breath.

Physical examination shall reveal the presence of cyanosis. Pulsus alternans, raised blood pressure levels, cardiomegaly and diffuse crepitations in the chest more marked at bases.

When this emergency develops during dental procedures the line of treatment shall be:

Step One - Terminate dental procedure.
Step Two - Position the patient in a sitting position.

Administer O2. Sedate the patient with Injection Morphine 15 mg subcutaneously stat. Monitor vital signs like pulse, blood pressure, respiratory rate.

Injection Aminophylline (0.24 g in 10 cc glucose) be administered intravenously slowly. If patient is previously not on digitalis then give Injection Digoxin 0.25-0.5 mg intramuscularly stat to be repeated after six to 8 hours depending on the clinical condition.

Injection Lasix 80 mg intravenously stat. Prophylactic cover of antibiotics (Injection Ampicillin 500 mg intravenously eight hourly).

Once the patient recovers from the acute episode, Cardiac reserve should be assessed and treatment instituted for the underlying cardiac disease such as hypertension, coronary heart disease, valvular heart disease. Once the cardiac condition is stabilized, after proper medication dental procedure can be carried out.

Hypertensive emergency. Often a patient who has hypertension but is not aware about it or it has not been detected creates problem when he/she comes for dental treatment. To obviate such complication or an emergency situation it is always better to check the blood pressure levels of every patient and take detailed history about hypertension related problems like anginal pain, headache and features of breathlessness.

In normotensive persons, stress accompanying dental procedures can elevate blood pressure levels. Main problem in hypertensives is increased bleeding during surgical procedures especially if blood pressure levels are not properly controlled. In hypertensives who are on medication, orthostatic hypotension may develop. Recognition of hypertension is by patients complaints of headache, dizziness, blurring of vision and by observing raised levels of blood pressure.

Hypertension as such has to be treated with adequate drugs. It is better to give a small dose of sedation night before the dental procedure (Diazepam 5 mg) to relieve stress and anxiety.

During dental procedure, monitor blood pressure levels. If there is acute rise of blood pressure, sublingual Nifedipine (5 mg) be given as an emergency measure. If bleeding occurs from the site of operation local application of adrenaline pack can be employed to control bleed. A haemostatic dressing placed within the socket, intra oral pressure packs, ice packs (outside) and avoidance of mouth rinses be advised. At the same time secretions from the throat be aspirated. If there is severe bleed patient may have to be hospitalized.

Hypotension. Fall in blood pressure may sometimes occur in the form of hypotension and may create problem. This occurs as a form of vaso vagal attack but sometimes it portends a serious condition like myocardial infarction, myocarditis. Patients who are on long term steroids and their adrenal glands are hypertrophied may suddenly develop adrenal crisis because of acute stress.

Hypotension should be suspected when in a patient while dental procedures are being carried out suddenly patient starts developing cold sweats, restlessness, confusion and even nausea and vomiting. Pulse will be thready and feeble. Heart rate may vary but sounds are feeble. Fall in blood pressure levels is evident, systolic levels going below 90 mmHg.

Once person develops hypotension, dental procedure be stopped immediately. Patient should be placed in a horizontal position on the bed. Foot end of the bed be raised. Aminister O_2 and vaso pressor drugs (Injection Mephetine 15 mg I/M stat). Start intravenous infusion and Injection Decadrone 8 mg intravenously be given stat and be repeated six hourly.

In the mean time try to find out the cause of hypotensive ciris. An emergency electrocardiogram be done to exclude cardiac insuffiency and arrhythmias. Enquire about any drugs (antihypertensives, beta blockers) the patient isalready on.

If the cause is either an myocardial infarction or

a cerebrovascular accident the treatment should be on those lines. Adrenal crisis requires urgent management (intravenous steroids, saline infusions). If the hypotension is not due to serious ailments, supportive measures generally suffice. Dental treatment should be started only after the patient has completely recovered.

Pain In chest. Sometimes an elderly person while getting dental procedures may complain of either heaviness or choking sensation in chest. This may be harbinger of an anginal pain or if the pain persists it might be an attack of myocardial infarction. An anginal pain is generally present in substernal region, radiates to the arms and shoulder. There is often a feeling of choking sensation but if it is due to myocardial infarction there are accompanying symptoms like cold sweats. The pain now becomes very severe and prolonged.

Enquire from the patient whether he is already on antianginal drugs like isosorbide dinitrate. Administer tablet Sorbitrate (10 mg) subingually. Discontinue the dental procedure. Patient be made to lie down in bed. Administer Injection Pethidine 50 mg or Injection Morphine 15 mg to relieve pain.

An urgent electrocardiogram be done to exclude acute myocardial infarction. If it is so then treatment has to be on that lines. To a large extent this type of emergency can he prevented. Any patient of angina should not be operated or dealt surgically till his/her angina is in stable condition and the electrocardiogram does not show any major abnormality.

Acute myocardial infarction. Acute myocardial infarction is a grave medical emergency and requires urgent medical management. A classical case of myocardial infarction has substernal discomfort, a choking or constricting sensation with pain radiating to the left arm and shoulder. This is often accompanied by cold sweats, a feeling of apprehension and anxiety.

Difficulty arises when in an occasional case the pain is primarily referred to the jaw or a patient may presentwith tooth ache. In such case the oro-dental cavity does not have any apparent infection or cause for this tooth or jaw ache. If one comes across an elderly person or those above the age of 50 with this unusual complaint, one should be very cautious. Often these patients are restless, apprehensive and occasionally breathless. Face may give an ashen grey appearance. It may be difficult to make an exact clinical diagnosis but at least one must be aware that this type of presentation can be due to coronary heart disease. An urgent electrocardiogram and a detailed history shall clinch the diagnosis. Often such patients have been mistakenly treated for tooth problem with dire consequences.

In addition a dental patient with previous history of coronary heart disease must be identified and patients cardiac status be assessed. Any risk involved with carrying out dental procedures must be weighed and risks involved must be explained to the patient and his/her relations.

Enquire about history of pain chest or heart attack and when it occurred. Whether the patient is on any drug (Aspirin, nitrates, beta blockers) and as to what is his cardiac status? Does the patient feel uncomfortable while going upstairs or walking for a short distance. Is the patients condition now well under control? Physical examination should include looking for any signs of congestive heart failure, cardiomegaly and presence of any murmurs in the heart (systolic murmur in cases with mitral incompetence). An electrocardiogram is a must for evidence of myocardial injury. Echocardiogram is helpful for assessing left ventricular dysfunction.

Physical fitness of the patient shall depend on absence of anginal pain and breathlessness during post myocardial infarction phase and patients ability to return to his/her daily routines and how early normal activity was resumed.

Dental therapy involves stress and can be an important cause of inducing stress in a case recovering after myocardial infarction.

In an acute case of myocardial infarction dental treatment has to be postponed and only conservative line of therapy followed. It is a good practice to postpone all procedures for at least three months since heart after myocardial infarction takes six to eight weeks to recover from the injury. Any major surgical work must be delayed for six months.

During dental work. Sometimes while dental procedures are being carried out in stable patient of coronary heart disease, because of stress an attack of acute myocardial infarction may occur. Immediately the procedure be stopped. Patient given pethidine or morphine to relieve pain. O_2 be administered immediately and further the patient be managed on lines of acute myocardial infarction.

Post myocardial infarction period. It requires careful handling. No dental procedures even seemingly innocous must be carried out during the next three months but preferably in the next six months. If there is dental infection or some other problems, manage it by oral antibiotics and analgesics.

Only emergency procedures in the post myocardial infarction period be considered and that too preferably in a hospital setting with electro-cardiographic monitoring. It is always preferable to try medications in all cases and only when there is no response to medical therapy then only any procedure be carried out and that too after taking all due precuations. No dental treatment be carried for very long period and its duration should vary with the patients level of tolerance.

Prevention. In any case with a history of coronary heart disease before instituting any dental treatment all pros and cons must be assessed.

It must be ensured that the patient is taking all the prescribed medicines. After cardiac status is stable, a night before a sedative be given to allay anxiety and tension from the patients mind. While carrying out the procedure, it should be done in the minimum possible time Do not tire the patient. At any sign of discomfort to the patient the precedure must be stopped. All emergency drugs (O_2, analgesics, nitrates, vasopressors) must be readily available.

Another important precaution to be considered is that many patients of myocardial infarction are on long term anticoagulant therapy. Very low levels of prothrombin time may create problem in the form of excess bleeding. It is preferable if prothrombin time is not less than 20 to 30 per cent of the normal levels. At this level dental surgery can be carried out but with care and caution. Despite the precautions taken if bleeding does occur then hemostatic dressing pack be placed at the site of dental procedure. Applying of ice packs outside the oral cavity and placing intra-oral packs may help. At the same time patient is advised not to rinse his/her mouth for the next 48 hours and only liquid or soft semi solid diet is permitted. Use of coagulants like vitamin K and antidotes to the anticoagulant therapy should be done under the advice of treating physician.

Cardiac arrest. It is a grave emergency and is characterised by the sudden stoppage of functioning of the heart. There is pump failure which may be reversible if prompt management is done and in time. If immediate intervention is not done death shall result.

Cardiac arrest is not very common in dental practice but occasionally a case especially of old myocardial infarction or hypertensive may develop cardiac arrest. It may be as a result of electro-mechanical dissociation because of use of drugs like local anaesthetics, and sedatives as well as narcotics. Sometimes severe haemorrhage and shock may precipitate it. It may also follow during general anaesthesia. Serious cardiac arrhythmias like ventricular tachycardia, ventricular fibrillation are important causes of cardiac stand still or asystole. When ventricular asystole occurs, there are no contractile movements of the myocardium and there is ventricular standstill.

Recognition. It is important to recognise cardiac arrest at the earliest. There is absence of carotid or femoral pulses. Patient is unresponse. Heart beat is not palpable and blood pressure becomes unrecordable. Further on it leads to absence of ventilation. There is loss of consciousness and respiration. Tissue hypoxia or anoxia develops rapidly leading to metabolic acidosis. Once such development takes place it is important to institute immediate resuscitative measures.

Management. Attempt should be made to revive the patient by doing cardiopulmonary resuscitation. The basic approach consists of A-B-C steps in which A stands for maintaining respiratory airways while B stands for reviving breathing and C for adequate circulatory support.

Cardiopulmonary resuscitation involves team work where a number of people including medical assistant and nursing staff have an equally important role to play. If cardiac arrest occurs when the patient is sitting on a dental chair and a procedure is being undertaken, immediately terminate the procedure and put the patient on a firm non-resistant surface.

Steps to be followed are:

Step I. Remove any dentures or foreign material from the oral cavity. Loosen the clothing especially round about the neck. To keep respiratory passages clear, lift the patients head by placing one hand behind the patients neck lifting it and the other hand on patients forehead tilting it backwards. This way the neck is extended and tongue does not fall back to obstruct the throat.

Other manouvre includes placing fingers behind the angle of the mandible, keeping head tilted backwards and forcing jaw forward. Both these methods are adopted to keep the respiratory passages patent. Remove secretions from the throat by constant suction. Introduce an airway.

Step II. Apply a thump on the heart. It should be delivered at the junction of middle and lower third of sternum. Idea is to stimulate cardiac contractility. Feel for the carotid pulse. If not felt then external cardiac massage be done manually by pressing firmly by both hands on the patients chest above the xiphoid process. Constant compression over the precordium is done at the rate of 60-80 per minute. It is important to do compression and release in a proper manner. Successful cardiac massage results in return of carotid pulsation.

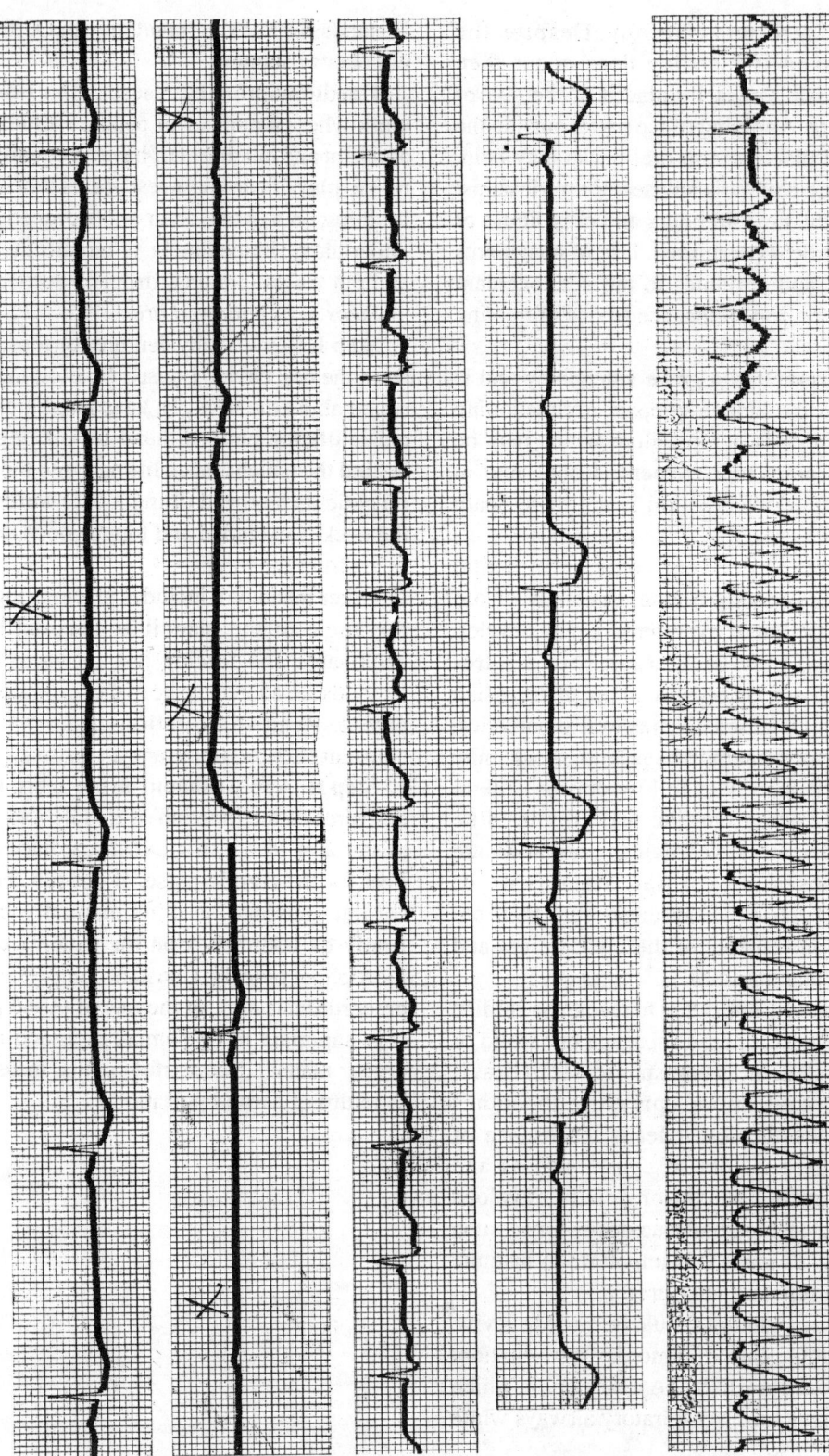

Fig. 12.1. Brady Arrhythmia. Producing sinus arrest, 1st two strips show severe degree of bradycardia producing periods of sinus arrest Inj. Atropine was administered intravenously. Heart rate increased but there was varying degree of block which soon manifested as complete heart block. Inj. Isoprenaline in infusion (5 mg. in 500 cc of 5% dextrose) was started. Patient developed ventricular tachycardia going on to ventricular flutter. At this stage isoprenaline was discontinued and lignocaine administered. Rhythm returned to sinus form.

Step III. Start respiratory resuscitation immediately. Mouth to mouth respiration be done immediately till an Ambu bag is available. It is advisable to pass an endotracheal tube and by means of a ventilator, positive pressure respiration with oxygen enriched air at rate of 10-12 litres/ minute is given.

Step IV. Start an intravenous infusion immediately. Administer sodium biocarbonate 100 ml intravenously (1 meq/kg) as a bolus dose rapidly, to be repeated after 10 minutes. This is to counteract metabolic acidosis.

Step V. Do cardiac monitoring by cardioscope/ electrocardiogram. If there is ventricular asystole give intracardiac epinephrine (1 ml of 1 in 1000 dilution) through third or fourth intercostal space on the right side of heart.

Epinephrine is given to restore electrical activity of the heart. If electrocardiogram shows ventricular tachycardia then administer Injection Lidocaine 100 mg as a bolus dose to be repeated after 10 minutes and half an hour and then maintain by an infusion at rate of 1 to 4 mg per minute.

If there is ventricular fibrillation then apply electrodes and a DC shock of 200 joules be administered immediately. Additional shocks of higher energy may be given if fibrillation is not controlled. Generally shocks upto 400 joules are sufficient. Once fibrillation disappears, heart resumes normal functioning. If fibrillation reappears, DC shock is repeated.

If cardiac arrest is due to bradyarrhythmias, then administer Injection Atropine 0.5 mg intravenously, to be repeated after five minutes till the pulse returns. When there is electrochemical dissociation of heart, administer calcium chloride or calcium gluconate (10 ml of 10% solution) Calcium is not to be given if patient is on digitalis previously.

Step VI. Monitor blood pressure levels. If levels are below 90 mmHg, dopamine infusion at the rate of 2-50 pg/kg/minute be started.

Step VII. Maintain A-B-C support. It should be continued till heart starts beating normally and respiration becomes normal.

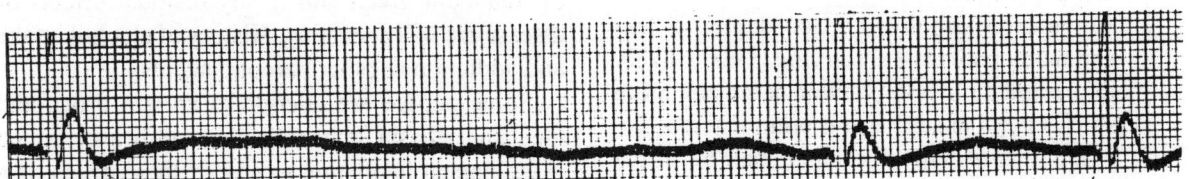

Fig. 12.2. Sinus arrest. This tracing is from a case of acute myocardial infarction showing periods of sinus asystole.

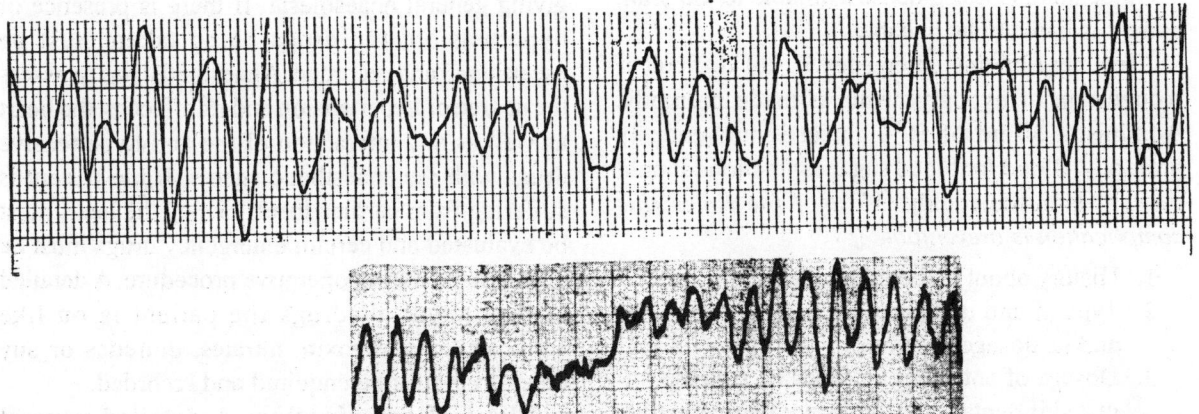

Fig. 12.3. Polymorph Ventricular Tachycardia degenerating to ventricular fibrillation.

Important precautions. Cardiopulmonary resuscitation must be done immediately since every second counts. Delay beyond four to six minutes in recovoery of the heart may result in irreversible brain damage. Once the patient has come out of the crisis, attempt should be made to identify the cause and cardiac status of the patient evaluated. Further treatment should be done keeping in mind the underlying illness.

Prevention. Cardiac arrest can be prevented if one does not undertake dental procedures without proper precuations in cardiac patients or those with decompensated cardiac reserve. In all such risky individuals dental procedures be carried out after complete evaluation and assessment.

Diabetic emergencies. In a case of diabetic who is on either oral antidiabetic drugs or insulin, there is danger of developing hypoglycaemia when the patient comes for dental procedures.

Factors which will induce hypoglycaemia are:

1. Patient takes normal dose of insulin or antidiabetic drug in the morning before coming for dental procedures.
2. Amount of carbohydrates consumed is less and many patients are starving. This is likely to precipitate hypoglycaemic coma and more so if general anaesthesia is administered.
3. Symptoms of hypoglycaemia shall be in the form of pallor, sweating, tremors, palpitation and marked weakness.

Since there is less glucose available to the brain patient is liable to be irritable.

Treatment of this emergency is not difficult if recognition of hypoglycaemia is made promptly. Administer 50 ml of 50% glucose intravenously promptly. Blood for blood sugar estimations should be sent simultaneously. *Most of the times this complication is preventable if*

1. History about diabetes is taken.
2. Type of anti diabetic drug patient already on and its dosage schedule.
3. Dosage of anti diabetic drugs be suitably adjusted if dental procedures are contemplated.
4. It is preferable to give no anti diabetic drug on the day the dental procedure is to be carried out. Give intravenously 10% glucose infusion neutralised by 25 units of soluble insulin at the time of procedure.

Further dosage of insulin is to be monitored depending on urine sugar and blood glucose levels.

EVALUATION OF A CASE FOR GENERAL ANAESTHESIA

Before administering general anaesthesia to any patient a complete history about any previous ailment, drug allergy, complete examination of the patient and relevant investigations should be carried out. At the same time patient must be prepared suitably both psychologically and medically for undergoing operative procedure. It is always advisable to admit the patient 48 hours before the operation so that proper assessment of the patients conditions can be arrived.

History. Take detailed history about any major ailment in the past and recently. Ascertain the type of treatment given and if any residual effects of disease are still persisting. History of alcohol intake and addiction to other narcotic agents.

Some people are allergic to certain drugs and local anaesthesia. It must be thoroughly ascertained if the person is allergic to any of these drugs. If a patient is chronic smoker, he/she is likely to have chronic cough and this has to be considered when giving general anaesthesia. If there is presence of hypertension, the drugs being taken must be ascertained and recorded. Anaesthetist has to assess the degree of hypertension and its effect on the heart as well as any interaction of the anti hypertensive drugs with the anaesthetic agents. If the patient is suffering from cardiac insufficiency the heart must be evaluated and certain emergency drugs must be kept at hand during operative procedure. A detailed history about all drugs the patient is on like anticoagulants, digoxin, nitrates, diuretics or any other drug must be enquired and recorded.

Physical examination. A detailed general physical examination must be done preoperatively. *In this:*

1. *Look for anaemia and state of nutrition.* Patient who is severely anaemic is not fit for general anaesthesia. Anaemia must be corrected before hand. If emergency operation is to be done, Blood transfusion must be administered.

2. *Pulse rate.* It should be between 60-80 beats per minute. If the pulse rate is either high or slow, cause must be found out.

3. Blood pressure must be evaluated carefully. Neither high or low blood pressure is desirable. An hypertensive must be treated before hand and blood pressure levels brought to normal or near normal levels.

   High blood pressure is an untoward symptom but if there are no complications accompanying such as cardiomegaly, renal or lung complications or features of left heart or congestive failure the anaesthesia can be given by controlling blood pressure levels. But if these complications are present then great caution has to be employed.

4. Lungs be examined for evidence of chronic bronchitis with or without emphysema and other lung diseases. Look for clubbing, cyanosis and emphysema. Patients respiratory functions must be evaluated. A chronic smoker is likely to be at disadvantage.

   A simple test is breath holding test, here the patient is instructed to breathe deeply and then close his mouth, compress his nose and hold his breath as long as possible. The average patient can hold his breath from twenty five to forty five seconds or more but if he is unable to do so and can not hold his breath for at least 15 seconds it means severe respiratory or cardiac insufficiency. The choice of anaesthesia in such patients has to be assessed carefully and during operation, **adequate** amount of oxygen supply must be available.

   In such patients it is desirable to institute breathing exercises for at least a week before operation and the patient is encouraged to continue with these exercises as soon as he regains consciousness. In this way many pulmonary complications are avoided. Breathing exercises programme must be carried out under the guidance of a physiotherapist with advice from the physician.

5. Abdomen be examined for hepatomegaly, splenomegaly, ascites and any organomegaly. Lymph glands in the body be palpated for evidence of any disease of reticuloendothelial system.

6. Bleeding tendencies must be looked into. History of bleed from any source after any simple injury or bruising be considered.

7. Oral cavity must he carefully examined and if any loose teeth are present or if there is any great degree of sepsis these should be taken care of before operation. In patients using dentures these must be removed before administering premedication since failure to do this may choke the patient.

8. Patient colour should be carefully examined and if any signs of anaemia or polycythaemia are present they must he attended to.

9. Urine should be carefully tested and if any evidence of diabetes is present, blood sugar estimations be done. Urine be examined not only for sugar but also for albumin and ketone bodies. Diabetes must be controlled before hand with insulin. In the presence of ketone bodies it is usual to institute 10 per cent glucose drip neutralising with 25 units of soluble insulin in each bottle. This infusion is given till urine is ketone free. It is preferable in any diabetic patient who is on oral antidiabetic drugs, to switch on to soluble insulin 48 hours before operation.

   On the day of operation, patient is put on 5% or 10% glucose drip neutralised with soluble insulin (1 unit of insulin for 2 g of glucose). After operation, patient has to be continued on insulin injections till the wound has healed. This may have to be carried out for 10-14 days. Once recovery is complete and patient is ambulatory he can be switched on to oral antidiabetic drugs.

10. If urine contains considerable amount of albumin this indicates renal pathology and anaesthetist in consultation with the physician

must evaluate the risks and the type of anaesthesia.

11. Heart size must be evaluated. Position of apex beat, presence of abnormal pulsations over the precordium and cardiac murmurs must be assessed.

12. Look for patients veins especially over the ankles and antecubital fossa. Suitable veins must be identified for intravenous purposes.

Investigations. *In every patient due for general anaesthesia following investigations be carried out:*

1. Haemoglobin to assess anaemia.

2. Total and differential leucocyte count.

3. Bleeding time (BT) and clotting time (CT) for bleeding disorders.

4. Platelet count:-Low platelet count indicates thrombocytopenia.

5. Complete urine examination for albumin, sugar, ketone bodies and presence of any casts and cells.

6. Blood urea.

7. Blood sugar (fasting and Post prandial) to exclude diabetes.

8. Prothrombin time for bleeding disorders.

9. X-ray heart (PA view) for heart size. It shall also assess any pathology in the lungs.

10. Electrocardiogram for any myocardial damage or insufficiency or presence of any arrhythmia.

11. Pulmonary function tests to evaluate the lung functions.

Preparation of the patient:

1. *Diet.* On the day of operation it is essential that the patient is on empty stomach. On the day before operation the diet should be light and easily digestible.

2. If the patient has not moved his bowels on the day of operation it is advisable to give a low bowel enema so that the bowels are empty at the time of operation.

3. Breathing exercises must be instituted a week before in those patients who have chronic cough.

4. People who are chronic smokers, tobacco in them not only acts as an irritant to the mucous membranes of the respiratory tract but also interferes with the smooth induction of anaesthesia. Heavy smokers cause excretion of thick mucous in the early morning hours and often this mucous is expelled by violent or vigorous coughing . This is not desirable. Smokers must stop smoking before hand and preferably for two to three weeks before general anaesthesia to prevent pulmonary complications during and after general anaesthesia.

5. In persons who are habitual drinkers of alcohol amount of alcohol must be decreased since people who are chronic alcoholics in them undue tolerance to anaesthetic drugs may be seen.

6. A sleeping drought is given night before so as to ensure good night sleep and allay anxiety.

7. Premedication is given on the day of operation and acts as a valuable help to the anaesthetist and helps in induction of general anaesthesia.

Contraindications to general anaesthesia. Though there are no absolute contra-indications to general anaesthesia but there are certain relative contraindications which may make the procedure of general anaesthesia serious risk.

1. Presence of shock, dehydration.

2. Very high or low levels of blood pressure.

3. Decompensated heart.

4. Presence of serious cardiac arrhythmias.

5. Any gross anatomical abnormality.

6. Chronic respiratory insufficiency.

7. Hepatic de-compensation/ chronic liver disease/portal cirrhosis.

8. Renal insufficiency/acute or chronic renal failure.

9. Diseases of central nervous system (meningitis/encephalitis).

10. Septicaemia.

11. Massive ascites.

12. Chronic respiratory obstruction.

DIETS IN VARIOUS DISEASE STATES

Diet forms an important part in the treatment of any disease besides various therapeutic measures employed. In planning diet for any sick person it is essential to keep the needs of the person in view as well as nutritional requirements and the malady from which the patient is suffering from. Diet advised should be based on the persons likes and dislikes, socioeconomic factors as well as the part of it being tasteful and palatable to take.

In this section general guidelines for various disease states are suggested and diet in any person should be planned keeping these broad outlines in view.

Diabetes mellitus. A diabetic diet has to he balanced one meeting a person's nutritional needs while keeping it within permissible caloric limits. It must help patient maintain his normal weight as per age, sex and height. Attempt should be made to maintain blood sugar levels as close to normal as possible.

Food should be wholesome, nutritious and palatable. Monotony in food must be avoided. Too much restrictions should not be enforced. It is a sane practice for a diabetic patient to take the same food as taken by other family members except for some modifications done keeping a diabetics needs in view.

Carbohydrates form major bulk of indian diet and are main source of energy. No exact rules can be laiddown for the total amount of carbohydrates since it shall depend on the patients age, weight, appetite and caloric requirements. On an average carbohydrates should make fifty percent of the total dietary caloric intake (carbohydrate content in diet varying from 120-300 g or more). This shall increase in growing children, young adolescents and thin undernourished insulin dependent diabetics. Carbohydrates with a low sugar content should form the main bulk. These should be equally distributed throughout the day. Small snacks in between main meals are given so as to minimize blood sugar

fluctuations. Food exchanges be employed to make the diet more flexible.

Protein intake should be sufficient to meet body's needs (10-15% of total energy intake). Fibre in the diet in the form of pulses, fruits cereals should he taken in plenty since these foods shall not only produce satiety but also help in lowering cholesterol levels.

Fats in a diabetic diet must be minimal (30-35% of total energy intake) and must be mainly from polyunsaturated and monounsautrated sources. Saturated fats must be taken in minimal amount. Salt intake should also be minimal and it is important in diabetics who have associated hypertension. As a general principle a diabetic must avoid foods with high sugar content (sweets, chocolate, puddings, gur, cakes, pastries, jams, squashes). Fruits like banana, dates, grapes, mango, vegetables (potatoes, arbi, zimikand, shakarkandi, kachalu, peas, beetroot), rice, maida articles, dry fruits, nuts and sweet alcoholic drinks.

Foods which can be freely permitted include green and leafy vegetables, Tomatoes, cucumber, radishes, melons, water melons, citrus fruits, unsweetened tea or coffee, soups, zeera water, jamun, fish, chicken, butter. milk and soda water.

A diabetic must take care to be sparing with food containing refined sugars and carbohydrates. A diabetic diet of 1200 calories shall consist of 150 g of carbohydrates, 50-60 g of proteins and 40 g of fats. This is the diet advised for obese non-insulin dependant diabetics while in insulin dependant diabetic, diet of 2100 calories (carbohydrates 255 g, proteins 85 g, fats 80 g) is prescribed. In a diabetic with ketosis the amount of protein in diet must be restricted.

Alcohol in diabetics is permitted in moderation but in patients on oral hypoglycaemic agents, caution must be employed because of their interaction with alcohol.

Cholesterol lowering diet. With the growing role of cholesterol in the causation of cardiovascular and gall bladder disorders, more stress is now being placed on cholesterol lowering diet. This diet means reduction of total fat intake particularly saturated fats and encouraging patient to take high fibre containing foods.

Patient should avoid butter, ghee, coconut oil, whole milk cream, mayonnaise, hydrogenated oils (Vanaspati) yogurt made with whole milk, sweets, pastries, chocolates, cakes, ice-cream, pies, Jams, liver, kidney, pork, red meat, egg yolk, sausages, tinned fish, prawns, horlick, cocoa, craft cheese, nuts of all kinds, drinking chocolate, rich gravies.

Foods which may be permitted liberally are fresh fruit juices (lime, orange) skimmed milk and curd, white of egg, chicken, fish (baked or boiled) green leafy vegetables. Clear soups, low fat yogurt and cheese. Plain and salted biscuits, whole grain cereals, marmalade and honey.

In addition patient must take minimum amount of poly and monounsaturated fats. Vegetables should preferably be taken either boiled or baked. Foods with high sugar content and low fibre diets be avoided. It is preferabe to restrict intake of alcoholic drinks of all types.

Diet in gastrointestinal disorders. Basic rule is to have clean nourishing energy building foods and to avoid rich fried andspicy foods. At the same time intake of tea, coffee, alcohol and cola drinks must be restricted. Fluid intake must be sufficient so that the patient does not suffer from dehydration. If a patient suffers from chronic abdominal problem, drinking water must be boiled, cooled and then taken.

Peptic ulcer. Strict dietary control is not necessary. It is advisable to take frequent small feeds. Excessive eating at one time must be avoided. Small milk feeds should be taken at frequent intervals. Diet should be soft bland, non-irritating, non-spicy. Raw under cooked or fibrous vegetables (cabbage, radish, tomatoes) fruits with skins, raw fruits, guava, pine apple, seasoned spicy meats, strong tea, coffee, alcoholic drinks, cakes, pastries, sauces and gravies must be avoided.

It is preferable that patient takes refined foods, well cooked and soft vegetables, potatoes, peas, cauliflower, beans, bananas, mangoes, chiku, sweet grapes, soft meats (chicken, fish) milk, cream, weak tea, custards, jellies, ice cream, sweet custard etc. Basic rule for an ulcer diet is to avoid any food that causes symptoms after ingestion.

Constipation. High fibre diet containing lot of roughage he taken. There should be liberal use of unrefined cereals (whole meal bread, legumes), fresh fruits, leafy and fibrous vegetables. Person must take liberal quantities of water, soup, fruit juices, salads etc. Refined foods like sweets, pastries, puddings, rice, bananas, white bread be avoided.

Coeliac disease. Basic aim in diet in cases of coeliac disease is to give food which is gluten free. Gluten free flour is available for making breads, biscuits, cakes and cereals.

Patient is permitted. Soya flour, rice, sago, arrowroot, maize, corn or rice based cereals, fresh fruits and vegetables, milk, cheese, nuts, tea, coffee, fruit juices, jams, marmalade, eggs, fish poutry.

Foods forbidden include. Wheat flour, rye, biscuits, cakes oat meal, barley, barley water and any food which may overtly contain gluten.

Steatorrhoea/malabsorption syndrome. Avoid all fried food, whole milk, cheese, cream, ice cream, soups, rich gravies, cakes, pies etc. Food primarily should be low fat and of high content of calcium. The items in such a diet include skimmed milk, lean meat, poultry, fish, soft vegetables, sweets and desserts (without fat) porridge, soft bread, potatoes, rice, cereals, margarine, jam, apple, banana, tomatoes, tea and coffee etc.

Diet in liver diseases. Patients with infective hepatitis can be given a normal diet but since they donot tolerate fats, so their intake has to be restricted. Food should be soft, palatable, containing good amount of easily assimilable carbohydrates (fruit juices, glucose, sweet biscuits, sweetened rice, sago) and adequate quantities of proteins. Fried and rich foods should be avoided. As appetite returns, a normal diet is gradually introduced.

For patients with cirrhosis of liver, high protein diet (eggs, fish, chicken, cereals, legumes, milk) along with fresh fruits, vegetables juices is prescribed. Diet should be low in sodium and only small amount of salt is permitted. Food items which contain good amount of sodium (tinned meats, frozen foods, nuts, potato chips, sausages, sauces) be avoided.

Diet in renal diseases. In patients with acute nephritis, diet mainly consists of carbohydrates and restricted amounts of proteins and fluids. For patients with progressive renal failure or uraemia proteins have to be restricted (0.6-0.8 g/kg body weight per day). Sodium in the amount of 50 mmol per day is permitted and potassium intake is also restricted if levels of serum potassium are high. Diet mainly consists of whole meal bread, marmlade or honey, small quantity of fish, fruits and vegetables. Milk about 200 ml per day is permitted. Patient can take good quantities of sugar, jam, honey, marmalade, tea and lemonade.

Cases of nephrotic syndrome shall require high protein (80 g of protein per day) and low sodium (60-80 mmol) as well as fats. Diet mainly consists of milk, cereals, fish, chicken, legumes, vegetables, puddings, custard and fresh fruits.

Salt restricted diets. These diets are advised in cases of congestive heart failure, generalized anasarca, ascites, hypertension and attempt made to restrict intake of sodium in the diet to bare essential (60-80 mmol/day). Foods which contain considerable amount of sodium must be restricted and these include.

Tinned fish, vegetable soups, sauces, chutneys salted nuts, potato chips, ham, bacon, sausages, dry fruits, chocolates. To make diet palatable in a patient on sodium restricted diet, vinegar, mustard, pepper and sodium free salt substitute can be used. But there is no need to restrict intake of tea and coffee. For those patients where salt has to be restricted to minimum quantity, in addition to above no salt is to be used for cooking purposes. All food stuffs like breakfast creals, milk, butter where salt is present in hidden form, their amount must be restricted.

Diet in fevers/typhoid fever. When a patient is having fever and there are features of toxaemia, diet should mainly consist of milk, tea and glucose water. As the condition improves, soft bread, custard, banana, soft cooked or boiled eggs, soups, mashed potatoes, boiled vegetables like green peas, cauliflower, french beans and vegetables puree are added. One should be slow in adding solid or semisolid foods in cases of typhoid since there is inflammation in peyer's patches in intestines and solid or hard food given in such people may produce intestinal perforation. So basic approach should he to provide adequate nutrition, fluid intake and satisfy the needs of the patient.

Selected Bibliography

1. Brain's Diseases of the Nervous System (ed) Donaghy, M. Eleventh edition. Oxford University Press. Oxford 2001.
2. Harrison's Priciples of Internal Medicine (Editors) Kasper, D.L.: Braunwald, E.: Hauser, S.L. Vol. I & II. 16th Edition McGraw Hill Co. New York, London 2005.
3. Hurst's 'The Heart' (Editors) Fuster, V.: Alexande, R.W.: Rourke, R.A. Vol. I & II Eleventh Edition. McGraw Hill Co. New York & London 2004.
4. Jones, F. Avery: Gummer, J.W.P.; Lennard Jone, J.E.: Clinical Gastroenterology. Blackwell Scientific Publication. Oxford & London.
5. Khosla, S.N.: Essentials of Medicine. CBS Publishers, New Delhi 2008.
6. Khosla, S.N.: Typhoid Fever. Atlantic Publishers. New Delhi 2008.
7. Kumar, P.: Clark, M.: Clinical Medicine, 5th Edition. W.B. Saunders & Co. Philadelphia & London 2003.
8. Malamed, F.S.: Handbook of Medical Emergencies in the Dental office. 3rd edition. C.V. Mosby Co. St Louis 1997.
9. Sherlock, S.: Dooley, J.: Diseases of Liver and Biliary System. Blackwell Scientific Publication Oxford 2002.
10. Shah, N. Siddharth (Editor) A.P.I. Textbook of Medicine (Vol. I & II). Association Physicians of India Bombay 2008.
11. Swashm, M.: Hutchison's Clinical Methods. W.B. Saunder's Co. London 1997.
12. Vakil, R.J.: Golwalla, A.F.: Clinical Diagnosis. Asia Publishing House. Bombay.

Appendix

Normal Serium Values

Albumin, Serum	3.0 - 5.5 g/dl
Acid Phosphatase	2.5 - 12.0 iu/liter
Alkaline Phosphatase	3 - 13 K.A. units1.5 - 4.0 Bodansky units
Alpha -1 antitrypsin	200 - 500 mg/dl
Amylase / Serum	2 - 10 units/litre
Bilirubin	0.4 - 1.5 mg/dl
Total	0.2-1.2mg/di
Direct	0 - 0.4 mg/dl
Calcium Serum	8.7 - 10.6 mg/dl
Carotene (Carotenoids)	50 - 300 µg/dl
Cholestrol	
Total Plasma Cholestrol	< 200 mg/dl
LDL Cholestrol	<130 mg/dl
HDL Cholestrol	>60 mg/dl
Creatine Phosphokinase	
Total	20 - 200 iu/litre
Isoenzymes	
MM Fraction	94 - 95%
MB Fraction	0-5%
BB Fraction	0-2%
Normal Values in	
Heart	80% MM 20% MB
Brain	100% BB
Skeletal muscle	95% MM 2% MB
Creatinine, Serum	
Male	0.7 - 1.5 mg/dl
Female	0.5 - 1.3 mg/dl
Folate, Serum	1.9 - 14.0 ng/ml
Gastrin	60 - 200 pg/ml

Glucose, Serum (Fasting)	60 -100 mg/dl
Globulins	2.0 - 3.2 g/dl
Immunoglobulin, Quantitation	
IgG	700 - 1500 mg/dl
IgA	70 - 400 mg/dl
IgM	30 - 250 mg/dl
IgD	0 - 40 mg/dl
Insulin, Fasting	6 - 26 μU/ml
Iodine Protein Bound	4 - 8 μg/dl
LDH, Serum	20 - 220 IU/litre
Magnesium, Serum	1.5 - 2.5 meq/litre
5' - Nucleotidase	0.3 - 3.2 Bodansky unit
Phosphorus, inorganic, serum	2.0 - 4.3 mg/dl
Potassium, plasma	3.1 - 4.3 meq/litre
Serum	3.5 - 5.2 meq/litre
Proteins, total, serum	5.0-8.0g/dl
Protein, electrophoresis	
Albumin	3.2 - 5.2 g/dl
Alpha - 1	0.6 - 1.0 g/dl
Alpha - 2	0.6-1.0g/dl
Beta	0.6 - 1.2 g/dl
Gamma	0.7 - 1.5 g/dl
SGOT (AST)	5 - 40 IU/litre
SGPT (ALT)	5 - 30 IU/litre
Sodium, serum	135 - 145 meq/litre
Triglycerides	20 - 150 mg/dl
Urea, nitrogen, Serum	10 - 38 mg/dl
Uric acid	
Male	2.5 - 7.5 mg/dl
Female	2.0 - 7 mg/dl
Vitamin A	0.15 - 0.60 μg/ml
Vitamin B$_{12}$	200 - 850 pg/ml

ENDOCRINOLOGICAL NORMAL VALUES

Adrenocortico trophin (ACTH)	
Serum	15 - 100 pg/ml
Cortisol,	
Serum	
Morning	5 - 25 μg/dl
Evening	< 10 μg/dl
Urine	20 - 70 μg/24 hrs.
Gastrin, serum	30 - 200 pg/ml
Growth hormone, serum	
Adult	<5mg/ml

Insulin, plasma (fasting)	6-20 µU/ml
17-Hydroxycorticosteroids	
(Urine)	
Male	2 - 12 mg/24 hrs.
Female	2 - 8 mg/24 hrs.
17-Ketosteroids	
(Urine)	
Children	0 - 2 mg/24 hrs.
Adolescents	0 - 18 mg/24 hrs.
Adult Male	8 - 18 mg/24 hrs.
Adult Female	5 - 15 mg/24 hrs.
Parathyroid hormone, serum	
C - Terminal	150 - 350 pg/ml
N - Terminal	230 - 630 pg/ml
Radio active iodine ($I^{13'}$) uptake	
(RAIU)	5% - 25% at 24 hrs.
Thyroid stimulating	
Hormone, serum (TSH)	<10 µU/ml (0.4 - 5 µU/ml)
Thyroxine, serum (T_4)	
Total	4 - 11 µg/dl
Free	0.8 - 2.4 ng/dl
Tri-Iodothyroxin (T_3), serum	70 - 190 ng/dl
Vanillylmandelic acid (VMA)	
Urine	1 - 8 mg/24 hrs.

NORMAL HAEMATOLOGICAL VALUES

Haemoglobin	
Men	13-16g/dl
Women	11 - 14.5 g/dl
Red blood cell	
Men	$4.1\text{-}6.6 \times 10^{12}/1$
Women	$3,5 - 4.5 \times 10^{12}/1$
PCV	
Men	40 - 54%
Women	35 - 47%
MCV (Mean corpuscular volume)	86 - 94 fl
MCH (Mean corpusular Haemoglobin)	28 -32 pg
MCHC (Mean corpuscular Haemoglobin concertation)	32 - 36 g/dl
Reticulocyles	0.2 - 2.5%

ESR	Male		0 - 10 mm Ist hour westergren
	Female		0 - 20 mm Ist hour westergren
White cells			
	Adults		$(5 - 10 \times 10^3 mm^3)$
Differential leucocyte count			
	Neutrophils		40 - 75%
	Lymphocytes		20 - 45%
	Monocytes		2 - 9%
	Eosinophils		1 - 5%
	Basophils		0 - 1%
Platelets			150,000 - 400,000 per mm^3
Osmotic fragility			
	Haemolysis begins		0.45 - 0.39% NaCl
	Haemolysis completed		0.33 - 0.30% NaCl
Bleeding Time			3.5 - 7.5 Min.
(Lee & White method)			
Prothrombin time			12 - 14 Secs.
Plasma fibrinogen			150 - 400 mg/ml
Partial thromboplastin time			20 - 40 Sec.
(PTT)			
Serum iron			60 - 160 µg/100ml
Total iron binding capacity			280 - 400 µg/100ml
(TIBC)			
Thrombin time			10 - 15 secs.
Fibrin degradation products			< 10 µg/ml

Volume	Male	Female
Blood	52 - 83 ml/kg	50 - 75 ml/kg
Plasma	25 - 43 ml/kg	28 - 45 ml/kg
Red cell	20-36m1/kg	19-31ml/kg

Coagulation factors

Factors II, V, VII, VIII, IX, X

XI & XII   60 - 100 per cent or 1.0 unit/ml

Bone marrow (Differential cell count)

Myeloid cells	56.7%
Neutrophil series	53.6%
Myeloblasts	0.3 - 5%
Promyelocytes	2.1 - 4.1%
Myelocyte	8.2 - 15.7%
Meta myelocyte	9 - 24%
Bands	9.5 - 15.3%
Segmental cells	7 - 30%
Eosinophilic precursors	0.5 - 3.0%
Eosinophils	0.5 - 4.0%

Basophil series	0.2 - 1.3%
Erythroid	25.6%
Pronormoblasts	0.2 - 1.3%
Basophil normoblasts	0.5 - 2.4%
Polychromatophilic	
Normoblasts	0.5 - 2.4%
Orthochromatic normoblasts	0.4 - 4.6%
Megakaryocytes	<0.1%
Lympho-reticular cells	
Lymphocytes	11.1- 23.2%
Plasma cells	0.4 - 3:9%
Reticulum cells	0.1 - 2%
Monocytes	0.5 - 5%
Myeloid/erythroid ratio	3:1 to 4:1

TESTS OF PULMONARY FUNCTION

	Men	Women
Forced vital capacity (FVC)	4.8 L	3.3 L
Forced expiratory volume	3.8 L	2.8 L
FEV/FVC	76%	77%
Maximal mid expiratory flow M.MF (FEF 25 - 27)	4.8 L/S	3.6 L/S
Maximal expiratory flow rate MEFR (FEF 200 - 1200)	9.4 L/S	6.1 L/S
Total lung capacity (TLC)	6- 7 L	5- 6 L
Function residual capacity (TLC)	2 - 3 L	2 - 3 L
Residual volume	1 2 L	1- 2 L
Inspiratory capacity (IC)	4.8 L	3.7 L
Expirarory reserve volume (ERV)	3.2 L	2.3 L
Vital capacity	1.7 L	1.4 L
Resistance to airflow		
Pulmonary resistance (RL)	< 3.0 H_2O/Sec/L	
Airways resistance (RAW)	< 2.5 cm H_2O/Sec/L	
Blood gases		
Arterial O_2 tension (PaO_2)	95 ± 5 mm Hg	
Arterial CO_2 tension ($PaCO_2$)	40 ± 2 mm Hg	
Arterial blood pH (pH)	7.40 ± 0.02	
Arterial bicarbonate (HCO_3)	24 ± 2 mmol/l	

CARDIOVASCULAR NORMAL VALUES

Normal pressures in the heart and great vessels
Right atrium	Mean 2.8 mm Hg (Range 1 - 5)
Left atrium	Mean 7.9 mm Hg (Range 2 - 12)

Right ventricle		Mean 2.5 mm Hg (Range 17 - 32)
Left ventricle		
Peak systolic		130 mm Hg (Range 90 - 140)
End diastolic		8.7 mm Hg (Range 5 - 12)
Pulmonary artery		Mean 15 mm Hg (Range 9 - 19)
Peak systolic		25 mm Hg (Range 17 - 32)
End diastolic		9 mm Hg (Range 4 - 12)
Cardiac output (Fick)		2.5 - 3.6 Litres/m^2 of body surface area per minute

Normal value of doppler echocardiographic measurements:

	Range	Mean
RVD (cm)	0.9 - 2.6	1.7
LVID (cm)	35 - 5.7	4.7
Post. L.V. wall thickness (cm)	0.6 - 1.1	0.9
I.V.S. wall thickness (cm)	0.6 - 1.1	0.9
Left atrial dimension (cm)	1.9 - 4.0	2.9
Aortic root dimension (cm)	2.0 - 3.7	2.7
Aortic valve separation (cm)	1.5 - 2.6	1.9
Aortic valve sepration (cm)	15 - 2.6	1.9
Mitral valve (EF slope)	> 7.0 mm/sec	
Mitral valve (DE amplitude)	> 20 mm	
Tricuspid flow (m/sec)	0.3 - 0.7	0.5
Pulmonary artery (m/sec)	0.6 - 0.9	0.75

URINE NORMAL VALUES

Generally colourless but it may change with fluid intake and diet.

Specific gravity	1.003 - 1.030
pH	4.6-8.0
Acidity	
Titratable	20-40meq/24 hr.
Proteins	
Qualitative	negative
Quantitative	10- 150mg/24hr
Glucose	
Qualitative	negative
Quantitative	16 - 300 mg/24 hr
Ammonia	30 - 50 meq/24 hr
Amylase	35 - 260 somogyi units/hr
Bence-jones proteins	negative
Bilirubin	negative
Calcium	< 7.5 meq/24 hr.
Chloride	120 - 240 meq/24 hr
Sodium	130 - 260 meq/24 hr (varies with dietary sodium intake)
Potassium	25 - 100 meq/24 hr
Creatine	

Male	0 - 40 mg/24 hr
Female	0 - 100 mg/24hr
Creatinine	15 - 25 mg/kg body weight/24hr
Phosphorus	0.8-2.0 g/24 hr
Porphobilinogen	
Qualitative	negative
Quantitative	0- 2.4 mg/24 hr
Porphyrins	
Coproporphyrin	50 - 250 µg/24 hr
Uroporphyrin	10 - 30 µg/24 hr
Uric Add	80 - 976 mg/24 hr
Urobilinogen	0.05 - 3.5 mg/24 hr

CEREBROSPINAL FULID/NORMAL. VALUES

Colour	Colourless
Pressure	7 - 20 cm Water
Proteins	
Lumbar	15 - 45 mg/dl
Cisternal	15 - 25 mg/dl
Ventricular	5 -15 mg/dl
Glucose	48 - 86 mg/dl
Chloride	110 - 129 meq/litre
Bilirubin	negative
Cells	0 - 5 mm^2 all Lymphocytes

ALIMENTARY TRACT FUNCTION TESTS

Gastric Secretion		
Volume		
	Fasting	20 - 100 ml/hr
	Nocturnal	< 800 ml/10 hr
Acid output		
BAO		
	Male	3.7 ± 2.1 meq/hr
	Female	2.2 ± 1.7 meq/hr
Stimulated after histamine		
	Male	23 ± 7 meq/hr
	Female	18 ± 5 meq/hr
Serum gastrin		< 150 pg/ml
DrXylose test		
(25 g D-Xylose/5g		> 5 g/5 hr (25 g D-Xylose dose)
D-Xylose after an 8 hr		
fast urine collected for		
5 hrs following ingestion)		> 1 g/5 hr (5 g D-Xylose dose)

Serum level (1 hr. after
        ingestion of D-Xylose)   > 25 mg/dl
Faecal fat estimation (Stool fat
on diet containing 50 - 80 g fat/day
for 4 days prior stools collection   < 6 g/24hr
Triolein breath test
5 $\mu C_1 C^{14}$ triolein adminstered
in 30 ml lipomul: breath   > 3.5 % of dose/hr
collection hourly for 6 hr
for measurement of breath $^{14}CO_2$

Index

255